Prostate and renal cancer, benign prostatic hyperplasia, erectile dysfunction and basic research

an update

Prostate and renal cancer, benign prostatic hyperplasia, erectile dysfunction and basic research

an update

The Proceedings of the VII Congress on Progress and Controversies
in Oncological Urology (PACIOU VII) and the
Seventh Congress of the Dutch Urological Association
Rotterdam, The Netherlands, October 2002

Edited by
Ch. H. Bangma and D. W. W. Newling

Co-Editors
J. L. H. R. Bosch, P. C. M. S. Verhagen, G. R. Dohle,
G. W. Jenster and F. H. Schröder

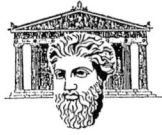

The Parthenon Publishing Group
International Publishers in Medicine, Science & Technology

A CRC PRESS COMPANY
BOCA RATON   LONDON   NEW YORK   WASHINGTON, D.C.

**Library of Congress
Cataloging-in-Publication Data**
Data available on application

British Library Cataloguing in Publication Data
Data available on application

ISBN 1-84214-196-1

Published in the USA by
The Parthenon Publishing Group
345 Park Avenue South, 10th Floor
New York, NY 10010
USA

Published in the UK and Europe by
The Parthenon Publishing Group
23–25 Blades Court
Deodar Road
London SW15 2NU
UK

Copyright © 2003 The Parthenon Publishing
Group

First published in 2003

Typeset by AMA DataSet, UK.
Printed and bound by Bookcraft (Bath) Ltd.,
Midsomer Norton, UK

Contents

Section 3   Basic research on prostate cancer

**Section 4   Translational research in prostate cancer: what is close to
                clinical practice?**

Section 5   Diagnosis and outcome in locally confined prostate cancer

Section 6   Prostate cancer, epidemiology, risk factors and outcomes per treatment

Section 7   Renal cancer

Section 8   Prostate cancer, locally advanced and node positive

Section 9   Advanced prostate cancer

List of Editors and principal contributors

F. Algaba
Fundació Puigvert
Universitat Autònoma de Barcelona
Pathology Section
Cartagena 340
08025 Barcelona
Spain

P. Alken
Urologische Universitätsklinik
Universität Heidelberg
Klinikum Mannheim
Theodor-Kutzer-Ufer 1–3
D-68135 Mannheim
Germany

W. Arap
MD Anderson Cancer Center
The University of Texas
1515 Holcombe Boulevard, Box 0427
Houston
Texas 77030
USA

Ch. H. Bangma
Department of Urology
Erasmus Medical Center Rotterdam
PO Box 2040
3000 CA Rotterdam
The Netherlands

P. Berthon
UroGene
4 rue Pierre Fontaine
91058 Evry-Genopole Cedex
France

M. H. Blanker
Department of General Practice
Erasmus Medical Center Rotterdam
PO Box 1738
3000 DR Rotterdam
The Netherlands

L. Boccon Gibod
Department of Urology and Pathology
Hôpital Armand
Trousseau
Paris 75018
France

J. L. H. R. Bosch
Department of Urology
Erasmus Medical Center Rotterdam
PO Box 2040
3000 CA Rotterdam
The Netherlands

A. O. Brinkmann
Department of Reproduction and
    Development
Erasmus Medical Center Rotterdam
PO Box 1738
3000 DR Rotterdam
The Netherlands

P. R. Carroll
Department of Urology, A610
University of California
San Francisco
California 94143
USA

Z. Culig
Department of Urology
University of Innsbruck
Anichstrasse 35
A-6020 Innsbruck
Austria

G. R. Cunha
Department of Anatomy and Urology
University of California
San Francisco
California 94143
USA

A. G. Dalgleish
Division of Oncology
Level 2 Jenner Wing
St. George's Hospital Medical School
Cranmer Terrace, Tooting
London SW17 0RE
UK

A. V. D'Amico
Joint Center for Radiation Therapy
Harvard Medical School
330 Brookline Avenue – 5th Floor
Boston
Massachusetts 02215
USA

L. J. Denis
Oncological Center Antwerp
Lange Gasthuisstraat 35–37
B-2000 Antwerp
Belgium

G. R. Dohle
Department of Urology
Erasmus Medical Center Rotterdam
PO Box 2040
3000 CA Rotterdam
The Netherlands

J. L. Donovan
Department of Social Medicine
University of Bristol
Canynge Hall
Bristol BS8 2PR
UK

D. S. Ernst
Tom Baker Cancer Centre
Alberta Cancer Board
1331–29 Street NW
Calgary T2N 4N2
Canada

M. L. Essink-Bot
Department of Public Health
Erasmus Medical Center Rotterdam
PO Box 1738
3000 DR Rotterdam
The Netherlands

L. Gooren
Division of Andrology; Department of
    Endocrinology
Vrije Universiteit Medical Center
PO Box 7057
1007 MB Amsterdam
The Netherlands

M. Graefen
Department of Urology
University Hospital Hamburg-Eppendorf
Martinistrasse 52
D-20246 Hamburg
Germany

K. Griffiths
Laurel Cottage
Castleton
Cardiff CF3 2UR
UK

M. Häggman
Department of Urology
Uppsala University Hospital
S-75185 Uppsala
Sweden

F. C. Hamdy
Academic Urology Unit
Royal Hallamshire Hospital, I Floor
Glossop Road
Sheffield S10 2JF
UK

H. Huland
Department of Urology
University Hospital Eppendorf
Martinistrasse 52
D-20246 Hamburg
Germany

L. Incrocci
Department of Radiation Oncology
Erasmus Medical Center Rotterdam
PO Box 5201
3008 AE Rotterdam
The Netherlands

P. Iversen
Department of Urology D-2112
Rigshospitalet
University of Copenhagen
Blegdamsvej 9
2100 Copenhagen
Denmark

D. Jacqmin
Service de Chirurgie Urologique
Hôpitaux Universitaires de Strasbourg
BP 426
F-67091 Strasbourg Cedex
France

G. W. Jenster
Department of Urology
Josephine Nefkens Institute Be 362a
Erasmus Medical Center Rotterdam
PO Box 1738
3000 DR Rotterdam
The Netherlands

O.-P. Kallioniemi
Medical Biotechnology Group
VTT Technical Research Center of Finland
   and University of Turku
PO Box 106
FIN 20521 VTT
Finland

D. Kirk
Department of Urology
Gartnavel General Hospital
1053 Great Western Rd
Glasgow G12 0YN
UK

Z. Kirkali
Department of Urology
Dokuz Eylül University School of Medicine
35340 Inciralti
Izmir
Turkey

L. Klotz
Division of Urology
Health Sciences Centre
Sunnybrook and Women's College
University of Toronto
2075 Bayview Avenue #MG 408
Toronto M4N 3M5
Canada

H. J. de Koning
Department of Public Health
Erasmus Medical Center Rotterdam
PO Box 1738
3000 DR Rotterdam
The Netherlands

G. P. Krestin
Department of Radiology
Erasmus Medical Center Rotterdam
PO Box 2040
3000 CA Rotterdam
The Netherlands

H. Lilja
Department of Clinical Chemistry
University Hospital Malmö
S-205 02 Malmö
Sweden

C. Logothetis
Department of Genitourinary Medical
   Oncology
MD Anderson Cancer Center
University of Texas, Box 0427
1515 Holcombe Boulevard
Houston
Texas 77030
USA

J. R. Masters
Institute of Urology
3rd Floor Research Laboratories
University College London
67 Riding House Street
London W1 7EJ
UK

E. J. H. Meuleman
Department of Urology
University Medical Center
PO Box 9101
6500 HB Nijmegen
The Netherlands

G. H. J. Mickisch
Center of Operative Urology Bremen
Robert-Koch-Strasse 34a
D-28277 Bremen
Germany

F. Montorsi
Department of Urology
Hospital San Raffaele
Via Olgettina 60
I-20132 Milan
Italy

R. P. Myers
Department of Urology
Mayo Clinic
Mayo Graduate School of Medicine
200 First Street SW
Rochester
Minnesota 55905
USA

M. A. Noordzij
Department of Urology
Erasmus Medical Center Rotterdam
PO Box 2040
3000 CA Rotterdam
The Netherlands

S. E. Oliver
Department of Social Medicine
University of Bristol
Canynge Hall
Bristol BS8 2PR
UK

J. J. M. Pel
Department of Urology
Sector Furore, Room Ee1630
Erasmus Medical Center Rotterdam
3000 DR Rotterdam
The Netherlands

D. P. Petrylak
Department of Urology
Columbia-Presbyterian Medical Center
161 Fort Washington Avenue
New York
New York 10032
USA

H. Porst
Urological Office
Neues Jungfernstieg 6a
D-20354 Hamburg
Germany

J. Rassweiler
Urology Clinic
Klinikum Heilbronn am Gesundbrunnen 20
D-74064 Heilbronn
Germany

J. C. Romijn
Department of Urology
Erasmus Medical Center Rotterdam
PO Box 1738
3000 DR Rotterdam
The Netherlands

F. H. Schröder
Department of Urology
Erasmus Medical Center Rotterdam
PO Box 2040
3000 CA Rotterdam
The Netherlands

C. N. Sternberg
Department of Medical Oncology
San Camillo and Forlanini Hospitals
Pavillion Cesalpini
Circonvallazione Gianicolense 87
I-00152 Rome
Italy

P. C. M. S. Verhagen
Department of Urology
Erasmus Medical Center Rotterdam
PO Box 2040
3000 CA Rotterdam
The Netherlands

A. N. Vis
Department of Urology
Erasmus Medical Center Rotterdam
PO Box 1738
3000 DR Rotterdam
The Netherlands

P. C. Walsh
Department of Urology
Johns Hopkins Hospital
Marburg 134, 600 N Wolfe Street
Baltimore
Massachusetts 21287
USA

Foreword

This is the seventh monograph in the series *Progress and Controversies in Oncologic Urology (PACIOU)*, reflecting the contribution of many speakers during the congress in October 2002 in Rotterdam, The Netherlands.

The congress was a great success for the nearly 600 participants. Although the retirement of Fritz Schröder from clinical practice overshadowed some of the activities, it was the high standard of the content of the presentations that impressed most.

For the first time, an update on basic research in prostate cancer is added to the recent progress in cancer of the prostate, the kidney, and in the field of benign prostatic hyperplasia and impotence. Basic research has developed tremendously during the last decades, and, for many of us readers, this source of changes for clinical practice is hard to follow. PACIOU will continue to highlight the importance of the close relationship between the laboratory and the clinic during the years to come, and educational sessions will be combined with the state of the art in research.

Thanks to the authors and co-editors, an interesting update has again been put together in a very short time-frame. We hope that this book serves the purpose of a reference for the next 2 years, after which PACIOU will once more be organized in the autumn of 2004 in Rotterdam.

Chris Bangma
Rotterdam, February 2003

Sexual health in the aging male

1

E. J. H. Meuleman

Introduction

Demographic studies show an increasing proportion of older people in developed countries. For example, during the past 100 years in The Netherlands the mean life expectancy has approximately doubled. This development is largely due to improved hygiene, reduction of newborn mortality and more effective therapy and prevention of acute diseases in older age. With larger numbers of people reaching advanced age, health problems as well as social and psychological problems of older men play an increasingly important role in clinical medicine and in research.

Sexual health

Erectile dysfunction is the most common sexual disorder among elderly men. Although most of the difficulties are mild and do not totally prevent intercourse, about 26% experience moderate to complete erectile dysfunction. The impact of this category of erectile dysfunction on sexual activity among men is marked, and it is obvious that these men seek treatment[1]. Data from the Massachusetts Male Aging Study show that the annual incidence of erectile dysfunction in men 40–69 years of age is 26 per 1000 (40–49 years: 12/1000; 60–69 years: 46/1000). In the Cologne Male Survey a prevalence of 19.2% was found, with a steep age-related increase[2]. Recently, the prevalence of erectile dysfunction and its influence on both quality of life and health care-seeking behavior was assessed in The Netherlands among men aged 40–79 years, together with their partners[3]. The prevalence of erectile dysfunction increased with age class. To the question regarding problems in achieving an erection, 13% of all men answered affirmatively (40–49 years:

6%; 50–59: 9%; 60–69: 22%; 70–79: 38%). All men aged 40–49 years of age with erectile dysfunction and 16% of men aged 70–79 with erectile dysfunction considered the symptom as bothersome. Thirty-four per cent of all men with erectile dysfunction and 16% of their spouses were dissatisfied with their sex life. Erectile dysfunction bears a strong correlation with general quality of life and comorbidity. However, it is noteworthy that the lack of a sexual partner appeared to be the most prevalent and serious sexual problem for men[4].

The incidence of erectile dysfunction increases with the presence of concomitant conditions such as diabetes mellitus, heart disease, hypertension, depression, pelvic surgery, negative mood, lack of self-esteem, problems with relationships or just inadequate sexual experience[5–8]. Vascular disease is thought to be the most common cause of organic erectile dysfunction, and it may be an early symptom of cardiac morbidity and mortality[4]. Greenstein and colleagues found a correlation between the severity of ischemic coronary disease and erectile dysfunction[9]. There is a corresponding above-average prevalence among men treated with cardiovascular drugs and antidepressants[10,11]. Moreover, lower urinary tract symptoms (LUTS) and current or previous medical treatment of benign prostatic hyperplasia correlate with the occurrence of sexual dysfunction. On closer examination, this co-occurrence is to be expected, since the prevalence of both conditions increases with age[12].

The likely world-wide increase in the prevalence of erectile dysfunction (associated with rapidly aging populations), combined with newly available and highly publicized medical treatments, will raise challenging policy issues in nearly all countries[13]. However, to date, only a minority of men with a sexual problem are seeking help, and not every man seeking help is a candidate for (symptomatic) medical treatment.

Even in an era in which sexual issues can be discussed straightforwardly, men are very secretive about their medical conditions, in particular those concerned with any aspect of sexual functioning. They try to avoid public clinics, preferring to visit private clinics. Sexual problems are concealed from general practitioners who, in The Netherlands, account for 80.8% of all sildenafil prescriptions (urologist: 13.8%; psychiatrist: 0.6%; gynecologist: 0.3%)[14]. In 1998, in The Netherlands only 25% of men with erectile dysfunction consulted a doctor, with a mean delay of 13 months, and men between 50 and 59 years of age account for the majority of filed prescriptions for sildenafil (34.1%). In a broader perspective, that men are less accustomed than women to receiving medical care may be the main reason for the so-called 'gender gap', i.e. the difference in life expectancy that is currently 7–8 years less for men than it is for women[15]. Based on the presumption that in 2025 about 322 million men world-wide will suffer from erectile dysfunction and only one in three will seek treatment, current projections estimate that 100 million men will opt for treatment[13].

Not every man presenting with erectile dysfunction is a candidate for symptomatic treatment. Because of the frequent association of sexual problems and aging, ample time should be taken to educate the patient about the alterations in sexual response with aging[16]. Sexual desire, penile rigidity and sensitivity decrease, and it takes longer for men to obtain an erection[17]. Erections become more dependent on direct physical stimulation of the penis and less responsive to visual, psychological or non-genital excitation. Aging also affects the ejaculatory phase of the sexual response. The orgasmic muscular contractions are fewer and less intense. There is a slow but gradual decline in semen volume per ejaculation; it usually takes longer to reach ejaculation and semen may dribble out at orgasm. The sensation of ejaculatory urgency is reduced, and intercourse may take place without ejaculation occurring on every occasion. The older man's refractory period during which he is unresponsive to further stimuli following orgasm gradually lengthens.

In the literature, there is much debate on the role of a declining androgen level as an independent factor in the declining sexual function of the aging male, and the desirability of testosterone supplementation. Reportedly, men with high testosterone levels are more likely to have higher levels of sexual activity, and men who desire sexual intercourse more than once a week have higher testosterone levels than men satisfied with a lower frequency[18]. Nevertheless, the correlation between testosterone levels and libido is poor, and the testosterone levels required to sustain normal sexual interest are apparently low[19]. In a screening program for the early detection of prostate cancer, Rhoden and colleagues found no correlation between total testosterone levels and erectile dysfunction, or its severity[20]. Currently, a multicenter study is being conducted in Europe to investigate the efficacy of testosterone supplementation in aging, testosterone-deficient males.

The physician treating men with erectile dysfunction should realize that it is frequently a sequela of a medical condition, such as vascular disease, or the use of pharmacological agents, and most treatments are rehabilitative, rather than curative[21,22]. Therefore, important aims of treatment should be adjustment of life-style and modification of risk factors where possible, such as use of medication, being overweight, smoking, alcohol consumption and lack of exercise[23]. In this holistic medical approach, the patient should be informed that daily life-style decisions and practices exert a profound impact on both short- and long-term health and quality of life. Scientific and medical advances over the past 5 years have consolidated the evidence that positive life-style measures are vitally important to good health. Medical professionals in general, and physicians in particular, occupy a uniquely powerful position from which to encourage patients to change their behaviors.

In fact, in many surveys, physician recommendations have been shown to be the leading reason why individuals change actions and behaviors. Unfortunately, a distinct minority of physicians wield this power wisely, if at all[24].

How does this knowledge relate to the field of sexual medicine? Although mid-life changes may be too late to reverse the effects of life-style on erectile function, there is no longer any serious doubt that early adoption of life-style changes may be the best approach to reducing the burden of erectile dysfunction on health and general well being[25], and that it is extremely important to educate men to remain as active as possible for as long as possible. The phrase 'use it or lose it' is particularly appropriate for the genitalia. This is a very important message that is not always welcomed by the aging population: the best way to prevent or to limit the signs of aging is to remain active.

Adjustment of life-style and risk modification

Medication

It is a general belief that medication-induced sexual dysfunction can significantly interfere with a patient's quality of life and lead to poor compliance[26]. Drugs that interfere with hormonal, monoaminergic, adrenergic and cholinergic mechanisms are associated with impaired sexual desire, erection or ejaculation. However, for several reasons it is extremely difficult to find convincing evidence that sexual problems are drug-related. First, not much is known about pharmacological mechanisms and the frequency of erectile dysfunction as a side-effect of medication. Furthermore, limited access to valid pharmacoepidemiological data is a major drawback. The authors of a recent comprehensive reference text *Drug-Induced Infertility and Sexual Dysfunction* were able to access information only in the public domain. Two valuable sources of data are not available in the public domain. These are databases collated by the Committee on Safety of Medicines (CSM) via the yellow card notification scheme, and those held by the pharma-ceuticals' manufacturers. Manufacturers have a reporting obligation to notify the CSM about serious or life-threatening adverse effects. Sexual dysfunction does not come into this category[27]. Moreover, when an association between drug consumption and a sexual dysfunction is present, confounding variables such as life-style and the use of other drugs may prevent conclusions about causality. Finally, patients may willingly report socially acceptable side-effects such as nausea, lethargy or headaches, but there is increasing evidence that they may not volunteer information about sexual dysfunction.

How, then, should one proceed when erectile dysfunction seems to be a side-effect of medication? A causal relationship may be suspected if the onset of erectile dysfunction coincides with the start of the medication. In the majority of cases, however, a causal relationship remains unclear. If strong suspicion remains, a change of medication, lowering of dosage or a 'drug holiday' may yield a positive result.

Obesity

The association between obesity and illness was initially alluded to by Hippocrates, who observed that 'When more food than is proper has been taken, it occasions disease'. In the Massachusetts Male Aging Study, being overweight (body mass index $\geq 28 \ kg/m^2$) almost doubled the incidence of erectile dysfunction at follow-up[28]. Obesity, defined as a body mass index (BMI) of over 30, is a condition that is reaching epidemic proportions not only in the developed but also in the developing world. The BMI is defined as body weight in kilograms divided by the square of height in meters. Normal weight is represented by a value between 18 and 25, while values between 25 and 30 indicate overweight. Obesity is associated with adverse lipid profiles, hypertension and diabetes, and may be independently associated with coronary heart disease[29,30]. Sixty-three per cent of men and 55% of women are overweight in the USA. Twenty-two per cent are grossly overweight, with a BMI over $30 \ kg/m^2$. The frequency of overweight is maximal between the ages of 50 and 60 years, and shows a subsequent tendency to decline slowly[31]. The prevalence of obesity has doubled in the past decade[32]. The consequences are serious. Approximately 80% of obese adults have at least one and 40% have two or more associated diseases such as diabetes, hypertension, cardiovascular disease, gall-bladder disease and cancer, and the morbidity of diseases of the locomotor system such as osteoarthrosis. The literature is unequivocal about the relationship between erectile dysfunction and obesity. Derby and colleagues found obesity status, regardless of follow-up weight loss, to be associated with erectile dysfunction[25].Chung and associates, however, demonstrated that obesity in itself is not an underlying risk factor, but does impose a risk by being associated with the development of vascular disease[33].

Smoking

There is a wealth of clinical and experimental evidence that smoking and erectile dysfunction are closely related. The risk of erectile dysfunction caused by atherosclerosis of the internal pudendal artery is one-third higher in smokers than in non-smokers[34]. Penile Doppler ultrasonographic studies in smokers and non-smokers show a reduced erectile response and a reduced increase in blood flow velocity in smokers following pharmacological stimulation[35], and heavy smokers have the fewest minutes of nocturnal tumescence and detumesce the fastest[36]. Moreover, smokers show not only lower penile brachial pressure index (BPI) values but also higher incidence of the incomplete response to papaverine injection than do non-smokers[37]. Animal experiments indicate that chronic smoking leads to age-independent decreases in penile nitric oxide synthase (NOS) activity and neuronal (n)NOS content[38]. In the Massachusetts Male Aging Study, cigarette smoking almost doubled the risk of developing moderate to severe erectile dysfunction at follow-up (24% vs. 14%). Cigar smoking and passive exposure to cigarette smoke also significantly predicted incident erectile dysfunction. Cigarette smoking has

been consistently, and in a dose-related manner, shown to be related to the development of atherosclerosis[39–41]. On the other hand, cigarette smoking has not been shown to be a potent risk factor for the sequelae of atherosclerosis in a population such as the Japanese, characterized by low serum cholesterol levels. These observations, in conjunction with results from studies that have shown a markedly decreased risk after quitting smoking, with the excess risk of atherosclerosis declining relatively quickly after quitting, suggest that smoking may act as a triggering agent, rather than a necessary and sufficient factor[42,43].

Passive exposure to secondary cigarette smoke has been associated with clinically manifest as well as subclinical atherosclerosis and carotid atherosclerosis through a number of pathophysiological mechanisms[44,45]. Although the relative risks associated with passive smoking are less than those attributed to direct inhalation, the large proportion of the population exposed to environmental tobacco smoke suggests that the adverse health consequences for a large number of persons may be affected by even small increases in the risk of coronary disease, as well as possibly selected cancers.

Alcohol

The effects of alcohol consumption were well known to Shakespeare, who commented in *Macbeth* that 'alcohol provokes the desire but takes away the performance'. Shakespeare's observations were based on anecdotal evidence, but have been confirmed in the laboratory setting. When penile erection and vaginal vasocongestion following visual erotic stimulation are measured, the subjective impression of sexual arousal is increased, while the objectively measured response is reduced following alcohol consumption[46,47]. Alcohol also causes orgasmic delay in women[48] and depresses testosterone concentrations in men following acute ingestion[49].

In the UK 27% of men drink more than the recommended limit of 3–4 units per day[50]. The effects of alcohol on sexual function can be divided into those that result from acute alcohol consumption by otherwise healthy individuals (social drinking), and those secondary to chronic alcoholism. The latter effects are not just caused by the pharmacological effects of ethanol, but are compounded by secondary systemic disturbances induced by alcohol, including liver disease, malnutrition and domestic disharmony. Consumption of alcohol has not been shown to lead to an increased risk of atherosclerosis, and a substantial body of evidence indicates that moderate alcohol intake is associated with a reduced risk of developing and dying from atherosclerosis. The majority of studies examining the association between alcohol use and atherosclerosis have suggested either a negative or a U-shaped relationship[51].

In chronic alcoholics, sexual dysfunction is related to the quantity, frequency and duration of drinking. Additionally, the drinking pattern appears to be of importance: heavy drinkers suffer more often from pancreatitis, esophageal varices, polyneuropathy or erectile dysfunction than do episodic drinkers. Thus, the drinking pattern, particularly frequent inebriation, has an influence on the occurrence of alcohol-related disorders[52]. One study showed that 59% of men attending an alcoholism program experienced erectile dysfunction, and 48% had difficulties with ejaculation during bouts of heavy drinking[53]. Chronic alcoholism may result in permanent impotence even after the complete cessation of drinking for many years[54].

Exercise

In a longitudinal survey ($n = 1156$, average follow-up 8.8 years), physical activity was associated with erectile dysfunction, with the highest risk among men who remained sedentary and the lowest among those who remained active or initiated physical activity. The results suggest that sedentary men may be able to reduce their risk of erectile dysfunction by adopting regular physical activity at a level of at least 200 kcal/day, which corresponds to walking briskly for 3.5 km[55]. In an Australian survey among 427 men over the age of 40, a history of vigorous exercise was protective against erectile dysfunction across all ages[56].

Symptomatic treatment

Up to the end of the 20th century, fewer than 10% of men sought treatment and, even within this apparently well-motivated group, a high treatment drop-out rate was routinely observed. It was hypothesized that drop-out occurred as the treatment options were relatively invasive/intrusive in nature or artificial, had associated risks, may be irreversible and were expensive. On this basis, it was anticipated that the general availability of effective oral therapeutics, such as sildenafil and apomorphine sublingual, would have a far-reaching impact on the management of male sexual health issues. To date, however, still the drop-out rate for symptomatic erectile dysfunction treatment (oral medication: 45%) (Souverein, personal communication) is high, and patient education and counselling remain the cornerstones in any erectile dysfunction treatment.

Preferred symptomatic treatment for erectile dysfunction in the Cologne Male Survey (mean age 51.8 years) comprised: oral treatment (73.8%), intraurethral prostaglandin E_1 (5.1%), intracavernosal injection therapy (4.7%), erection devices (5.8%), surgery (8.2%) and implantation of a penile prosthesis (2.4%); 46.2% of the men indicated that they were willing to contribute €25 monthly to their treatment. In patients above the age of 65 years (mean 69.5 years) the most popular initial treatment choices are injection therapy (30.3%), vacuum device (27.0%) and oral medication (20.2%)[57].

Conclusion

Erectile dysfunction is a common disorder among elderly men: the annual incidence of erectile dysfunction in men 60–69 years of age is 46 per 1000 men. The incidence of erectile dysfunction increases with age and the presence of concomitant conditions such as diabetes mellitus, heart disease, hypertension, depression, negative mood, lack of self-esteem, problems with relationships or just inadequate sexual experience. Although there is a wealth of information regarding risk factors contributing to the development of erectile dysfunction, and given that current symptomatic treatments are invasive, costly or have unproved long-term benefits, in daily practice too little attention is paid to the modification of risk factors and secondary prevention. A more physically active life-style, quitting smoking, reduction of overweight and a moderate alcohol intake may be viewed as integral components of a comprehensive erectile dysfunction risk reduction program. Given the high drop-out rates for symptomatic erectile dysfunction treatment, patient education and counselling are the cornerstones in any treatment of erectile dysfunction.

References

1. Koskimäki J, Hakama M, Huhtala H, Tammela TLJ. Effect of erectile dysfunction on frequency of intercourse: a population based prevalence study in Finland. *J Urol* 2000;164:367–70
2. Braun M, Wassmer G, Klotz T, Reifenrath B, Mathers M, Engelmann U. Epidemiology of erectile dysfunction: results of the Cologne Male Survey. *Int J Impotence Res* 2000;12:305–11
3. Meuleman EJH, Donkers LHC, Robertson C, Keech M, Boyle P, Kiemeney LALM. Erectiestoornis: prevalentie en invloed op de kwaliteit van leven: het Boxmeer-onderzoek. *Ned Tijdschr Geneeskd* 2001;145:576–81
4. Goldstein I. The mutually reinforcing triad of depressive symptoms, cardiovascular disease, and erectile dysfunction. *Am J Cardiol* 2000;86 (Suppl 2A):41F–5F
5. Johannes CB, Araujo AB, Feldman HA, Derby CA, Kleinman KP, McKinlay JB. Incidence of erectile dysfunction in men 40 to 69 years old: longitudinal results from the Massachusetts Male Aging Study. *J Urol* 2000;163:460–3
6. Araujo AB, Durante R, Feldman HA, Goldstein I, McKinlay JB. The relationship between depressive symptoms and male erectile dysfunction: cross-sectional results from the Massachusetts Male Aging Study. *Psychosom Med* 1998;60:458–65
7. Ventegodt S. *Resultater fra livskvalitctsundersøgelsen af 4626 31–33 årige danskere født på Rigdshospitalet 1959–1961 [Quality of life among 4626 31–33-year-olds]*. Copenhagen: Forskningcentrets Forlag
8. Mitchell WB, Marten DiBartolo P, Brown TA, Barlow DH. Effects of positive and negative mood on sexual arousal in sexually functional males. *Arch Sex Behav* 1998;27:197–207
9. Greenstein A, Chen J, Miller H, Matzkin H, Villa Y, Braf Z. Does severity of coronary disease correlate with erectile dysfunction? *Int J Impotence Res* 1997;9:123–26
10. Feldman HA, Goldstein I, Hatzichristou DG, Krane RJ, McKinlay JB. Impotence and its medical and psychosocial correlates: results of the Massachusetts Male Aging Study. *J Urol* 1994;151:54–61
11. Melman A, Gingell JC. The epidemiology and pathophysiology of erectile dysfunction. *J Urol* 1999;161:5–11
12. Souverein PC, Egberts ACG, Sturkenboom MCJM, Meuleman EJH, Leufkens HGM, Urquhart J. The Dutch cohort of sildenafil users: baseline characteristics. *J Urol* 2001;165:219
13. Aytac IA, McKinlay JB, Krane RJ. The likely worldwide increase in erectile dysfunction between 1995 and 2025 and some possible policy consequences. *BJU Int* 1999;84:50–6
14. Read S, King M, Watson J. Sexual dysfunction in primary medical care: prevalence, characteristics and detection by the general practitioner. *J Public Health Med* 1997;19:387–91
15. Lunenfeld B. Aging male [Editorial]. *Aging Male* 1998;1:1–7
16. Schiavi RC. Sexuality and aging. In Melman A, ed. *Impotence*. Philadelphia: WB Saunders, 1995: 711–26
17. Verwoerdt A, Pfeiffer E, Wang HS. Sexual behavior in senescence. Patterns of sexual activity and interest. *Geriatrics* 1969;24:137–54
18. Schiavi RC, Schreiner-Engel P, Mandeli J, Schanzer H, Cohen E. Healthy aging and male sexual function. *Am J Psychiatry* 1990;147:766–71
19. Davidson JM, Chen JJ, Crapo L, Gray GD, Greenleaf WJ, Catania JA. Hormonal changes and sexual functioning in aging men. *J Clin Endocrinol Metab* 1983;57:71–7

20. Rhoden EL, Teloken C, Mafessoni R, Vargas Souto CA. Is there any relation between serum levels of total testosterone and the severity of erectile dysfunction. *Int J Impotence Res* 2002; 14:167–71

21. Meuleman E, Broderick G, Meng Tan H, Montorsi F, Sharlip I, Vardi Y. Clinical evaluation and the doctor–patient dialogue. In Jardin A, Wagner G, Khoury S, Guiliano F, Padma-Nathan H, Rosen R, eds. *Erectile Dysfunction*. Plymouth, UK: Plymbridge Distributors Ltd, cservs@plymbridge.com, 2000:115–38

22. Gooren LJG. Quality-of-life issues in the aging male. *Aging Male* 2000;3:185–89

23. Guay AT. Erectile dysfunction. Are you prepared to discuss it? *Postgrad Med* 1995;97:127–30, 133–5, 139–40

24. Rippe JM. Preface. In Rippe JM, ed. *Lifestyle Medicine*. Malden, MA: Blackwell Science, 1999:XXIII

25. Derby CA, Mohr BA, Goldstein I, Feldman HA, Johannes CB, McKinlay JB. Modifiable risk factors and erectile dysfunction: can lifestyle changes modify risk? *Urology* 2000;56:302–6

26. Fossey MD, Hamner MB. Clonazepam-related sexual dysfunction in male veterans with PTSD. *Anxiety* 1994–95;1:233–6

27. Forman R, Gilmour White S, Forman N. Preface. *Drug-Induced Infertility and Sexual Dysfunction*. Cambridge, UK: Cambridge University Press, 1996:IX

28. Feldman HA, Johannes CB, Derby CA, *et al.* Erectile dysfunction and coronary risk factors: prospective results from the Massachusetts Male Aging Study. *Prev Med* 2000;30:328–38

29. Van Itallie TB. Health implications of overweight and obesity in the United States. *Ann Intern Med* 1985;103:983–88

30. Hubert HB, Feinleib M, McNamara PM, *et al.* Obesity as an independent risk factor for cardio-vascular disease: a 26 year follow-up of participants in the Framingham Heart Study. *Circulation* 1983;67:968–77

31. Gooren LJG. Visceral obesity, androgens and the risks of cardiovascular disease and diabetes mellitus. *Aging Male* 2001;4:30–8

32. Must A, Spandano J, Coackley EH, Field AE, Colditz G, Dietz WH. The disease burden associated with overweight and obesity. *J Am Med Assoc* 1999;282:1523–9

33. Chung WS, Sohn JH, Park YY. Is obesity an under-lying factor in erectile dysfunction? *Eur Urol* 1999;36:68–70

34. Rosen MP, Greenfield AJ, Walker TG, *et al.* Cigarette smoking: an independent risk factor for atherosclerosis in the hypogastric–cavernous arterial bed of men with arteriogenic impotence. *J Urol* 1991;145:759–63

35. Vidal Moreno JF, Moreno Pardo B, Jimenez Cruz JF. Assessment of tobacco impact on penile vascularization with echo-Doppler and intra-cavernous injection. *Actas Urol Esp* 1996;20: 365–71

36. Hirshkowitz M, Karacan I, Howell JW, Arcasoy MO, Williams RL. Nocturnal penile tumescence in cigarette smokers with erectile dysfunction. *Urology* 1992;39:101–7

37. Aoki M, Kumamoto Y. Analyses of factors contributing to the erectile dysfunction with aging by nocturnal penile tumescence, penile blood pressure index and papaverine test. *Nippon Hinyokika Gakkai Zasshi* 1990;81:1633–41

38. Xie Y, Garban H, Ng C, Rajfer J, Gonzales CNF. Effect of long term passive smoking on erectile function and penile nitric oxide synthase in the rat. *J Urol* 1997;157:1121–6

39. US Department of Health and Human Services. *The health consequences of smoking: cardiovascular disease. A report of the Surgeon General*. Publ. no. USDHHS (PHS) 84–50204. Washington, DC: USDHHS,1983

40. Bartecchi CE, MacKenzie TD, Schrier RW. The human costs of tobacco use. *N Engl J Med* 1994;330:907–12

41. MacKenzie TD, Bartecchi CE, Schrier RW. The human costs of tobacco use. *N Engl J Med* 1994;330:975–80

42. Ockene JK, Kuller LH, Svedsen KH, Meilahn E. The relationship of smoking cessation to coronary heart disease and lung cancer in the multiple risk factor intervention trial. *Am J Public Health* 1990;80:954–8

43. Wilhelmson C, Elmfeldt D, Vedin JA, *et al.* Smoking and myocardial infarction. *Lancet* 1975;1:415–20

44. Diex-Roux AV, Nieto FJ, Cromstock GW, *et al.* The relationship of active and passive smoking to carotid atherosclerosis 12–14 years later. *J Chron Dis* 1978;24:425–32

45. Howard G, Wagenknecht HG, Burke GL, *et al.* Cigarette smoking and progression of athero-sclerosis: the Atherosclerosis Risk in Communities (ARIC) Study. *J Am Med Assoc* 1998;279: 119–24

46. Wilson GT, Niaura RS, Adler JL. Alcohol, selective attention and sexual arousal in men. *J Stud Alcohol* 1985;46:107–15

47. Buffum J. Pharmacosexology: the effects of drugs on sexual function. *J Psychoactive Drugs* 1998; 14:5–14

48. Wilson GT, Lawson D. Effects of alcohol on sexual arousal in women. *J Abnormal Psychol* 1976;85:489–97

49. Mendelson JH, Mello NK, Ellingboe J. Effects of acute alcohol intake on pituitary gonadal hormones in normal males. *J Pharmacol Exp Ther* 1977;202:676–82

50. British Heart Foundation. *Coronary heart disease statistics*. London, UK: BHF, 1997:1–25

51. Aronson Friedman L, Kimball AW. Coronary heart disease mortality and alcohol consumption in Framingham. *Am J Epidemiol* 1986;124:481–9

52. Wetterling T, Veltrup C, Driessen M, John U. Drinking pattern and alcohol-related medical disorders. *Alcohol Alcoholism* 1999;34:330–6

53. Mandell W, Miller CM. Male sexual dysfunction as related to alcohol consumption: a pilot study. *Alcoholism Clin Exp Res* 1983;7:65–9

54. Smith CG, Arch RH. Drug abuse and reproduction. *Fertil Steril* 1987;48:355–73

55. Pate RR, Pratt SN, Blair SN, *et al.* Physical activity and public health: a recommendation from the Centers for Disease Control and Prevention and the American College of Sports Medicine. *J Am Med Assoc* 1995;273:402–7

56. Pinnock CB, Stapleton AM, Marshall VR. Erectile dysfunction in the community: a prevalence study. *Med J Aust* 1999;171:353–7

57. Finelli A, Hirshberg ED, Radomski SB. The treatment choice of elderly patients with erectile dysfunction. *Geriatr Nephrol Urol* 1998;8:15–19

Determinants of sexual function in the aging male

J. L. H. R. Bosch

2

The prevalence of erectile dysfunction has recently been studied in various countries in Europe and other continents. However, determinants of erectile dysfunction on a population level have been studied only in a handful of these surveys[1-4]. An example of a survey in which both prevalence and determinants of erectile dysfunction have been studied is the Krimpen study. In this study, the prevalence rates of erectile dysfunction and its determinants, and the level of concern about the dysfunction, were studied in a population-based sample of men aged 50 years or over in Krimpen aan den IJssel, a commuter town of about 28 000 inhabitants, near Rotterdam[5].

The investigated group consisted of 1688 men aged 50–78 years. They were studied by means of self-administered questionnaires, and measurements at a health center and a urology out-patient clinic. The study population represented a 50% response to an invitation to participate.

The prevalence of severe erectile dysfunction (i.e. erections of severely reduced rigidity or no erections) increased from 3 to 26% between the age groups of 50–54 and 70–78 years. Complete absence of erections was rare before the age of 65. One-third of men suffering from severe erectile dysfunction were concerned about the dysfunction, compared with only 8% of men with mild dysfunction (i.e. erections with reduced rigidity). In the same age strata, the prevalence of significant ejaculatory dysfunction (i.e. ejaculations with significantly reduced volume or no ejaculations) increased from 3 to 35%. The percentage of men who reported to be sexually active also decreased with increasing age, but was still surprisingly high at 69% between 70 and 78 years. Men without marital partners, and men with erectile or ejaculatory dysfunction, were sexually less active than other men in the same age strata. In sexually active men, 17–28% did not have normal erections, indicating that, in older age groups, normal erections are not an absolute prerequisite for a sexually active life. In general, men were less concerned about ejaculatory dysfunction than about erectile dysfunction. Since only a minority of men in the total population were concerned about the dysfunction, the term 'changed function' might be better than 'dysfunction'.

Recently, we conducted a systematic review of studies on the prevalence of erectile dysfunction in the general population[6]. Accepted guidelines for the reporting of systematic reviews were adhered to. We identified 23 studies, described in 35 articles, that met the inclusion criteria; of these studies, five, 15, two and one were from the USA, Europe, Asia and Australia, respectively. Six studies provided information on all 11 pre-specified methodological items; on average 1.8 items were missing. The reported prevalence rates varied from 2% in men younger than 40 years up to 93% in men older than 80 years. Comparison of prevalence rates is hampered by large methodological differences among the studies. The most important differences are the definition of erectile dysfunction and the type of questionnaire used to measure erectile dysfunction in the various studies. It is obvious that these two issues will have an important impact on the prevalence rates. Even if there is no true difference in prevalence between two populations, then still the apparent difference could be quite large if different definitions and different questionnaires are used. In general, the more items a questionnaire contains, the greater is the chance that an individual man will score an 'abnormal' answer on one of the questions. Furthermore, some studies are conducted only in men who are sexually active or who have a partner available; such studies may underestimate the prevalence of erectile dysfunction.

Traditionally, erectile dysfunction has been associated with several factors[7] :

(1) Cardiovascular disease, including myocardial infarction, coronary artery disease, hypertension, hyperlipidemia, cerebrovascular accident. The incidence of erectile dysfunction in men with heart disease and hypertension may be double that found in men without these problems[8]. Indeed erectile dysfunction itself is often a microvascular disease. It has been postulated that erectile dysfunction might be a precursor of more serious vascular disease states. This hypothesis, however, has not yet been proven in a prospective study.

(2) Cigarette smoking and substance abuse including alcohol abuse. An overall effect of smoking is not obvious. Smoking increases the risk for erectile dysfunction in men who have been treated for cardiovascular problems or hypertension. The effects of alcohol are less certain. In smaller quantities alcohol may be protective against vascular disease.

(3) Diabetes. Particularly those men who have vascular, neurological and/or nephrological complications of diabetes mellitus are more likely to suffer from erectile dysfunction.

(4) Surgical or non-surgical pelvic organ trauma can lead to vascular or neural damage. Spinal cord injury or cauda equina syndrome may also cause impotence. Wellknown iatrogenic causes include radical prostatectomy, colorectal surgery and aortoiliac vascular surgery. These factors play a minor role on a population level.

(5) Drugs, particularly antidepressants, antipsychotics, drugs that can lower the blood pressure (antihypertensives), antiarrhythmics and drugs that have endocrine effects such as antiandrogens, steroids and hormone replacement therapy.

(6) Chronic diseases such as chronic obstructive pulmonary disease (COPD), and renal, hepatic, hormonal and neurological disorders.

(7) Psychological factors such as depression, and relationship or marital problems including problems of sexual technique. In the Massachusetts Male Aging Study, however, depression and anger were not associated with incident erectile dysfunction, but new cases were more likely to occur among men who exhibited a submissive personality[9].

Table 1 summarizes the findings of four studies[1–4] that analyzed determinants of erectile dysfunction on a population level. Most of these studies looked at the different factors only in a univariate fashion. The Krimpen study was an exception to this pattern; the following factors were taken into account in a multivariate logistic regression analysis: age, body mass index, symptoms of benign prostatic hyperplasia (lower urinary tract symptoms, LUTS), smoking, COPD, history of cardiac complaints, lower level of education, hypertension (World Health Organization-2 definition), diabetes mellitus, previous prostate operation, alcohol consumption. The following factors were statistically significant independent determinants of severe erectile dysfunction in the multivariate analysis: age, smoking, obesity, level of education, LUTS and treatment for cardiovascular problems as well as COPD.

The parameter 'population attributable risk' (PAR) takes into account the prevalence of a certain risk factor in the general population. In the total population, the PAR was greatest for LUTS and obesity.

Table 1 Determinants of erectile dysfunction (ED) in four population-based studies[1-4]

Risk factors for ED	Krimpen study	Cologne study	Italian study	MMA Study
Marital status	–	0	–	0
Level of education	+	0	+	0
Age	+	+	+	+
Body mass index	+	0	0	–
LUTS	+	+	0	0
Smoking habits	+	–	+	–
Alcohol	–	–	–	+
COPD	+	0	0	0
Cardiovascular	+	0	+	+
Hypertension	–	+	+	0
Diabetes mellitus	–	+	+	+
Medications	–	0	0	0
Pelvic surgery	–*	+	+	0
Depression	0	0	0	+

*In the Krimpen study pelvic surgery is limited to prostate surgery; +, indicates that the factor was a significant determinant; –, indicates that the factor was not a determinant; 0, indicates that the factor was not taken into account in the analysis; MMA, Massachusetts Male Aging; LUTS, lower urinary tract symptoms; COPD, chronic obstructive pulmonary disease

References

1. Blanker MH, Bohnen AM, Groeneveld FPMJ, *et al.* Correlates for erectile and ejaculatory dysfunction in older Dutch men: a community-based study. *J Am Geriatr Soc* 2001;49:436–42
2. Braun M, Wassmer G, Klotz T, Reifenrath B, Mathers M, Engelmann U. Epidemiology of erectile dysfunction: results of the 'Cologne Male Survey'. *Int J Impotence Res* 2000;12:305–11
3. Parazzini F, Menchini Fabris F, Bortolotti A, *et al.* Frequency and determinants of erectile dysfunction in Italy. *Eur Urol* 2000;37:43–9
4. Feldman HA, Goldstein I, Hatzichristou DG, Krane RJ, McKinlay JB. Impotence and its medical and psychosocial correlates: results of the Massachusetts Male Aging Study. *J Urol* 1994;151:54–61
5. Blanker, MH, Bosch JLHR, Groeneveld FPMJ, Bohnen AM, Prins A, Hop WCJ. Erectile and ejaculatory dysfunction in a community-based sample of men aged 50–78 years: prevalence, concern and relation to sexual activity. *Urology* 2001;57:763–8
6. Prins J, Blanker MH, Bohnen AM, Thomas S, Bosch JLHR. Prevalence of erectile dysfunction: a systematic review of population-based studies. *Int J Impotence Res* 2002;in press
7. Jardin A, Wagner G, Khoury S, Giuliano F, Padma-Nathan H, Rosen R. *Recommendations of the International Scientific Committee on the Evaluation and Treatment of Erectile Dysfunction.* Paris: Health Publications, 2000
8. Johannes CB, Araujo AB, Feldman HA, Derby CA, Kleinman KP, McKinlay JB. Incidence of erectile dysfunction in men 40 to 69 years old: longitudinal results from the Massachusetts Male Aging Study. *J Urol* 2000;163:460–3
9. Araujo AB, Johannes CB, Feldman HA, Derby CA, McKinlay JB. Relation between psychosocial risk factors and incident erectile dysfunction: prospective results from the Massachusetts Male Aging Study. *Am J Epidemiol* 2000;152:533–41

Impact of radical prostatectomy and primary radiotherapy for localized prostate cancer on quality of life

3

M. L. Essink-Bot, I. J. Korfage and H. J. de Koning

Introduction

External-beam radiotherapy (EBRT) and radical prostatectomy (RP) have been the most common primary treatments for localized prostate cancer. There is no convincing evidence available to show that either treatment is more effective in saving quantity of life than the other. A recent report of a trial comparing RP and expectant management showed a significant reduction of prostate cancer mortality after RP, but a trial comparing RP and EBRT is not yet available[1]. Quality of life (QoL) issues become decisive in this situation.

Among the first QoL studies of primary treatment for localized prostate cancer, that of Litwin and colleagues found no differences in general QoL between groups of men who had previously been treated by RP or EBRT, but the groups differed from men without prostate cancer regarding sexual, urinary and bowel function[2]. Fowler and associates also reported similar general QoL and different patterns of side-effects in men after EBRT and RP[3]. The findings of such cross-sectional studies need to be confirmed by prospective longitudinal comparative studies, preferably randomized controlled clinical trials. Prospective observational cohort studies provide the next best information: if a pretreatment assessment is included, it is to some extent possible to adjust the results after RP or EBRT for pretreatment differences between treatment groups in terms of background characteristics (e.g. age), disease characteristics (e.g. cancer stage) and functional aspects of QoL (e.g. urinary or sexual function).

We conducted a search of the published literature to identify observational cohort studies with a pretreatment assessment comparing QoL in RP and EBRT. The designs and results have been compared with each other and with those of the Prostate Cancer Outcomes Study, a large population-based observational study with a retrospective pretreatment assessment[4].

Methods

Quality of life

Health-related QoL is the variable complementary to survival in studies of patient outcome. QoL is commonly defined as physical, psychological and social functioning and well-being. Medical and clinical variables (such as tumor stage and symptoms) are indispensable for the interpretation of QoL scores.

The common approach to empirical QoL assessment includes combining generic and condition-specific measures. Generic measures determine QoL in general terms, thus allowing for comparisons across disease (including 'no disease') and treatment groups. The Short Form-36 (SF-36) is an example of a generic QoL measure. The specific consequences of localized prostate cancer and its various treatments are in the areas of urinary, bowel and sexual functioning. Prostate cancer-specific QoL measures address these areas, preferably in terms of functioning and experienced bother. Typically, a variable such as 'urinary functioning' is measured by multiple items that are combined into a scale score. This approach is psychometrically superior to single-item questions, because a more reliable overall score is provided. However, the interpretation of such a scale score depends on the item content of the scale.

Literature search

We performed a PubMed search in May 2002. We used the following search strategy: 'Prostatic neoplasms [majr] AND quality of life [majr] AND Prostatic Neoplasms/therapy [majr] AND 1998/1/1 [mhda]:2002/5/29[mhda]'. This resulted in 111 references.

Two of the authors (M.L.E.-B., I.J.K.) independently selected on the basis of the abstracts the articles that met the following criteria:

(1) Empirical QoL study of patients with localized prostate cancer, comparing treatment by RP or EBRT in the same study;

(2) Prospective longitudinal design, including a pretreatment assessment of at least sexual and urinary function, or, in a population-based study, at least a retrospective pretreatment assessment;

(3) Included generic and prostate cancer-specific QoL assessments in follow-up;

(4) Published in English.

Five published cohort studies were identified[5–9]. Because most of these appeared to refer to relatively small and selected patient samples, the Prostate Cancer Outcomes Study was added[4].

Selected studies

The study reported by Talcott's group included 287 from 398 eligible American men with localized prostate cancer diagnosed in 1990–94. These men were treated at various centers, including non-teaching hospitals. We used mainly two publications from this study. The 1998 publication focused on comparing frequencies of urinary, bowel and sexual dysfunction before and after RP and EBRT until 12 months after the start of treatment[10]. In the article published in 1999 the relationship between generic QoL (SF-36) scores and the occurrence of urinary, bowel or sexual dysfunction was analyzed in a subsample of 125 men from the original cohort[5]. Table 1 provides further details.

Schapira and colleagues reported a study including 122 men (from 274 eligible; response rate 45%) with localized prostate cancer, recruited from four academically affiliated US hospitals, treated with RP, EBRT or expectant management. Differences in change scores over time in prostate cancer-specific scale scores and SF-36 scale scores between treatment groups were analyzed, with adjustments for age, comorbidity, and other covariates[6].

The article of Galbraith and co-workers reported a cohort selected from a US tertiary care facility. Five groups of patients were included of 24–59 men each: watchful waiting, prostatectomy, conventional EBRT, proton-beam radiotherapy and combined conventional–proton-beam EBRT. The statistical methods are not quite clear, but consisted mainly of comparisons of SF-36 scale scores and prostate cancer-specific scale scores per two treatment groups per assessment moment[7].

Lee and associates compared the QoL after RP, EBRT and interstitial brachytherapy in a prospective cohort study among 90 patients treated at a US teaching hospital in 1998–99. Analysis focused on QoL (as measured mainly with the Functional Assessment of Cancer Therapy (FACT) scales) changes over time within each treatment group, but included a covariance analysis with adjustment for age, tumor characteristics, baseline QoL scores and other confounders[8].

Our group reported on the first part of the ongoing Rotterdam QoL study that started in 1996, hence representing the only European study. The Rotterdam QoL study is a side study to the European Randomized Screening for Prostate Cancer (ERSPC) trial[11], and aims at providing a detailed description of the QoL effects of primary treatments for localized prostate cancer, to enable inclusion of these

Table 1 Characteristics of published studies of quality of life (QoL) in localized prostate cancer. The first five are cohort studies with a pretreatment assessment. The last column refers to a population-based longitudinal study with a retrospective pretreatment assessment

Characteristic	Talcott[5,10]	Schapira[6]	Galbraith[7]	Lee[8]	Madalinska[9]	Potosky[4]
Total n reported	125[5]/279[10]	122	185	90	278	1591
n RP	125	42	59	23	107	1156
n EBRT	135	51	96	23	171	435
Age (years): mean (range)	RP 61 (41–72) EBRT 68 (49–86)	RP 64 (58–68) EBRT 73 (68–75)	RP 65 EBRT (68–71) (3 types)	RP 61 EBRT 69	RP 63 (50–73) EBRT 68 (50–82)	? (55–74) RP 48% > 65, EBRT 78% > 65
TNM stage (%) T1	RP/EBRT 18/20	RP/EBRT 55/43	not reported	RP/EBRT 83/52	RP/EBRT 17/11	not reported
T2	RP/EBRT 73/60	RP/EBRT 45/57		RP/EBRT 17/48	RP/EBRT 67/61	
PSA at enrolment: median/mean	RP 8.2/15.3 EBRT 8.3/13.0	RP 7.6* EBRT 7.1*	RP 9.8† EBRT 14.1–22.8†	RP 6.2* EBRT 8.1*	RP 8.2/5.6 EBRT 15.2/8.7	RP 28% PSA >10 ng/ml, EBRT 36% >10
Assessments	pre-Tx, 3 m, 12 m	pre-Tx, 3 m, 12 m	pre-Tx, 6 m, 12 m, 18 m	pre-Tx, 1 m, 3 m, 12 m	pre-Tx, 6 m, 12 m	6 m, 12 m, 24 m
Generic QoL measures	SF-36	SF-36	SF-36, QLI	FACT-G	SF-36, EQ-5D	SF-36 (5 scales)
Prostate cancer-specific QoL measures	SWOG (PTSS?)	UCLA PCI	PTSS (SWOG)/ BSRI-S	FACT-P, IPSS	UCLA PCI + sex items	urinary, sexual and bowel function and bother scales

*Median; †mean; RP, radical prostatectomy; EBRT, external-beam radiotherapy; TNM, tumor, nodes, metastasis; PSA, prostate-specific antigen; Tx, treatment; m, months; SF-36, Short Form-36; QLI, Quality of Life Index; FACT-G, Functional Assessment of Cancer Therapy – General form; EQ-5D, EuroQoL measure for health-related quality of life; SWOG, Southwest Oncology Group; PTSS, Prostate Treatment Specific Symptoms Measure; UCLA PCI, University of California, Los Angeles Prostate Cancer Index; BSRI-s, Bem Sex-role Inventory – Short form; FACT-P, Functional Assessment of Cancer Therapy – Prostate cancer form; IPSS, International Prostate Symptom Score

effects in the overall evaluation of population-based prostate cancer screening. Data from 278 (of 299) patients treated in Erasmus MC (University Hospital Rotterdam) or one of three general Rotterdam hospitals by RP or EBRT in 1996–98 were included in the analysis reported by Madalinska and colleagues. This analysis focused on post-treatment differences between the treatment groups, using covariance analysis with age and baseline QoL as covariates[9].

The Prostate Cancer Outcomes Study (PCOS)[4,12,13] aimed at obtaining longitudinal, community-based estimates of health outcomes in men diagnosed with prostate cancer. From their various publications, we refer mainly to that by Potosky and co-workers[4]. A total of 5672 US men with biopsy-proven prostate cancer in 1994–95 were eligible for the PCOS. Of them, 62% ($n = 3533$) participated in surveys at 6, 12 and 24 months after diagnosis. The 6-month survey included retrospective questions on urinary, bowel and sexual functioning 'just before' the prostate cancer diagnosis. All assessments included current urinary, bowel and sexual functioning, and five SF-36 scales. Data from 1591 men aged 55–74 years were used for the comparison of RP ($n = 1156$) and EBRT ($n = 435$). This study compared health status outcomes at 24 months after diagnosis with statistical correction (propensity score) for pretreatment differences between treatment groups in age, baseline functioning, race, comorbidity and educational attainment.

Results

Characteristics of the studies

Table 1 indicates study characteristics and some characteristics of the patients included in the five cohort studies. In all studies, EBRT patients were older than RP patients. Mean age of the RP patients ranged from 61 in Talcott's and Lee's studies to 65 in Galbraith's study. Schapira's study included the oldest EBRT group. Patients in the studies published by Lee and Schapira showed more favorable distributions of TNM (tumor, nodes, metastasis) stages than did the other studies.

Symptoms

Frequencies of selected single symptoms of urinary, bowel and sexual dysfunction were reported in four studies. For Table 2 we selected symptom variables from the reports that seemed to be defined similarly across studies, but we cannot be sure that definition differences partly explain different results.

Wearing of incontinence pads was infrequent preceding treatment for localized prostate cancer. One year after treatment, the frequency was higher among RP patients (27% (PCOS)–44% (Schapira)) than among patients treated with EBRT (1% (PCOS)–8% (Schapira and Madalinska)).

Bowel urgency preceding treatment was somewhat more frequent than wearing of urine pads. Twelve months after treatment, bowel urgency was reported more often in EBRT (28% (Talcott)–36% (PCOS)). Erectile dysfunction was more frequent than urinary leakage or bowel urgency preceding treatment, and it was uniformly more frequent among patients who were to undergo EBRT (reflecting probably partly that EBRT patients were older). Preceding treatment, the percentages of men reporting erectile dysfunction ranged from 12% (Madalinska) to 35% (Schapira) in the RP group, and 26% (Madalinska) to 61% (Schapira) in the EBRT group. At 12 months after treatment, the frequency of erectile dysfunction was higher among RP patients (72% (PCOS)–93% (Talcott)) than among EBRT patients (52% (Madalinska)–75% (Schapira)).

Prostate cancer-specific QoL

The University of California, Los Angeles (UCLA) Prostate Cancer Index (PCI) was employed in the studies reported by Schapira and Madalinska. It includes scales on urinary, bowel and sexual function, complemented by items on the level of bother in each of these areas. Madalinska's group used items on sexual functioning and bother from another source[14]. The PCOS study used PCI-like scales. Talcott did not use scales, and Lee's and Galbraith's studies employed other prostate cancer-specific scales.

Table 2 Frequencies (percentages) of selected urinary, bowel and sexual dysfunction symptoms pretreatment and at 12 and 24 months (m) after treatment

Study	Wearing pads*			Bowel urgency[†]			Erectile dysfunction[‡]		
	Pre	12 m	24 m	Pre	12 m	24 m	Pre	12 m	24 m
Talcott[10]									
RP	3	35	—	7	6	—	32	93	—
EBRT	1	5	—	1	28	—	45	67	—
Schapira[6]									
RP	2	44	—	not	not	—	35	89	—
EBRT	4	8	—	reported	reported	—	61	75	—
Madalinska[9]									
RP	3	35	—	7	6	—	12	87	—
EBRT	1	8	—	11	30	—	26	52	—
PCOS									
RP[4,12]	2	27	28	—	—	15	16	72	80
EBRT[4,13]	2	1	3	20	36	36	42	54	62

*Talcott: 'wearing pads'; Schapira: 'use of ≥ 1 pad a day for control of urine'; Madalinska: 'use of ≥ 1 pad a day for control of urine'; Prostate Cancer Outcomes Study (PCOS): 'wearing pads to stay dry'
[†]Talcott: 'bowel urgency or tenderness (at least mild)'; Madalinska: 'bowel urgency(> 3 stools a day), a few times a week or more often'; PCOS: 'frequency of urgent bowel movements, some days or almost every day'
[‡]Talcott: 'no erections or erections usually inadequate for sexual intercourse'; Schapira: 'not having an erection firm enough for sexual intercourse'; Madalinska: '(almost) always problems with getting erections; sum of numbers of men reporting being sexually active and having erectile problems, and of numbers of men reporting not being sexually active because of erectile problems'; PCOS: 'erections not firm enough for sexual intercourse'

Numerical comparison of scale scores from different studies is difficult if different scales were used. Furthermore, some studies that used the PCI reported figures adjusted for, for example, age, whereas others reported unadjusted figures or difference scores. Therefore, comparison across studies was limited to verbal interpretation of the results.

All studies found good urinary function preceding treatment. At 12 months, urinary function had declined significantly in all RP groups studied, and the amount of bother experienced was significant. Urinary functioning in the EBRT groups was generally reported as little changed. Bowel functioning was generally good preceding treatment. At 12 months, bowel functioning had declined in the EBRT groups, but not in the RP groups. Preceding treatment, sexual dysfunction was more common than urinary or bowel dysfunction. Although not all men with sexual dysfunction after treatment reported high bother scores, the amount of bother owing to sexual dysfunction was significant, especially in the RP groups.

Subgroup analyses on the level of bother experienced by men with erectile problems after treatment but with good erectile function preceding treatment were not reported in the selected studies.

Generic QoL

The SF-36 was employed in five of the six studies selected, hence providing theoretically good opportunities for comparison. However, direct comparison of scale scores on the basis of published figures was not possible owing to different reporting of the results.

Madalinska and Schapira reported pretreatment SF-36 scores per treatment group. RP patients were healthier and younger than EBRT patients, and this was reflected by better generic SF-36 scores preceding treatment. Madalinska concluded that the EBRT group's scores were similar and the RP group's scores better than age- and sex-adjusted reference scores from the Dutch general population.

The studies from Galbraith, Madalinska, Talcott (SF-36), Lee (FACT scales) and Potosky (five SF-36 scales) reported analyses of differences in generic QoL after treatment between the RP and EBRT groups, with adjustment for baseline characteristics (age in all studies; baseline QoL in Madalinska and Lee; tumor characteristics and/or various demographic characteristics in Lee, Talcott and PCOS). Only Madalinska found significant differences between the treatment groups, for four SF-36 scales (Role–Physical, Bodily Pain, General Health Perceptions, Role–Emotional), all with better scores for the RP group. In the other studies differences were statistically insignificant after adjustment for baseline characteristics.

Schapira and Lee additionally tested between-group differences in score patterns over time. Schapira found no significant differences in change scores between the RP and the EBRT groups. Lee found in both groups significant (but similar) decreases in functional and physical well-being, but increases in emotional well-being. Analyses of within-group changes over time from the Rotterdam QoL study were not yet published.

Talcott's group used the SF-36 data from their study to analyze the relationship between generic QoL (SF-36 scale scores) and symptoms (sexual, urinary or bowel)[5]. In a cross-sectional analysis, five out of eight scales registered diminished scores in men with urinary, bowel or sexual dysfunction. From their longitudinal analyses it appeared that SF-36 scores in the mental, role performance and social domains of men who had no lasting side-effects of primary treatment *improved* from baseline to 12 months after the start of treatment, whereas the scores of men with side-effects remained stable. Scores in the physical domain were stable for both groups. Despite this complicated pattern, the observed changes in SF-36 scores were rather small.

Discussion

We are aware that our comparison of published cohort studies of QoL in localized prostate cancer may not do justice to the special qualities of each individual study. These studies were designed to provide answers to specific research questions, not for mutual comparability. However, the comparison adds to the body of knowledge and provides guidelines for further investigations.

With the necessary precautions regarding dissimilarities in definitions and selection of patients, about 30% of men in the available empirical cohort studies reported wearing urinary incontinence pads 12 months after surgery. When asked specifically, urinary incontinence was perceived as a problem. Symptoms of incontinence were infrequent after EBRT. However, the case may be that EBRT patients experience other urinary symptoms rather than leakage, especially irritative symptoms. The original UCLA PCI has been extended with items on, for example, urinary urgency to accommodate for this omission[15]. Twelve months after EBRT, approximately 30% of men experienced bowel problems. Sexual function showed the biggest decline, especially in RP. At 12 months after RP, only about 10% of men reported erections firm enough for intercourse. Many, although not all, men with sexual dysfunction after treatment for prostate cancer reported this as a major problem. Whether urinary dysfunction after treatment causes more or less bother than either bowel or sexual dysfunction is not clear, because the studies did not provide separate figures for the groups with good function preceding treatment but with dysfunction afterwards. Cross-sectional studies showed a relatively strong association between bowel dysfunction and bowel bother, and a somewhat less strong association between urinary dysfunction and bother, whereas sexual dysfunction is a relatively weak predictor of sexual bother[16,17].

At 12 months, the total side-effects of EBRT seem to be less frequent and less burdensome than those of RP. However, there is evidence to suggest that the situation at 12 months can be subject to change[4,7,16,18]. Side-effects of RP may still improve, and side-effects of EBRT can become incident or get worse after 12 months. We need results from prolonged follow-up studies, such as the Rotterdam study[19].

Most studies reported differences in urinary, bowel and sexual functioning and associated bother between RP and EBRT, but these were not reflected by generic QoL differences between the groups. If between-group differences in generic scores were found, these were attributable to pretreatment differences between the treatment groups, especially in age. Moreover, changes in generic QoL over time from pretreatment to 12 months afterwards appeared to be small, if any. On the basis of these findings, generic QoL scores in localized prostate cancer patients have been regarded as rather uninformative, but this conclusion may be premature.

First, the observation that generic QoL 12 months after treatment for localized prostate cancer is generally good is in accordance with common knowledge. These men seem to function relatively well. They may have symptoms of urinary, bowel or sexual dysfunction, but in general they can live with these. Naturally, this is not meant to trivialize the side-effects of primary treatment.

Second, men may have adapted to their situation. They may regard the side-effects of treatment as 'all in the bargain', as the price paid for the treatment they underwent to get rid of their prostate cancer and to improve their chances of survival.

Third, we may use the wrong measure for determining generic QoL. We say that the effects of prostate cancer treatment on generic QoL are small, which is in fact generic QoL *as defined by the SF-36* and similar measures. The situation may be similar to that of the mythical Pygmalion, who mistook the marble statue of the girl he loved for 'the real thing'. If urinary, bowel or sexual dysfunction has an effect on generic QoL, the question is whether the SF-36 is able to pick it up. On inspection of the SF-36 items, it is not quite clear which are relevant for respondents to express the effects of physical symptoms other than pain. And respondents are asked to rate limitations 'as a result of your physical health'–but whether, as an example, men who complete the questionnaire generally regard urinary or sexual dysfunction as an element of their physical health is not known. Qualitative research of the meaning of SF-36 items to respondents, as ongoing in the Rotterdam QoL study, may provide some answers.

From scarce longitudinal analyses in the data from the selected studies there is the suggestion of an improvement of mental health between the pretreatment assessment and 12 months later, with stable general physical functioning. This suggested finding focuses on the fact that the pretreatment assessment is not a real 'baseline' assessment. At the time of the pretreatment assessment the men had recently been told the diagnosis of prostate cancer. The two events (being diagnosed with cancer and the subsequent primary treatment) probably both have their specific effects afterwards. We hypothesize that the real stressor is the diagnosis, not the treatment, and that the treatment reduces the distress. In the Rotterdam QoL study this hypothesis is being investigated by including a pre-diagnosis QoL assessment in the screening phase.

References

1. Holmberg L, Bill-Axelson A, Helgesen F, *et al.* A randomized trial comparing radical prostatectomy with watchful waiting in early prostate cancer. *N Engl J Med* 2002;347:781–9

2. Litwin MS, Hays RD, Fink A, *et al.* Quality-of-life outcomes in men treated for localized prostate cancer. *J Am Med Assoc* 1995;273:129–35

3. Fowler FJJ, Barry MJ, Lu-Yao G, Wasson JH, Bin L. Outcomes of external-beam radiation therapy

for prostate cancer: a study of Medicare beneficiaries in three surveillance, epidemiology, and end results areas. *J Clin Oncol* 1996;14:2258–65

4. Potosky AL, Legler J, Albertsen PC, *et al.* Health outcomes after prostatectomy or radiotherapy for prostate cancer: results from the Prostate Cancer Outcomes Study. *J Natl Cancer Inst* 2000; 92:1582–92

5. Clark JA, Rieker P, Propert KJ, Talcott JA. Changes in quality of life following treatment for early prostate cancer. *Urology* 1999;53:161–8

6. Schapira MM, Lawrence WF, Katz DA, McAuliffe TL, Nattinger AB. Effect of treatment on quality of life among men with clinically localized prostate cancer. *Med Care* 2001;39:243–53

7. Galbraith ME, Ramirez JM, Pedro LW. Quality of life, health outcomes, and identity for patients with prostate cancer in five different treatment groups. *Oncol Nurs Forum* 2001;28:551–60

8. Lee WR, Hall MC, McQuellon RP, Case LD, McCullough DL. A prospective quality-of-life study in men with clinically localized prostate carcinoma treated with radical prostatectomy, external beam radiotherapy, or interstitial brachytherapy. *Int J Radiat Oncol Biol Phys* 2001; 51:614–23

9. Madalinska JB, Essink-Bot ML, de Koning HJ, Kirkels WJ, van der Maas PJ, Schroder FH. Health-related quality-of-life effects of radical prostatectomy and primary radiotherapy for screen-detected or clinically diagnosed localized prostate cancer. *J Clin Oncol* 2001;19:1619–28

10. Talcott JA, Rieker P, Clark JA, *et al.* Patient-reported symptoms after primary therapy for early prostate cancer: results of a prospective cohort study. *J Clin Oncol* 1998;16:275–83

11. de Koning HJ, Auvinen A, Berenguer Sanchez A, *et al.* Large-scale randomized prostate cancer screening trials: program performances in the European Randomized Screening for Prostate Cancer trial and the Prostate, Lung, Colorectal and Ovary trial. *Int J Cancer* 2002;97:237–44

12. Stanford JL, Feng Z, Hamilton AS, *et al.* Urinary and sexual function after radical prostatectomy for clinically localized prostate cancer: the Prostate Cancer Outcomes Study. *J Am Med Assoc* 2000;283:354–60

13. Hamilton AS, Stanford JL, Gilliland FD, *et al.* Health outcomes after external-beam radiation therapy for clinically localized prostate cancer: results from the Prostate Cancer Outcomes Study. *J Clin Oncol* 2001;19:2517–26

14. Korfage IJ, Essink-Bot ML, Madalinska JB, Kirkels WJ, Litwin MS, de Koning HJ. Measuring disease specific quality of life in localized prostate cancer: the Dutch experience. *Qual Life Res* 2003;in press

15. Wei JT, Dunn RL, Litwin MS, Sandler HM, Sanda MG. Development and validation of the expanded prostate cancer index composite (EPIC) for comprehensive assessment of health-related quality of life in men with prostate cancer. *Urology* 2000;56:899–905

16. Litwin MS, Flanders SC, Pasta DJ, Stoddard ML, Lubeck DP, Henning JM. Sexual function and bother after radical prostatectomy or radiation for prostate cancer: multivariate quality-of-life analysis from CaPSURE. Cancer of the Prostate Strategic Urologic Research Endeavor. *Urology* 1999;54:503–8

17. Bacon CG, Giovannucci E, Testa M, Glass TA, Kawachi I. The association of treatment-related symptoms with quality-of-life outcomes for localized prostate carcinoma patients. *Cancer* 2002;94:862–71

18. Litwin MS, Pasta DJ, Yu J, Stoddard ML, Flanders SC. Urinary function and bother after radical prostatectomy or radiation for prostate cancer: a longitudinal, multivariate quality of life analysis from the Cancer of the Prostate Strategic Urologic Research Endeavor. *J Urol* 2000;164: 1973–7

19. Korfage IJ, Essink-Bot ML, Kirkels WJ, de Koning HJ, Schroder FH. Long-term health-related quality of life in localized prostate cancer. *Qual Life Res* 2002;11:623

Sexual function before and after radical retropubic prostatectomy: a prospective analysis

4

G. R. Dohle, Y. D. Dubbelman, S. F. M. Broersen, M. F. Wildhagen and F. H. Schröder

Introduction

Radical prostatectomy has been associated with a loss of sexual potency in the majority of cases, owing to injury to the autonomic cavernous nerves. Since introduction of the anatomical approach to the neurovascular bundles by Walsh and Donker[1], nerve-sparing radical prostatectomy has become the operation of choice in potent and sexually active men with organ-confined prostate carcinoma. Numerous reports of recovery of sexual potency after a nerve-sparing radical prostatectomy have been published since, showing a high rate of potency after the operation in a selected group of patients[2,3]. Most of these studies, however, have involved sexually active young patients with early-stage cancer and low cancer volume. In contrast, studies from community practices have shown a much lower rate of potency after radical prostatectomy[4,5], questioning the feasibility of the nerve-sparing procedure in general urological practice.

We performed a prospective study, analyzing sexual function by means of a standardized interview in 770 patients before and after radical retropublic prostatectomy (RRP). Furthermore, we studied psychosexual and vascular function in 48 men before and after the operation using combined psychosexual testing and color Doppler ultrasound.

Material and methods

All men, candidates for RRP, were interviewed by questionnaire, including items on sexual activity, sexual function, percentage of erection during sexual activity, spontaneous erections, orgasm and desire. The questionnaires also requested information on age of the patient, preservation of the neurovascular bundles, pathological stage of the tumor, incontinence and urethral strictures.

The first interview was held during intake, 6 weeks to 3 months before the operation. Subsequent interviews were carried out every 3 months after the procedure in the first year of follow-up and every 6 months in the following years. Evaluation was performed after at least 1 year of follow-up. Results relating to sexual function were correlated with the outcome of surgery. Potency was defined as the ability to have unassisted intercourse.

To evaluate the psychosexual and vascular factors involved in RRP we carried out a study of 48 men, using the international index of erectile function (IIEF) questionnaire, psycho-physiological testing, including visual erotic stimulation with vibratory stimulation, and color Doppler ultrasound with intracavernosal injection of 0.25 mg of a mixture of papaverine and phentolamine (R/Androskat; Byk Cosmopharma, The Netherlands). These investigations were performed prior to the operation and 3 months after the RRP.

Results

Before the operation, 80% of the men were sexually active and had orgasms. Erectile dysfunction was already present in 12%. Sexual desire was low or absent in 12% of the men. After a bilateral nerve-sparing radical prostatectomy potency was preserved in 29%, after a unilateral nerve-sparing prostatectomy potency was preserved in 19% and in only 10% after a non-nerve-sparing procedure. An age-related decline in potency was found after the operation: of the men younger than 60 years 38% were still potent, between 60 and 65 years 29% and between 65 and 70 years only 19%. Erections were totally absent in 16% of the patients; 55% (irrespective of the type of operation) of the men remained sexually active after the operation. Only 17% of the patients successfully used pharmacological therapy such as sildenafil for improvement of sexual function. Orgasm was absent in 34% of the men after the procedure. No correlation was found with pathological tumor stage. Incontinence was strongly related to sexual activity: 77% of the continent patients were sexually active versus only 20% of the incontinent men.

The psychosexual and vascular evaluation showed a highly significant decrease in erectile function, orgasm and sexual satisfaction. Table 1 gives results of the IIEF questionnaire carried out in 48 men before and after RRP. Only sexual desire and arousal remained unchanged after the operation. The amount of erection decreased from 73 to 50% during visual erotic stimulation with vibratory stimulation and a low dose of intracavernosal injection. Maximal penile tumescence decreased from 29 to 20 mm (Table 2).

Color Doppler ultrasound investigations showed no significant changes in arterial cavernous flow after the operation, compared with before the RRP (Table 3). Resistance index was slightly decreased, indicating corpus cavernosum insufficiency, which was already present before the operation. Although vascular abnormalities were

Table 1 International index of erectile function (IIEF) score before and 3 months after radical retropubic prostatectomy (RRP): range of score for each item is indicated

	Mean score before RRP	Mean score 3 months after RRP	p Value
Erectile function (1–30)	21.1 ± 9.4	5.4 ± 4.4	< 0.0001
Coital satisfaction (0–15)	8.5 ± 4.6	2.0 ± 3.2	< 0.0001
Orgasm (0–10)	7.8 ± 3.7	2.8 ± 3.2	< 0.0001
Libido (2–10)	6.4 ± 1.6	5.7 ± 2.2	0.073
Total sexual satisfaction (0–10)	7.1 ± 2.8	3.9 ± 3.0	< 0.0001

Table 2 Results of psychosexual evaluation before and after radical retropubic prostatectomy (RRP)

	Mean score before RRP	Mean score 3 months after RRP	p Value
Sexual excitement (0–6)	3.59 ± 1.21	3.38 ± 1.52	0.4
Amount of erection (%)	73 ± 21	50 ± 27	< 0.0001
Tumescence increase (mm)	29.76 ± 10.1	20.49 ± 10.3	< 0.0001

Table 3 Results of color Doppler ultrasound investigations of the penis

	Before RRP	3 Months after RRP	p Value
Peak systolic flow velocity (cm/s)	45.5 ± 13.4	41.9 ± 13.5	0.079
End diastolic flow velocity (cm/s)	8.9 ± 2.95	9.4 ± 4.71	0.174
Resistance index	0.80 ± 0.07	0.77 ± 0.09	0.525

RRP, radical retropubic prostatectomy

encountered in some men, they were already present before the RRP.

Discussion

In a general urological practice, the mean age of patients undergoing a radical prostatectomy is 60–70 years. Before the operation, potency is reported in 67–84% of cases[6,7]. Selection criteria for performing a nerve-sparing radical prostatectomy are: normal erection before the operation and organ-confined disease.

In most studies a selection of patients are presented; usually, only those men who were potent before the operation and who had a nerve-sparing radical prostatectomy are evaluated. From most studies it is impossible to determine the results for the total group of operated patients. Fowler and colleagues[4] reported on a sample of Medicare patients who underwent radical prostatectomy in various institutions in the USA. From their survey it was concluded that in only 11% of patients were erections sufficient for intercourse. It is unknown how many of these 855 patients had a nerve-sparing radical prostatectomy. More recently, Schover and associates[5] performed a postal survey of 1236 men after RRP, and concluded that only 13% of men had reliable firm erections and another 8% of men were achieving erections with medical aids. This probably reflects the results for sexual function after RRP in a general urological practice.

From two large series[3,8] it can be estimated how many of the total group of operated patients were potent after the operation. Geary and colleagues[8] evaluated 459 men who were operated on between 1983 and 1991 and found potency in 51 cases (11%).

In most series, a correlation has been found between the number of spared neurovascular bundles and the recovery of potency: in cases of bilateral nerve-sparing radical prostatectomy, potency was reported in 31–76%; in cases of uni-lateral nerve-sparing radical prostatectomy, recovery of erection occurred in 13–56%. Catalona and associates[3] reported on 1870 patients operated on between 1983 and 1997, and found potency in 68% of men who

underwent a bilateral nerve-sparing procedure and 47% potency after a unilateral nerve-sparing prostatectomy.

The outcome related to potency after the operation is mainly determined by age and the number of neurovascular bundles saved during surgery[2]. Since advanced tumor stage usually coincides with wide excision of one or both neurovascular bundles, potency rates in these cases are limited. In practice, in many patients a nerve-sparing procedure is not achieved, and potency is usually lost.

The best results are achieved in younger patients with organ-confined disease[2,3]. Also, sexual activity before the operation has good prognostic value[8]. In most series, the number of spared neurovascular bundles is the most important prognostic factor. Other related factors are: age, tumor stage, cancer volume, incontinence and strictures. In 12% of cases, recovery of erections appeared after a follow-up of 1 year. In non-nerve-sparing radical prosta-tectomy, potency recurred in 0–17%[2,6].

Radical prostatectomy may also affect orgasm, in terms of total absence or reduced intensity, or even pain. We found orgasm to be absent in 34% after the operation, and reduced intensity was reported by 30% of men and pain by 9%[9].

We have reviewed articles on the etiology of impotence after radical prostatectomy; neuro-genic factors appear to be the most common explanation for this feature. Arguments in favor of a neurogenic cause are: clear relationship to the number of spared neurovascular bundles, absence of a history of vascular disease in most cases and a good response to low doses of intracavernosal treatment.

A vascular component has been suggested in studies using duplex scanning before and after nerve-sparing radical prostatectomy. A decrease in peak systolic flow velocity and diameter of the cavernosal arteries was determined in 8/20 cases by Abosief and colleagues[7]. An explan-ation for this decrease was found in the cadaveric dissections of Breza and co-workers[10], who found accessory pudendal arteries in 7/10 cases originating from the obturator artery, the inferior vesical artery or the superior vesical artery. These accessory pudendal arteries are found anterolateral to the prostatic surface and are usually injured during dissection. They supply additional blood to the cavernous bodies. In two cases in the above study, the accessory pudendal artery was the main supply to the penis. Kim and colleagues[11] also found decreased penile blood flow on color Doppler ultrasound after radical prostatectomy, especially on the side where the nerve bundle had been sacrificed. These differences, however, were not statistically significant. Also, no evidence for veno-occlusive dysfunction was found after radical prostatectomy in the ten studied cases. Polascik and Walsh[12] reported the presence or absence of accessory pudendal arteries in a series of 835 radical prostatectomies and found the accessory artery present in only 4% of cases. Preservation of the accessory pudendal artery did not significantly increase potency rates.

Diagnostic investigations into erectile failure are limited by the available treatment options. In practice, a goal-directed approach as proposed by Lue[13] is effective in most cases. Invasive diagnostic procedures should be performed only if they influence therapy choice.

The management of erectile failure after radical prostatectomy focuses primarily on pharmacological treatment, such as sildenafil and intracavernosal injection therapy. The efficacy of sildenafil after a nerve-sparing RRP averages 30–47%. This therapy is usually ineffective after a non-nerve-sparing procedure.

Both papaverine–phentolamine mixtures and prostaglandin E_1 are effective treatments in 60–85% of cases. Vacuum devices have also been applied successfully after radical prostatectomy. The combination of these therapies with sexual counselling increases acceptance by the patient and his partner, and provides better long-term results. In cases of therapy failure, a penile prosthesis can be offered.

Conclusions

Nerve-sparing radical prostatectomy preserves potency in 31–76% of cases of sexually active men with organ-confined disease. However, in most cases of radical prostatectomy a nerve-sparing procedure is not performed, and potency is usually lost. Prognostic factors for recovery of sexual potency are: number of spared neurovascular bundles, age, sexual activity before the operation, tumor stage, incontinence and strictures.

The etiology of impotence following radical prostatectomy is multifactorial, but neurogenic factors play a major role. Vascular factors may play a substantial role in selective cases, where accessory internal pudendal arteries are the major supply for the cavernous bodies.

Color Doppler ultrasound appears to be the most reliable diagnostic test for impotence after radical prostatectomy. Some men will respond to sildenafil after a nerve-sparing procedure, and most patients respond well to intracavernosal injections, probably indicating a mainly neurogenic cause of erectile dysfunction.

Acknowledgement

We would like to thank Mrs W. A. Phillips-Bolle and Mrs A. M. Schoen-Verkerk for their accurate maintenance of the radical prostatectomy database.

References

1. Walsh PC, Donker PJ. Impotence following radical prostatectomy: insight into aetiology and prevention. *J Urol* 1982;128:492–7

2. Walsh PC. Radical prostatectomy for localized prostate cancer provides durable cancer control with excellent quality of life. *J Urol* 2000;163:2030–1

3. Catalona WJ, Carvalhal GF, Mager DE, Smith DS. Potency, continence and complication rates in 1870 consecutive radical retropubic prostatectomies. *J Urol* 1999;162:433–8

4. Fowler FJ, Barry MJ, Lu-Yao G, Roman A, Wasson J, Wennberg JE. Patient-reported complications and follow-up treatment after radical prostatectomy. *Urology* 1993;42:622–9

5. Schover LR, Fouladi RT, Warnecke CL, *et al.* Defining sexual outcome after treatment for localized prostate carcinoma. *Cancer* 2002;15:1773–85

6. Davidson PJT, Van Den Ouden D, Schroeder FH. Radical prostatectomy: prospective assessment of mortality and morbidity. *Eur Urol* 1996;29:168–73

7. Abosief SR, Shinohara K, Breza J, Narayan P. Role of penile vascular injury in erectile dysfunction after radical prostatectomy. *Br J Urol* 1994;73:75–82

8. Geary ES, Dendinger TE, Freiha FS, Stamey TA. Nerve sparing radical prostatectomy: a different view. *J Urol* 1995;154:145–9

9. Steineck G, Helgesen F, Adolfson J, *et al.* Quality of life after radical prostatectomy or watchful waiting. *N Engl J Med* 2002;347:790–6

10. Breza J, Abosief SR, Orvis BR, Lue TF, Tanago EA. Detailed anatomy of penile neurovascular structures: surgical significance. *J Urol* 1989;141:437–43

11. Kim ED, Blackburn D, McVary KT. Post-radical prostatectomy penile blood flow: assessment with color Doppler ultrasound. *J Urol* 1994;152:2276–9

12. Polascik TJ, Walsh PC. Radical retropubic prostatectomy: the influence of accessory pudendal arteries on the recovery of sexual function. *J Urol* 1995;153:150–2

13. Lue TF. Impotence: a patient's goal-directed approach to treatment. *World J Urol* 1990;8:67–74

Effects of endocrine treatment: can libido and sexual function be preserved?

5

P. Iversen, I. Melezinek and A. Schmidt

Introduction

Quality of life for men with prostate cancer is receiving increasing attention and, acknowledging that endocrine therapy remains conceptually a palliative treatment, many patients view preservation of quality of life as an equally important goal of therapy as prolongation of survival[1]. The issue of quality of life is further emphasized by the moves to initiate endocrine therapy earlier in the course of the disease and in younger men.

Sexuality is an important aspect of quality of life, particularly in middle-aged men but also for a majority of elderly men[2,3]. However, loss of libido and erectile dysfunction are frequent sequelae of the diagnosis and treatment of prostate cancer[4,5]. Among 401 men with prostate cancer, 71% experienced a loss of libido after surgery or medication (prostatectomy, radiotherapy, hormonal therapy with goserelin, buserelin or leuprolide alone or in combination with flutamide, bicalutamide or nilutamide, and orchidectomy) and, overall, approximately two-thirds of those questioned would prefer their level of sexual activity to be higher[5]. Indeed, sexual functioning is sufficiently important to some older men that, if they were diagnosed with prostate cancer, they would trade some reduction in survival time for maintained sexual function. In a sample of 50 men (mean age 58 years), 68% were willing to exchange a 10% or greater advantage in 5-year survival, to maintain sexual potency[6]. Likewise, Mazur and Hickman[7] found that, of 230 men (mean age 65 years), 67% would trade a 14% survival advantage to prevent impotence, while Helgason and colleagues[4] found that only 38%

of a group of 299 men would unconditionally accept a treatment with a 50% risk of impotence.

Sexual interest, often referred to as sexual desire or sexual drive, is difficult to define[8], and we have not been able to find a precise definition in the sexological literature. In recent studies investigating the use of the non-steroidal antiandrogen bicalutamide in prostate cancer, sexual interest was assessed in a validated quality of life questionnaire[9] by scoring the response to three questions addressing 'interest in sex', 'if the patient felt sexually attractive' and, finally, 'whether others find the patient sexually attractive'[10–15].

The decline in sexual interest and activity in prostate cancer patients may be caused by a multiplicity of factors including the psychological impact of the diagnosis, the disease itself and its treatment[5]. In advanced prostate cancer, androgen deprivation is the mainstay of treatment, and has traditionally been achieved by either medical or surgical castration alone or in some cases in combination with an antiandrogen as combined androgen blockade (CAB). Both these approaches to treatment are associated with a loss of libido and erectile capability in more than 80% of patients[5,16–19].

In men for whom their sexuality is important, a decrease in sexual interest and/or erectile capability can result in psychological distress, difficulties with relationships and loss of self-esteem[5]. Indeed, Helgason's group[4] found that the decline in sexual function (including sexual desire, erectile capacity and orgasm pleasure) was the most common cause of disease-related stress in men with prostate cancer. While erectile dysfunction can be effectively treated[20,21], there are no recognized effective therapies for loss of sexual interest[21]. However, in the absence of sexual interest, the treatment of sexual dysfunction becomes less relevant and, therefore, hormonal treatments for advanced prostate cancer that spare sexual interest are needed.

Monotherapy with a non-steroidal antiandrogen is an emerging treatment option for men with prostate cancer[22]. There is a widespread perception that non-steroidal antiandrogens have less impact on sexual interest and function than do other treatments for advanced prostate cancer. This review presents data on sexual interest and function obtained from clinical studies of the three non-steroidal antiandrogens (bicalutamide, flutamide and nilutamide) as monotherapy, focusing particularly on bicalutamide which has been the most extensively evaluated in randomized, controlled studies in this setting. All three agents are indicated for treatment of metastatic carcinoma of the prostate in combination with castration. In addition, bicalutamide (150 mg/day) has been approved as a monotherapy treatment for locally advanced prostate cancer in some countries, and further approvals are expected.

Theoretical basis for preservation of sexual interest and function with non-steroidal antiandrogens

The relationship between hormones and sexual behavior in man is complex and poorly understood[23]. However, the fact that androgen deficiency, as in men who have undergone medical or surgical castration, generally causes loss of sexual interest and potency[16,18,24,25] implies that maintenance of testosterone levels is important for normal sexual activity.

The non-steroidal antiandrogens antagonize the effects of androgens, of both testicular and adrenal origin, at the receptor level. They also block the negative feedback mechanism regulating testosterone action at the hypothalamus and pituitary gland, thereby increasing plasma luteinizing hormone (LH) and, consequently,

testosterone concentrations. A moderate increase in estrogen is also observed owing to the higher concentrations of androgens available for aromatization. Details of studies of the effects of the non-steroidal antiandrogens on serum testosterone in prostate cancer patients are presented in Table 1[26–35]. Flutamide and bicalutamide have similar effects; there are currently few data on nilutamide. In general, serum testosterone concentrations increase by a mean of 50–100%, with peak concentrations occurring after 1–9 months; the effects do not appear to be dose-related over the range of doses studied[30]. Testosterone concentrations, although elevated, remain within the normal range. It is suggested that this is because the increased concentration of estradiol limits increases in LH secretion[29].

Any benefits of the non-steroidal antiandrogens for sexual interest and function are unlikely to be explained as a direct result of the maintenance of normal testosterone levels, because the hypothalamic androgen receptors must be blocked to some extent as demonstrated by the rising LH concentrations. Animal experiments suggest that the compounds responsible for sexual drive in man are metabolites of testosterone (such as estrogens after the peripheral conversion of testosterone by aromatase), acting either directly or by modifying neural androgen metabolism[36–44]. These pathways would be unaffected by the non-steroidal antiandrogens, which, therefore, offer theoretical benefits over castration with respect to sexual behavior.

Assessment of sexual interest/function in prostate cancer patients

An accurate assessment of the changes in sexual interest and function following the different treatment options for advanced prostate cancer and how patients feel about these changes is necessary, so that patients and their physicians may select the treatment that best meets the patients' needs. However, the design of studies of the sexual aspects of quality of life in elderly men with a potentially life-threatening disease presents a number of difficulties.

Table 1 The effect of non-steroidal antiandrogens on serum testosterone levels in prostate cancer patients

Reference	Non-steroidal antiandrogen	n	Increase in total testosterone	Time to peak increase	Comments
Migliari et al.[26]	bicalutamide 50 mg	5	—	—	mean levels at 6 months were 59% above baseline. The majority of increase was seen within 8 weeks
Soloway et al.[27]	bicalutamide 50 mg	32	median 90%	4 weeks	remained elevated through 48 weeks of treatment
Chodak et al.[28]	bicalutamide 50 mg	243	median 65%	9 months	median levels remained within normal range throughout the 24-month study
Verhelst et al.[29]	bicalutamide 150 mg	23	mean 96%	4 weeks	mean values did not exceed normal limits. Increase occurred in all but one patient. At 24 weeks, levels remained 66% above baseline
Tyrrell et al.[30]	bicalutamide 10–200 mg	390	—	4–12 weeks	increases within the normal range. No dose-related effect (increases at 3 months ranged from 25% at 10 mg/day, to 83% at 30 mg/day and 77% at 200 mg/day)
Lund and Rasmussen[31]	flutamide 750 mg	20	mean 44%	1 month	returned to baseline at 12 months
Delaere and van Thillo[32]	flutamide 750 mg	32	—	6 months	59% increase seen within 1 month. Further increases seen in patients (n = 16) followed for at least 6 months. In patients still in study at 9 and 12 months (n = 7 and 4, respectively), levels remained slightly above baseline
Boccon-Gibod et al.[33]	flutamide 750 mg	104	50%	3 months	decreased over time, but remained 25% above baseline at 24 months
Brufsky et al.[34]	flutamide 750 mg	20	—	—	mean increase of 77% after 4.9–29.4 weeks
Decensi et al.[35]	nilutamide 300 mg	26	mean about 45%	3 months	38% increase seen within 1 month

First, it is common for patients with advanced prostate cancer, particularly those over 75 years of age, to have relatively low levels of interest/function before study entry. In the pivotal trials of bicalutamide 150 mg/day monotherapy[10,11], approximately 50% of patients had no sexual interest at study entry (data on file), while Boccon-Gibod and colleagues[33] reported that they were unable to assess the impact of flutamide on sexual function because the vast majority of patients (mean age about 73 years) were impotent before the initiation of treatment. Additionally, some patients may have experienced erectile difficulties before the diagnosis of prostate cancer or following previous therapy (prostatectomy or radiotherapy).

Second, sexual function is a difficult parameter to assess in clinical trials owing to the lack of a clear definition of erectile functioning[45] and the lack of standardized methodology. Although the measurement of nocturnal penile tumescence (NPT) and rigidity, a widely accepted method of differentiating between organic and psychogenic sexual dysfunction[46,47], correlates well with actual functioning in small studies in prostate cancer patients[4,26], it is not practical for use in large trials. Furthermore, sexual function should not be assessed only objectively; patients' feelings about changes in function also need to be examined.

A further problem in assessing both sexual function and interest is that many elderly men find it difficult to discuss sexual issues with their physician. For example, 22% of patients enrolled in one of the phase III trials of bicalutamide 150 mg/day versus CAB refused to respond directly to physician questioning[48].

Finally, as castration is currently the standard therapy for advanced prostate cancer, studies of new therapies tend to have an open design. There are, however, difficulties in interpreting data on sexual interest/function obtained from such open trials, as patients, informed that regimens containing castration are likely to result in loss of sexual activity, will consider these events less severe or report them less frequently, as they were expected.

The problems inherent to assessing sexual function in prostate cancer patients are illustrated by the failure of a study specifically designed to compare bicalutamide 150 mg/day with medical castration with goserelin acetate (Zoladex®) to draw definitive conclusions on the relative effects of the two treatments on sexual interest and function. This was due to the large proportion of patients who were protocol violations (68% of patients), that is they were thought not to demonstrate sufficient evidence of sexual function at entry to the trial as they did not have at least one qualifying episode of NPT (a rigidity of > 60% for at least 10 min) per night (data on file). Such a large proportion of protocol violations may have affected the power of the trial analyses. Data from the Derogatis Interview of Sexual Functioning-Male (DISF-M) questionnaire[49] used in this trial did not give consistent evidence of the level of sexual function of patients at entry to the trial (data on file). Thirty-eight men with locally advanced prostate cancer and aged between 46 and 73 years were recruited to this double-blind study and randomized to bicalutamide 150 mg/day ($n = 17$) or goserelin acetate 3.6 mg every 28 days ($n = 21$). The primary end-points were mean penile rigidity assessed by NPT, and sexual function and interest assessed by the DISF-M questionnaire[49]. There were no significant differences in either treatment group in the change from baseline in mean penile rigidity. Results from the DISF-M questionnaire showed

that patients who received bicalutamide 150 mg/day had less change from baseline in sexual function on all dimensions of the questionnaire than that of patients who received goserelin acetate 3.6 mg. However, the difference between the two groups did not reach statistical significance.

Effect of non-steroidal antiandrogens on sexual interest and function

Nilutamide

Published clinical experience with nilutamide monotherapy is limited to a single open uncontrolled study in which 26 patients with metastatic prostate cancer were treated with nilutamide 100 mg three times daily[35] and studied for 10 months. Sexual potency in this study was assessed by patient interview only. Fifteen of the men claimed to be potent before treatment, of whom seven (47%) maintained libido and potency on nilutamide; libido and potency were completely abolished in five patients (33%) and attenuated in the remaining three (20%). Of the seven men in whom potency was maintained on nilutamide, all four who were subsequently switched to a luteinizing hormone-releasing hormone (LH-RH) agonist experienced a loss of libido and erectile function.

Flutamide

Flutamide has been used more widely as a monotherapy for advanced prostate cancer than has nilutamide. The majority of published data are from relatively short, small, open studies, involving patients with metastatic disease. Only one small ($n = 104$) study of flutamide monotherapy versus castration has been published[33], in which median time to progression and overall survival at 69 months were similar for the two treatments. There are no comparative data on the effects of treatment on sexual parameters, as the majority of patients were impotent before study entry. Three small pilot studies have also investigated the combination of the 5α-reductase inhibitor finasteride with flutamide[34,50,51]. This combination resulted in a mean reduction in serum prostate-specific antigen (PSA) levels of > 90%. Details of changes in sexual interest and/or function in these studies and in trials of flutamide monotherapy are presented in Table 2[31,32,34,50–59]; data were obtained by patient self-reporting or direct patient questioning with the exception of the study by Brufsky's group[34], which used a patient-completed questionnaire. In several of these studies, around two-thirds of previously sexually potent men retained potency during

Table 2 Summary of data on sexual interest and function in published studies of flutamide monotherapy for advanced prostate cancer

Reference	Patients receiving flutamide (n)	Daily dose	Changes in sexual interest	Changes in sexual function
Airhart et al.[52]	14	750–1500 mg	no change	no data
Sogani et al.[53]	72	750 mg	—	32/37 (87%) retained potency, although some decline in nine of these; potency loss took 3–34 months. Two previously impotent patients regained potency
Johansson et al.[54]	15	750 mg	80% maintained libido	80% maintained potency
Lund and Rasmussen[31]	20	750 mg	no change	no change
Prout et al.[55]	52	750 mg	—	13/21 (62%) previously potent men retained potency, 5/31 (16%) previously impotent men regained potency
Pavone-Macaluso et al.[56]	37	750 mg	—	6/9 (67%) retained normal sexual performance, 1/18 regained some sexual performance
Delaere and van Thillo[32]	40	750 mg	decreased in five patients to varying degrees	10/15 (67%) of men who were sexually potent before treatment retained potency, although in five of these potency was reduced
Dudov and Todorov[57]	15	750 mg	39% reported impaired libido	34% reported impaired/absent erections
Chang et al.[58]	44	750 mg	—	decline in function in eight patients (18%)
Schröder et al.[59]	147	750 mg	—	78% lost sexual activity and 80% lost erections
Fleshner and Trachtenberg[50]	22	375–750 mg*	diminished or total loss of libido in three (14%) patients	total loss of morning erections in one patient (5%)
Ornstein et al.[51]	13	750 mg*	—	potency preserved in 66% of men
Brufsky et al.[34]	20	750 mg*	maintained initially in 18 of the 19 (95%) men with good libido at baseline. At last follow-up, good libido still maintained in 12 men	of the 11 who were completely potent before treatment, nine (82%) men initially retained complete potency. At median 16.4 months follow-up, 6/11 men were potent and 2/11 were partially potent

*Patients also received finasteride

treatment with flutamide; a small proportion of previously impotent men regained sexual function on flutamide. There are fewer data on sexual interest, but it appears to be preserved in a similar proportion of patients. The results of the large randomized study of Schröder and colleagues (European Organization for Research and Treatment of Cancer (EORTC) protocol 308929)[59] are a notable exception to the other results presented in Table 2[31,32,34,50-58]. This study compared flutamide and the steroidal antiandrogen cyproterone acetate (CPA) in M1 prostate cancer patients with good prognostic factors. The authors found that the decreases in sexual function and activity with flutamide were surprisingly large (Table 2)[31,32,34,50-59], and although less pronounced, the decreases were not statistically different from those observed with CPA. Contributing to the apparent discrepancy could be the long follow-up in the EORTC study (in excess of 2 years). Furthermore, the patients receiving flutamide were significantly older with a median age of 73 years versus 69 in the CPA group. Still, these results are unexpected given that CPA exhibits pronounced progestogenic effects, thereby reducing gonadotropin secretion and testosterone synthesis[60]. Consequently, CPA has previously been reported to be associated with a severe suppression of libido and loss of erectile potency, the incidence of which is comparable to that seen following castration[61].

Flutamide has also been investigated in benign prostatic hyperplasia (BPH). Results on changes in sexual function in these studies confirm the findings in advanced prostate cancer patients. In a double-blind, placebo-controlled, dose–response study involving 372 men aged 42–88 years (mean 66 years) with BPH[62], sexual dysfunction was reported by a small proportion (3–8%) of each treatment group after 24 weeks, with no significant difference between the groups. In a smaller ($n = 87$), open, placebo-controlled study, none of the BPH patients (mean age 65 years) reported impotence after treatment with flutamide 750 mg/day for periods of up to 6 months[63].

Studies using bicalutamide 50 mg/day

In the initial studies of bicalutamide monotherapy in metastatic prostate cancer patients, a 50-mg daily dose (the dose otherwise used as a component of CAB) was compared in an open manner with castration (surgical or medical)[12,13,28]. Since these open, randomized, multicenter trials had a similar design, pooling of the data was possible. An overview analysis of these studies involving a total of more than 1000 patients with metastatic prostate cancer revealed that there was a median survival difference between the treatments of approximately 3 months, favoring castration[14]. Therefore, in subsequent studies in prostate cancer patients, bicalutamide monotherapy was evaluated at 150 mg/day, rather than at 50 mg/day.

In all three studies in which the bicalutamide 50-mg dosage was used, quality of life was assessed using a self-administered questionnaire[9]. When the data were pooled, the scores for sexual interest and function were superior in the bicalutamide group[14]. In the largest of the studies involving 486 men[28], sexual interest and function were maintained with bicalutamide for up to 3 months, with a slight decline thereafter. In contrast, in the castration group there was a decline in both parameters within 1 month and there was a significant difference between the treatments, favoring bicalutamide 50 mg/day, at 1, 3 and 6 months for sexual interest and at 1 and 3 months for sexual function.

Sexual function has also been assessed objectively in patients receiving bicalutamide 50-mg/day monotherapy. Using continuous monitoring of penile tumescence and rigidity on multiple nights in five men (mean age 61 years) with advanced prostate cancer, Migliari and associates[26] found that 6 months' therapy with bicalutamide 50 mg/day had no effect on the number of tumescence episodes, tumescence duration, maximal change in penile circumference or duration of rigidity. Only one of the patients (20%) reported a decrease in sexual desire and libido.

Bicalutamide 50-mg/day monotherapy has also been evaluated in three double-blind, placebo-controlled studies in a total of 126 BPH patients over 24 weeks[64,65] (data on file). Although these studies used different questionnaires to assess sexual parameters, findings were consistent across the studies, with all three concluding that retention of both sexual interest and function was comparable in the bicalutamide and placebo groups; these data are in agreement with the findings on flutamide in BPH[62,63]. A further analysis of data from the largest of these studies in patients with high sexual interest and high sexual function at baseline showed that the impact of bicalutamide on both parameters was similar to that of placebo (data on file). It is interesting to note that even with placebo there was a decline in sexual interest and some loss of sexual function in these patients over time.

Studies of bicalutamide 150 mg/day

Subsequent bicalutamide monotherapy studies were conducted using 150 mg/day. Two large phase III studies comparing bicalutamide 150-mg/day monotherapy with castration (orchidectomy or the LH-RH agonist goserelin acetate) in 1453 patients with locally advanced (M0) or metastatic (M1) prostate cancer had an identical design, to permit a combined analysis. In the pooled analysis of 480 M0 patients after a median follow-up of 6.3 years with 56% deaths, there was no overall difference in survival or time to progression with bicalutamide 150 mg/day compared with castration[15]. Two smaller open European studies[48,66] have compared bicalutamide 150 mg/day with CAB in patients with advanced disease. The study population ($n = 220$) of Boccardo's group[48] comprised approximately equal proportions of locally advanced and metastatic patients, whereas the 235 patients enrolled by Chatelain and colleagues[66] mainly had metastatic disease at entry. Survival data in these trials are not currently mature, but indicate that CAB is not more effective than bicalutamide 150-mg/day monotherapy.

Quality of life, including sexual interest and function, was an important outcome measure in all four of these phase III trials, and these studies attempted to overcome some of the difficulties in assessing sexual function described above. Several analyses focused specifically on patients with sexual interest and/or function at study entry. In addition, although there is no universally accepted health-related quality of life instrument for prostate cancer patients, all four phase III studies used the same validated questionnaire, covering ten domains including sexual interest and function[9], which was completed in private by the patient, although Boccardo's group[48] also used direct questioning.

As described above, the two largest monotherapy studies of bicalutamide 150 mg/day had an identical design to permit a pooled analysis. Separate analyses of quality of life data were performed at 12 months for locally advanced and metastatic patients[10,11].

Of the 480 patients with locally advanced disease at entry, 337 responded to questions on changes in sexual interest during the 12-month period. The combined analysis at 12 months showed that bicalutamide was associated with a significant advantage for sexual interest compared with castration ($p = 0.029$), although a decrease was recorded in both groups[11] (Figure 1). The reduction in the mean score for the sexual interest dimension was 23% for bicalutamide 150 mg/day and 47% for castration. After the first month of treatment, the decrease in sexual interest was slightly greater in patients receiving castration. After that, patients treated with castration experienced a further

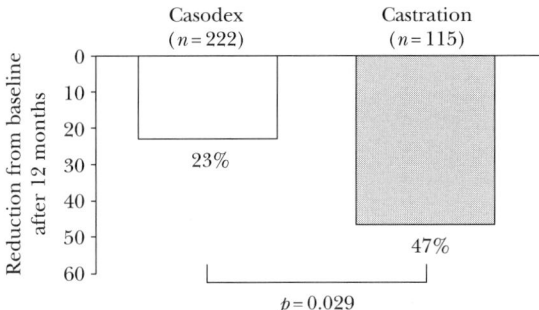

Figure 1 Percentage reduction from baseline in sexual interest after 12 months' treatment: bicalutamide (Casodex®) 150 mg daily versus castration in patients with locally advanced M0 prostate cancer

decline, unlike patients receiving bicalutamide. This is consistent with the fact that following medical castration (which was used in 86% of the castration group) testosterone concentrations, after an initial increase (flare), decrease to within the castrate range within 21 days[67]. A dramatic and sustained fall in sexual interest follows the reduction in testosterone concentrations. In contrast, the reduction in sexual interest with bicalutamide 150 mg/day occurs after the diagnosis has been established and changes little over time. Thus, the benefits of bicalutamide 150 mg/day over castration are evident within a month and are maintained for at least 12 months.

Approximately 50% of M0 patients in both treatment groups had no sexual interest at study entry. Further analyses were therefore performed on data (last value carried forward (LVCF) analysis) provided by only those patients with some degree of interest at baseline (i.e. those who had scope for deterioration). This allowed assessment and comparison of changes in sexual interest of the two treatments. Since it takes some time for castrated patients to lose their interest in sex, using this type of analysis was not expected to produce any bias against castration. In this exploratory analysis, the benefit for bicalutamide 150 mg/day was even more pronounced than in the overall study population[68]. Of those patients with sexual interest at study entry who responded to the specific question on sexual interest ($n = 198$), 64% of the bicalutamide group still had some interest in sex during the 12 months compared with only 30% of the castration group ($p < 0.01$). Similarly, 71% and 42% of the bicalutamide and castration groups, respectively, still felt they had some sexual attractiveness ($p < 0.01$; $n = 147$). Patients receiving bicalutamide 150 mg/day as monotherapy were also more likely still to feel that others found them to have some sexual attractiveness (71% vs. 52%; $n = 141$), although the difference did not reach statistical significance (Figure 2).

Similar results were obtained when patients with metastatic disease at study entry were analyzed, although the differences between the bicalutamide 150-mg/day and castration treatment groups were not as great as for the patients with less advanced disease[10] (data on file). At 12 months, data from the 210 men answering

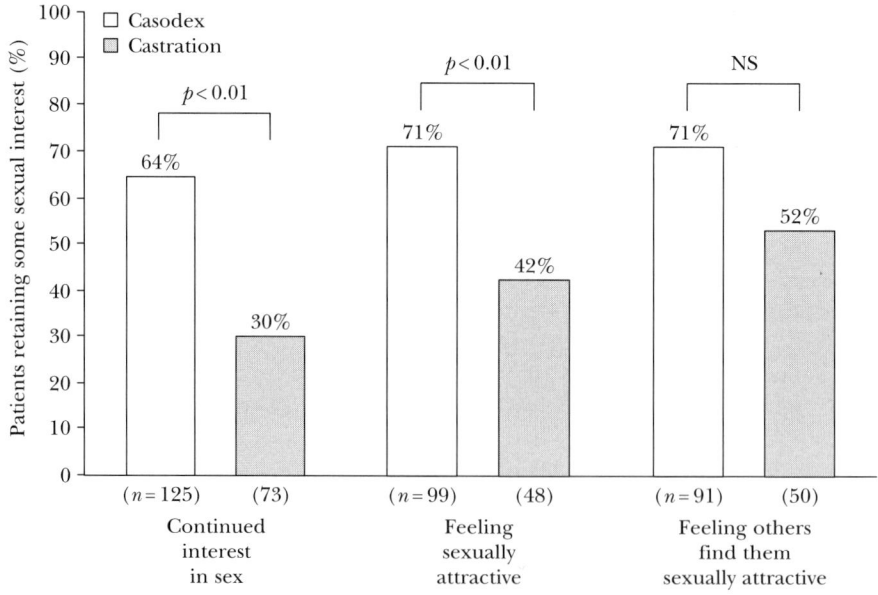

Figure 2 Sexual interest of patients with locally advanced M0 prostate cancer after 12 months' treatment: bicalutamide 150 mg versus castration. NS, not significant

questions on the sexual interest dimension showed that sexual interest was maintained to a significantly greater extent with bicalutamide 150 mg/day than with castration ($p = 0.041$), with a difference between the groups apparent at 1 month. As with the locally advanced disease group, a significant proportion of patients (56%) had no sexual interest at study entry. In exploratory analyses, excluding these patients (data on file), there was a clear difference ($p < 0.01$) between treatment groups with respect to the proportion of patients retaining some sexual interest (67% vs. 40%; LVCF analysis). Differences were also apparent for feeling sexually attractive and feeling that others found them sexually attractive, although these were not significant.

A smaller number of patients in these two studies answered questions on sexual function at 12 months, and statistical analyses could not be undertaken. In the locally advanced patients ($n = 70$), sexual function was reduced by 18% from baseline in the bicalutamide 150-mg/day group and by 37% in the castration group[68] (Figure 3). The reduction in sexual function in the castration group was lower than expected, and this may have been because patients who lost sexual function were less likely to answer the relevant question (which was asked after the question on sexual interest) than the minority of patients who had some sexual function remaining.

The results of the two phase III studies of bicalutamide 150-mg/day monotherapy versus

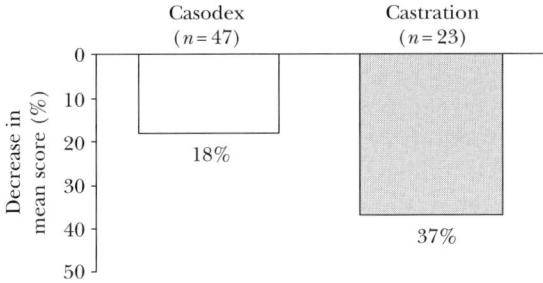

Figure 3 Percentage reduction from baseline in sexual function after 12 months' treatment: bicalutamide 150 mg versus castration in patients with locally advanced M0 prostate cancer

CAB support the above findings[48,66]. In the study of Boccardo's group[48], of those responding to direct physician enquiry who had normal libido and erections at entry, significantly more patients treated with bicalutamide 150 mg/day retained sexual interest during follow-up (median 38 months) than in the CAB group (40% vs. 15%; $p = 0.01$). Similarly, the proportion of patients who maintained their erectile capability was greater in the bicalutamide 150-mg/day group than in the CAB group (31% vs. 7%; $p = 0.002$). Responses to the quality of life questionnaire, which was completed by 130 men, showed significant ($p \leq 0.05$) differences for sexual interest, favoring bicalutamide, at 2, 6 and 9 months[69]. In the other study[66], there was also a non-significant trend in favor of bicalutamide 150 mg/day with respect to sexual interest over the first 24 months of treatment.

As mentioned above, the interpretation of data on sexual interest and function from open studies in which castration is a comparator can be difficult. However, data on bicalutamide have also been obtained from two blinded studies (data on file), the results of which are consistent with those described above.

In the first of these, the impact of bicalutamide on sexual interest and function was evaluated using the EORTC quality of life questionnaire in a randomized, double-blind phase IIb study versus chlormadinone acetate 100-mg/day monotherapy in 109 Japanese patients with locally advanced (36%) or metastatic (64%) prostate cancer (data on file); chlormadinone is a steroidal progestogen with antiandrogenic properties, widely used for the treatment of prostate cancer in Japan. In this study, the daily dose of bicalutamide was 80 mg, which, based on weight-adjusted plasma bicalutamide concentrations, is a dose pharmacologically equivalent to 150 mg in Western patients (data on file). Of the bicalutamide-treated patients with some sexual interest at study entry ($n = 28$), 64% retained sexual interest and 77% maintained sexual function after 3 months' treatment.

Bicalutamide 150 mg/day was also compared with flutamide 750 mg/day in a randomized single-blind study involving 148 patients with locally advanced disease (data on file). Quality of life was assessed using the Rotterdam symptom questionnaire, which includes a question on sexual interest. At 12 weeks, 72% of bicalutamide patients and 68% of flutamide patients showed no worsening in their responses concerning sexual interest, compared with baseline. This result for flutamide is consistent with previously published data (Table 2)[31,32,34,50–59].

The Scandinavian Prostatic Cancer Group study 6 (SPCG-6) is part of the large bicalutamide Early Prostate Cancer Program, and included a total of 1218 men with early non-metastatic prostate cancer, of whom slightly more than 80% had not undergone therapy of primary curative intent (i.e. were otherwise candidates for watchful waiting). Patients were randomized beween bicalutamide monotherapy 150 mg daily and placebo. A first preliminary analysis of time to progression is just about to be published[70]. Sexual function was assessed using a shortened version of the Golombok and Rust Inventory of Sexual Satisfaction (GRISS) questionnaire, which was completed by the patient at baseline and at 12, 24, 36 and 48 weeks after randomization (Table 3). This questionnaire comprised six questions, two addressing the frequency of sexual activity and four concerning erectile function. The questions were answered in a semiquantitative manner (never, rarely, some-

times, etc.), allowing a numerical score to be assigned for the purposes of analysis. The proportion of men retaining some sexual activity and function (which could be less than at baseline) and the proportion maintaining sexual activity and function (the same or higher than at baseline) were calculated.

The results of the GRISS questionnaire obtained at 24 and 48 weeks after randomization are presented in Figures 4 and 5. At 48 weeks, 78% of patients in the placebo group retained some sexual activity as opposed to 63% in the bicalutamide group. Corresponding figures for maintenance of sexual activity were 48% and 31%. With respect to sexual function, 85% of placebo patients retained some sexual function at 48 weeks compared with 75% of patients in the bicalutamide arm, while 53% and 35%, respectively, maintained their pretreatment level of sexual function. Thus, while a higher proportion of patients retain and maintain sexual activity and function after randomization to placebo than to bicalutamide, the differences are relatively small, with the majority of patients retaining some sexual activity and function after treatment with bicalutamide.

Conclusions

Quality of life issues are increasingly influencing treatment choices in prostate cancer patients, and sexuality is an important component of quality of life for many middle-aged and older men. Sexual interest is a prerequisite for sexual activity and cannot be effectively treated, whereas in patients with sexual interest, erectile dysfunction can be managed in a variety of ways. Lack of sexual interest, therefore, should be regarded as a greater problem than erectile dysfunction.

The impact of the currently available hormonal therapies on sexual interest and function varies, and therefore may be an important consideration when selecting therapy for specific patients with advanced disease. Loss of libido and sexual function are frequently experienced after medical or surgical castration. The data presented in this

Table 3 The GRISS (Golombok–Rust Inventory of Sexual Satisfaction) shortened version questionnaire used in the Scandinavian Prostatic Cancer Group study 6 (SPCG-6)[70] to assess sexual activity (questions 1 and 2) and sexual function (questions 3–6). Possible answers are: never, hardly ever, occasionally, usually, always

(1) Do you have sexual intercourse more than twice a week?
(2) Are there weeks in which you don't have sex at all?
(3) Do you become easily sexually aroused?
(4) Do you fail to get an erection?
(5) Do you get an erection during foreplay with your partner?
(6) Do you lose your erection during intercourse?

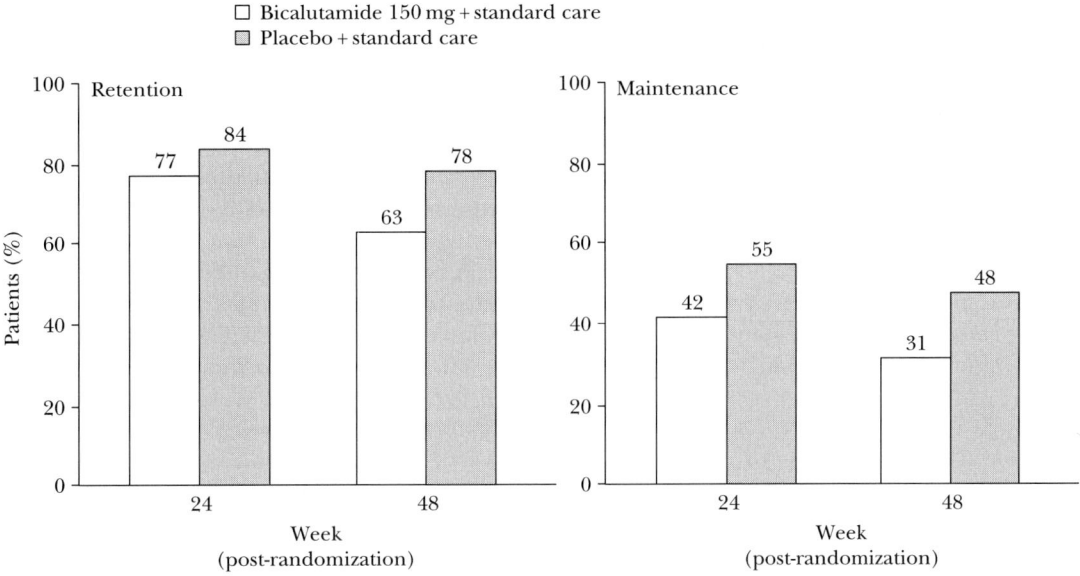

Figure 4 Sexual activity as assessed by the GRISS (Golombok–Rust Inventory of Sexual Satisfaction) questionnaire in men treated with bicalutamide 150 mg daily compared with placebo at 24 and 48 weeks after start of treatment relative to baseline. For definition of 'retention' and 'maintenance' see text

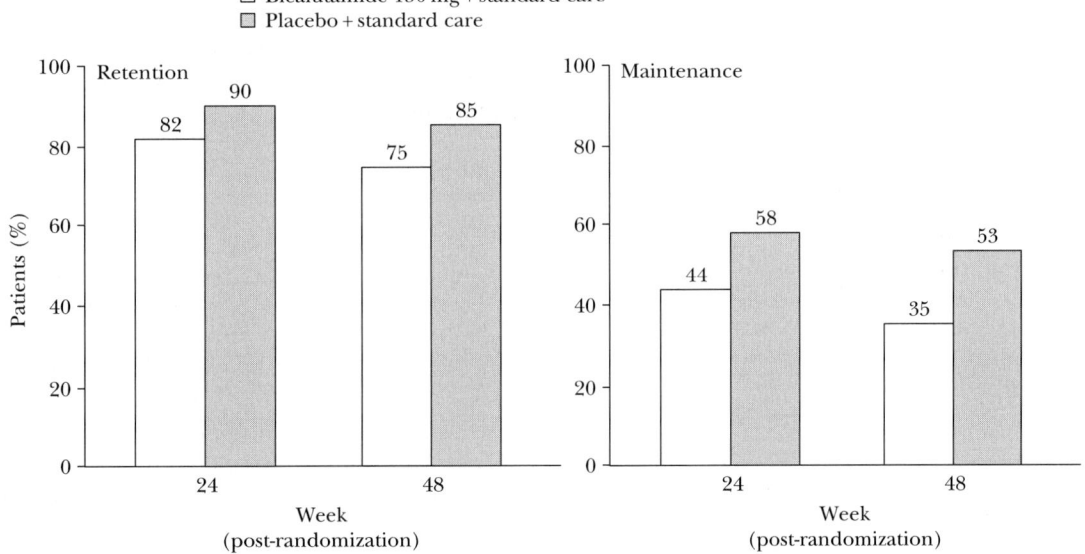

Figure 5 Sexual function as assessed by the GRISS (Golombok–Rust Inventory of Sexual Satisfaction) questionnaire in men treated with bicalutamide 150 mg daily compared with placebo at 24 and 48 weeks after start of treatment relative to baseline. For definition of 'retention' and 'maintenance' see text

review confirm the widespread perception that monotherapy with a non-steroidal anti-androgen offers benefits over castration with respect to preservation of libido and sexual potency. Overall, approximately two-thirds of patients with locally advanced or metastatic prostate cancer retain sexual interest following treatment with non-steroidal antiandrogens, a significantly greater proportion than after medical or surgical castration. Sexual function is also maintained to a greater extent than following castration. These findings are consistent for the two most studied non-steroidal antiandrogens (bicalutamide and flutamide), in groups at different disease stages (locally advanced and metastatic), in both open and blinded studies, and using different methods of evaluation. Bicalutamide 150 mg/day has been the most extensively investigated non-steroidal antiandrogen, and findings on sexual interest are consistent in patients with both locally advanced and metastatic prostate cancer. In a placebo-controlled study in early, non-metastatic prostate cancer, a slightly smaller fraction of patients treated with bicalutamide 150-mg monotherapy maintain, or retain some, sexual activity and function after 48 months when compared with placebo. However, the difference is small. Longer follow-up seems warranted. Bicalutamide appears to be a useful treatment option for men with advanced prostate cancer who wish to remain sexually active.

References

1. Crawford ED, Bennett CL, Stone NN, et al. Comparison of perspectives on prostate cancer. Analyses of survey data. *Urology* 1997;50: 366–72

2. Pfeiffer E. Sexuality in the aging individual. *J Am Geriatr Soc* 1974;22:481–4

3. Persson G. Sexuality in 70 year old urban population. *J Psychosom Res* 1980;24:335–42

4. Helgason AR, Adolfsson J, Dickman P, et al. Waning sexual function – the most important disease-specific distress for patients with prostate cancer. *Br J Cancer* 1996;73:1417–21

5. Kirby RS, Chodak GW, Watson A, Newling DWW. Prostate cancer and sexual function. *Prost Cancer Prost Dis* 1998;1:179–84

6. Singer PA, Tasch ES, Stocking C, et al. Sex or survival: trade-offs between quality and quantity of life. *J Clin Oncol* 1991;9:328–34

7. Mazur DJ, Hickman DH. Patient preferences. Survival vs. quality-of-life considerations. *J Gen Intern Med* 1993;8:374–7

8. Ackerman MD, D'Attilio JP. Male psychogenic sexual dysfunction: sex and behaviour therapy. In Singer C, Weiner WJ, eds. *Sexual Dysfunction. A Neuro-Medical Approach.* Armonk, NY: Futura Publishing, 1994:229–44

9. Cleary PD, Morrissey G, Oster G. Health-related quality of life in patients with advanced prostate cancer: a multinational perspective. *Qual Life Res* 1995;4:207–20

10. Tyrrell CJ, Kaisary AV, Iversen P, et al. A randomised comparison of 'Casodex' (bicalutamide) 150 mg monotherapy versus castration in the treatment of metastatic and locally advanced prostate cancer. *Eur Urol* 1998;33:447–56

11. Iversen P, Tyrrell CJ, Kaisary AV, et al. Casodex (bicalutamide) 150-mg monotherapy compared with castration in patients with previously untreated nonmetastatic prostate cancer: results from two multicentre randomized trials at a median follow-up of 4 years. *Urology* 1998;51: 389–96

12. Kaisary AV, Tyrrell CJ, Beacock C, Lunglmayr G, Debruyne F. A randomised comparison of monotherapy with Casodex 50 mg daily and castration in the treatment of metastatic prostate carcinoma. *Eur Urol* 1995;28:215–22

13. Iversen P, Tveter K, Varenhorst E. Randomised study of Casodex 50 mg monotherapy vs. orchidectomy in the treatment of metastatic prostate cancer. *Scand J Urol Nephrol* 1996;30:93–8

14. Bales GT, Chodak GW. A controlled trial of bicalutamide versus castration in patients with advanced prostate cancer. *Urology* 1996;47:38–43

15. Iversen P, Tyrrell CJ, Kaisary AV. Bicalutamide ('Casodex') 150 mg monotherapy compared with castration in patients with non-metastatic locally advanced prostate cancer: 6.3 years' follow-up. *J Urol* 2000;164:in press

16. Rousseau L, Dupont A, Labrie F, Couture M. Sexuality changes in prostate cancer patients receiving antihormonal therapy combining the antiandrogen flutamide with medical (LHRH agonist) or surgical castration. *Arch Sex Behav* 1988;17:87–98

17. Ferrari P, Castagnetti G, Ferrari G, et al. Combination treatment in M1 prostate cancer. *Cancer* 1993;72(Suppl):3880–5

18. Lucas MD, Strijdom SC, Berk M, Hart GAD. Quality of life, sexual functioning and sex role

identity after surgical orchidectomy in patients with prostatic cancer. *Scand J Urol Nephrol* 1995; 29:497–500

19. Fossa SD, Woehre H, Kurth K-H, *et al.* Influence of urological morbidity on quality of life in patients with prostate cancer. *Eur Urol* 1997; 3(Suppl 3):3–8

20. Sharlip ID. Evaluation and nonsurgical management of erectile dysfunction. *Urol Clin North Am* 1998;25:647–59

21. Meinhardt W, Kropman RF, Vermeij P. Comparative tolerability and efficacy of treatments for impotence. *Drug Safety* 1999;200: 133–46

22. Boccon-Gibod L. Are non-steroidal anti-androgens appropriate as monotherapy in advanced prostate cancer? *Eur Urol* 1998;33: 159–64

23. Nickel JC, Morales A, Condra M, Fenemore J, Surridge DH. Endocrine function in impotence: incidence, significance and cost-effective screening. *J Urol* 1984;132:40–3

24. Salmimies P, Kockott G, Pirke KM, *et al.* Effects of testosterone replacement on sexual behaviour in hypogonadal men. *Arch Sex Behav* 1982;11: 345–53

25. Buffum J. Pharmacosexology update: prescription drugs and sexual function. *J Psychoact Drugs* 1986;18:97–106

26. Migliari R, Muscas G, Usai E. Effect of Casodex on sleep-related erections in patients with advanced prostate cancer. *J Urol* 1992;148: 338–41

27. Soloway MS, Schellhammer PF, Smith JA, Chodak GW, Kennealey GT. Bicalutamide in the treatment of advanced prostatic carcinoma: a phase II multicenter trial. *Urology* 1996; 47(Suppl 1A):33–7

28. Chodak G, Sharifi R, Kasimis B, Block NL, Macramalla E, Kennealey GT. Single agent therapy with bicalutamide: a comparison with medical or surgical castration in the treatment of advanced prostate carcinoma. *Urology* 1995;46: 849–55

29. Verhelst J, Denis L, Van-Vliet P, *et al.* Endocrine profiles during administration of the new non-steroidal anti-androgen Casodex in prostate cancer. *Clin Endocrinol* 1994;41:525–30

30. Tyrrell CJ, Denis L, Newling D, *et al.* Casodex 10–200 mg daily, used as monotherapy for the treatment of patients with advanced prostate cancer. *Eur Urol* 1998;33:39–53

31. Lund F, Rasmussen F. Flutamide versus stilboestrol in the management of advanced prostatic cancer: a controlled prospective study. *Br J Urol* 1988;61:140–2

32. Delaere KPJ, van Thillo EL. Flutamide monotherapy as primary treatment in advanced prostatic carcinoma. *Semin Oncol* 1991;18:13–18

33. Boccon-Gibod L, Fournier G, Bottet P, *et al.* Flutamide versus orchidectomy in the treatment of metastatic prostate carcinoma. *Eur Urol* 1997;32:391–6

34. Brufsky A, Fontaine-Rothe P, Berlane K, *et al.* Finasteride and flutamide as potency-sparing androgen-ablative therapy for advanced adeno-carcinoma of the prostate. *Urology* 1997;49: 913–20

35. Decensi AU, Boccardo F, Guarneri D, *et al.* for the Italian Prostatic Cancer Project. Monotherapy with nilutamide, a pure nonsteroidal antiandrogen, in untreated patients with metastatic carcinoma of the prostate. *J Urol* 1991;146:377–81

36. Crews D, Morgentaler A. Effects of intracranial implantation of oestradiol and dihydro-testosterone on the sexual behaviour of the lizard *Anolis carolinensis*. *J Endocrinol* 1979; 82:373–81

37. Thompson DL, Pickett BW, Squires EL, Nett TM. Sexual behavior, seminal pH and accessory sex gland weights in geldings administered testosterone and(or) estradiol-17 beta. *J Anim Sci* 1980;51:1358–66

38. Dykeman DA, Katz LS, Foote RH. Behavioral characteristics of beef steers administered estradiol, testosterone and dihydrotestosterone. *J Anim Sci* 1982;55:1303–9

39. Dohanich GP, Clemens LG. Inhibition of estrogen-activated sexual behaviour by androgens. *Horm Behav* 1983;17:366–73

40. Sodersten P, Eneroth P, Hansson T, *et al.* Activation of sexual behaviour in castrated rats: the role of oestradiol. *J Endocrinol* 1986; 111:455–62

41. De Bruijn M, Broekman M, van der Schoot P. Sexual interactions between estrous female rats and castrated male rats treated with testosterone proprionate or estradiol benzoate. *Physiol Behav* 1988;43:35–9

42. Watson JT, Adkins-Regan E. Testosterone implanted in the preoptic area of the male Japanese quail must be aromatized to activate copulation. *Horm Behav* 1989;23:432–47

43. Rasia-Filho AA, Peres TM, Cubilla-Gutierrez FH, Lucion AB. Effect of estradiol implanted in the corticomedial amygdala on the sexual behavior of castrated male rats. *Braz J Med Biol Res* 1991;24:1041–9

44. Wood RI. Estradiol, but not dihydrotestosterone, in the medial amygdala facilitates male hamster sex behavior. *Physiol Behav* 1996;59:833–41

45. Robinson JW, Dufour MS, Fung TS. Erectile functioning of men treated for prostate carcinoma. *Cancer* 1997;79:538–44

46. Schvartzman P. The role of nocturnal penile tumescence and rigidity monitoring in the evaluation of impotence. *J Fam Pract* 1994;39:279–82

47. Levine LA, Lenting EL. Use of nocturnal penile tumescence and rigidity in the evaluation of male erectile dysfunction. *Urol Clin North Am* 1995;22: 775–88

48. Boccardo F, Rubagotti A, Barichello M, *et al.* Bicalutamide monotherapy versus flutamide plus goserelin in prostate cancer patients. Results of an Italian prostate cancer project (PONCAP) study. *J Clin Oncol* 1999;17:2027–38

49. Derogatis LR. The Derogatis Interview for Sexual Functioning; an introductory report. *J Sex Marital Ther* 1997;23:291–304

50. Fleshner NE, Trachtenberg J. Combination finasteride and flutamide in advanced carcinoma of the prostate: effective therapy with minimal side effects. *J Urol* 1995;154:1642–5

51. Ornstein DK, Rao GS, Johnson B, Charlton ET, Andriole GL. Combined finasteride and flutamide therapy in men with advanced prostate cancer. *Urology* 1996;48:901–5

52. Airhart RA, Barnett TF, Sullivan JW, *et al.* Flutamide therapy for carcinoma of the prostate. *South Med J* 1978;71:798–801

53. Sogani PC, Vagaiwala MR, Whitemore WF. Experience with flutamide in patients with advanced prostatic cancer without prior endocrine therapy. *Cancer* 1984;54:744–50

54. Johansson JE, Andersson SO, Beckman KW, Lingardh G, Zador G. Clinical evaluation of flutamide and estramustine as initial treatment of metastatic carcinoma of prostate. *Urology* 1987;29:55–9

55. Prout GR, Keating MA, Griffin PP, Schiff SF. Long term experience with flutamide in patients with prostatic carcinoma. *Urology* 1989; 34(Suppl 4):37–45

56. Pavone-Macaluso M, Pavone S, Serretta V, Daricello G. Antiandrogens alone or in combination for treatment of prostate cancer: The European experience. *Urology* 1989; 34(Suppl 4):27–36

57. Dudov A, Todorov D. Goserelin vs. flutamide in previously untreated advanced prostate cancer (APC). *Can J Infect Dis* 1995;6:396c (abstr 3034)

58. Chang A, Yeap B, Davis T, *et al.* Double blind randomized study of primary hormonal treatment of stage D2 prostate carcinoma: flutamide versus diethylstilbestrol. *J Clin Oncol* 1996;14: 2250–7

59. Schröder FH, Collette L, de Reijke TM, *et al.* Prostate cancer treated by anti-androgens: is sexual function preserved? *Br J Cancer* 2000; 82:283–90

60. Vogelzang NJ, Kennealey GT. Recent developments in endocrine treatment of prostate cancer. *Cancer* 1992;70(Suppl 4):966–76

61. Jacobi GH, Altwein JE, Kurth KH, Basting R, Hohenfellner R. Treatment of advanced prostatic cancer with parenteral cyproterone acetate: a phase III randomised trial. *Br J Urol* 1980;52:208–15

62. Narayan P, Trachtenberg J, Lepor H, *et al.* A dose response study of the effect of flutamide on benign prostatic hyperplasia: results of a multicenter study. *Urology* 1996;47:497–504

63. Stone NN, Clejan S, Smith JA, *et al.* Treatment of benign prostatic hypertrophy with flutamide. *Eur Urol* 1990;18(Suppl 1):24

64. Eri LM, Tveter KJ. A prospective, placebo-controlled study of the antiandrogen Casodex as treatment for patients with benign prostatic hyperplasia. *J Urol* 1993;150:90–4

65. Eri LM, Tveter KJ. Safety, side effects and patient acceptance of the antiandrogen Casodex in the treatment of benign prostatic hyperplasia. *Eur Urol* 1994;26:219–26

66. Chatelain C, Fourcade RO, Delchambre J. Bicalutamide (Casodex) versus combined androgen blockade: open French multicentre trial in patients with metastatic prostate cancer. *Br J Urol* 1997;80(Suppl 2):283 (abstr 1111)

67. Dijkman GA, del Morale PF, Plasman JW, *et al.* A new extra long acting depot preparation of the LHRH analogue Zoladex. First endocrinological and pharmacokinetic data in patients with advanced prostate cancer. *J Steroid Biochem Mol Biol* 1990;37:933–6

68. Iversen P. Quality of life issues relating to endocrine treatment options. *Eur Urol* 1999; 36(Suppl 2):20–6

69. Rubagotti, Boccardo F, Canobbio L, *et al.* Evaluation of quality of life of prostate patients during up front therapy with either Casodex monotherapy or goserelin plus flutamide. *Proc Am Soc Clin Oncol* 1998;17:341 (abstr 1315)

70. Iversen P, Tammela TLJ, Vaage S, *et al.*, SPCG-6 study group. Bicalutamide (Casodex) 150 mg versus placebo as immediate therapy either alone or as adjuvant to standard care for early non-metastatic prostate cancer. First report from the Scandinavian Prostatic Cancer Group study 6. *Eur Urol* 2002;in press

Oral therapy

6

H. Porst

Introduction

Until 1998, effective pharmacotherapy of erectile dysfunction was limited to intra-cavernous self-injection therapy and trans-urethral therapy with alprostadil (MUSE™), the latter with clearly less efficacy. The approval of sildenafil marked a breakthrough in the conservative treatment of erectile dysfunction and revolutionized completely the manage-ment of this disease. With the availability of effective oral therapy, the management of erectile dysfunction became more and more an issue for the general or family practitioner, and meanwhile more than 70% of all Viagra™ prescriptions are provided by non-urologists. One major negative consequence of this development is that many physicians have given up any diagnostic screening in these patients, and are limiting their activities more or less to pure prescription of the medication. The urologist, who was for a long time the first referral for erectile dysfunction patients, should continue to underline his expertise in this field by providing a thorough diagnostic work-up of patients comprising medical and sexual history, somatic examination, laboratory tests, including testosterone, prolactin and serum glucose, and intracavernosal pharmaco-testing with 10–20 µg alprostadil combined with Doppler/duplex sonography of the cavernous arteries. In this connection, systolic peak flow velocities < 25 cm/s are indicative of an arteriogenic etiology, and should prompt the urologist to refer the patient for a further cardiovascular screening, as a considerable subset of these patients are suffering from generalized athero-sclerosis and therefore are at risk of coronary or cerebral artery disease.

Diagnosis-oriented therapy of erectile dysfunction

Based on the diagnosis, principally four main categories of erectile dysfunction patients may be discriminated.

Psychogenic (functional) erectile dysfunction In these patients all diagnostic tests result in a normal outcome. These patients may be treated by sexual counselling if available, or any oral drug therapy such as yohimbine, apomorphine sublingual or a phosphodiesterase-5 (PDE-5) inhibitor.

Endocrinological erectile dysfunction Depending on the underlying endocrinological disorder, these patients are primarily managed by testosterone replacement therapy, prolactin inhibitors, dehydroepiandrosterone (DHEA) or specific treatment of any other endo-crinological disorder. In the case that after 2–3 months of specific endocrinological inter-vention no improvement of erectile dysfunction is reported by the patient, additional erectile dysfunction-specific medications (apomorphine sublingual, PDE-5 inhibitor) are added.

Predominant organic erectile dysfunction In these patients, yohimbine or apomorphine sub-lingual have proved to be mostly ineffective; therefore, PDE-5 inhibitors are the first choice.

Arteriogenic erectile dysfunction and/or three or more cardiovascular risk factors As these patients are at risk of coronary heart disease and other manifestations of atherosclerosis, it is advisable to subject them to a thorough cardiovascular assessment before prescription of any erectile dysfunction-specific medication.

Clinical profile of oral erectile dysfunction-specific drugs

Yohimbine

Yohimbine is the main alkaloid from the bark of the Central African coryanthe johimbehe tree. It is a central α_2-adrenoceptor blocker with a 50–100 times higher activity on presynaptic receptors than on postsynaptic adrenoceptors. Besides its central site of action, it is said to act also on the α_2-adrenoceptors of the penile arteries and on presynaptic α_2-adrenoceptors localized on α_1-adrenoceptors of sympathetic nerve terminals in the cavernous smooth muscle cell[1]. With these sites of action the main effects of yohimbine are attributed to a decrease of the sympathetic tone and, thus, facilitation of erection. The efficacy and safety of yohimbine have been analyzed in numerous studies. A meta-analysis of seven large yohimbine studies revealed a superiority to placebo, which prompted the authors to state that there is a rationale for using this drug in appropriate cases of erectile dysfunction[2]. On the other hand, the Clinical Guidelines Panel on Erectile Dysfunction of the American Urological Association came to the conclusion that the data currently available on yohimbine do not allow any recommendations for a standard treatment of erectile dysfunction with this drug, which in particular applies to cases of organic erectile dysfunction[3]. Finally, yohimbine has been reported to be effective in orgasmic disorders, i.e. delayed ejaculation or orgasm[4]. According to personal experience, prescribing yohimbine makes sense only in patients without any major organic factors. The doses used are 5–10 mg three times daily for 2 months, or alternatively 10–15 mg as needed 1–1.5 h prior to coitus.

Apomorphine sublingual

Apomorphine sublingual is a central dopamine receptor agonist with effects on D_1 and D_2 receptors. The drug has been marketed in Europe since June 2001 in 2- and 3-mg tablets. The efficacy and safety of 2, 3 and 4 mg apomorphine were investigated in an open-label, dose-optimizing study involving 863 patients (mean age 58 years, range 31–78). In this broad-spectrum population with 44% of patients suffering from hypertension, 23% from diabetes and 17% from coronary heart disease, the global efficacy rate was 56.3%, defined as a significant improvement in the ability to achieve an erection[5]. A meta-analysis of three multi-center, double-blind apomorphine studies with doses of 1, 4, 5 and 6 mg in a total of 1472 patients, with 28% of them suffering from hypertension, showed the following success rates (successful coitus per application) as compared with placebo: 45% vs. 35% ($p < 0.001$) for the 2-mg dose, 48% vs. 29% ($p < 0.001$) for the 4-mg dose, 51% vs. 27% ($p < 0.001$) for the 5-mg dose and 64% vs. 32% ($p < 0.001$) for the 6-mg dose[6].

The results of a recently published study[7] of apomorphine comparing the efficacy of 3 and 4 mg in various patient subgroups are given in Table 1. As encountered also in other apomorphine trials, nausea was the most common dose-dependent drug-related adverse event, with incidence rates of 1% (2 mg), 15% (4 mg), 24% (5 mg) and 29% (6 mg), compared with 2% of patients on placebo.

Further side-effects reported in conjunction with the application of apomorphine are dizziness, somnolence, increased sweating, yawning, headache and asthenia. Syncope was a rare but typical side-effect of apomorphine and had a global incidence rate of 0.8–1%. In dose-titration studies of 2–3–4 mg, the incidence rate was only 0.1% with an initial dose of 2 mg as compared with 1.4% when starting with the 4-mg dose. In apomorphine sublingual–alcohol interaction studies, ingestion of 0.6 g/kg ethanol before administration of 6 mg apomorphine resulted in a significant reduction of blood pressure in some patients[8].

All studies of apomorphine published to date, involving more than 5000 documented patients, allow the following final conclusions. Success rates (erection firm enough for coitus)

Table 1 Results of a randomized, double-blind, cross-over study of apomorphine (Apo) 3 mg vs. placebo and apomorphine 3 mg vs. 4 mg. Data from reference 7

	Percentage of erections firm enough for intercourse							
	Apo 3 mg vs. placebo				Apo 3 mg vs. 4 mg			
Concomitant disease	n	Baseline	Placebo	3 mg	n	Baseline	3 mg	4 mg
CHD	14	13%	28%	42%	10	17%	49%	40%
Hypertension	74	22%	32%	44%**	24	18%	45%	46%
Diabetes	27	21%	29%	39%***	8	19%	28%	36%
BPH	44	18%	34%	50%*	16	18%	44%	40%

*$p = 0.008$, **$p = 0.001$, ***$p = 0.017$; CHD, coronary heart disease; BPH, benign prostatic hyperplasia

were between 45% for the 2-mg and 64% for the 6-mg dose. In all apomorphine studies, relatively high placebo success rates (25–42%) were striking. Nausea is the most common side-effect with apomorphine sublingual, occurring in about 10% for the currently marketed doses of 2 and 3 mg. Meanwhile, apomorphine sublingual has been marketed for more than 16 months in Europe in 2- and 3-mg doses, and it has been shown that this drug cannot compete with sildenafil. The low sales rates of apomorphine throughout Europe, with shares of only 4–6% of the entire erectile dysfunction drug market, mirror the low acceptance rate of this drug. This is primarily due to its low efficacy rate. Prescription of this drug can only be recommended in patients in whom a relevant organic etiology of erectile dysfunction is excluded by means of intracavernous pharmaco-testing and Doppler/duplex sonography.

Phosphodiesterase inhibitors

The phosphodiesterase (PDE) system currently includes 11 isoenzyme families, with further subcategories. In the human corpus cavernosum 14 PDE isoforms have been found, and among them the PDE-5 family holds a dominant position[9]. It is well known that both 3'5'-cyclic adenosine monophosphate (cAMP) and 3'5'-cyclic guanosine monophosphate (cGMP) are generated in the corpus cavernosum while erection is in process, and these second messen-gers are responsible for the decrease in intracellular Ca^{2+} concentrations resulting in relaxation of cavernous smooth musculature and, thus, erection. Physiologically, cAMP and cGMP are broken down to the biologically inactive AMP and GMP. In addition to PDE-5, the PDE-3 and -4 enzymes have also been found in the corpus cavernosum. Whereas PDE-5 influences cGMP metabolism, PDE-3 and -4 have an impact exclusively on cAMP metabolism. Generally speaking, PDE inhibitors prevent cleavage of the second messengers cAMP and cGMP in dependence of the targeted PDE, and thus lead to an intracellular increase of cAMP or cGMP concentration which, in turn, supports the erection process (Figure 1).

Sildenafil (Viagra™)

Sildenafil was first synthesized in 1989, and was originally intended for use in the treatment of coronary heart disease (CHD) or hypertension. However, its effects on CHD turned out to be only marginal, but patients involved in these trials reported considerable improvement in their erectile function. Thus, sildenafil was investigated further for the indication of erectile dysfunction, and has become a 'blockbuster' since 1998 when it was first approved in the USA. Meanwhile, more than 20 million patients have been treated with this drug, and its share in the erectile dysfunction market is around 90%. Its global efficacy in various patient groups[10] is summarized in Table 2.

Table 2 provides convincing evidence of the high efficacy of sildenafil in broad-spectrum erectile dysfunction populations.

All studies of sildenafil published to date show a dose-dependency of the drug-related adverse events. For example, in one of the very first sildenafil trials, the drug-related side-effect profile was as follows[11]:

Headache Placebo 6%, sildenafil 25 mg 14%, 50 mg 21% and 100 mg 30%;

Flushing Placebo 1%, sildenafil 25 mg 13%, 50 mg 27% and 100 mg 20%;

Dyspepsia Placebo 1%, sildenafil 25 mg 3%, 50 mg 11% and 100 mg 16%;

Nasal congestion Placebo 2%, sildenafil 25 mg 1%, 50 mg 3% and 100 mg 11%;

Visual disturbances Placebo < 1%, sildenafil 25 mg 2%, 50 mg 6% and 100 mg 9%.

Since the marketing of sildenafil, numerous reports, mostly in the mass media and not in the peer-reviewed scientific literature, have been published speculating on the cardiovascular safety profile of this drug. Meanwhile, many investigations have been completed, all focusing on whether sildenafil has any detrimental effects on coronary blood flow or myocardial contractility in patients with an increased cardiovascular risk profile, including patients on multimodal antihypertensive medications.

The results of these investigations can be summarized as follows. Sildenafil increased the coronary perfusion reserves by 13% in patients with CHD[12] and increased endothelium-mediated vasodilatation and perfusion in patients with chronic heart failure[13]. In all placebo-controlled trials of sildenafil, the incidence of serious cardiovascular events was not higher in the population treated with sildenafil compared with the placebo groups. In conclusion, to date, there is no evidence that sildenafil is responsible for any serious cardiovascular events, provided that contraindications such as concomitant nitrate or nitric oxide donor medications have been thoroughly considered.

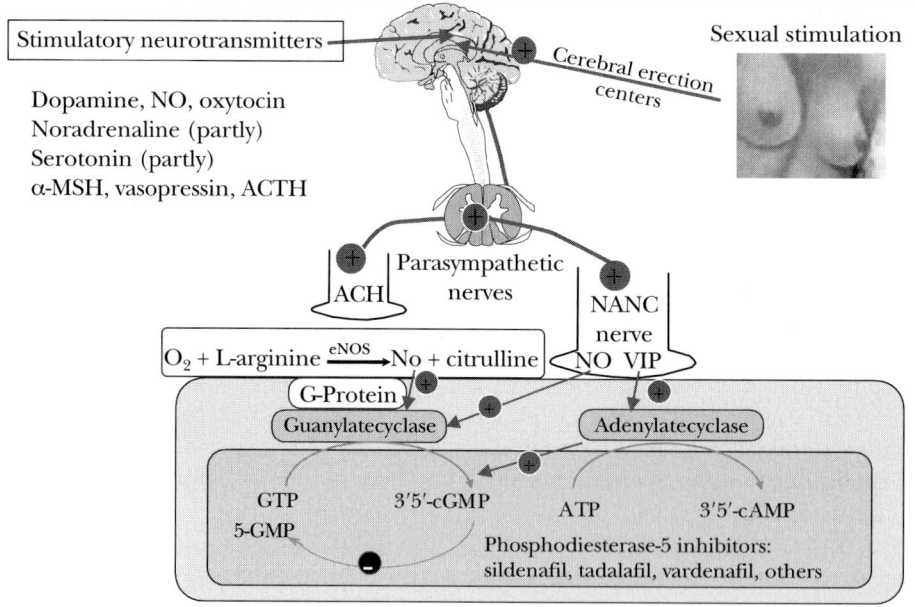

Figure 1 Pharmacological basics in the treatment of erectile dysfunction with phosphodiesterase-5 (PDE-5) inhibitors. NO, nitric oxide; MSH, melanocyte-stimulating hormone; ACTH, adrenocorticotropic hormone; ACH, acetylcholine; eNOS, endothelial nitric oxide synthase; GTP, guanosine triphosphate; cGMP, cyclic guanosine monophosphate; NANC, non-adrenergic, non-cholinergic; VIP, vasoactive intestinal peptide; ATP, adenosine triphosphate; cAMP, cyclic adenosine monophosphate

Table 2 Efficacy of sildenafil (Viagra™) in various patient groups. Data (and additional references) from reference 10

| Author | n | Subgroup | Improved erections (GAQ) | | IIEF (change from baseline) | | | |
| | | | | | Question 3 | | Question 4 | |
			Placebo	Active	Placebo	Active	Placebo	Active
Blonde, 2000	152	diabetes I	18%	59%	11%	78%	20%	100%
	822	diabetes II	17%	63%	31%	100%	20%	100%
	1693	non-diabetes	26%	83%	20%	95%	22%	111%
Kloner, 2000	1218	hypertension	20%	70%		not reported		
Rendell, 1999	250	diabetes I/II	10%	56%	12.5%	82%	33%	93%
Olsson, 2000	224	CHD	24%	71%	22%	105%	20%	120%
Conti, 1999	357	CHD	20%	70%		not reported		
Rosen, 1999	146	depression	20%	82%	37%	131%	43%	179%
Giuliano, 1999	178	spinal cord inj.	10%	80%	10%	95%	9%	134%
Schmid, 2000	41	spinal cord inj.	NA	93%		not reported		
Maytom, 1999	27	spinal cord inj.	7%	75%		not reported		
Wagner, 1999	2240	non-elderly < 65 years	23%	75%	10%	80%	12%	100%
	742	elderly > 65 years	17%	67%	6%	82%	14%	114%
Fowler, 1999	217	multiple sclerosis	24%	89%		not reported		
Chen, 2001	35	dialysis	NA	80%		not reported		

CHD, coronary heart disease; GAQ, Global Assessment Question; NA, not available; IIEF, International Index of Erectile Dysfunction

Tadalafil (Cialis™)

Tadalafil is a novel PDE-5 inhibitor developed by the biotechnology company ICOS Corp. in Bothell, USA. Meanwhile, the drug has attained an approval letter from the Food and Drug Administration (FDA), and its marketing is expected in the second half of 2003 in the USA, whereas in Europe the drug was approved just recently. In contrast to sildenafil and vardenafil, the molecular structure of tadalafil is quite different. This may be the reason that the compound cannot be considered a pure PDE-5 inhibitor but a combined PDE-5/11 inhibitor, because in therapeutic doses as well as PDE-5 also PDE-11 is inhibited. In this connection, it should be mentioned that PDE-11 is found in relevant concentrations in the testicle, the heart, the pituitary and the prostate. At present it is not clear what the ultimate physiological function of PDE-11 is, and whether inhibition of this enzyme would have any importance in terms of these organs. A further important difference from other PDE-5 inhibitors is the

pharmacokinetics of this new drug, which shows a half-life of 17.5 h, more than four times longer than that of the competitors. In very recent studies it has been proven that this drug also has statistically significant efficacy after 36 h, with 60% completed attempts for intercourse as compared with only 30% after placebo[14].

The integrated data of five placebo-controlled, double-blind randomized trials with 1112 patients enrolled, many of them with diabetes and/or hypertension, showed a clear dose-dependent efficacy with 75% success rates (completed coitus) with the 20-mg dose (Figure 2)[15].

In these five trials, the drug-related adverse events were more or less comparable with those related to the other two PDE-5 inhibitors. With the highest dose (20 mg) of tadalafil, the side-effect rate > 2% was as follows:

Headache 14% vs. 6% after placebo;

Dyspepsia 10% vs. 2% after placebo;

Back pain 6% vs. 5% after placebo;

Myalgia 5% vs. 2% after placebo;

Nasal congestion 5% vs. 4% after placebo;

Flushing 4% vs. 2% after placebo.

Different from sildenafil, tadalalfil has nearly no impact on retinal PDE-6, which is mirrored by a very low rate of visual disturbances (< 1%) in the clinical trials.

Considering all the data on tadalafil available to date, there is no doubt that this new PDE-5 inhibitor represents a real alternative to sildenafil, and will challenge this drug.

Vardenafil (Levitra™)

Vardenafil is also a novel PDE-5 inhibitor developed by Bayer GmbH, Leverkusen, Germany. Meanwhile, this drug has also received an approval letter from the FDA, and

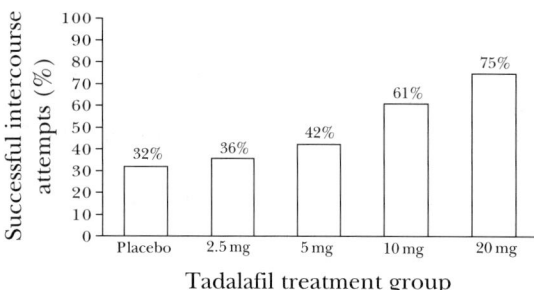

Figure 2 Results of integrated phase III analyses with tadalafil (Cialis™): five double-blind, placebo-controlled trials ($n = 1112$), diabetes mellitus, coronary heart disease, post-myocardial infarction included; based on question 3 of the sexual encounter profile (SEP 3), successful intercourse with completion. Data from reference 15

its marketing can be expected by 2003 in both the USA and Europe.

Compared with sildenafil, the molecular structure of vardenafil shows at first glance only minor differences. However, these minor differences may be responsible for the fact that, *in vitro*, the biochemical potency of vardenafil, mirrored by its IC_{50} (inhibitory concentration giving 50% maximal) for PDE-5, is nine times higher than that of sildenafil. Therefore, in clinical use, doses of vardenafil yielding comparable efficacy rates to sildenafil are five times lower. In addition, the pharmacokinetics of vardenafil reveals a very short T_{max} (time to maximum concentration) allowing the shortest time of onset of erection among all three competing PDE-5 inhibitors. Details of the pharmacokinetics of all three PDE-5 inhibitors are summarized in Table 3[16–18].

In a very large placebo-controlled, double-blind randomized phase IIb trial, the efficacy and safety of vardenafil was assessed in a mixed erectile dysfunction population involving 601 patients. About one-third each suffered from psychogenic, mixed or organogenic erectile dysfunction, respectively, and also about one-third each from mild, moderate or severe erectile dysfunction according to the erectile function domain of the International Index of Erectile Dysfunction (IIEF). In terms of the most relevant efficacy parameter, question 3 of the sexual encounter profile (SEP), which includes penetration and erection maintenance ability, all three vardenafil doses (5,10 and 20 mg) yielded efficacy rates between 70 and 75%[20] (Figure 3). The most frequently reported side-effects in this trial are summarized in Table 4.

Table 3 Clinical profiles of phosphodiesterase-5 (PDE-5) inhibitors. Pharmacokinetics of the PDE-5 inhibitors sildenafil, vardenafil and tadalafil. Data from references 16–19

Parameter	Sildenafil 100 mg	Vardenafil 20 mg	Tadalafil (IC-351) 20 mg
T_{max}(h)	1.16 ± 0.99	0.660 (0.250–3.0)	2.0
$T_{1/2}$(h)	3.82 ± 0.84	3.94 ± 1.31	17.5
C_{max}(ng/ml)	327 ± 236	20.9 ± 1.83	378
AUC (ng × h/ml)	1963 ± 859	74.5 ± 1.82 (μg × h/l)	8066 (μg × h/l)

T_{max}, time to maximum concentration; $T_{1/2}$, half life; C_{max}, maximum concentration; AUC, area under the curve; IC, inhibitory concentration

In a further phase III trial in diabetics involving 452 patients, with 20 mg vardenafil, the success rates were as follows[21]:

Global Assessment Question (GAQ improvement of erections) 72%;
Successful intercourse (penetration SEP 2) 64%;
Successful completion of intercourse (maintenance of erection SEP 3) 54%.

Conclusions

Sildenafil (Viagra™) marked without any doubt a breakthrough in the management of erectile dysfunction and revolutionized the treatment of

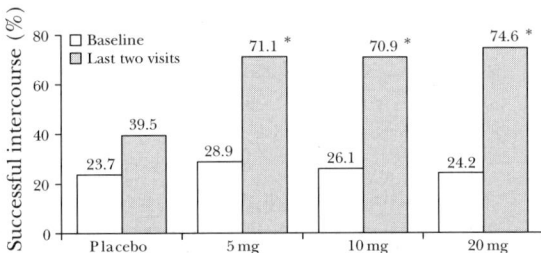

Figure 3 Results (successful intercourse with completion) of the first large phase IIb trial with vardenafil: efficacy results, patient diary/maintenance, 'did your erection last long enough to complete sexual intercourse with ejaculation?' Data from reference 20. *$p < 0.001$ vs. placebo

this disorder. Meanwhile, more than 20 million patients have been treated world-wide with sildenafil, which bears witness to the success of this drug. Despite this impressive success, it is obvious that sildenafil does not have all the features of an ideal impotence drug as, in the long term, 40–50% of all patients discontinue sildenafil medication for various reasons.

It is fair to state that the new PDE-5 inhibitors are, from the perspective of efficacy as measured by questions 3 and 4 of the IIEF or by questions 2 and 3 of the SEP, comparable to sildenafil but differ in terms of pharmacokinetics and intensity of side-effects. To date, no data are available from direct head-to-head comparison trials between these three PDE-5 inhibitors, but such trials are under way. There is no question that all three PDE-5 inhibitors are safe and effective, and the future will show us which drug is preferred by couples.

Owing to its low efficacy, compared with the PDE-5 inhibitors, apomorphine sublingual will not play a major role in the future, but its use in so-called psychogenic (functional) erectile dysfunction patients may represent a reasonable alternative. It remains to be seen whether other centrally or peripherally acting drugs may challenge the PDE-5 inhibitors in the future.

Table 4 Results*of the first large phase IIb trial with vardenafil. Data from reference 20

Adverse event (AE)	Placebo (n = 152)	5 mg (n = 147)	10 mg (n = 141)	20 mg (n = 150)
Headache	6 (3.9%)	10 (6.8%)	12 (8.5%)	23 (15.3%)
Flushing	1 (0.7%)	15 (10.2%)	16 (11.3%)	17 (11.3%)
Dyspepsia	0	1 (0.7%)	4 (2.8%)	10 (6.7%)
Rhinitis	5 (3.3%)	7 (4.8%)	4 (2.8%)	11 (7.3%)
AE leading to premature discontinuation	2 (1.3%)	7 (4.8%)	2 (1.4%)	1 (0.7%)

*Number of patients out of the safety population (all those who took at least one dose of placebo or vardenafil) who experienced one AE at any time over the 12-week treatment period at any severity at 5% or greater in any treatment arm and higher than with placebo

References

1. Saenz de Tejada I. Commentary on mechanisms for the regulation of penile smooth muscle contractility. *J Urol* 1995;153:1762
2. Ernst E, Pittler MH. Yohimbine for erectile dysfunction: a systematic review and meta-analysis of randomized clinical trials. *J Urol* 1998;146:433–6
3. Montague DK, Barada JH, Belker AM, *et al.* Clinical Guidelines Panel on Erectile Dysfunction: summary report on treatment of organic erectile dysfunction. *J Urol* 1996;156:2007–11
4. Adeniyi AA, Andrews HD, Helal MA *et al.* Yohimbine in orgasmic dysfunction. *Int J Impotence Res* 2000;12(Suppl 5):S7
5. Auerbach S, Agre K, Buttler S, *et al.* Efficacy and safety of escalating doses of 2, 3 and 4 mg apomorphine SL in the treatment of patients with erectile dysfunction. *Int J Impotence Res* 2000;12:22
6. Padma-Nathan H, Agre K, Fromm S, *et al.* Efficacy of apomorphine SL vs. placebo for erectile dysfunction in patients with hypertension. *Int J Impotence Res* 2000;12:45
7. Dula E, Bukofzer S, Perdok R, *et al.* Double-blind, cross-over comparison of 3 mg apomorphine SL with placebo and with 4 mg apomorphine SL in male erectile dysfunction. *Eur Urol* 2001;39:558–64
8. Argiolas A, Hedlund H. The pharmacology and clinical pharmacokinetics of apomorphine SL. *BJU Int* 2001;88(Suppl 3):18–21
9. Stief CG, Taher A, Truß M, *et al.* Die Phosphodiesterase-Isoenzyme des humanen Corpus cavernosum penis und deren funktionelle Bedeutung. *Akt Urol* 1995;26:22–4
10. Porst H. *Manual der Impotenz.* Bremen:UNI-MED Verlag, 2000
11. Goldstein I, Lue TF, Padma-Nathan H, *et al.* Oral sildenafil in the treatment of erectile dysfunction. *N Engl J Med* 1998;338:1397–404
12. Herrmann H, Chang G, Klugherz BD, *et al.* Hemodynamic effects of sildenafil in men with severe coronary artery disease. *N Engl J Med* 2000;342:1622–6
13. Katz SD, Balidemaj K, Homma S, *et al.* Acute type 5 phosphodiesterase inhibition with sildenafil enhances flow-mediated vasodilation in patients with chronic heart failure. *J Am Coll Cardiol* 2000;36:845–51
14. Porst H, Rosen R, Padma-Nathan H, *et al.* Tadalafil allows men with erectile dysfunction to have successful intercourse up to 36 hours postdose. *Int J Impotence Res* 2002;14(Suppl 3):S104
15. Brock G, McMahon C, Cherr KK, *et al.* Efficacy and safety of tadalafil for the treatment of erectile dysfunction: results of integrated analyses. *J Urol* 2002;168:1332–6
16. *Viagra Product Monography.*
17. Klotz T, Sachse R, Heidrich A, *et al.* Vardenafil increases penile rigidity and tumescence in erectile dysfunction patients: a Rigiscan and pharmacokinetic study. *World J Urol* 2001;19:32–9
18. Ferguson KM. Basic science, PDE inhibitors and preclinical development. Presented at the *Global Medical Conference: New management options for patients with erectile dysfunction,* Indianapolis, USA, June 1, 2001
19. Bischoff E, Niewohner U, Haning H, *et al.* The inhibitory selectivity of vardenafil on bovine and human recombinant phosphodiesterase isoenzymes. *Int J Impotence Res* 2001;13(Suppl 4):S41
20. Porst H, Rosen R, Padma-Nathan H, *et al.* The efficacy and tolerability of vardenafil, a new, oral, selective phosphodiesterase type 5 inhibitor, in patients with erectile dysfunction: the first at-home clinical trial. *Int J Impotence Res* 2001;13:192–9
21. Goldstein J, Young JM, Fischer J, *et al.* Vardenafil, a new highly selective PDE 5 inhibitor improves erectile function in patients with diabetes mellitus. Presented at the *American College of Clinical Pharmacology Meeting,* Tampa, USA, October 2001: abstr 279E

Intracavernosal injection therapy for erectile dysfunction: an update

7

F. Montorsi, A. Salonia, A. Briganti, G. Zanni, F. Dehó, L. Barbieri and P. Rigatti

Introduction

The management of patients with erectile dysfunction has recently been grouped into three different levels[1]. Initially, patients should be advised to control every clinical abnormality or life-style factor associated with a higher risk of erectile dysfunction. Usually, this first step alone is not able to cause a significant improvement of the patient's erectile function, and first-line therapy is considered. This includes oral pharmacotherapy, use of a vacuum device or psychosexual therapy. The majority of patients who are currently seen for erectile dysfunction are prescribed either sildenafil or apomorphine sublingual, the two drugs that are officially marketed. This happens because the efficacy and safety of the oral approach have been clearly established, and because most patients would rather undertake a therapy that is simple to use. Patients who do not respond to oral therapy are considered for second-line treatment, which includes intraurethral or intracavernosal administration of vasoactive drugs. To date, it has been rare to prescribe one of the second-line therapies when choosing treatment for the first time: this used to happen when sildenafil was the only oral drug on the market, as patients using nitrates had a definite contraindication to the use of sildenafil. A second patient category might be represented by those requesting a fast response that could not be obtained with sildenafil; however, apomorphine sublingual is characterized by a fast onset of action, and may represent an effective solution for these patients[2]. In conclusion, intraurethral and intracavernosal therapies are currently used almost exclusively in patients who fail to respond to oral therapy; however, when counselling the patient with erectile dysfunction on the treatment options available, every alternative should be extensively detailed at the first office visit.

The aim of this article is to review the latest results obtained with these therapeutic options, and to demonstrate the correct approach to patients candidate for these therapies.

Intracavernosal injection therapy

When a patient is considered a potential candidate for vasoactive injection therapy, the characteristics of the treatment are extensively explained along with the potential limitations and adverse effects. He is asked to read and sign a detailed informed consent. Patients with a history of hemoglobinopathy, bleeding diathesis, Peyronie's disease or idiopathic priapism are excluded from treatment. In addition, patients with poor manual dexterity, poor visual acuity or morbid obesity, or those in whom a transient hypotensive episode may have a deleterious effect (e.g. unstable cardiovascular disease and transient ischemic attack), are not ideal candidates for this treatment. Finally, patients with serious psychiatric disorders or patients who might misuse or abuse this therapy should be excluded from treatment.

The first phase of the pharmacological erection program consists of dose titration of the drug or mixture used for injections. Patients are placed in the sitting position on the examination couch during each injection and kept in this position for 30 min. Systemic blood pressure is recorded as baseline in the event of syncope, and to check for hypertension. The right side (lateral aspect) of the penis is cleansed with an alcohol swab. The first injection is then performed with a very small amount of either the drug or the mixture. The needle is inserted by a quick jab up to the hilt of the needle so that the tip of it reaches the centre of the right corpus cavernosum. Injections must not be performed on the dorsal and ventral aspect of the penis, to avoid damage to the dorsal neurovascular bundle of the penis and the urethra, respectively. Immediately after injection, the base of the penis is squeezed firmly between the right thumb and index finger, while the accessible portion of the penis is massaged for up to 5 min by squeezing it laterally along the length of the shaft between the left thumb, and index and middle fingers, thus distributing the drug throughout the pendulous shaft. Patients are then left alone to watch an erotic video and they are invited to masturbate without ejaculation to optimize sexual stimulation. The erectile response is then assessed by the physician and the patient. The dose of the injected drug or mixture is considered adequate when it produces an erection equal to 50–75% of the maximal erectile response reported by the patient. If a patient reaches a maximal rigid erection during the titration phase in the clinic, a lower dose is suggested for home use as the erectile effect induced by the drug or mixture during sexual activity is usually greater than that observed under laboratory conditions. If the first injection does not produce a satisfactory erectile response (that is, less than 50% of the maximal potential response), the patient is re-injected after at least 24 h and the dose is slightly increased. The titration process proceeds until the optimal dose is identified or the maximal injected volume is reached. At our clinic, three versions of a four-drug mixture composed of papaverine, phentolamine, alprostadil and atropine sulfate are used, and 0.05 ml is usually injected first. We subsequently use 0.05-ml increments[3,4]. If after the injection a full rigid erection persists for longer than 1 h, 20–40 µg of adrenaline is injected intracorporeally to obtain complete detumescence. Appropriate electrocardiographic and blood pressure monitoring are used during this procedure. Patients are contacted by telephone the next day to verify

persistence of detumescence. After the appropriate dose of the drug or mixture has been determined, patients watch the thorough demonstration of both a conventional insulin syringe and an automatic self-injection system (Disetronic pen®; Medis, Milan, Italy) (Figure 1) with which multiple injections can be performed, thus avoiding the maneuvers needed before each injection performed with the insulin syringe (preparation of the syringe, needle and appropriate amount of the drug)[5]. The pen consists of a capsule that is screwed together with the adaptor after inserting the filled glass cartridge. The needle is then screwed into the adaptor. The glass cartridge consists of a rubber piston and a conus in front, which is closed with a cap. The cartridge set contains a pull rod and a needle in addition to the glass cartridge (Figure 2). To fill the cartridge, the pull rod is screwed into the thread of the rubber piston and, after removing the cap, the needle is stuck upon the conus. The glass cartridge volume is 3 ml. At our clinic the cartridge is filled with a four-drug vasoactive mixture, which is described in detail below[6,7]. As the average volume of mixture used at each injection by our patients is below 0.2 ml, every cartridge has a drug load that is usually enough for 8–10 injections. We supply 29-gauge needles for injections. To prepare the pen for injection, the adaptor is first removed from the capsule. The full glass cartridge is then inserted into the capsule with the conus pointing forward. The adaptor is screwed firmly into the capsule. The needle is removed from the blister and screwed together with the cap into the adaptor. The needle cap is pulled out and, while the pen

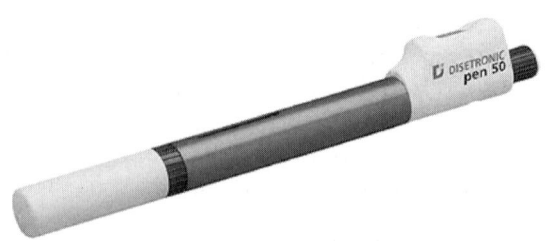

Figure 1 Self-injection system Disetronic pen in use at our institution

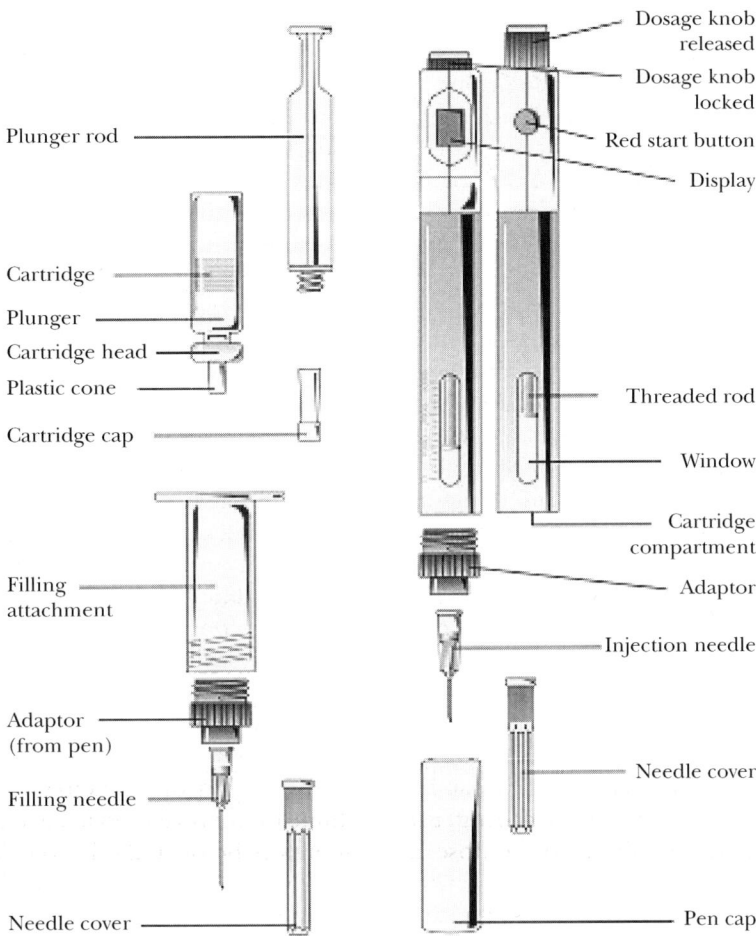

Figure 2   Components of the Disetronic system

with the needle is held pointing upwards, the knob is pressed slowly until it reaches the top. Some drops of liquid should come out, but if this does not occur the knob is turned clockwise for approximately 2–3 clicks and is slowly pressed until it stops. The knob is slowly released, drops are shaken off and the cap is put into the adaptor. To inject the drug, the needle is inserted into the corpus cavernosum and the pen knob is gently depressed until it stops. Two models of this system are currently available, which differ only in the volume (20 or 50 μl) of liquid released with every click of the knob. We currently use 20 μl for pure psychogenic and neurogenic patients, and 50 μl for vasculogenic cases.

Patients are instructed to limit injection use to three times a week, with no more than one injection in any 24-h period. They are also taught to inject the right and left cavernous body alternately. Patients are then warned to return immediately to the emergency room if erection persists for longer than 3 h. Patients are also told to refrigerate the drug or mixture, if it contains prostaglandin E_1, and to examine the drug or solution for changes in color or the formation of a precipitate.

Patients are reassessed once a month for the first 2 months, and subsequently every 3 months. At each follow-up visit, injection frequency, duration and consistency of erections, and patient satisfaction are recorded. The penis is carefully examined for nodules, hematomas or areas of induration. Liver function is assessed every 6 months. Penile ultrasonography is performed to verify any clinical findings on digital palpation of the penis.

Results and complications of vasoactive intracavernous injection therapy

The follow-up of approximately 4000 patients treated world-wide with papaverine alone or in combination with phentolamine has been published[8], in addition, long-term results with intracavernous injection therapy based on prostaglandin E_1 have been reported[9–14]. Reported side-effects have included hematomas, burning pain after injection, urethral damage, cavernositis or local infections, fibrotic changes of the corpora cavernosa, curvature and prolonged erections or priapism. Recently, Beal and Mears[15] reported a case of a penile lymphoma following local injection for erectile dysfunction. The two most important complications are prolonged erections and localized fibrotic changes of the corpora cavernosa. Prolonged erections are usually encountered during the dose titration phase, and have been reported in 2–15% of patients treated[8,9]. The development of painless fibrotic nodules within the corpora cavernosa may lead to penile curvature. This problem has been reported in 1.5–60% of patients treated for 1 year[8,9]. We believe that most of the fibrotic nodules occur in patients who inject themselves very frequently (multiple traumas to the corporeal tissue) and who do not compress the injection site for a sufficient amount of time, with the subsequent development of intracavernous hematomas.

The role of intracavernosal vasoactive therapy in promoting a return of spontaneous erections is controversial. An increase in the frequency of spontaneous erections and a decreased need for treatment is a common finding during follow-up of intracavernous vasoactive injection therapy. It has been demonstrated that the chronic use of prostaglandin E_1 intracavernous injections is able to improve cavernosal artery function markedly as shown by color Doppler sonography[16]. The improved hemodynamic response seen in patients chronically injecting themselves may be explained on a microvascular level. It has been shown that the long-term administration of vasoactive agents in monkeys causes hypertrophy of sinusoidal smooth muscle at the ultrastructural level. Both papaverine and prostaglandin E_1 lead to a hypertrophic response, but papaverine results in a combination of hypertrophy, atrophy and fibrosis, whereas with prostaglandin E_1 the normal cellular architecture is preserved. With the sinusoidal muscle 'toned up' after long-term self-injection with prostaglandin E_1, the efficiency of sinusoidal smooth muscle action may improve, leading to the observed increase in cavernosal artery flow. In addition, it has been shown that prostaglandin E_1 may improve the hemodynamic response partly by promoting neovascularization[16]. This issue remains controversial, as Wespes and colleagues[17] were unable to demonstrate any significant changes of the intracavernous structure following long-term treatment with intracavernosal alprostadil. In this study, a total of ten patients underwent biopsy of the corpora cavernosa before and after a 3-year treatment with alprostadil (overall, 150–250 injections per patient). No histological difference was observed with classic staining. A reduction was noted in the percentage of intracavernous smooth muscle after treatment in two of five patients on the side of injection, but there was no difference with the other corpus cavernosum. No difference was observed in the percentage of intracavernous smooth muscle between both corpora in the five patients with biopsies performed only after treatment. A recent study by Brock and associates[18] supported the contention that long-term intracavernosal alprostadil therapy acts on the penile smooth muscle to improve the erectile response, and promotes the return of spontaneous erection. In this study, 70 men with a stable heterosexual partner entered the titration phase, and the effective alprostadil dose was determined before entry into the 12-month self-treatment home phase. Duplex ultrasonography was used to measure the peak systolic velocity and diameter of the cavernosal arteries throughout the study. An effective dose was established for 67 (96%) of the 70 men (median dose of alprostadil 15 µg). During the home phase, 94% of men responded to alprostadil and the median dose remained unchanged. Complete duplex ultrasound data were obtained in 38 men, and showed significant increases in post-injection peak systolic velocity in both cavernosal arteries ($p < 0.001$ at 12 months) and between the pre-injection and post-injection cavernosal arterial diameters ($p = 0.0001$) compared with baseline. Reports of a return of spontaneous erections increased throughout the study compared with baseline (37%, 26 of 70) and were confirmed by interview for 46 (85%) of 54 men with available data overall. The issue of the curative effects of intracavernosal injection therapy yet remains clinically controversial, as in another study nocturnal penile tumescence activity remained unchanged after long-term intracavernous injection use[19]. In this study, Maniam and co-workers enrolled 19 men with organic erectile dysfunction; all patients underwent nocturnal penile tumescence testing before and after alprostadil-based intracavernous injection therapy of at least 6 months in duration. A five-item questionnaire was used to assess subjective changes in erectile activity over time. In this study, mean time on intracavernous injection therapy was 2.4 years and mean injection frequency was 3.7 times monthly. Nine patients believed that unaided erection improved after intracavernosal injection, and six achieved intercourse without injection who were unable to do so before injection. However, no statistically significant changes were noted in any of the five objectively measured nocturnal penile tumescence parameters.

Clinical experience with approved agents

Papaverine

Papaverine hydrochloride is an opium alkaloid that acts on a post-receptor level via the inhibition of phosphodiesterase, leading to an accumulation of cyclic adenosine monophosphate (cAMP), which attenuates the α_1 receptor-mediated contraction of the smooth muscle cell, possibly by interfering with calcium ion mobilization. This drug facilitates erection by relaxation of smooth muscles in the sinusoids and by dilatation of helicine arteries[20]. Doses ranging from 10 to 60 mg are usually given when papaverine is used as a single agent. At present, however, papaverine is usually used in combination either with phentolamine alone or with phentolamine and prostaglandin, to increase the overall erectogenic effect and reduce toxicity.

It is well known that intracavernous injections of papaverine may induce corporeal fibrosis. This is thought to be due to the acidity of papaverine solutions (pH ranging from 3 to 4), which, unfortunately, cannot be corrected by the use of a buffer because the papaverine solution precipitates at a pH > 5.

Papaverine is extensively metabolized in the liver, and papaverine-induced hepatotoxicity in the form of an increase of liver transaminases and drug-induced hepatitis has been reported[21]. A recent study has demonstrated that, to avoid side-effects, the single injection dose of papaverine should not exceed 4.5 mg[22]. Reported efficacy rates with dosage between 30 and 110 mg varied between 27 and 78% and were dependent on dosage and the patient population investigated[23]. A literature analysis of 19 publications that included 2181 patients overall demonstrated that papaverine produced an average response rate of 61% in in-office testing[23]. The most important side-effects were priapism in 3–18.5%, which occurred mostly during the titration phase. Fibrotic alterations were seen in 5–30% of patients, with an average of 5.7% in 15 retrospective studies[23]. Owing to safety concerns, monotherapy with papaverine has been discontinued in most industrialized countries. However, because of its considerably low cost, self-injection monotherapy with papaverine still continues in many developing countries.

Phentolamine and papaverine–phentolamine combination

Phentolamine mesylate is an α_1- and α_2-adrenergic receptor blocking agent that dilates arterial vessels and abolishes sympathetic inhibition of erection. Lack of effect on venous return by intracavernous phentolamine has been demonstrated in both animal and human studies[24]. Since a single intracavernous phentolamine injection does not produce a satisfactory erectile response, the drug is not used alone but in combination with papaverine and prostaglandin E_1[3,4,6]. The most frequently used doses of phentolamine are listed in Table 1. The most common side-effects observed after intravenous administration of phentolamine are orthostatic hypotension and tachycardia. The combination of papaverine–phentolamine is marketed in several European countries (Androskat™): this solution has a pH which varies between 3.1 and 3.5 and is stable for 2–3 years. Combining the cyclic nucleotide cAMP–cyclic guanosine monophosphate (cGMP)-accumulating effects of papaverine and the α-adrenoceptor blocking effects of phentolamine results in an increased average response rate of up to 60–70% observed during in-office testing. With home use, response rates as high as 90% have been reported[26]. The global efficacy rate of this combination as evaluated in large retrospective studies is 68.5%[23]. Frequent side-effects were similar to those of papaverine. Priapism was

reported in 6–15% and fibrosis in an average 12% of patients treated[10,23].

Prostaglandin E_1 (alprostadil)

Prostaglandin E_1 has α blocking properties mediated through a membrane receptor, and relaxes the cavernous and arteriolar smooth muscle while causing restriction of venous outflow. Prostaglandin E_1 produces full erections at doses as low as 2.5 µg. When used as a single agent, the maximal injected dose usually ranges from 30 to 40 µg. Prostaglandin E_1 is the most widely used component of multidrug vasoactive mixtures, which permit a reduction in the doses of each single agent, thus reducing side-effects.

In contrast to papaverine or to the papaverine–phentolamine combination, large world-wide prospective studies have been conducted in accordance with good clinical practice guidelines for both alprostadil preparations (alprostadil sterile powder, Caverject™, and alprostadil alfadex, Viridal™ or Edex™), and long-term follow-up of 4–5 years is available[27,28]. A review of these large studies shows that the efficacy rate of alprostadil during in-office titration varied between 70 and 75% in more than 10 000 patients[13,23]. In a variety of prospective self-injection trials, the success rates (defined as successful penetration per injection) varied between 89 and 96%[29]; this is higher than any reported efficacy rate among all the available marketed vasoactive drugs[30]. The positive effect of alprostadil injections on quality of life has been demonstrated[31]. Clinical and self-reported measurements were used to assess physiological and psychological status at baseline, and at 3, 6, 12 and 18 months for 579 patients who entered the self-injection phase of an open-label, flexible-dose clinical trial. Quality of life was measured using the Center for Marital and Sexual Health Sexual Functioning Questionnaire, which focuses on the psychosocial and physical dimensions of erectile dysfunction, the Brief Symptom Inventory, which measures mental health and the Duke Health Profile, which measures general quality of life. It was clear from this study that clinical improvements in erectile function

Table 1 Six vasoactive mixtures for intracavernous injection therapy

	Amount of drug in solution					
	1*	2*	3†	4‡	5‡	6‡
Prostaglandin E_1 (µg)	100	200	30	80	200	300
Papaverine (mg)	300	300	150	80	240	300
Phentolamine (mg)	10	20	5	20	20	20
Atropine (mg)	0	0	0	3	3	3
Saline (ml)	0	0	2.4	0	0	0

*Reference 3; †reference 25; ‡mixtures currently used at our institution

due to alprostadil therapy were associated with improvements in sexual activity, sexual satisfaction and overall mental health.

Recently, Heaton and co-workers[32], in an open-label, flexible dose-escalating study, assessed the high efficacy and safety of intracavernosal alprostadil for the treatment of erectile dysfunction in more than 300 men suffering from either type I or type II diabetes mellitus. The authors established the effective alprostadil dose for the patients by titration at the clinic, and trained them fully in the self-injection techique prior to entry into a 6-month self-treatment home-phase trial. During the home phase, Heaton and co-workers reported that, in this population, a satisfactory erectile response (i.e. penile rigidity adequate for intercourse and lasting up to 60 min) was achieved after 99% of injections in both type I and type II diabetic men, with a median dose of 20 µg (range 2.5–60). Treatment was generally well tolerated with a low incidence of penile pain (24%). Regarding diabetic patients complaining of severe erectile dysfunction, it has been recently shown by Perimenis and colleagues[33] that, even if they initially respond to a moderate dosage of prostaglandin E_1 (PGE$_1$,); over time they can need increasing dosages of PGE$_1$ or a mixture of PGE$_1$ and papaverine. Indeed, doses of PGE$_1$ or mixtures of PGE$_1$ and papaverine had to be increased over time (PGE$_1$ from 17.5 to 20 µg and papaverine from 0.9 to 16 mg, throughout the 7 years of follow-up; $p < 0.002$), after Rigiscan® had been used for objective determination of the initial dosage. Overall, in 18 diabetic patients followed-up regularly for 7 years after they had begun self-injections, interestingly, it was found that compliance with the treatment was significantly higher, compared with a control group (i.e. 22 non-diabetic men) ($p = 0.001$). This was for many reasons, such as higher familiarity with the self-injection treatment (especially in those with type I diabetes mellitus), low response to oral agents making them more likely to accept injections as the only cure and fewer options in the case of intracavernosal therapy failure. Although self-injections were generally safe and well-tolerated, Perimenis and colleagues observed a decrease in the frequency of injections particularly in diabetic patients, but without any statistically significant difference in comparison with the control group. Moreover, in the diabetic population, alprostadil showed a higher grade of effectiveness than sildenafil[34]. Nevertheless, therapy with intracavernosal alprostadil is more invasive, has more severe side-effects (such as pain) and needs accurate instructions for self-injection[34].

A patient category of particular interest to urologists is represented by those undergoing a radical prostatectomy. Early use of intracavernous agents aimed at promoting erections during the immediate postoperation period has been shown to enhance the recovery of spontaneous erections[35]. We recently[36] reported data concerning our experience in terms of subsequent therapy by means of intracavernosal injection and sildenafil in 85 preoperatively potent patients (mean age 59 years, range 47–63 years) with clinically localized prostate cancer, who underwent a bilateral nerve-sparing radical retropubic prostatectomy (bilateral NSRRP). Patients were subdivided into two groups and were subsequently treated with the following protocols: group 1 ($n = 45$), three intracavernosal injections of alprostadil per week for 3 months followed by oral sildenafil as needed for 3 months; group 2 ($n = 40$), oral sildenafil as needed starting 3 months after the procedure. At the end of the injection phase (3-month follow-up), 27/45 (60%) of patients in group 1 were able to achieve vaginal penetration at least once versus 4/40 (10%) patients in group 2. Twenty per cent (9/45) and 50% (20/40) of group-1 and -2 patients, respectively, were able to obtain spontaneous penile tumescence, while 20% (9/45) and 40% (16/40) in groups 1 and 2, respectively, did not report any erectile activity. At the 6-month follow-up, sildenafil as needed allowed 82% (37/45) of group-1 patients to penetrate their partner compared with 52% (21/40) of group-2 patients ($p < 0.001$). Eleven per cent (5/45) and 30% (12/40) of group-1 and -2 patients were able to obtain penile tumescence, respectively. The erectile dysfunction inventory treatment satisfaction (EDITS) score (73.5 vs. 66.5) and the International Index Erectile Function (IIEF) erectile function domain score (25 vs. 20) were significantly greater in group 1 than in group 2 ($p < 0.01$). Sildenafil was used at the 25-, 50- and 100-mg dose by 14%, 28% and 58% and 0%, 18% and 82% of group-1 and group-2 patients, respectively ($p < 0.001$). The proportion of successful attempts was 61% in group 1 and 43% in group 2 ($p < 0.01$). We concluded that the early use of intracavernosal injection therapy with alprostadil in preoperatively fully potent patients undergoing NSRRP significantly enhances the subsequent response to sildenafil as needed, compared with the response seen in sildenafil users who have not used early prophylactic injections.

The most frequently reported adverse effect of prostaglandin E_1 intracavernous injections is local corporeal pain, which occurs in 13–80% of patients and is dose-related (occurring more frequently at doses greater than 15 µg). Three hypotheses have been suggested to explain pain. First, the pain is related to the acidity of the injected agent, as has been described with local anesthetics; second, the pain is caused by pharmacologically induced vasodilatation and represents vascular pain; third, the pain is caused by the direct activation of pain receptors via prostaglandin E_1. To avoid this adverse effect, 7.5% sodium bicarbonate or 20 mg procaine should be added to the prostaglandin E_1 solution[37,38].

Side-effects seen with alprostadil treatment include the above-mentioned penile pain, priapism, which is almost uniquely seen during the dose titration phase, and corporeal fibrosis, which is encountered in 7.5–11.7% of patients during the course of the 4–5 years of long-term follow-up. Between 33 and 47% of penile fibroses healed spontaneously, suggesting that the incidence of persistent penile fibroses in patients on long-term self-injection therapy is between 5 and 7%[28–30].

Moxisylyte

Moxisylyte is known to be a competitive norepinephrine antagonist, acting on post-synaptic α_1 receptors. *In vivo* it clearly decreases the spontaneous activity, amplitude and tone of the contractions of cavernous smooth muscle in dogs, and it relaxes *in vitro* norepinephrine-contracted corporeal smooth muscle strips[39]. Intracavernous injection of 10, 20 or 30 mg of moxisylyte is able to induce an adequate erection for intercourse in 85% of patients[40]. The most interesting characteristic of this drug is its very low rate of adverse effects including priapism (< 1%) and fibrosis (< 2%). However, in all published moxisylyte trials, clinically relevant reductions in blood pressure accompanied by orthostatic symptoms and dizziness were described in 5–8% of patients[41].

Vasoactive intestinal peptide–phentolamine combination

As vasoactive intestinal peptide (VIP) alone injected intracavernosally in volunteers did not result in rigid erections, a combination of VIP and phentolamine was developed for self-injection therapy[42]. In a large prospective trial with 289 patients, 77% responded with grade-3 erections, considered by the investigators to be sufficient for intercourse[43]. In this study, two priapisms (0.6%) were observed. In a large UK multicenter study, an efficacy rate consistently higher than 80% was seen in all patients categories, irrespective of the etiology of the disease; however, the total drop-out rate was 65%, and was thus considerably higher than in all other alprostadil injection trials[30]. The greatest advantage of the Invicorp™ preparation is its high availability in a ready-for-use automatic single injection device equipped with a 29-gauge needle[44,45].

Clinical experience with agents under investigation

Calcitonin gene-related peptide

Calcitonin gene-related peptide (CGRP) relaxes smooth muscle cells by hyper-polarization via potassium channel opening and cAMP stimulation. In patients, intracavernous injections of CGRP induced dose-related increases in penile arterial inflow, cavernous smooth muscle relaxation and cavernous outflow occlusion, and an erectile response. In the literature, CGRP (5 μg) has been used in combination with PGE$_1$ (10 μg) in patients who did not respond to the combination papaverine–phentolamine, including patients with hemodynamically proven veno-occlusive dysfunction[46,47]. Full erections were obtained in more than 70% of patients. No significant complications were seen with this drug at low doses; however, facial flush and hypotension were reported at higher doses (25 μg)[46,47]. Owing to the limited number of patients treated to date and to the short follow-up, CGRP is not yet suggested as a first-choice drug to be used in all candidates for injection therapy, but should be considered when PGE$_1$ or other drugs alone fail to produce a full erectile response.

Linsidomine

Linsidomine chloridrate is the active metabolite of the antianginal drug molsidomine, and is believed to liberate nitric oxide non-enzymatically (nitric oxide donor), which, in turn, stimulates guanylate cyclase leading to an increase in the intracellular concentration of cGMP. Linsidomine also hyperpolarizes the cell membrane by influencing the sodium–potassium pump, thus rendering the smooth muscle cell less responsive to adrenergically mediated contraction. Linsidomine has been tested with a single injection dose of 1 mg, and in these conditions its effectiveness was comparable to the combination of papaverine and phentolamine[48], while the injection of 20 μg of PGE$_1$ produced greater erectile effects than linsidomine in the majority of patients[49]. In addition, linsidomine did not prove to be effective in the treatment of patients with corporeal veno-occlusive dysfunction[50].

No adverse effects including pain, priapism or corporeal fibrosis have been reported after injection of linsidomine. The drug safety profile and its low cost make linsidomine an appealing drug for patients responding to the combination papaverine–phentolamine.

Sodium nitroprusside

Sodium nitroprusside (SNP), a nitric oxide donor similar to SIN-1, was evaluated in a comparative trial with alprostadil. In a total of 95 patients, 49% responded with partial and 15% with complete rigidity to 300–400-mg doses of nitroprusside compared with 54% and 20%, respectively, after 20 μg alprostadil. With nitroprusside doses of 600 mg, global response rates of 84% were achieved. Because alprostadil produced better response rates and sodium nitroprusside was incriminated by hypotonic blood pressure reactions in up to 15% of patients, this compound did not enter the phase of multicenter trials[51].

More recently, Fu and colleagues[52] studied the effect of intracavernous SNP (300 μg) or a control drug mix (papaverine 30 mg + phentolamine 1 mg) on penile erection. They reported that SNP was able to facilitate both relaxation of the penile smooth muscle and penile erection (i.e. the hardness of the penis was scored above 100 as evaluated by the Virag[53] method; $p < 0.05$) without significant side-effects. In this series, SNP was not associated with either pain or priapism, and the authors concluded that it might be used in patients affected by erectile dysfunction who experience pain and priapism with papaverine–phentolamine.

Atropine

The use of atropine sulfate in pharmacological erection programs was first reported by Virag and associates[54]. It is now known that atropine sulfate in low doses (10^{-8} mol/l) blocks muscarinic receptors, thereby diminishing cholinergic inhibition of the adrenergic and cholinergic excitation of the non-adrenergic, non-cholinergic neuroeffector systems controlling neurogenic corporeal smooth muscle relaxation. However, in large pharmacological doses (10^{-3} mol/l), atropine causes release of endothelium-derived relaxing factor, which has recently been identified as a neurotransmitter involved in penile erection.

Atropine has never been suggested for single drug injections, but has always been included in multidrug vasoactive mixtures. Recently, however, Sogari and co-workers[55] have questioned the actual adjunctive role of atropine when added to trimix and used in the pharmacological erection test. At our clinic, 3 mg of atropine sulfate is part of a four-drug mixture (Table 1).

Forskolin

Treatment of human corpus cavernosum smooth-muscle cells with forskolin (0.1–10 μmol/l) produced an increase in cAMP synthesis in a concentration-dependent manner[25]. Forskolin is a direct adenylate cyclase activator, which has been used as a intracavernosal vasoactive agent in the management of vasculogenic impotence. Forskolin-induced adenylyl cyclase activity was markedly augmented by PGE$_1$ and its metabolite, PGE$_0$[55]. Recently, Kim and co-workers[56] tried to assess the potential cross-regulation of cyclic nucleotides in human corpus cavernosum. Incubation of primary cultures of human corpus cavernosum smooth muscle cells with either the nitric oxide donor SNP (10 nmol/l) or the phosphodiesterase type 5 (PDE-5) inhibitor sildenafil (50 nmol/l) produced little or no change in the intracellular cGMP levels. Incubation with both SNP and sildenafil produced marked increases in cGMP. Interestingly, incubation of cells with forskolin or PGE$_1$ produced significant enhancement of cGMP accumulation. These data seemed to demonstrate that cAMP up-regulates intracellular levels of cGMP, in part, by inhibition of PDE-5. Moreover, the authors noted that cGMP down-regulated cAMP synthesis via a mechanism requiring G-protein coupling of adenylyl cyclase. These observations may have important implications in the utility of pharmacotherapeutic agents targeting cyclic nucleotide metabolism for the treatment of erectile dysfunction.

From a clinical point of view, Mulhall and colleagues[57] investigated 31 patients with erectile dysfunction with, overall, 61% of them reporting improvement in rigidity and/or erection duration using intracavernosal forskolin (98 μg/ml), papaverine (29 mg/ml), phentolamine (0.98 mg/ml) and PGE$_1$.

Multiple drug mixtures

The association of multiple vasoactive drugs is designed to utilize the synergistic effect derived from the different mechanisms of action which produce the erectogenic effects. None of the drugs mentioned above are able to produce a full erectile response in all types of impotent patients candidate for the pharmacological erection program. Patients with severe penile vascular impairments, especially those with marked veno-occlusive dysfunction of the corpora cavernosa, are poor responders to single drug intracavernous vasoactive injection therapy. In addition, adverse effects observed during intracavernous pharmacotherapy are mainly drug-related, owing to the chemical composition of the drug itself, to the total dose of the drug used for a single injection and to the overall volume injected. In contrast, the association of multiple vasoactive drugs produces a full erectile response in more than 90% of patients with an average volume of injected mixture and an extremely limited drug dose.

The effectiveness of trimix vasoactive drug intracavernous injections has recently been evaluated in elderly men complaining of erectile dysfunction[58]. Richter and co-workers[58], indeed, observed a statistically significant association between the results obtained after the injection of a mix of papaverine + phentolamine + PGE$_1$ as compared with PGE$_1$ alone (χ^2 with two degrees of freedom:34.666; $p \leq 0.001$) in elderly men (mean age 67.1 years, range 63–85 years) with erectile dysfunction of organic origin. A functional erection was obtained in 74.7% after the trimix as compared with 48.3% treated with PGE$_1$ alone. The authors concluded that injection therapy with vasoactive drugs can be considered a treatment of choice in elderly men suffering from organic impotence because it is safe, hardly invasive and highly effective.

The most frequently used combinations are given in Table 1[13,59,60]. It is generally agreed in the literature that these multidrug combinations achieve the greatest rate of responders with the lowest rate of complications. However, the main drawback of multidrug injection therapy is that none of these pharmacological combinations has been approved by the National Health Care Authorities (the only exception being the combination papaverine–phentolamine in some European countries) and that they subsequently have to be prepared by the hospital pharmacy as they are not available on the market. It is the present authors' personal feeling that the only patients who may not be treated by multidrug preparations are those requiring a very limited amount of a single conventional drug. However, in our practice, we prefer to use a multidrug mixture (prepared in three different versions: mild, normal, strong) in each patient entering the pharmacological erection program. Patients with pure psychogenic or neurogenic impotence are treated with the mild mixture, patients with mild vasculogenic impotence are treated with the normal mixture and patients with significant cavernosal artery occlusive disease or corporeal veno-occlusive dysfunction are treated with the strong mixture. The mean ($\pm$ SE) volume per injection used by our first 600 patients treated was 0.21 ± 0.09 ml, 0.18 ± 0.05 ml and 0.20 ± 0.04 ml for the mild, normal and strong mixtures, respectively.

Intracavernosal injection therapy versus sildenafil treatment

The advent of sildenafil has revolutionized the management of patients with erectile dysfunction, as oral therapy has progressively gained the position of first-line option among the patient's choices. In a large, multicenter study[61], patients with erectile dysfunction of various etiologies who had been under treatment with alprostadil for at least 6 months and who were reporting satisfactory erections with intracavernosal treatment were switched to sildenafil, starting at the dose of 50 mg which was then titrated according to the patient's needs. At the end of a 12-week treatment with sildenafil, 69% of patients elected to con-

tinue to use the oral treatment. The EDITS questionnaire was used to compare treatment satisfaction in both groups, and similar results were found. However, alprostadil injections achieved a higher rate of erections resulting in intercourse, compared with sildenafil. Hatzichristou and colleagues[62] evaluated patient preference with regard to sildenafil and injection therapy in a group of impotent men on intracavernous injection therapy for more than a year. In phase 1 of this study, the efficacy of sildenafil 50 and 100 mg was determined with home use. In phase 2, responders to sildenafil were asked to use the preferred dose orally for a month and choose intracavernous injection or sildenafil. In phase 3, patients were asked to continue either treatment for 3 more months. Of 155 men who had been on intracavernous injection therapy for at least 1 year, 74.8% responded to sildenafil during study phase 1. After 1 month of treatment, 61.2% of responders preferred to continue with the oral drug, 26.7% returned to intracavernous injections and 12.1% used each drug alternately. Three months later, 63.8% of responders preferred oral treatment and 32.8% chose intracavernous injection, while 3.4% continued to use each treatment alternately. These studies showed that patients on intracavernous injection therapy should be given the option to try sildenafil, as most of them will ultimately elect to use oral treatment. It is also clear that a significant subset of patients, however, will decide to use injections most of the time or at least sporadically.

An interesting issue is related to sildenafil non-responders. Shabsigh and associates[63] studied patients who did not respond to an open-label trial of sildenafil at doses up to 100 mg. These patients entered an alprostadil alfadex in-office titration phase, to determine the optimal dose of the drug up to 40 μg, which was then used during a 6-week home trial. The alprostadil alfadex use at home resulted in improvements related to questions 3 and 4 of the IIEF in 89.6% and 85.1% of patients, respectively. The most common side-effect seen with alprostadil alfadex use was penile pain (29.4%). This study clearly demonstrated that the majority of sildenafil failures can be salvaged by intracavernosal alprostadil therapy.

The opposite finding was also demonstrated by McMahon and colleagues[64], who studied 93 patients who failed to respond to a home trial with high-dose alprostadil or trimix. Thirty-four per cent of these patients responded to sildenafil (the majority at the 100-mg dose). Another 47.5% of patients responded to the combination sildenafil–injection therapy. The most interesting finding of this study is the evidence that combining sildenafil and intracavernosal injection therapy may salvage a significant proportion of patients who fail injections alone.

Recently, Israilov and co-workers[65] showed that treatments with intracavernous injections of increasingly complex combinations of vasoactive drugs in patients with cardiovascular diseases who failed or had contraindications for sildenafil treatment are immediately effective in 94.3%, and effective after 1 year in 96% of patients treated. Overall, localized treatment with intracavernous injections seems to be effective, acceptable and generally well-tolerated in men with cardiovascular disease.

Sildenafil injection therapy

Using rat and rabbit models, Seo and colleagues[66] noted that there is a significant synergism on rabbit, cavernosal smooth muscle relaxation when sildenafil is combined with forskolin, sodium nitroprusside, VIP or phentolamine in rabbits, and when combined with PGE_1 in rats. Therefore, these results suggest potentially effective combined therapies of sildenafil and intracavernosal PGE_1, forskolin or VIP, or oral phentolamine for patients with erectile dysfunction who have no success after monotherapy with these agents.

McAuley and co-workers[67] investigated whether intracavernosal injection of sildenafil causes penile erection in the absence of active neurogenic input. They noted that, in the absence of pelvic nerve stimulation, the magnitude and duration of the intracavernosal pressure increase in a dose-dependent fashion in response to intracavernosal sildenafil in the rabbit, suggesting that intracavernosal sildenafil can cause vascular smooth muscle relaxation and penile erection by a mechanism independent of the classical nitric oxide/cGMP pathway.

Intraurethral therapy

A novel approach derived from transdermal application is transurethral drug delivery, which allows the transfer of drugs from the urethra directly into the corpora cavernosa. In a retrograde urethrogram study using contrast media with the proximal urethra constricted, Vardi and colleagues demonstrated vascular communications between the spongiosal and cavernosal compartments[68]. Their study documented the ability to transfer the drug by vascular communications from the corpora spongiosa (urethra) to the cavernosal spaces. All the intraurethral drugs for erection are postulated to work by this transfer mechanism.

Trials comparing intracavernosal versus intraurethral therapy

Intracavernosal injection therapy with alprostadil seems to offer a better efficacy profile than the intraurethral route with the same drug. Shabsigh and colleagues[69] performed a crossover, randomized, open-label multicenter study in 111 patients with erectile dysfunction of at least 6 months' duration, which compared the efficacy, safety and patient preference of intracavernous injections of alprostadil alfadex (EDEX™) with MUSE™ plus optional ACTIS™ (venous flow controller). The study showed that more EDEX than MUSE administrations resulted in an erection sufficient for sexual intercourse (82.5% versus 53.0%), and that significantly more patients using EDEX achieved at least one erection sufficient for sexual intercourse (92.6% versus 61.8%, $p < 0.001$). Patient and partner satisfaction was greater with EDEX, while overall adverse events were similar with both treatments. Porst[70] reported similar results in 103 unselected patients treated with MUSE at doses up to 1000 µg and intracavernous alprostadil up to 20 µg. There was a significant difference in cavernosal artery end-diastolic velocity at duplex examination performed after administration of either intraurethral or intracavernosal alprostadil, showing that the former treatment was not able to induce complete smooth muscle relaxation. Interestingly, side-effects, namely penile pain, were greater in the MUSE-treated patients. The finding that intracavernosal alprostadil is able to produce erections with better rigidity as compared with intraurethral alprostadil has also been shown by other investigators[71,72]. However, MUSE has been reported to be effective in 58% of patients who did not previously respond to intracavernosal injections of alprostadil[71-73].

Conclusions

At present, oral pharmacotherapy represents the first-line option for the majority of patients with erectile dysfunction. Patients who do not respond to oral therapy or those who are not eligible for this treatment are considered for second-line treatments which include intracavernosal injections, intraurethral suppositories or topicals. Intracavernosal injection therapy seems to be associated with the highest efficacy within this group; however, the major limitation of this approach is represented by its high attrition rate.

In a recent review article by Lue and colleagues[74] it has been shown that, among the pharmacological treatment options available for erectile dysfunction, intracavernous injection therapy remains the most effective, although the drop-out rate is high. However, proper evaluation of every patient should be performed so that a number of potentially life-threatening causes of erectile dysfunction cannot be over-looked.

References

1. Jardin A, Wagner G, Koury S, *et al.*, eds. *Recommendations of the 1st International Consultation on Erectile Dysfunction.* Plymouth: Plymbridge Distributors 2000:711–26
2. Dula E, Keating W, Siami PF, *et al.* Efficacy and safety of six dose and dose optimization regimen of sublingual apomorphine versus placebo in men with erectile dysfunction. The Apomorphine Study Group. *Urology* 2000;56:130–5
3. Montorsi F, Guazzoni G, Rigatti P, *et al.* Pharmacological management of erectile dysfunction. *Drugs* 1995;50:465–79
4. Montorsi F, Guazzoni G, Bergamaschi F, *et al.* Four-drug intracavernous therapy for impotence due to corporeal veno-occlusive dysfunction. *J Urol* 1993;149:1291–5
5. Montorsi F, Guazzoni G, Bergamaschi F, *et al.* Intracavernous vasoactive pharmacotherapy: the impact of a new self-injection device. *J Urol* 1993;150:1829–32
6. Montorsi F, Guazzoni G, Bergamaschi F, *et al.* Effectiveness and safety of multidrug intracavernous therapy for vasculogenic impotence. *Urology* 1993;42:554–8
7. Montorsi F, Guazzoni G, Bergamaschi F, *et al.* Clinical reliability of multi-drug intracavernous vasoactive pharmacotherapy for diabetic impotence. *Acta Diabetol* 1994;31:1–5
8. Zentgraf M, Baccouche M, Junemann KP. Diagnosis and therapy of erectile dysfunction using papaverine and phentolamine. *Urol Int* 1988;43:65–8
9. Linet OI, Neff LL. Intracavernous prostaglandin E_1 in erectile dysfunction. *Clin Invest* 1994;72:139–49
10. Porst H. Current perspectives on intracavernosal pharmacotherapy for erectile dysfunction. *Int J Impot Res* 2000;12(Suppl 4):S91–100
11. Leungwattanakij L, Flynn V, Hellstrom WJG. Intracavernosal injection and intraurethral therapy for erectile dysfunction. *Urol Clin North Am* 2001;28:343–54
12. Baniel J, Israilov S, Engelstein D, *et al.* Three-year outcome of a progressive treatment program for erectile dysfunction with intracavernous injections of vasoactive drugs. *Urology* 2000;56:647–52
13. Spahn M, Manning M, Juenemann KP. Intracavernosal therapy. In Carson CC, Kirby RS,

Goldstein I, eds. *Textbook of Erectile Dysfunction.* Oxford: Isis Medical Media, 1999:345–53

14. Hatzichristou DG, Pescatori ES. Current treatments and emerging therapeutic approaches in male erectile dysfunction. *BJU Int* 2001; 88(Suppl 3):11–17

15. Beal K, Mears JG. Short report: penile lymphoma following local injections for erectile dysfunction. *Leuk Lymphoma* 2001;42:247–9

16. Marshall GA, Breza J, Lue TF. Improved hemodynamic response after long-term intracavernous injection for impotence. *Urology* 1994; 43:844–7

17. Wespes E, Sattar AA, Noel JC, *et al.* Does prostaglandin E_1 therapy modify the intracavernous musculature? *J Urol* 2000;163:464–6

18. Brock G, Mai Tu L, Linet O. Return of spontaneous erection during long-term intracavernosal alprostadil (Caverject) treatment. *Int J Impotence Res* 2001;57:536–41

19. Maniam P, Seftel A, Corty E, *et al.* Nocturnal penile tumescence activity unchanged after long-term intracavernous injection therapy. *J Urol* 2001;165:830–3

20. Wang Q, Large WA. Modulation of noradrenaline-induced membrane currents by papaverine in rabbit vascular smooth muscle cells. *J Physiol (Lond)* 1991;439:501–12

21. Andersson KE, Holmquist F, Wagner G. Pharmacology of drugs used for treatment of erectile dysfunction and priapism. *Int J Impotence Res* 1991;3:155–72

22. Meinhardt W, Lycklama AAB, Kropman RF, *et al.* Comparison of a mixture of papaverine, phentolamine and prostaglandin E_1 with other intracavernous injections. *Eur Urol* 1994;26: 319–21

23. Porst H. The rationale for PGE_1 in erectile failure: a survey of world-wide experience. *J Urol* 1996;155:802–15

24. Wespes E, Rondeux C, Schulman CC. Effect of phentolamine on venous return in human erection. *Br J Urol* 1989;63:95–7

25. Traish AM, Moreland RB, Gallant C, *et al.* G-protein-coupled receptor agonists augment adenylyl cyclase activity induced by forskolin in human corpus cavernosum smooth muscle cells. *Recept Signal Transduct* 1997;7:121–32

26. Witjes WPJ. The efficacy and acceptance of intracavernous autoinjection therapy with the combination of papaverine/phentolamine. A prospective multicenter trial in 60 patients. *Int J Impotence Res* 1992;4:65–72

27. Linet OI, Ogrinc FG and Alprostadil Study Group. Efficacy and safety of intracavernosal alprostadil in men with erectile dysfunction. *N Engl J Med* 1996;334:873–7

28. Linet OI, Ogrinc FG. Penile fibrosis during 18 months of intracavernosal therapy with alprostadil (Caverject™). *Int J Impotence Res* 1996;8:D85

29. Linet OI. Long-term safety of Caverject™ (alprostadil S.PO, PGE_1) in erectile dysfunction (ED). *Int J Impotence Res* 1998;10:S37

30. Porst H. Intracavernous alprostadil alfadex – an effective and well tolerated treatment for erectile dysfunction. Results of a long-term European Study. *Int J Impotence Res* 1998;10:225–31

31. Willke RJ, Glick HA, McCarron TJ, *et al.* Quality of life effects of alprostadil therapy for erectile dysfunction. *J Urol* 1997;157:2124–8

32. Heaton JPW, Lording D, Liu S-N, *et al.* Intracavernosal alprostadil is effective for the treatment of erectile dysfunction in diabetic men. *Int J Impotence Res* 2001;13:317–21

33. Perimenis P, Gyftopoulos K, Athanasopoulos A, *et al.* Diabetic impotence treated by intracavernosal injections: high treatment compliance and increasing dosage of vaso-acting drugs. *Eur Urol* 2001;40:398–402

34. Montorsi F, Guazzoni G, Strambi LF, *et al.* Recovery of spontaneous erectile function after nerve-sparing radical retropubic prostatectomy with and without early intracavernous injections of alprostadil: results of a prospective, randomized trial. *J Urol* 1997;158:1408–10

35. Lepore G, Nosari I. Efficacy of oral sildenafil in the treatment of erectile dysfunction in diabetic men with positive response to intracavernosal injection of alprostadil. *Diabetes Care* 2001;24: 409–11

36. Montorsi F, Salonia A, Barbieri L, *et al.* The subsequent use of I.C. alprostadil and oral sildenafil is more efficacious than sildenafil alone in nerve sparing radical prostatectomy. *J Urol* 2002;167(Suppl):A1098

37. Moriel EZ, Rajfer J. Sodium bicarbonate alleviates penile pain induced by intracavernous injections for erectile dysfunction. *J Urol* 1993; 149:1299–300

38. Schramek P, Plas EG, Hubner WA, *et al.* Intracavernous injection of prostaglandin E_1 plus procaine in the treatment of erectile dysfunction. *J Urol* 1994;152:1108–10

39. Imagawa A, Kimura K, Kawanishi Y. Effect of moxisylyte hydrochloride on isolated human penile corpus cavernosum tissue. *Life Sci* 1989;44:619–23

40. Costa P, Sarrazin B, Bressolle F, *et al.* Efficiency and side effects of intracavernous injections of moxisylyte in impotent patients: a dose-finding study versus placebo. *J Urol* 1993;149: 301–5

41. Costa P, Iacovella JA, Bouvet AA. Efficacy and tolerability of moxisilite and placebo injected intracavernously in patients with erectile dysfunction (ED): a multicenter, double-blind study. *J Urol* 1997;157(Suppl):203

42. Dinsmore WW, Alderdice DK. Vasoactive intestinal polypeptide and phentolamine mesylate administered by autoinjector in the treatment of patients with erectile dysfunction resistant to other intracavernosal agents. Br J Urol 1998;81:437–40

43. Hackett G. The results of a 6 month multi-center placebo-controlled study of Invicorp™ in the treatment of nonpsychogenic erectile dysfunction. J Urol 1998;159:240

44. Dinsmore WW, Gingell C, Hackett G, et al. Treating men with predominantly non-psychogenic erectile dysfunction with intra-cavernosal vasoactive intestinal polypeptide and phentolamine mesylate in a novel auto-injector system: a multicentre double-blind placebo-controlled study. Br J Urol 1999;83:274–9

45. Sandhu D, Curless E, Dean J, et al. A double blind, placebo controlled study of intracavernosal vasoactive intestinal polypeptide and phento-lamine mesylate in a novel auto-injector for the treatment of non-psychogenic erectile dysfunction. Int J Impotence Res 1999;11:91–7

46. Truss MC, Becker AJ, Thon WF, et al. Intra-cavernous calcitonin gene-related peptide plus prostaglandin E_1: possible alternative to penile implants in selected patients. Eur Urol 1994; 26:40–5

47. Stief CG, Wetterauer U, Schaebsdau F, et al. Calcitonin gene-related peptide: a possible role in human penile erection and its therapeutical application in impotent patients. J Urol 1991;146: 1010–14

48. Stief CG, Holmquist F, Djamilian M, et al. Preliminary results with the nitric oxide donor linsidomine chloridrate in the treatment of human erectile dysfunction. J Urol 1992;148: 1437–40

49. Porst H. Prostaglandin E_1 and the nitric oxide donor linsidomine for erectile failure: a diag-nostic comparative study of 40 patients. J Urol 1993;149:1280–3

50. Wegner HEH, Knispel HH. Effect of nitric oxide-donor, linsidomine chloridrate, in treat-ment of human erectile dysfunction caused by venous leakage. Urology 1993;42:409–11

51. Martinez-Pineiro L. Preliminary results of a comparative study with intracavernous sodium nitroprusside and prostaglandin E_1 in patients with erectile dysfunction. J Urol 1995;153: 1487–90

52. Fu Q, Yao DH, Jiang YQ. A clinical comparative study on effects of intracavernous injection of sodium nitroprusside and papaverine/phentolamine in erectile dysfunction patients. Asian J Androl 2000;2:301–3

53. Virag R, Frydman D, Legman M, et al. Intra-cavernous injection of papaverine as a diagnosis and therapeutic method in erectile failure. Angiology 1984;35:79–84

54. Virag R, Shoukry K, Floresco J, et al. Intra-cavernous self-injection of vasoactive drugs in the treatment of impotence: 8-year experience with 615 cases. J Urol 1991;145:287–91

55. Sogari PR, Teloken C, Vargas Souto CA. Atropine role in the pharmacological erec-tion test: study of 228 patients. J Urol 1997; 158:1760–3

56. Kim NN, Huang Y, Moreland RB, et al. Cross-regulation of intracellular cGMP and cAMP in cultured human corpus cavernosum smooth muscle cells. Mol Cell Biol Res Commun 2000;4: 10–14

57. Mulhall JP, Daller M, Traish AM, et al. Intra-cavernosal forskolin: role in management of vasculogenic impotence resistant to standard 3-agent pharmacotherapy. J Urol 1997;158: 1752–8

58. Richter S, Vardi Y, Ringel A, et al. Intracavernous injections: still the gold standard for treatment of erectile dysfunction in elderly men. Int J Impo-tence Res 2001;13:172–5

59. Govier FE, McClure RD, Weissman RM, et al. Experience with triple-drug therapy in a pharma-cological erection program. J Urol 1993;150: 1822–4

60. Valdevenito R, Melman A. Intracavernous self-injection pharmacotherapy program: analysis of results and complications. Int J Impotence Res 1994;6:81–91

61. Giuliano F, Montorsi F, Mirone V, et al. Switching from intracavernous prostaglandin E_1 injection to oral sildenafil citrate in patients with erectile dysfunction: results of a multi-center European study. The Sildenafil Multicenter Study Group. J Urol 2000;164:708–11

62. Hatzichristou D, Apostolidis A, Tzortzis V, et al. Sildenafil versus intracavernous injection therapy: efficacy and preference in patients on intracavernous injection for more than 1 year. J Urol 2000;164:1197–200

63. Shabsigh R, Padma Nathan H, Gittleman M, et al. Intracavernous alprostadil alfadex is effective and safe in patients with erectile dysfunction after failing sildenafil. Urology 2000;55:477–80

64. McMahon CG, Samali R, Johnson H. Treatment of intracorporeal injection non-response with sildenafil alone or in combination with triple agent intracorporeal injection therapy. J Urol 1999;162:1992–8

65. Israilov S, Niv E, Livne PM, et al. Intracavernous injections for erectile dysfunction in patients with cardiovascular disease and failure or contra-indications for sildenafil citrate. Int J Impotence Res 2002;14:38–43

66. Seo KK, Kim SC, Jun IO, et al. Synergistic effects of sildenafil on relaxation of rabbit and rat

cavernosal smooth muscles when combined with various vasoactive agents. *BJU Int* 2001; 88:596–601

67. McAuley IW, Kim NN, Min K, *et al.* Intracavernosal sildenafil facilitates penile erection independent of the nitric oxide pathway. *J Androl* 2001;22:623–8

68. Vardi Y, Saenz de Tejada I. Functional and radiologic evidence of vascular communication between the spongiosal and cavernosal compartments of the penis. *Urology* 1997;49:749–52

69. Shabsigh R, Padma-Nathan H, Gittleman M, *et al.* Intracavernous alprostadil alfadex is more efficacious, better tolerated, and preferred over intraurethral alprostadil plus optional ACTIS: a comparative, randomised, crossover, multi-center study. *Urology* 2000;55:109–13

70. Porst H. Transurethral alprostadil with MUSE™ vs. intracavernous alprostadil – a comparative study in 103 patients with erectile dysfunction. *Int J Impotence Res* 1997;9:187–92

71. Shokeir AA, Alserafi MA, Mutabagani H. Intracavernosal versus intraurethral alprostadil: a prospective randomised study. *Br J Urol* 1999; 83:812–15

72. Werthman P, Rajfer J. MUSE therapy: preliminary clinical observations. *Urology* 1997;50: 809–11

73. Engel JD, McVary KT. Transurethral alprostadil as therapy for patients who withdrew from or failed prior intracavernous injection therapy. *Urology* 1998;51:687–92

74. Lue TF, Lee KL. Pharmacotherapy for erectile dysfunction. *Chin Med J* 2000;113:291–8

Mechanisms and prevention of erectile dysfunction after radiotherapy for prostate cancer

8

L. Incrocci

Introduction

In recent years, the number of patients diagnosed with prostate cancer has increased dramatically[1,2], owing to the widespread use of prostate-specific antigen (PSA) testing and the possibility for cure of early disease. Standard treatments for prostate cancer are radical prostatectomy, external-beam radiotherapy, brachytherapy, hormonal therapy and observation. The choice of treatment depends on tumor staging, the patient's age and co-morbidity, and the urologist's and patient's preferences. A commonly ignored or not properly addressed aspect is the impact of prostate cancer therapy on the patient's future sexual functioning[3].

Evaluation of erectile dysfunction: definition and methodology

The National Institutes of Health (NIH) consensus on erectile dysfunction defined impotence as: 'the consistent inability to attain and maintain a penile erection sufficient to permit satisfactory sexual activity'[4]. Furthermore, the rigidity of erections, presence of spontaneous daytime erections and morning/night erections are also important issues. In most published studies, authors have used the general terms potency or impotence without giving a proper operational definition[5,6]. Only in some articles has a detailed definition been provided[5,6]. The most practical and rapid way to evaluate erectile dysfunction is by using a questionnaire. The various questionnaires reported in the published literature have fairly often been limited to a few items, and incorporated into a more general questionnaire on the toxicity of radiation treatment[5,6]. In articles from the 1970s and 1980s, only rates of potency or impotence are mentioned, without reference to the methodology used. More recently an international questionnaire, the International Index of Erectile Function (IIEF), has been introduced[7]. The IIEF has been translated and validated in many countries, and offers the possibility of making comparisons between studies.

Incidence of erectile dysfunction after radiotherapy

Articles from the 1970s dealt with the introduction of radiotherapy for prostate cancer in the pre-PSA era. Until then, surgery was the mainstay of treatment as prostate cancer was considered to be relatively radioresistant. Erectile dysfunction incidence was reported in up to 41%[5,6]. In the 1980s, radiotherapy was delivered using megavolt energies. Post-radiotherapy erectile dysfunction was mentioned in most studies, with frequencies ranging from 11 to 73%[5,6]. The 1990s were characterized by PSA testing and by the three-dimensional (3D) conformal techniques. The use of more fields, and shaped blocks, a computer planning system and 3D treatment plans resulted in smaller treatment volumes. Only a few prospective studies from the 1990s dealt specifically with sexual functioning after radiotherapy. Rates of erectile dysfunction varied from 7 to 72%.

Incidence of erectile dysfunction after brachytherapy

Brachytherapy was originally introduced not only to limit the detrimental effects of radiotherapy on bowel and urinary function, but also to help preserve sexual function. Rates of erectile dysfunction after brachytherapy alone were usually lower than after radiotherapy alone[5]. In studies from the 1970s, rates of erectile dysfunction ranged from 0 to 25%, being highest when brachytherapy was used in combination with radiotherapy, and in the 1980s from 8 to 61%[5]. In the 1990s, in studies using iodine-125, palladium-103 or both, the erectile dysfunction rate ranged from 2 to 51%. The highest rates, ranging from 25 to 89%, were reported in studies combining a temporary iridium-192 implant with subsequent radiotherapy[5].

Mechanisms of post-radiation erectile dysfunction

In the 1980s, Goldstein and associates[8] performed a detailed study of 23 patients treated with radiotherapy for prostate cancer, to understand the etiology of post-radiation erectile dysfunction. Nocturnal penile tumescence testing, bulbocavernous reflex latency, perineal electromiography, penile Doppler ultrasonography and endocrine screening of the hypothalamic–pituitary–gonadal axis were carried out. Subjects were considered potent if they could develop an erection sufficiently rigid for vaginal penetration and sustain it until ejaculation[8]. Before radiotherapy, 15 patients met the criteria for potency; 14 months after radiotherapy, they all complained of a worsening in erectile function. Neurological examinations were normal, while penile Doppler evaluation was abnormal in all 15 patients. Selective pudendal arteriography performed in two subjects revealed occlusive vascular disease within the pelvic radiation field. Mittal[9] published a study of penile circulation, before and 6–9 months after radiotherapy, and its effect on erectile function in six patients who were potent before radiotherapy. Penile circulation was measured using the penile brachial index (PBI) and penile flow index (PFI); no statistically significant differences between pre- and post-radiation values were found. The author concluded that penile circulation was not abnormal after radiation, and that the etiology of erectile dysfunction was a more complex mechanism not directly attributable to vascular damage as previously suggested[8,9]. A major criticism of the above study could be that evaluation at 6–9 months after radiation is presumably too early to detect damage to vessels, and also that PBI and PFI are now obsolete tests. Zelefsky and Eid[10] evaluated 98 patients who became impotent after radiotherapy or radical prostatectomy. Median time from radiation to evaluation was 14 months. The penis was scanned with duplex ultrasound before, and after, an intracavernosal injection of prostaglandin. Among radiotherapy patients, 32% had cavernosal dysfunction (abnormal cavernosal distensibility with a normal penile peak blood flow) and 63% had arteriogenic dysfunction (peak penile blood flow rates less than 25 cm/s). Neurogenic dysfunction was found in 3% of the radiotherapy and in 12% of the prostatectomy group. The authors concluded that the predominant etiology of post-radiation erectile dysfunction was arteriogenic[10]. Fisch and co-workers[11] evaluated the effect of the radiation dose to the bulb of the penis on erectile function in 21 patients, at 2 years after treatment. A strong dose-volume relationship with the likelihood of remaining potent after radiotherapy was observed. Patients who received 70 Gy or more to 70% of the bulb of the penis appeared to be at very high risk of developing post-radiotherapy erectile dysfunction. Similar results were reported after brachytherapy[12]. (Figure 1 shows the relationship between radiation fields and the corporal bodies.) DiBiase and colleagues[13] postulated that brachytherapy-related impotence might be due to excessive radiation to the neurovascular bundles. The authors made a detailed calculation of the administered dose to these regions. Merrick and colleagues[14], using the same methodology as DiBiase and co-workers[13], found no significant difference in the mean

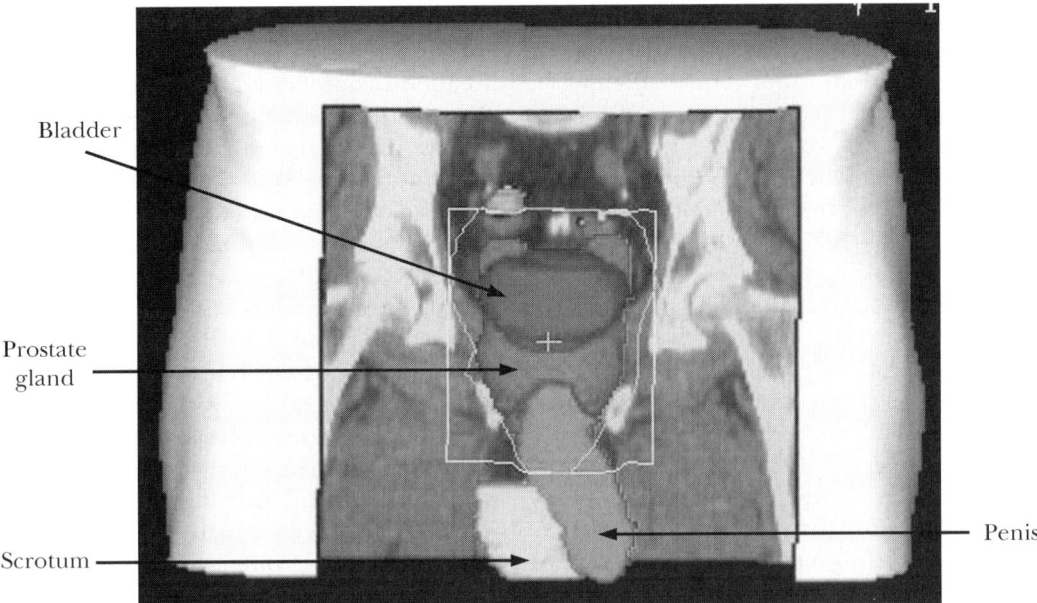

Figure 1 Anteroposterior radiation field and its relation to the penis

dose to the neurovascular bundles between potent and impotent men, between the two isotopes ^{125}I and [103]Pd or between radiotherapy- and non-radiotherapy-containing regimens, after a follow-up time of 37 months[14]. Although no test is currently available to assess cavernous nerve autonomic function, one animal study suggested that a decrease in nitric oxide synthase-containing nerve fibers in the corpora cavernosa may contribute to post-radiation erectile dysfunction[15]. Age, comorbidity and a history of transurethral resection of the prostate (TURP) did not always correlate positively with post-radiation erectile dysfunction[5,6]. Tumor stage and hormone manipulation was not found to influence rates of erectile dysfunction in most studies, while total radiation dose was sometimes found to be correlated with dysfunction rates[5,6]. It is very important to determine the patient's pre-treatment sexual functioning because up to 60% of patients may have some erectile difficulties before radiotherapy, and these are more likely to become fully impotent after treatment[5,6]. The time elapsed between radiation therapy and erectile dysfunction evaluation also has to be considered. It is not possible to draw final conclusions when the evaluation is done at 6–12 months after radiotherapy or brachytherapy because it takes at least 18–24 months for erectile dysfunction occurrence to reach a maximum[5,6,16,17].

Prevention of post-radiation erectile dysfunction

Prevention is a difficult matter. If one accepts the hypothesis that radiation induces vascular damage, then decreasing the dose to pelvic vascular structures could decrease erectile dysfunction rate. Both conventional and conformal radiotherapy techniques seem to result in the same rates of dysfunction[18]. However, a relationship between radiation field size and sexual function (i.e. the smaller the field size, the better the sexual functioning) has also been reported[16]. Nevertheless, prospective studies with large series of patients, and the use of standardized validated questionnaires, have to confirm these findings. Conformal techniques using shaped blocks do not appear to spare the neurovascular bundles, as these are always entirely in the high-dose prostate field. No reliable data are available, however, to correlate doses in this region with the occurrence of erectile dysfunction after radiotherapy[5,6]. Furthermore, special radiation beams (such as proton, pion and neutron) have been reported to have detrimental effects on potency, similar to those reported for the more commonly used photon beams[5].

Recently, intensity modulated radiotherapy (IMRT) techniques have been introduced. IMRT is an advanced 3D conformal technique that uses a computerized treatment plan optimization with an inverse technique, and intensity-modulated radiation beams with dynamic multi-leaf collimator. IMRT was introduced in the treatment of prostate cancer in 1996, resulting in a significantly lower incidence of rectal toxicity[19]. A comparison of 3D conformal radiotherapy and IMRT plans in ten patients with prostate cancer showed a significantly lower radiation dose to the corporal bodies in favor of the IMRT techniques (Sethi and colleagues, personal communication). However, currently, there are no data on the use of IMRT and erectile dysfunction. Because of a strong relationship between radiation dose in the penile bulb and erectile dysfunction[11,12], it seems warranted to limit this dose to prevent post-radiation dysfunction.

Therapy for post-radiation erectile dysfunction

To our knowledge, only two articles were published on therapy for post-radiation erectile dysfunction, before sildenafil citrate (Viagra®) was introduced, indicating the efficacy of intra-cavernosal injection (ICI) of phentolamine–papaverine[20] and of penile implants[21]. With the availability of sildenafil, these methods of therapy are losing popularity. The efficacy of sildenafil after radiotherapy in open-label studies was reported in up to 90% of patients[22–25], but it was less effective in the only double-blind study recently performed[26]. Sildenafil improved erections significantly, compared with placebo; 55% of patients had successful intercourse using sildenafil. Ninety per cent of patients needed the 100-mg dose,

and side-effects were mild or moderate[26]. Sildenafil has been found to be effective in 80% of patients complaining of erectile dysfunction after transperineal ultrasound-guided brachytherapy, with or without radiotherapy[27], and in 62% in another study[28]. The latter authors found no differences in the efficacy of sildenafil between patients treated by brachytherapy alone and brachytherapy combined with radiotherapy, but patients who were not on a neoadjuvant androgen-deprivation regimen responded significantly better to sildenafil[28]. Also, sildenafil taken at bedtime has been found to increase nocturnal erectile activity significantly, especially in older patients, and in patients with vasculogenic erectile dysfunction[29]. We hypothesize that sildenafil given during, and for some months after, radiotherapy could somehow prevent or minimize the vascular deterioration that usually follows radiation.

Currently, new drugs for erectile dysfunction such as the central agent apomorphine, and a new class of phosphodiesterase inhibitors (tadalafil, vardenafil), are under evaluation; they might be effective in treating post-radiation dysfunction.

Conclusions

Before final conclusions can be drawn on the incidence of post-radiation erectile dysfunction a correct methodology is mandatory. The definition of (im)potence advocated by the NIH should always be used, and erectile dysfunction evaluation should be standardized by using, prospectively, validated questionnaires on quality of life and sexual functioning. One should wait at least 18–24 months when erectile dysfunction occurrence reaches a maximum, and remains stable further on. Although arterial damage seems to be the main cause of erectile dysfunction after radiotherapy, a multifactorial etiology must be considered, taking into account comorbidity, previous TURP, drugs and, more importantly, pre-treatment erectile function. Conformal techniques using shaped blocks do not appear to spare the neurovascular bundles. Radiation dose to the penile bulb seems important in developing post-radiation erectile dysfunction. The recently introduced IMRT techniques result in a decrease of dose to the penile bulb, but there are no data so far on its relationship with post-radiation erectile dysfunction.

Patients need to be correctly informed on the anatomy of the prostate, on the possible sequelae of radiation on their functioning and about the currently available effective treatments for erectile dysfunction (sildenafil, intracavernosal injections, vacuum devices and erection prostheses).

Acknowledgement

Professor A. K. Slob is thanked for his critical reading of the manuscript, and his continuous support.

References

1. Greenlee RT, Hill-Harmon MB, Thun M. Cancer statistics, 2001. *CA Cancer J Clin* 2001;51:15–36

2. Jensen OM, Esteve J, Moller H, *et al.* Cancer in the European Community and its member states. *Eur J Cancer* 1990;26:1167–256

3. McCammon KA, Kolm P, Main B, *et al.* Comparative quality-of-life analysis after radical prostatectomy or external beam radiation for localized prostate cancer. *Urology* 1999;54:509–16

4. National Institutes of Health. NIH consensus development panel on impotence. *J Am Med Assoc* 1993;270:83–90

5. Incrocci L, Slob AK, Levendag PC. Sexual (dys)function after radiotherapy for prostate cancer: a review. *Int J Radiat Oncol Biol Phys* 2002;52:681–93

6. Incrocci L, Slob AK. Incidence, etiology, and therapy for erectile dysfunction after external beam radiotherapy for prostate cancer. *Urology* 2002;60:1–7

7. Rosen RC, Riley A, Wagner G, *et al.* The International Index of Erectile Function (IIEF). A multidimensional scale for assessment of erectile dysfunction. *Urology* 1997;49:822–30

8. Goldstein I, Feldman MI, Deckers PJ, *et al.* Radiation-associated impotence. *J Am Med Assoc* 1984;251:903–10

9. Mittal B. A study of penile circulation before and after radiation in patients with prostate cancer and its effect on impotence. *Int J Radiat Oncol Biol Phys* 1985;11:1121–5

10. Zelefsky MJ, Eid JF. Elucidating the etiology of erectile dysfunction after definitive therapy for prostatic cancer. *Int J Radiat Oncol Biol Phys* 1998;40:129–33

11. Fisch BM, Pickett B, Weinberg V, *et al.* Dose of radiation received by the bulb of the penis correlates with risk of impotence after three-dimensional conformal radiotherapy for prostate cancer. *Urology* 2001;57:955–9

12. Merrick GS, Wallner K, Butler WM, *et al.* A comparison of radiation dose to the bulb of the penis in men with and without prostate brachytherapy-induced erectile dysfunction. *Int J Radiat Oncol Biol Phys* 2001;50:597–604

13. DiBiase SJ, Wallner K, Tralins K, *et al.* Brachytherapy radiation doses to the neurovascular bundles. *Int J Radiat Oncol Biol Phys* 2000;46:1301–7

14. Merrick GS, Butler WM, Dorsey AT, *et al.* A comparison of radiation dose to the neurovascular bundles in men with and without prostate brachytherapy-induced erectile dysfunction. *Int J Radiat Oncol Biol Phys* 2000;48:1069–74

15. Carrier S, Hricak H, Lee S, *et al.* Radiation-induced decrease in nitric oxide synthase-containing nerves in the rat penis. *Radiology* 1995;195:95–9

16. Beard CJ, Propert KJ, Rieker PP, *et al.* Complications after treatment with external-beam irradiation in early-stage prostate cancer patients: a prospective multiinstitutional outcomes study. *J Clin Oncol* 1997;15:223–9

17. Turner SL, Adams K, Bull CA, *et al.* Sexual dysfunction after radical radiation therapy for prostate cancer: a prospective evaluation. *Urology* 1999;54:124–9

18. Nguyen LN, Pollack A, Zagars GK. Late effects after radiotherapy for prostate cancer in a randomized dose–response study: results of a self-assessment questionnaire. *Urology* 1998;51:991–7

19. Zelefsky MJ, Fuks Z, Happersett L, *et al.* Clinical experience with intensity modulated radiation

therapy (IMRT) in prostate cancer. *Radiother Oncol* 2000;55:241–9

20. Pierce LJ, Whittington R, Hanno PM, *et al.* Pharmacologic erection with intracavernosal injection for men with sexual dysfunction following irradiation: a preliminary report. *Int J Radiat Oncol Biol Phys* 1991;21:1311–14

21. Dubocq FM, Bianco FJ Jr, Maralani SJ, *et al.* Outcome analysis of penile implant surgery after external beam radiation for prostate cancer. *J Urol* 1997;158:1787–90

22. Zelefsky MJ, McKee AB, Lee H, *et al.* Efficacy of oral sildenafil in patients with erectile dysfunction after radiotherapy for carcinoma of the prostate. *Urology* 1999;53:775–8

23. Kedia S, Zippe CD, Agarwal A, *et al.* Treatment of erectile dysfunction with sildenafil citrate (Viagra) after radiation therapy for prostate cancer. *Urology* 1999;54:308–12

24. Weber DC, Bieri S, Kurtz JM, *et al.* Prospective pilot study of sildenafil for treatment of post-radiotherapy erectile dysfunction in patients with prostate cancer. *J Clin Oncol* 1999;17:3444–9

25. Valicenti RK, Choi E, Chen C, *et al.* Sildenafil citrate effectively reverses sexual dysfunction induced by three-dimensional conformal radiation therapy. *Urology* 2001;57:769–73

26. Incrocci L, Koper PCM, Hop WCJ, *et al.* Sildenafil citrate (Viagra) and erectile dysfunction following external-beam radiotherapy for prostate cancer. A randomized, double-blind, placebo-controlled, cross-over study. *Int J Radiat Oncol Biol Phys* 2001;51:1190–5

27. Merrick GS, Butler WM, Lief JH, *et al.* Efficacy of sildenafil citrate in prostate brachytherapy patients with erectile dysfunction. *Urology* 1999; 53:1112–16

28. Potters L, Torre T, Fearn PA, *et al.* Potency after permanent prostate brachytherapy for localized prostate cancer. *Int J Radiat Oncol Biol Phys* 2001;50:1235–42

29. Montorsi F, Maga T, Ferini Strambi L, *et al.* Sildenafil taken at bedtime significantly increases nocturnal erections: results of a placebo-controlled study. *Urology* 2000;56: 906–11

Evaluation and management of lower urinary tract symptoms related to benign prostate disease: the contribution of the International Continence Society - 'Benign Prostatic Hyperplasia' study

9

J. L. Donovan

Introduction

The International Continence Society-'Benign Prostatic Hyperplasia' (ICS-'BPH') study was initiated following the First World Health Organization (WHO) Consultation on benign prostatic hyperplasia (BPH) in 1991. At this meeting, there was no formal acknowledgement of the role of urodynamics in the assessment of men presenting with lower urinary tract symptoms (LUTS), which were then typically described as 'prostatism' or 'clinical BPH', and the seven-item American Urological Association (AUA) symptom score was adopted as the International Prostate Symptom Score (IPSS)[1]. There were concerns that such a short symptom score did not cover the range of problematic symptoms experienced by patients, and that many urologists relied upon symptom ascertainment alone to select patients for invasive therapies, despite evidence that LUTS had poor diagnostic specificity. In addition, there were suggestions that urodynamic studies could be used to identify patients with obstruction who might be more suitable for invasive treatments, thus leading to better patient selection and outcome, particularly in the context of increasing diversification of technologies for the treatment of LUTS. In this context, the ICS-'BPH' study was established.

A number of things have now changed. In particular, there is general consensus that the IPSS is not diagnostic, and acceptance that urodynamic studies have a role in the evaluation of men with LUTS. There has also been a marked change in the use of terminology in this area. In particular, the term 'prostatism' has been rejected and there is considerable care now in the use of 'BPH'. BPH tends now to be reserved for histological diagnosis, with LUTS used to describe lower urinary tract symptoms, BPE (benign prostatic enlargement) an enlarged prostate found on digital or ultrasound examination, and BPO (benign prostatic obstruction) the diagnosis of obstruction confirmed by urodynamic studies[2]. The title of the ICS-'BPH' study was thus soon outdated, and so inverted commas were used to denote the difficulties surrounding the term 'BPH'[3]! In the sections that follow, the methods and major findings from the ICS-'BPH' study are presented and their contribution evaluated.

Methods of the ICS-'BPH' study

The main aims of the ICS-'BPH' study were:

(1) To investigate the relationships between the results of urodynamic studies and a wide range of urinary symptoms;

(2) To produce a valid and reliable symptom, sexual function and quality of life

questionnaire, including, if possible, a scored short form for use in clinical practice and research;

(3) To undertake an observational study of outcome of treatments according to current clinical practice around the world;

(4) To compare methods of pressure–flow analysis to establish the 'optimum' method of diagnosing bladder outlet obstruction.

These aims were addressed in three phases:

Phase I International, multicenter observational study collecting baseline data on LUTS and their impact on quality of life, sexual function, uroflowmetry and urodynamic studies;

Phase II International, multicenter observational study of outcome approximately 12 months following treatment;

Phase III Evaluation of treatments in randomized trials, e.g. CLasP study.

Urologists from around the world were invited to recruit consecutive patients over 45 years of age with LUTS presumed to be of benign origin who could complete a frequency–volume chart and questionnaire and undergo uroflowmetry and urodynamics. Men with significant urological disease, unfit for treatment or taking medication active on the lower urinary tract were excluded.

The ICS-'BPH' study questionnaire was designed to be self-completed. It was developed in English and then professionally translated into 15 other languages (Danish, Dutch, Finnish, French, French Canadian, German, Israeli, Italian, Japanese, Norwegian, Portuguese, Spanish, Swedish, Taiwanese, Turkish). Each translation was re-translated and checked by a lay advisor or national coordinator prior to use. In the ICS*male* questionnaire, men are asked to record each urinary symptom according to one of five grades from 'never' through 'occasionally', 'sometimes' and 'most of the time' to 'all of the time'. Immediately beneath each question concerning the prevalence of the symptom follows a question referring to the degree of problem or bother caused by each of the symptoms graded from 'not a problem' through 'a bit of a problem' or 'quite a problem' to 'a serious problem'. The majority of symptoms are presented in this format, with the exception of the more specific items of frequency, nocturia and acute retention which are couched in terms of numbers. In addition, there are seven specific questions concerning quality of life (ICS*QoL*), including three fixed format questions, two global quality of life questions and two open-ended questions. Patients in the UK also completed the generic health status instruments: Short Form 36 (SF-36)[4] and EuroQol[5]. Sexual function was explored using four questions (ICS*sex*). Each patient was also asked to keep a 7-day frequency–volume chart recording times of micturitions and incontinent episodes.

An assessment was made of the patient's prostate size by digital rectal examination (in grams) or by transrectal ultrasound (in cubic centimeters). Three flow rate measurements were requested for each patient, with the assessment of residual urine by ultrasound after each void. Urodynamic studies were recorded at the time of investigation by the clinician on the ICS-'BPH' study patient information record, and the urodynamic trace was photocopied to be analyzed centrally. The investigator was asked to judge whether the patient was unobstructed, had classical obstruction, questionable obstruction or another diagnosis. All data forms were returned centrally for processing and analysis using Statistical Analysis System (SAS) and Stata software.

Findings

Findings from the ICS-'BPH' study have focused on a wide range of issues concerned with the evaluation and management of LUTS related to benign prostate disease, particularly in the areas of LUTS and their impact on quality of life, issues around sexual function, the use of uroflowmetry and urodynamics, and strategies for the management of men with LUTS. Each of these areas is considered below after the presentation of the main results from the three phases.

Results from phases I, II and III of the ICS-'BPH' study

In phase I, the final number of eligible patients recruited was 1271 from 12 countries, with the largest contributions being 391 from The Netherlands, 214 from the UK, 129 from Germany and 105 from Japan. Of the patients, 20% were under 60 years of age and 34% over 70 years; 18% were unobstructed, 22% mildly obstructed and 60% obstructed according to urodynamic studies[3]. In phase II, 355 men from 15 of the original centers in nine countries were followed up approximately 12 months after receiving treatment according to routine clinical practice. Of these, 32% received transurethral resection of the prostate (TURP), 29% drug therapies, 20% conservative management, 9% minimally invasive therapies and 10% 'other'[6].

To date, phase III has involved the CLasP (Conservative management, non-contact Laser and TURP)-linked randomized controlled trials in the UK. In total, 570 men were randomized, 148 between laser therapy and TURP for acute urinary retention[7], 82 between laser therapy and TURP for chronic urinary retention[8] and 340 between laser, TURP and conservative management for uncomplicated LUTS[9].

ICS-'BPH' study questionnaire

A major output from the ICS-'BPH' study has been the study questionnaire. This contains three separate sections: ICSmale, including 22 questions measuring 20 urinary symptoms, with 19 sub-questions concerned with the degree of problem that they cause; ICSQol, seven questions relating to the impact on quality of life; and ICSsex, four questions concerned with sexual function and related problems.

The ICSmale questionnaire was shown to be valid and reliable in studies undertaken on the 1271 patients included in the phase I study[10].

The questionnaire was shown to be easy to complete; to detect the expected differences between older and younger men and men in the community compared with men in urology clinics; and to have high internal consistency and excellent levels of test–retest reliability[10]. In a further study, it was shown to have sensitivity to expected differences in outcome between different treatments[6].

The ICSmale questionnaire was used to investigate levels of urinary symptoms among men in the community and attending urology clinics. In the community, among 423 men over 40 years of age in a Leicestershire general practice, it was found that common symptoms included terminal dribble, hesitancy, intermittency and urgency, each with prevalences close to or in excess of 50%[11]. While symptoms of incontinence were relatively rare (urge incontinence, the most common, was reported by 20%), these symptoms, as well as frequency and nocturia, were reported to be the most problematic – 'at least a bit of a problem' – among 40–92%[11].

Among urology clinic attenders in phase I of the ICS-'BPH' study, the most prevalent symptoms were again found to be those related to voiding (such as reduced stream, intermittency and hesitancy), all reported by more than 80% of these men[12]. Such symptoms, however, were relatively well tolerated by men, with indications that they caused 'a bit of a problem' only among 40%. Symptoms causing the greatest reported problems were those of incontinence, identified as problematic by 80% or more. Interestingly, only a moderate relationship was found between prevalence and bothersomeness[12].

The international nature of the ICS-'BPH' study enabled the investigation of country variations in LUTS. It was found that country of origin was significantly associated with the prevalence of ten of the 20 symptoms in ICSmale, even after adjusting for potential confounders including sociodemographic variables[13]. The degree of problem caused by the symptoms also varied by country, but only significantly so for two symptoms (straining to start and hesitancy)[13].

CONFIDENTIAL
ICS*male*SF QUESTIONNAIRE

We would like to find out about your urinary symptoms and we are very grateful that you can help us by filling in this questionnaire.

Please answer each question, thinking about the **symptoms you have experienced in the last month.**

You will see that some questions ask how often you have a symptom:

Occasionally	=	**less than one third of the time**
Sometimes	=	**between one and two thirds of the time**
Most of the time	=	**more than two thirds of the time**

Please put a tick in one box for each question ☑

V1 Is there a delay before you can start to urinate?

never	0
occasionally	1
sometimes	2
most of the time	3
all of the time	4

V2 Do you have to strain to <u>continue</u> urinating?

never	0
occasionally	1
sometimes	2
most of the time	3
all of the time	4

V3 Would you say that the strength of your urinary stream is...

normal	0
occasionally reduced	1
sometimes reduced	2
reduced most of the time	3
reduced all of the time	4

V4 Do you stop and start more than once while you urinate?

never	0
occasionally	1
sometimes	2
most of the time	3
all of the time	4

V5 How often do you feel that your bladder has not emptied properly after you have urinated?

never	0
occasionally	1
sometimes	2
most of the time	3
all of the time	4

ICS*male*VS: sum scores V1–V5 [ ][ ]

Figure 1   The International Continence Society male short-form (ICS*male*SF) questionnaire

I1 Do you have to rush to the toilet to urinate?

never ☐ 0
occasionally ☐ 1
sometimes ☐ 2
most of the time ☐ 3
all of the time ☐ 4

I2 Does urine leak before you can get to the toilet?

never ☐ 0
occasionally ☐ 1
sometimes ☐ 2
most of the time ☐ 3
all of the time ☐ 4

I3 Does urine leak when you cough or sneeze?

never ☐ 0
occasionally ☐ 1
sometimes ☐ 2
most of the time ☐ 3
all of the time ☐ 4

I4 Do you ever leak for no obvious reason and without feeling that you want to go?

never ☐ 0
occasionally ☐ 1
sometimes ☐ 2
most of the time ☐ 3
all of the time ☐ 4

I5 Do you leak urine when you are asleep?

never ☐ 0
occasionally ☐ 1
sometimes ☐ 2
most of the time ☐ 3
all of the time ☐ 4

I6 How often have you had a slight wetting of your pants a few minutes after you had finished urinating and had dressed yourself?

never ☐ 0
occasionally ☐ 1
sometimes ☐ 2
most of the time ☐ 3
all of the time ☐ 4

ICS*male*IS: sum scores I1-I6 ☐☐

Figure 1 *Continued*

More recently, a scored short-form (SF) of the ICS*male* questionnaire has been developed using standard psychometric and other statistical analyses to allow the easier assessment of symptoms particularly within randomized trials and other studies[14]. The ICS*male*SF includes 11 items in two factors: five items are added together to produce a voiding score (ICS*male*VS) and six items added together to produce an incontinence score (ICS*male*IS) (Figure 1). These questions were selected after parallel analyses to ensure the inclusion of items that were problematic, sensitive to change and clustered according to factor analyses[14]. The authors advise that frequency, nocturia and quality of life should also be assessed, but through the use of separate questions or frequency–volume charts[14].

The findings about individual LUTS and the degree to which they caused problems for individuals were significant in their time for a number of reasons. The publication of results on individual LUTS rather than a single score allowed the assessment of the prevalence and impact of each symptom. Thus, the contribution of symptoms that had previously been neglected because they did not fall under the umbrella of 'prostatism' or symptoms supposedly not associated with 'BPH', such as incontinence, could be seen for the first time. This work also contributed to the body of work that indicated the need to measure the degree of problem caused by LUTS and take this into account, rather than just relying on simple symptom prevalence. Problems caused by LUTS were shown not to be directly related to simple prevalence within the ICS-'BPH' study, and common (supposedly 'BPH') symptoms were not the most problematic. The need to take an interest in problems as well as prevalence was further confirmed by the apparently greater stability of problems compared with symptom prevalence, in terms of both age and country of origin, and their critical role in determining whether men attended services or not. Thus, the final scored version of the ICS*male*SF was derived taking an interest in symptoms that were problematic and sensitive to outcome, as well as conforming to standard psychometric

and other statistical tests. The resultant questionnaire contains two scored parts, one including the usual 'BPH' questions associated with voiding, but also an incontinence part that includes the most problematic symptoms[14].

Impact of LUTS on quality of life

In addition to an interest in the degree of problem caused by urinary symptoms (see above and reference 12), the ICS-'BPH' study also investigated the impact of LUTS on quality of life. The ICS*QoL* questionnaire included two open-ended questions and five that could be included in a scored form: interference in life by LUTS, feelings about spending the rest of life with current LUTS, length of time with LUTS, and the need to change clothes or reduce drink intake because of LUTS. The questionnaire was shown to be easily completed by community-based men and urology patients constituting phase I of the ICS-'BPH' study[15]. Items confirmed expected relationships between the community and clinic populations, with each other and other individual LUTS[15]. They also exhibited good test–retest reliability, but levels of internal consistency were relatively low, suggesting that the items should not be combined in a score but used separately to assess issues of impact on quality of life[15].

The impact of LUTS on quality of life among the men in the ICS-'BPH' study was considerable, with 80% reporting some interference in their lives, 49% that they reduced their drink intake to reduce their LUTS, 23% that they had to change their clothes because of urinary leakage and 54% that they would be unhappy to spend the rest of their lives with their current LUTS[15]. In the ICS*male*SF, the authors suggest that the single question on interference with life should be added to all studies so that assessment of the impact of LUTS on quality of life can be included[14].

Issues around sexual function and activity

The conventional view up to the mid-1990s was that sexual function declined with increasing age and that, while it was not adversely affected by LUTS, it could be affected by some treatments, particularly TURP[1]. Both these aspects have been addressed as part of the ICS-'BPH' study.

During the developmental work for the study questionnaire, issues of sexual function were often raised by men during interviews, and so questions were devised to address this important issue. The ICSsex questionnaire comprised four questions about erectile function, ejaculation function, pain/discomfort on ejaculation and whether sex life was perceived to be spoilt by LUTS[16]. Men in phase I of the ICS-'BPH' study ($n = 1271$) and 423 community-based men completed the ICSsex questionnaire. Sexual dysfunction was found to be common in the community and clinic men, with age-standardized prevalences of over 50% for reduced erections and ejaculation[16]. Men were extremely bothered by sexual dysfunction, although there was a negative trend with age. In the clinic men, 46% reported that their sex lives were spoilt by LUTS, compared with 8% of community-based men, and significantly raised odds ratios of sexual dysfunction were found in those with LUTS, particularly symptoms of incontinence[16]. It was thus concluded that sexual dysfunction is associated with LUTS, is of concern to affected men and should be taken into account when managing 'BPH'[16].

Up to the early 1990s, there was a general consensus that TURP caused sexual dysfunction, particularly retrograde ejaculation (in up to 75%), and impotence (over 13%) according to a systematic review[17], results that were broadly confirmed in small-scale randomized trials. Less invasive therapies, such as laser, had been shown in some small-scale trials to result in lesser levels of sexual dysfunction[18,19]. However, one larger-scale trial indicated similar levels of impotence following surgery and watchful waiting[20]. In the CLasP study, we had the opportunity to investigate sexual dysfunction using the ICSsex questionnaire at baseline and follow-up in 340 men following randomization to non-contact laser therapy, TURP or conservative management[21]. Erectile and ejaculatory dysfunction were common and problematic at baseline in these men, and showed the expected trends with aging. After treatment, reduced ejaculation was reported in all groups, but was not significantly worse after TURP than after laser therapy[21]. Erectile function was actually significantly improved after TURP, and no difference was found between TURP and laser therapy. In addition, TURP was significantly better at relieving pain or discomfort on ejaculation than the other treatments[21]. There was also no difference between the groups in the reporting of new cases of sexual dysfunction following treatment[21]. Thus, compared with laser therapy, TURP appears to have a beneficial effect on sexual function, particularly erectile function and reducing pain/discomfort, and so older men who need treatment for LUTS and want to retain or improve sexual function should consider TURP as an option[21].

These studies have been particularly important in raising the profile of research in sexual functioning in older men. In both cases, the studies produced evidence that challenged the existing consensus, which was based largely on observational data collected using unstandardized questionnaires, in studies conducted often without collecting baseline values. The ICSsex questionnaire has shown itself to be a robust and useful brief measure of sexual dysfunction.

Role of urodynamics

A major aim of the ICS-'BPH' study was to investigate the role of urodynamic studies in patient evaluation. Each patient had up to three free urine flow measurements, with the highest maximum flow used for analysis, and then pressure and flow studies according to ICS standards. Patients' bladders were filled at 50 ml/min; intravesical and intra-abdominal pressure were measured; detrusor pressure was derived by electronic subtraction. From the voiding phase, the maximum urinary flow rate and detrusor pressure were recorded and then plotted onto a Schäfer nomogram (Lin-PURR) to quantify obstruction from 0 (no obstruction) to 6 (severe obstruction)[22].

At baseline, 933 patients had complete data for urodynamics and LUTS, and 18% were unobstructed, 22% mildly obstructed and 60%

obstructed. There were no clear relationships between individual or groups of LUTS as reported in the ICS*male* questionnaire and urodynamic variables[22]. Comparing those with obstruction and those without, there was a significantly higher prevalence of urgency and urge incontinence in those with obstruction, matching the low (but significant) correlation with detrusor pressure and Lin-PURR category[22].

It was also possible to investigate the relationships between uroflow variables and LUTS. At baseline, 83% of patients performed at least two simple flow studies. Maximum urinary flow rate was significantly lower in those with urodynamically diagnosed obstruction ($p < 0.001$) and was also negatively correlated with obstruction grade[23]. A threshold value of < 10 ml/s had a positive predictive value of 70% for obstruction, and a value of < 15 ml/s of 67%[23].

This part of the study confirmed with large numbers that there was little or no relationship between symptoms and urodynamic measures, and thus that these two forms of measurement assess different aspects of the same clinical condition[22]. It also showed that while uroflowmetry cannot replace urodynamics, it can provide valuable information about diagnosis additional to reported LUTS[23]. The results from these articles also made it clear that it would not be possible to develop the ICS*male* questionnaire so that would assist in the diagnosis of obstruction, and that both clinical and patient-based methods of measurement would be required to build up a complete picture of a patient's condition.

Strategies for managing LUTS and benign prostatic disease

In phase II, 355 men from 15 of the original centers in nine countries were followed up approximately 12 months after receiving treatment according to routine clinical practice. These data provide an interesting snapshot of treatments used routinely in various parts of the world in the early 1990s. In phase II of the ICS-'BPH' study, 32% received TURP, 29%

drug therapies, 20% conservative management, 9% minimally invasive therapies and 10% 'other'[6]. There were significant differences between countries, with patients in Italy, Denmark, Australia, Japan and the UK tending to undergo surgical treatments, and patients from The Netherlands, Portugal, Israel and Germany having more conservative treatment ($p < 0.0001$)[6]. The ICS*male* questionnaire was able to detect differences between the treatments: for patients who underwent TURP, 15 LUTS were highly statistically significantly better at follow-up than at baseline ($p < 0.0001$), compared with five LUTS at the same level in those who received drug therapies, four LUTS for minimally invasive therapies, and no significant differences found in those undergoing watchful waiting[6].

To date, phase III has involved the CLasP-linked randomized controlled trials in the UK. In total, 570 men were randomized, 148 between laser therapy and TURP for acute urinary retention[7], 82 between laser therapy and TURP for chronic urinary retention[8] and 340 between laser, TURP and conservative management for uncomplicated LUTS[9]. These studies have all confirmed the superiority of TURP over laser therapy in each of these patient groups in terms of improving LUTS and maximum urinary flow, but have also shown that TURP resulted in greater levels of complications and longer hospital stay compared with laser[7–9]. Among men with uncomplicated LUTS, conservative management did not result in any deterioration in their condition or greater treatment failure compared with the other groups, albeit over the relatively short (7.5 months) follow-up period[9]. Further analyses of the symptom and quality of life impact of these treatments are currently under way.

Discussion

The ICS-'BPH' study was a multidisciplinary, multicenter and international research project. It involved collaboration between researchers and clinicians in 12 countries and had a challenging protocol. The study was established to address concerns about the ways in which men with troublesome urinary symptoms of benign origin were being evaluated and treated in the early 1990s. In particular, these concerns focused around the increasing reliance upon symptom assessment, often using unstandardized measures or relying upon questionnaires that included only symptoms related to voiding, and the increasing use of surgical and new technological approaches to management. The ICS-'BPH' study was initiated by urologists with a strong interest in the role of urodynamics in the assessment and outcome of patients with benign prostatic disease, and it was this interest that initially drove the study. All collaborating clinicians agreed to include consecutive eligible men and to carry out full urodynamic studies. In addition, it was felt necessary to develop a new questionnaire to allow the inclusion of as wide a range of LUTS as possible, and also to include questions on sexual function and quality of life.

The study was thus a considerable undertaking, and relied on much goodwill from collaborators and participants. The strengths of the study derived particularly from its size, international nature and multidisciplinarity. Several major weaknesses need to be acknowledged, however. The study was observational in nature, so very many biases that cannot be easily accounted for may be present. There were considerable (often statistically significant) differences between patients recruited in the different countries, and while these contributed to the breadth of the study could have introduced a number of biases. It was not clear, for example, why such differences should have arisen, or whether there were subtle and different perceptions of the meaning of questionnaire items between different cultures. The contributions from different countries were not balanced, and some countries contributed very many patients (e.g. The Netherlands) and others very few. Only a limited number of centers participated in phase II of the study, and this part of the study could

provide only a snapshot of management strategies in these countries and a way of assessing the responsiveness of the ICS-'BPH' study questionnaire to outcome. Phase III of the study included only randomized trials and, thus far, only three linked trials have been completed. These trials were based only in the UK, but have produced findings that are probably generalizable more widely.

One of the most important outputs from the ICS-'BPH' study was the study questionnaire: ICS*male*[10] and ICS*male*SF[14] to evaluate LUTS, ICS*sex*[16] for sexual function and ICS*QoL*[15] for impact on quality of life. These questionnaires have all been shown to be valid, reliable and responsive to outcome, and are now available to be used freely. The most valuable findings from the questionnaire were the importance of investigating the problems caused by symptoms as well as their simple prevalence, and the need to include assessment of the impact of LUTS on quality of life in general and sexual activity in particular. The discovery of the relationship between LUTS and sexual function[16], and that TURP may have a beneficial effect on sexual function[21], were important contributions to the literature.

The size of the ICS-'BPH' study and the wide-ranging ICS*male* questionnaire enabled detailed investigation of the relationships between LUTS and the findings of uroflowmetry and urodynamics. It allowed closure of the issue about potential relationships between these clinical findings and reported LUTS: that there were no clear patterns and that both were thus important but separate. Finally, the study contributed to the change in terminology in this area, particularly the greater care that needed to be taken with the term 'BPH'.

The ICS-'BPH' study thus made a contribution to the changing picture in evaluation and management of LUTS and 'BPH' during the 1990s. How many of the study's findings will be remembered in the future will be for others to judge.

Acknowledgements

ICS-'BPH' Study Steering Committee: Paul Abrams, Jean J. M. C. H. de la Rosette, Werner Schäfer, Jenny Donovan.

ICS-'BPH' Study contributors: Professor Barbalias, Professor Bosch, Mr Chapple, Dr Dabhoiwala, Dr Frimodt-Moller, Dr Gajewski, Dr Höfner, Dr Kalomiris, Dr Kinn, Dr Kondo, Dr Matos-Ferreira, Dr Mendes Silva, Dr Millard, Dr Nissenkorn, Dr Nordling, Dr Osawa, Dr Porru, Dr Rentzhog, Dr Schick, Dr Thüroff, Dr Tong-Long Lin, Dr Walter. Educational grants were provided by SmithKline Beecham, Merck Sharp and Dohme, Bard, Pfizer, Yamanouchi and Laboratories Debat.

CLasP study group: Professor Donovan, Professor Neal, Professor Abrams, Professor Peters, Ms Sara Brookes, Mr Essenhigh, Mr Hall, Mr Hamdy, Mr Hinchcliffe, Mr Powell, Mr Ramsden, Mr Feneley, Mr Gillatt, Mr Gingell, Mr Timoney, Mr Greene, Mr Mellon, Mr Thorpe, Ms Linda Kelly, Ms Esther Bartlett, Ms Julie Ellis-Jones, Ms Deborah Nevin and Ms Hazel Kay. The CLasP study was funded by the South West and Northern Regional NHS Research and Development Directorates. Bard UK provided the laser fibers.

References

1. Cockett AT, Aso Y, Denis L, *et al.* World Health Organization Consensus Committee recommendations concerning the diagnosis of BPH. *Prog Urol* 1991;1:957–72

2. Abrams P. New words for old: lower urinary tract symptoms for 'prostatism' [Editorial]. *Br Med J* 1994;308:929–30

3. Abrams P, Donovan JL, De La Rosette JJMC. The ICS-'BPH' study: background, aims and methodology. *Neurourol Urodynam* 1997;16: 79–92

4. Brazier J, Harper R, Jones NMB, *et al.* Validating the SF-36 health survey questionnaire: new outcome measure for primary care. *Br Med J* 1992;305:160–4

5. The EuroQol Group. *EQ-5D User Guide.* Rotterdam: The EuroQol Group, 1996

6. Donovan JL, Brookes ST, De La Rosette JJMC, *et al.* The responsiveness of the ICSmale questionnaire to outcome: evidence from the ICS-'BPH' study. *BJU Int* 1999;83:243–8

7. Chacko KN, Donovan JL, Abrams P, *et al.* Transurethral resection of the prostate or laser therapy for men with acute retention of urine: the CLasP study. *J Urol* 2001;166:166–70

8. Gujral S, Abrams P, Donovan JL, *et al.* A prospective randomised trial comparing transurethral resection of the prostate and laser therapy for men with chronic retention of urine: the CLasP study. *J Urol* 2000;164:71–6

9. Donovan JL, Peters TJ, Neal DE, *et al.* A randomised controlled trial comparing transurethral resection of the prostate, laser therapy and conservative management in men with symptoms associated with benign prostatic enlargement: the CLasP study. *J Urol* 2000;164:65–70

10. Donovan JL, Abrams P, Peters TJ, *et al.* The ICS-'BPH' study: the psychometric validity and reliability of the ICS*male* questionnaire. *Br J Urol* 1996;77:554–62

11. Jolleys JV, Donovan JL, Nanchahal K, Peters TJ, Abrams P. Urinary symptoms in the community: how bothersome are they? *Br J Urol* 1994;74:551–5

12. Peters TJ, Donovan JL, Kay HE, *et al.* The International Continence Society 'Benign Prostatic Hyperplasia' study: the bothersomeness of urinary symptoms. *J Urol* 1997;157:885–9

13. Witjes WPJ, de la Rosette J, Donovan JL, *et al.* The ICS-'BPH' study: international differences in lower urinary tract symptoms and related bother. *J Urol* 1997;157:1295–300

14. Donovan JL, Peters TJ, Abrams P, Brookes ST, De La Rosette JJMC, Schäfer W. Scoring the ICS*male*SF questionnaire. *J Urol* 2000;164: 1948–55

15. Donovan JL, Kay HE, Peters TJ, *et al.* Using ICSQoL to measure the impact of lower urinary tract symptoms on quality of life: evidence from the ICS-'BPH' study. *Br J Urol* 1997;80:712–21

16. Frankel SJ, Donovan JL, Peters TJ, *et al.* Sexual dysfunction in men with lower urinary tract symptoms. *J Clin Epidemiol* 1998;51:677–85

17. McConnell JD, Barry MJ, Bruskewitz RC, *et al. Benign Prostatic Hyperplasia: Diagnosis and*

Treatment. Clinical Practice Guideline. Rockville, MD: US Department of Health and Human Services, Agency for Health Care Policy and Research, 1994

18. Graversen PH, Gasser TC, Wasson JH, Hinman F Jr, Bruskewitz RC. Controversies about indications for transurethral resection of the prostate. *J Urol* 1989;141:475–81

19. Anson K, Nawrocki J, Buckley J, *et al.* A multicentre, randomized, prospective study of endoscopic laser ablation versus transurethral resection of the prostate. *Urology* 1995;46:305–10

20. Wasson JH, Reda DJ, Bruskewitz RC, Elinson J, Keller AM, Henderson WG. A comparison of transurethral surgery with watchful waiting for moderate symptoms of benign prostatic hyperplasia. *N Engl J Med* 1995;332:75–9

21. Brookes ST, Donovan JL, Peters TJ, Abrams P, Neal DE. Sexual dysfunction in men after treatment for lower urinary tract symptoms: evidence from randomised controlled trial. *Br Med J* 2002;324:1059–64

22. De La Rosette JJMC, Witjes WPJ, Schäfer W, *et al.* Relationships between lower urinary tract symptons and bladder outlet obstruction: results from the ICS-BPH study. *Neurourol Urodynam* 1998;17:99–108

23. Reynard JM, Yang Q, Donovan JL, *et al.* The ICS-'BPH' study: uroflowmetry, lower urinary tract symptoms and bladder outlet obstruction. *Br J Urol* 1998;82:619–23

Distinguishing nocturnal polyuria from benign prostatic hyperplasia-related nocturia: simple algorithms for general and urological practice

10

M. H. Blanker and J. Prins

Introduction

Nocturia is a common and often bothersome symptom in older men[1,2]. Nocturia may result in sleep disturbance, daytime fatigue and a lower level of general well-being, and is a risk factor for night-time falls[3–5]. Many physicians consider nocturia a sign of increased nocturnal urine production[6], which may represent a pathological condition reflective of congestive heart failure, venous stasis or hormonal changes with aging, or of lower urinary tract symptoms[4,7–9].

Before answering the question how nocturnal polyuria can be distinguished from other benign prostatic hyperplasia (BPH)-related causes of nocturia, various definitions and normal values need to be considered. In these considerations, data from the Krimpen study have been used as reference. In the Krimpen study, data from 1688 men were collected by way of self-administered questionnaires, a 3-day frequency–volume chart and additional measurements[10]. The questionnaire included the International Prostate Symptom Score (IPSS)[11] and questions on history of chronic disease, smoking habits, alcohol consumption and current medication use. Measurements at a health center and urology out-patient department included blood pressure, serum prostate-specific antigen (PSA), digital rectal examination (DRE), prostate volume by means of transrectal ultrasound (TRUS), uroflowmetry and post-voiding residual measurement. To exclude men with prostate carcinoma, biopsies were taken according to a protocol, based on DRE, PSA and TRUS[10].

Data on normal values for nocturnal voiding frequency and nocturnal urine production were derived from the frequency–volume charts of the participants[2,6,12,13].

Definitions and normal values

Nocturnal voiding frequency

Data from the Krimpen study illustrate clearly that nocturnal voiding frequency increases with advancing age[2]. More than 75% of men aged 50 years and older have at least one nocturnal voiding episode. Two or more episodes are present in 30% of men aged 50–54 years and in 60% of those 70–78 years old, while three or more episodes are reported in 5% and 20%, respectively (Table 1). So, one and two nocturnal voidings may be considered normal in older men, and attention should be focused on three or more voidings.

Nocturnal polyuria

Various definitions for 'nocturnal polyuria' have been suggested, but their use is hampered by a number of problems[8,9,14–19]. In general, the suggested definitions of 'abnormal' were not based on normal distributions and were not properly validated[6,13].

In definitions using nocturnal voided volumes only (for example nocturnal urine output divided by body weight[18], and nocturnal urine volume exceeding two standard deviations of

Table 1 Reference values for nocturnal voiding frequency in older men derived from frequency–volume charts (see also reference 2)

Number of nocturnal voiding episodes	Percentage of men				
	50–54 years	55–59 years	60–64 years	65–69 years	70–78 years
Zero	24.3	25.3	11.8	8.7	11.1
One	46.2	42.0	46.2	36.3	29.6
Two	24.7	28.4	31.3	40.3	37.8
Three or more	4.8	4.3	10.7	14.7	21.5

the mean of controls[9,15]) it is assumed that volumes voided at night are produced during the night. This assumption may lead to an over-estimation of nocturnal urine production and, therefore, seems incorrect.

Most definitions of 'nocturnal polyuria' (for example urine voided during sleep being over 35% of the total urine volume) refer to a day/night ratio in urine production[8,16]. Although mathematically related, the nocturnal urine production and day/night ratio show only poor agreement: men with a significantly increased nocturnal urine production can easily have a normal day/night ratio, whereas men with a normal nocturnal urine production can have a significantly disturbed day/night ratio. When analyzing nocturnal voiding frequency, attention should be focused on urine production during the night-time.

The Krimpen study provided normal values for nocturnal urine production[13]; for men aged 50–78 years, the mean nocturnal urine production was 60 ml/h (standard deviation 33 ml/h). Nocturnal urine production was significantly higher in elderly men: the difference between men aged 50–54 and 70–78 years was 13 ml/h. Nocturnal urine production was also significantly higher in men with 24-h polyuria (defined as a total voided volume exceeding 2500 ml), which may have resulted from habitually high fluid intake. Men who smoked had a slightly lower nocturnal urine production. Prostate volume, post-void residual and reduced urinary flow rate (Q_{max} less than 15 ml/s) appeared not to be related to nocturnal urine production in multivariate analyses[13].

Asplund and colleagues suggested using the cut-off value of 54 ml/h for increased nocturnal urine production[17]. This value was based on the mean nocturnal diuresis of men aged 25–35 years, participating in a previous study described by Kirkland and associates[17,20]. It seems illogical to use these younger subjects as reference for older men, as nocturnal urine production depends on age.

Based on the analyses of the Krimpen study, a cut-off value of 90 ml/h is suggested for the definition of nocturnal polyuria[6]. This value showed the best characteristics in predicting increased nocturnal voiding frequency (both two or more and three or more episodes). It should be stressed, however, that even this new definition predicts nocturnal voiding frequency only reasonably. Moreover, about one-third of men with 'increased' nocturnal urine production also have 24-h polyuria, most probably explaining the increased production[6].

Definitions of BPH

Clinical BPH is mostly defined by the concept clarified by Hald[21], in which the presence of lower urinary tract symptoms (LUTS), prostate enlargement and bladder outflow obstruction were considered together. Nocturnal voiding frequency appeared to be clearly related to clinical BPH (defined as IPSS greater than 7, prostate volume greater than 30 ml and maximum urinary flow rate less than 15 ml/h)[2]. When analyzing the separate parameters, however, it appeared that prostate volume was not related to nocturnal voiding frequency, whereas decreased urinary flow rate was related to two or more nocturnal voidings, but not to three or more voidings[2]. For these reasons, the parameters included in the definition of clinical

BPH should be considered separately, when analyzing nocturia.

Validity of collected data in clinical practice

In the out-patient clinic assessment of men with nocturia, two tools are mainly available for collecting information on voiding frequency and urine production: history-taking and the frequency–volume chart.

The main advantage of history-taking is that it provides instant information. The main disadvantage of history-taking is that it may be subject to recall bias[22]. Patients may underestimate or overestimate their nocturnal voiding frequency. In fact, only poor agreement has been shown between history-taking and prospectively collected data[2]. Another disadvantage of history-taking is that it provides no information on the voided volumes and urine production.

Frequency–volume charts have proved to be easy-to-use, low-cost and valid tools, not subject to recall bias, for collecting data on voiding frequency and voided volumes in a patient's natural environment[2,12,23–26]. Therefore, the use of frequency–volume charts is the preferred method for data collection on voiding frequencies and urine production.

To evaluate nocturnal voiding frequency properly, the recordings on a frequency–volume chart should cover at least one complete night. So, two consecutive days of recording may be sufficient. On the chart, patients should also record the times of sleeping and rising, as use of these sleeping hours is by far the most accurate way of judging nocturnal voiding frequency[2].

Daily practice: algorithm

Patients may visit their physician presenting nocturia as the main symptom, because of its bothersomeness or a fear of underlying pathology. In other patients, physicians may question the presence of nocturia as a sign of increased nocturnal urine production, which may represent a pathological condition reflective of congestive heart failure, venous stasis or hormonal changes with aging, or of lower urinary tract symptoms.

Physicians should first recognize that information on voiding frequency obtained from history-taking is inaccurate[2]. Whenever evaluation of nocturnal voiding frequency is necessary, frequency–volume charts should be used.

Frequency–volume chart instructions

The patient should be instructed to complete the chart for at least two consecutive days; each micturition should be collected in a measuring cup and recorded in deciliters (dl). A more precise recording (for example in ml) seems unnecessary for this purpose. Recording of the voided volumes in 1-h time units is sufficient. If the volume of one void was not measured, the patient should place a cross on the chart. Next, the patient should be instructed to record their bedtime and time of rising.

Interpretation of frequency–volume charts

In Figure 1, an algorithm for frequency–volume chart interpretation is illustrated. When using this flow diagram, it becomes unnecessary to estimate all further suggested measures. Interpretation of the frequency–volume chart may take 1 or 2 min, but it will provide important information.

First, nocturnal and diurnal voiding frequency are read from the chart. For this purpose, the patient-recorded sleeping times must be used. Nocturnal voiding frequency should be compared with reference values for the age of the patient (Table 1).

Second, the hourly urine production should be estimated, according to the method described by van Mastrigt and Eijskoot[27]: urine production is assumed constant between two voids, and hourly urine production can be estimated as the volume of each micturition divided by the number of hours that passed since the previous micturition[27]. In this approach, volumes voided during the night do not necessarily count as nocturnal urine production.

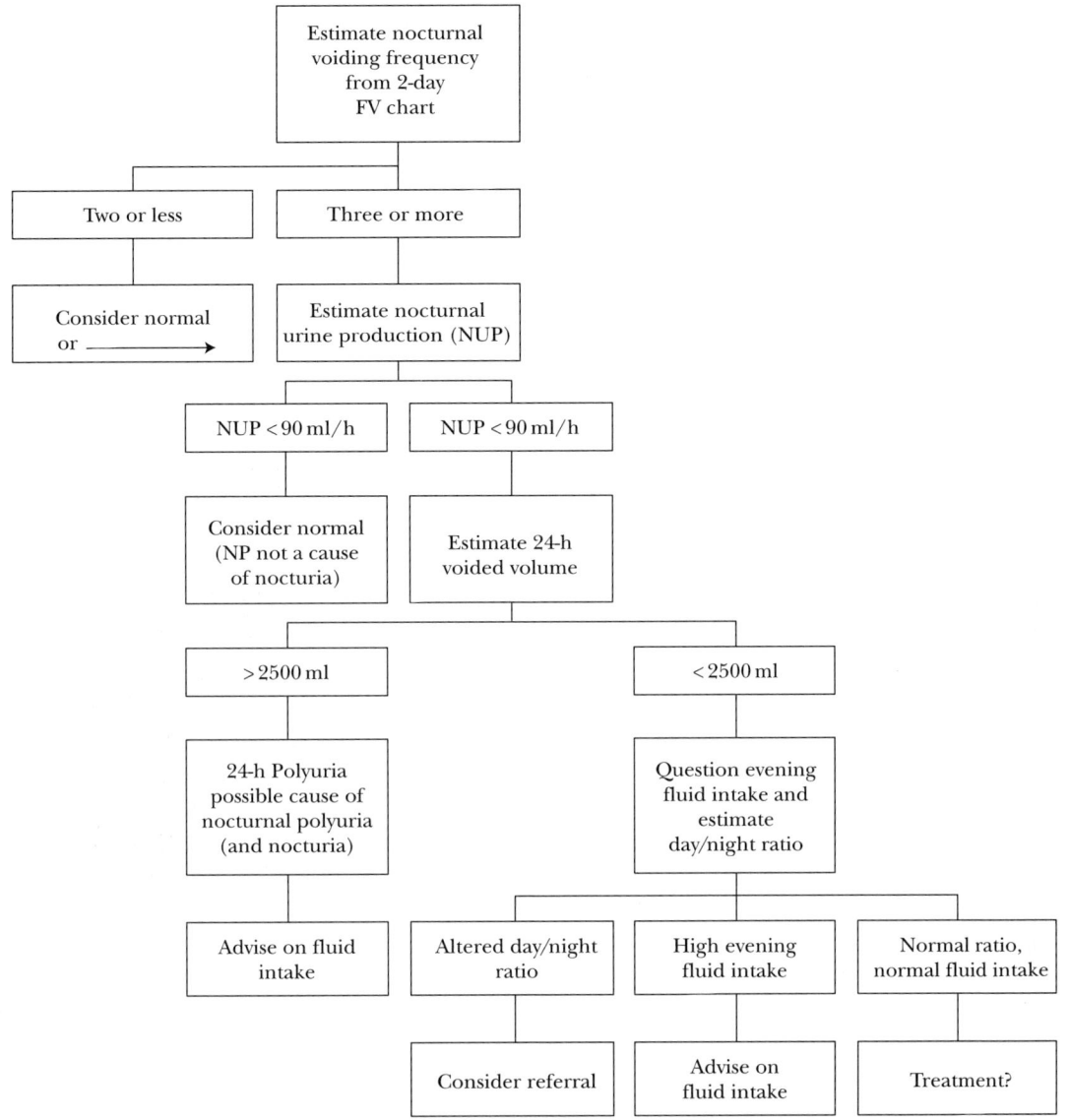

Figure 1 Algorithm for evaluation of patient with increased nocturnal voiding frequency. FV, frequency–volume; NP, nocturnal polyuria

Mean nocturnal urine production can be estimated as the average urine production during nightly hours. If nocturnal urine production is less than 90 ml/h, it should be considered normal[6]: in such cases, nocturnal polyuria is not a cause of increased nocturnal voiding frequency. If nocturnal urine production exceeds 90 ml/h, the physician should estimate the 24-h voided volume, as nocturnal urine production is significantly higher in men with 24-h polyuria (voided volume greater than 2500 ml)[6]. Moreover, about one-third of men with nocturnal urine production greater than 90 ml/h have 24-h polyuria. In these men, reducing the total fluid intake may be the first approach in dealing with nocturia.

If no 24-h polyuria exists, but nocturnal urine production is greater than 90 ml/h, additional information should be collected on fluid intake during the evening hours by questioning the patient. The recording of fluid intake by patients is difficult, time-consuming and often inaccurate, and is therefore not advised as a standard procedure.

Finally, the urine production day/night ratio may be considered as a measure of the circadian urine production rhythm[13]. It should be recognized that an altered day/night ratio is not a sign of urological disease, but a possible sign of internal disease, such as heart failure or venous stasis. In the case of a clearly altered pattern, urologists should consider referral to a general practitioner or the internal medicine outpatient clinic for further evaluation. Alterations of the circadian pattern are seen in elderly men (aged 65 years and over), and this should be taken into account[6].

When nocturnal polyuria is present without 24-h polyuria, an altered day/night ratio or a high fluid intake during the evening, a clear explanation of the increased nocturnal urine production is lacking. Treatment of such patients might be desired, but, to date, no appropriate treatment is available.

Other causes of nocturia

As well as considerations of nocturnal urine production, one should evaluate bladder outflow on uroflowmetry and prostate size on DRE or TRUS as routine urological work-up, and as possible urological parameters of nocturia. The latter parameter (prostate volume) in itself, however, is not related to changes in nocturnal urine production and nocturnal voiding frequency[2,6]. Reduced urinary flow rate and nocturnal polyuria may occur together in one patient; the presence of one does not rule out the presence of the other factor as a possible cause of nocturia.

Other reported causes of nocturia are the use of diuretics and awakenings for other reasons such as sleep disorders or anxiety[2,4]. History-taking should reveal these causes.

References

1. Weiss JP, Blaivas JG. Nocturia. *J Urol* 2000;163: 5–12
2. Blanker MH, Bohnen AM, Groeneveld FP, *et al.* Normal voiding patterns and determinants of increased diurnal and nocturnal voiding frequency in elderly men. *J Urol* 2000;164:1201–5
3. Asplund R, Aberg H. Health of the elderly with regard to sleep and nocturnal micturition. *Scand J Prim Health Care* 1992;10:98–104
4. Barker JC, Mitteness LS. Nocturia in the elderly. *Gerontologist* 1988;28:99–104
5. Stewart RB, Moore MT, May FE, *et al.* Nocturia: a risk factor for falls in the elderly. *J Am Geriatr Soc* 1992;40:1217–20
6. Blanker MH, Bernsen RMD, Bosch JLHR, *et al.* Relation between nocturnal voiding frequency and nocturnal urine production in older men: a population-based study. *Urology* 2002;60:612–16
7. Brendler CB. Evaluation of the urologic patient. In Walsh PC, Retik AB, Stamey TA, *et al.*, eds. *Campbell's Urology.* Philadelphia: WB Saunders, 1998:134

8. Weiss JP, Blaivas JG, Stember DS, *et al.* Nocturia in adults: etiology and classification. *Neurourol Urodyn* 1998;17:467–72
9. Matthiesen TB, Rittig S, Norgaard JP, *et al.* Nocturnal polyuria and natriuresis in male patients with nocturia and lower urinary tract symptoms. *J Urol* 1996;156:1292–9
10. Blanker MH, Groeneveld FPMJ, Prins A, *et al.* Strong effects of definition and nonresponse bias on prevalence rates of clinical benign prostatic hyperplasia: the Krimpen study of male urogenital tract problems and general health status. *BJU Int* 2000;85:665–71
11. Barry MJ, Fowler FJ Jr, O'Leary MP, *et al.* The American Urological Association symptom index for benign prostatic hyperplasia. The Measurement Committee of the American Urological Association. *J Urol* 1992;148:1549–57
12. Blanker MH, Groeneveld FP, Bohnen AM, *et al.* Voided volumes: normal values and relation to lower urinary tract symptoms in elderly men, a community-based study. *Urology* 2001;57:1093–8

13. Blanker MH, Bernsen RMD, Bosch JLHR, *et al.* Normal values and determinants of circadian urine production in older men: a population-based study. *J Urol* 2002;168:1453–7

14. Reynard JM, Cannon A, Yang Q, *et al.* A novel therapy for nocturnal polyuria: a double-blind randomized trial of frusemide against placebo. *Br J Urol* 1998;81:215–18

15. Matthiesen TB, Rittig S, Mortensen JT, *et al.* Nocturia and polyuria in men referred with lower urinary tract symptoms, assessed using a 7-day frequency–volume chart. *BJU Int* 1999;83:1017–22

16. Saito M, Kondo A, Kato T, *et al.* Frequency–volume charts: comparison of frequency between elderly and adult patients. *Br J Urol* 1993;72:38–41

17. Asplund R, Sundberg B, Bengtsson P. Desmopressin for the treatment of nocturnal polyuria in the elderly: a dose titration study. *Br J Urol* 1998;82:642–6

18. Homma Y, Yamaguchi O, Kageyama S, *et al.* Nocturia in the adult: classification on the basis of largest voided volume and nocturnal urine production. *J Urol* 2000;163:777–81

19. Weiss JP, Blaivas JG, Stember DS, *et al.* Evaluation of the etiology of nocturia in men: the nocturia and nocturnal bladder capacity indices. *Neurourol Urodyn* 1999;18:559–65

20. Kirkland JL, Lye M, Levy DW, *et al.* Patterns of urine flow and electrolyte excretion in healthy elderly people. *Br Med J (Clin Res Ed)* 1983;287:1665–7

21. Hald T. Urodynamics in benign prostatic hyperplasia: a survey. *Prostate Suppl* 1989;2:69–77

22. Coughlin SS. Recall bias in epidemiologic studies. *J Clin Epidemiol* 1990;43:87–91

23. Abrams P, Klevmark B. Frequency volume charts: an indispensable part of lower urinary tract assessment. *Scand J Urol Nephrol Suppl* 1996;179:47–53

24. Larsson G, Victor A. Micturition patterns in a healthy female population, studied with a frequency/volume chart. *Scand J Urol Nephrol Suppl* 1988;114:53–7

25. Neilson D. The accuracy of the frequency–volume chart: comparison of self-reported and measured volumes [Letter; Comment]. *Br J Urol* 1998;82:776–7

26. Siltberg H, Larsson G, Victor A. Frequency/volume chart: the basic tool for investigating urinary symptoms. *Acta Obstet Gynecol Scand Suppl* 1997;166:24–7

27. van Mastrigt R, Eijskoot F. Analysis of voided urine volumes measured using a small electronic pocket balance. *Scand J Urol Nephrol* 1996;30:257–63

Practical application of non-invasive tests to grade outflow obstruction and bladder contractility: the end of classical urodynamics?

11

J. J. M. Pel, J. W. N. C. Huang Foen Chung and R. van Mastrigt

Introduction

In most aging males, the prostate enlarges, which may obstruct the urethra that it surrounds. As a result, flow rate may be reduced, voiding becomes more frequent and the risk of residual urine in the bladder after voiding increases. A weakly contracting detrusor, however, also reduces the flow rate. To differentiate between the causes of impaired voiding, bladder pressure needs to be measured. The International Continence Society (ICS) has provided a provisional method for diagnosing obstruction on the basis of bladder pressure measured via catheters in the bladder and rectum. The invasiveness of these measurements, however, limits the clinical applicability of this test and, moreover, scientific research. The development of simple, non-invasive and inexpensive measurement devices could lower the threshold for practical application of urodynamic testing.

The Sector Furore of the Erasmus MC develops new measurement methods to assess bladder function. Recently, an external condom catheter was developed to measure bladder pressure non-invasively. This article presents an overview of the development of this condom-type catheter. It was tested in a group of healthy male volunteers and patients with lower urinary tract symptoms (LUTS). The results of these measurements clarify the merits and limitations of this new technique for both clinical and scientific application.

Condom-type catheter: development and validation

Previous studies showed that, on the basis of a combination of isovolumetric bladder pressure and maximum flow rate, classification of bladder outlet obstruction (BOO) is possible[1]. We developed an external condom catheter to measure this pressure non-invasively[2]. Instead of measuring the pressure of the urethra proximally (using a transurethral catheter positioned in the bladder), the pressure of the urethra is measured distally (in the condom). This change of measurement location reduces the risk of damaging and infecting the bladder and urethral wall. The catheter consists of an incontinence condom connected to a tube, a valve and a pressure transducer (Figure 1). The condom is adjusted to the penis, and taped with laboratory film to increase its stiffness and to prevent leakage of urine. When a volunteer or patient voids in the condom, the flow rate is interrupted by closing the tube with the valve. During this interruption, the condom is pressurized. A pressure transducer measures this pressure in the condom, p_{condom}. In theory, when the urethra is open, the maximum condom pressure equals the isovolumetric bladder pressure. During this test, the pressure and flow rate signals are displayed on a computer screen. Parameters such as maximum signal values are calculated automatically from the signals using self-written Matlab® programs.

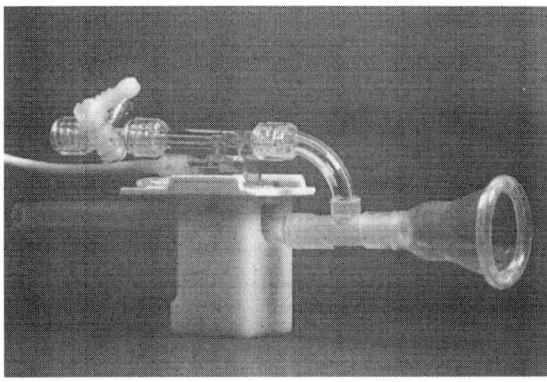

Figure 1 External condom catheter made to measure bladder pressure non-invasively. Reproduced with permission

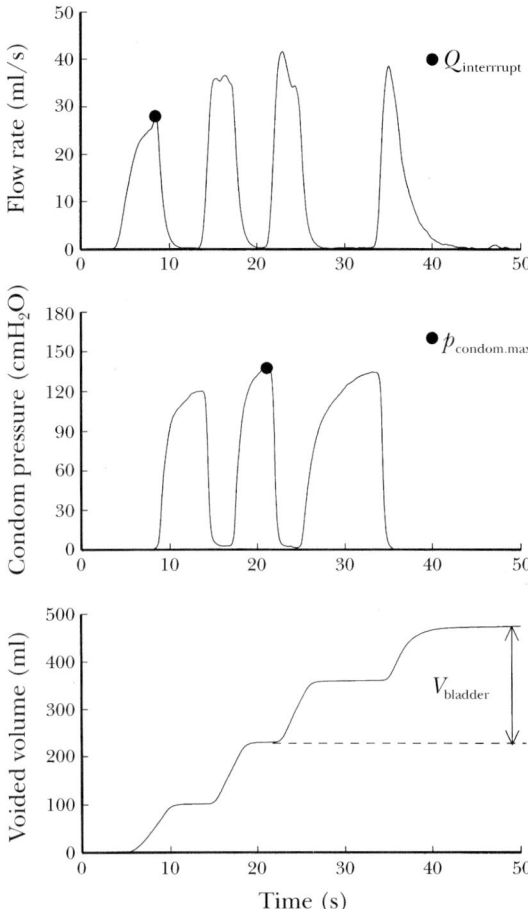

Figure 2 An example of repeated condom pressure measurement in a healthy volunteer. Voided volume (lowest panel), condom pressure (middle panel) and flow rate (top panel) are plotted as a function of time. $Q_{interrupt}$, interrupt flow rate; $p_{condom.max}$, highest condom pressure; $V_{bladder}$, bladder volume during interruption

Validation of condom pressure

The method was first tested in a group of healthy volunteers. All were able to apply the condom and the laboratory film correctly. None of them showed inhibition of flow rate after a single interruption of the stream, so that more than one pressure reading could be taken in one voiding. Figure 2 shows an example of such repeated pressure measurement. Upon interruption of the flow rate (top panel), the condom quickly filled with urine and the pressure increased to a maximum value (middle panel). The flow rate just prior to the *first* interruption, ~27 ml/s, was called the interrupt flow rate, $Q_{interrupt}$. After the pressure reached a maximum value, the valve was opened to continue voiding. In this example, the condom pressure was measured three times. The highest condom pressure, $p_{condom.max}$, of 135 cmH$_2$O was measured during the second interruption. To test whether this pressure depended on the bladder volume, we calculated bladder volume during the interruption, $V_{bladder}$, as the difference between the total voided volume and the voided volume at $p_{condom.max}$ (see lowest panel). On average, we found that the condom pressure values measured depended significantly on bladder volume. The highest condom pressure was found at approximately 52% of the maximum bladder volume[3]. As bladder volumes differ strongly between individuals, repeated interruptions in one voiding are necessary to correct the condom pressures for the volume dependence.

In a group of patients with LUTS, we tested how well condom pressure reflects bladder pressure. First, all patients underwent a standard pressure–flow study (PFS). On the basis of this test with catheters in the bladder and rectum, patients were classified as non-obstructed, equivocal or obstructed using the provisional ICS method for definition of obstruction[4]. Then, in a second procedure, the condom catheter was adjusted to the penis leaving the transurethral catheter *in situ*. After filling the bladder, the transurethral catheter was connected to a pressure transducer to measure the bladder pressure simultaneously with the condom pressure. Figure 3 shows an example, with the interrupted flow rate in the top panel and the simultaneously measured pressures in the lower panel. The interrupt flow rate was about 7 ml/s. During the second interruption, the maximum pressures were measured and both correlated well ($\sim$135 cmH$_2$O).

The difference in pressure $p_{bladder} - p_{condom.max}$ was plotted against the mean pressure $(p_{bladder} + p_{condom.max})/2$ for each patient (Figure 4). The median value of the pressure difference was 11 cmH$_2$O (50th centile). The borders of agreement were chosen at the 10th and 70th centiles. This means that the interval included 20% of measurements with a difference between bladder and condom pressure

higher than the median value, and 40% of measurements with less than the median value. The borderline values were -4.0 cmH$_2$O and 23.8 cmH$_2$O. On the basis of the invasive pressure–flow test, the patients were stratified into two groups: a combined non-obstructed and equivocal group, and an obstructed group. It was found that the bladder and condom pressures correlated better in the combined group of non-obstructed and equivocal patients than in the group of obstructed patients. Still, the less accurate pressure readings in obstructed patients were, on average, higher than those measured in the combined group. This suggests that a classification of BOO on the basis of a combination of condom pressure and flow rate may be possible. This is further explored in the section on clinical application below.

Condom-type catheter: limitations and improvement

Patients and volunteers were asked not to strain during voiding. Despite this encouragement, some patients still did. In this small group, we observed that in some cases the relatively high abdominal pressure was not reflected in the pressure measurement in the condom. Obviously, in these cases straining led to closure of the urethra, which resulted in an unreliable pressure reading in the condom. We therefore

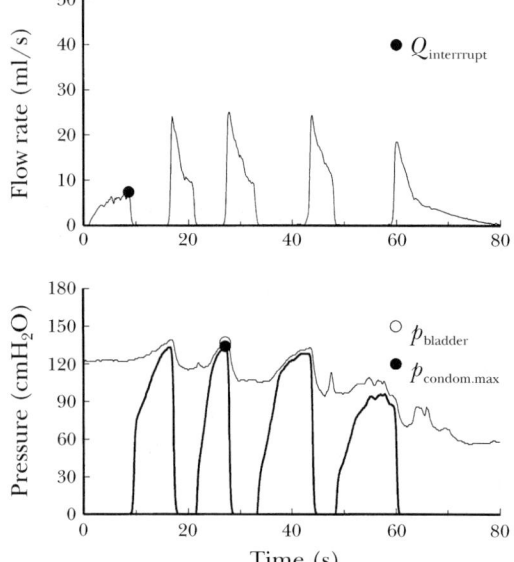

Figure 3 Flow rate (top panel) and simultaneously measured bladder pressure (thin line; transurethral catheter) and condom pressure (thick line) in an obstructed patient (lower panel). Maximum bladder pressure, $p_{bladder}$, and condom pressure, $p_{condom.max}$, are high and correlate well. Interrupt flow rate $Q_{interrupt}$ is about 8 ml/s

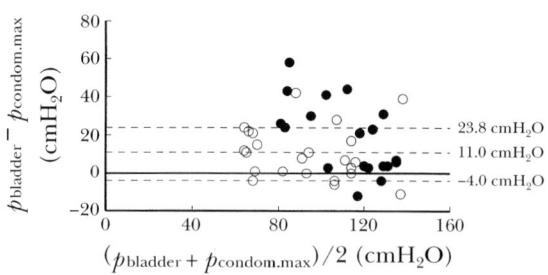

Figure 4 Difference between simultaneously measured bladder pressure, $p_{bladder}$, and condom pressure, $p_{condom.max}$, in a combined group of non-obstructed and equivocal patients (open circles) and a group of obstructed patients (closed circles) plotted as a function of the mean of both values

concluded that this test could only be done in those who void without straining. Furthermore, a too low flow rate at the moment of interruption prolongs the filling of the condom, which increases the risk of sphincter contraction or detrusor inhibition and, thus, an unreliable pressure reading in the condom. For a successful condom pressure measurement, it is therefore necessary that the condom is quickly filled and pressurized. The time necessary to reach the maximum condom pressure depends mainly on the flow rate. We reanalyzed the data of the group of patients in whom the bladder and condom pressure were simultaneously measured to calculate a minimum flow rate value, above which the condom pressure accurately represented the bladder pressure. To this end, we extended the difference plot of Figure 4 (Figure 5, top panel). The lower panel of Figure 5 shows the inverse cumulative percentage of patients outside the borderlines

as a function of $Q_{interrupt}$. When this graph is read from right to left, every time a case falls outside the reliability interval, this percentage increases. At a flow rate value less than 5.4 ml/s, 50% of the patients are outside the interval. This flow rate value was therefore chosen as a cut-off flow rate value above which the condom pressure accurately reflects the bladder pressure.

Redesigning the catheter

Each time the valve is closed, the condom needs to be filled with urine to reach a maximum pressure. This filling of the condom takes time, and has an impact on the accuracy of the measurement as explained above. The measurement would be more efficient and accurate if this (re)filling of the condom could be omitted. To achieve this, we developed a variable outflow resistance catheter. It consists of an incontinence condom connected to a set of three outflow tubes and a pressure transducer (Figure 6). Remotely controlled pneumatic valves are used to interrupt the flow of urine through each tube. This new condom-type catheter was designed to maintain a small pressure in the condom during voiding, called a

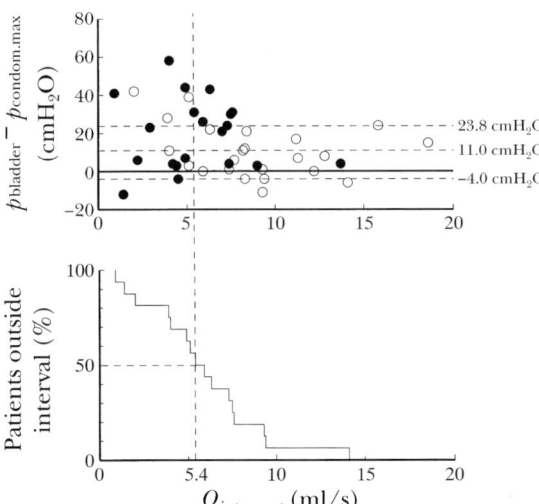

Figure 5 Difference between bladder pressure, $p_{bladder}$, and condom pressure, $p_{condom.max}$, measured in non-obstructed and equivocal patients (open circles) and obstructed patients (closed circles) as a function of the interrupt flow rate, $Q_{interrupt}$ (top panel). Borders of the reliability interval are the median value $\pm$ 14 cmH$_2$O. In the lower panel, the cumulative percentage of patients outside this interval (counted from right to left) is plotted against the interrupt flow rate. From this plot, a flow rate cut-off value of 5.4 ml/s is derived

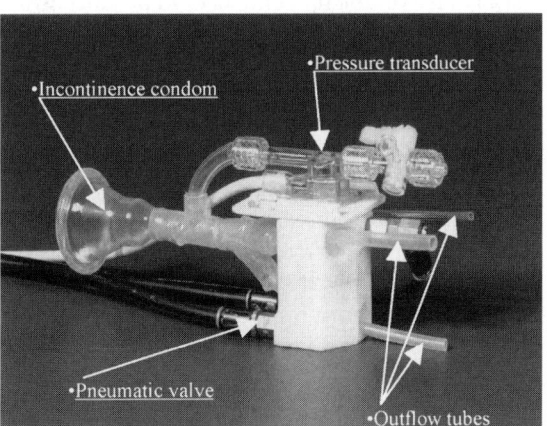

Figure 6 The variable resistance catheter is made to maintain a small pressure in the condom during voiding. In this way, the filling time of the condom during interruption of the flow rate was reduced. This improved the accuracy of the pressure reading in the condom. Reproduced with permission

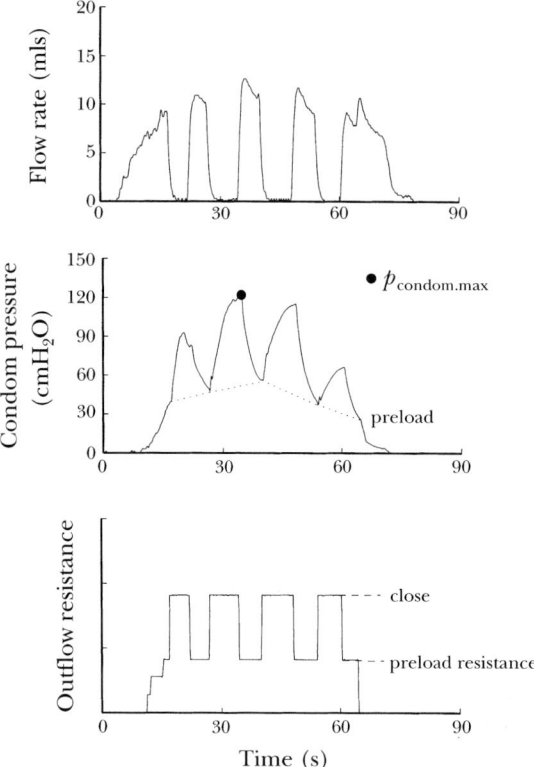

Figure 7 An example of measurement using the variable resistance catheter. Outflow resistance was stepwise increased to a preload resistance. As a result, the pressure in the condom increased to a preload value. Flow rate was repeatedly interrupted to measure maximum condom pressure, $p_{condom.max}$ and to test bladder volume dependence. Reproduced with permission from reference 6

preload[5,6]. When voiding starts, the catheter is set to a small outflow resistance (Figure 7). As a result, the condom fills partly with urine, and the pressure in it increases to a preload value. Superimposed on this preload, repeated isovolumetric pressure measurements are made by closing all tubes. When, after each measurement, the preload outflow resistance is restored, the condom remains partly filled with urine, which reduces its filling time during the next interruption. A second advantage of the preload is that it enables the investigator to monitor a

sphincter contraction (a sudden drop in condom pressure) or detrusor inhibition (a gradual decrease of the pressure) and even the bladder volume dependence.

Practical application of the condom-type catheter

After testing the condom-type catheter in a group of healthy volunteers and patients, we concluded that, for successful bladder pressure measurement in the condom, the free flow rate must exceed 5.4 ml/s and straining must be avoided. It is therefore recommended that a free flow rate measurement is carried out first to evaluate the urinary stream. If this measurement meets the requirements, then a pressure measurement can be made without the use of catheters in the bladder and rectum. As mentioned, the invasiveness of classical urodynamics limits clinical testing and scientific research. The measurement of bladder pressure non-invasively opens up new possibilities for clinical tests and population-based research.

For instance, the condom-type catheter may be used as a new classification tool to identify BOO in patients. To explore this possibility, we constructed a nomogram based on flow rate and condom pressure[7]. Again, we reanalyzed the data of patients who first underwent an invasive pressure–flow test followed by a non-invasive test. Among five strategies, we tested a classification on the basis of the maximum flow rate, Q_{max}, alone (strategy I) and a combination of maximum flow rate and maximum condom pressure (strategy II). The selected patient population for the non-invasive test had a wide variety of urological symptoms ranging from BOO to incontinence. We found that, in this population, all patients voiding with a maximum flow rate smaller than 4.5 ml/s were obstructed and all those voiding with a maximum flow rate higher than 13.8 ml/s were non-obstructed. Thirty per cent of the patients could thus be correctly classified. To classify BOO in the remaining 70% of patients,

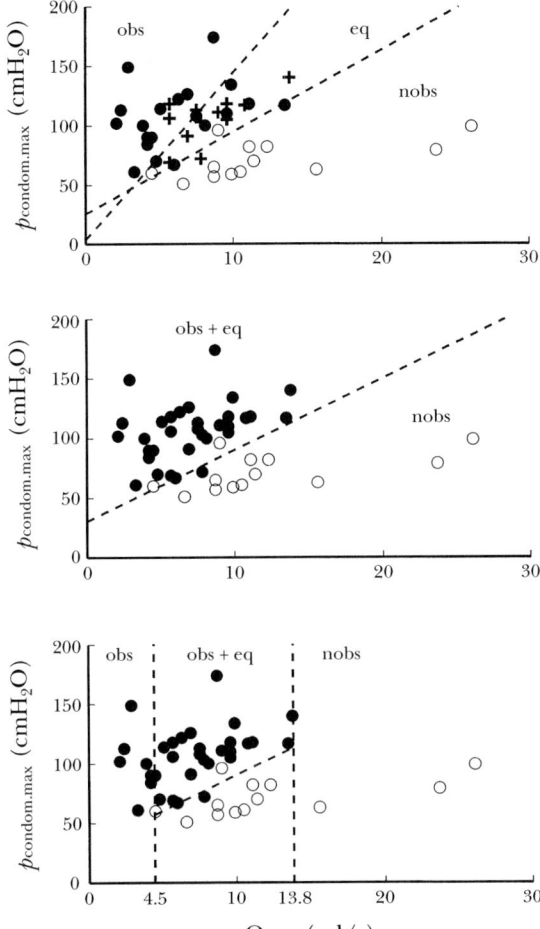

Figure 8 In the top panel, the maximum condom pressure, $p_{condom.max}$, is plotted versus the maximum flow rate, Q_{max}, in non-obstructed (open circles), equivocal (plus symbols) and obstructed patients (closed circles). Classification lines were calculated using logistic regression to separate obstructed (obs) from equivocal (eq) and equivocal from non-obstructed (nobs) patients. The lowest panel shows a two-step approach: patients with a maximum flow rate less than 4.5 ml/s or higher than 13.8 ml/s are diagnosed by flow rate alone. The remaining patients are classified using a combination of maximum flow rate and a separately measured maximum condom pressure. Reproduced with permission from reference 7

measurement of bladder pressure was necessary. In the second strategy, we plotted for each patient $p_{condom.max}$ versus Q_{max} (Figure 8, top panel). Logistic regression was used to calculate separation lines between non-obstructed

(open circles) and equivocal (plus symbols) and between equivocal and obstructed patients (closed circles). In this way, 73% of all patients could be correctly classified. However, the equivocal zone was delineated by crossing lines, indicating that three independent classification zones cannot be constructed. We therefore attempted to join two classification zones. As the $p_{condom.max}$ values measured in the equivocal and obstructed group were significantly higher than those in the non-obstructed group (Mann–Whitney U test: $p < 0.05$), we combined the equivocal patients with the obstructed patients. We recalculated a separation line between this combined group of patients and the non-obstructed patients, and found that the overall success rate was increased by 20% to 93% (Figure 8, middle panel). A combination of both strategies resulted in a two-step approach: patients voiding with a $Q_{max} < 4.5$ ml/s and $Q_{max} > 13.8$ ml/s were classified by flow rate alone. The remaining patients were classified using a combination of maximum flow rate and a separately measured maximum condom pressure (lowest panel). Using this strategy, 93% of our patients could be correctly classified non-invasively.

Clinical application

To evaluate the newly constructed non-invasive obstruction nomogram, we tested a small group of patients who underwent a transurethral resection of the prostate (TURP). The day before the TURP, patients were asked to drink about half a liter of water to produce two separate voidings. We first measured the free flow rate to evaluate the urinary stream. Patients who strained (severely) during this test were not included in the study. Next the condom pressure was measured and evaluated. Both measurements were repeated 6 weeks after surgery. To visualize the urodynamic changes after the TURP, we plotted for each patient the maximum condom pressure versus the maximum free flow rate (Figure 9, top panel). A thin line connects the measurements before and after TURP. In one patient (labelled (A)), the flow rate and the condom pressure

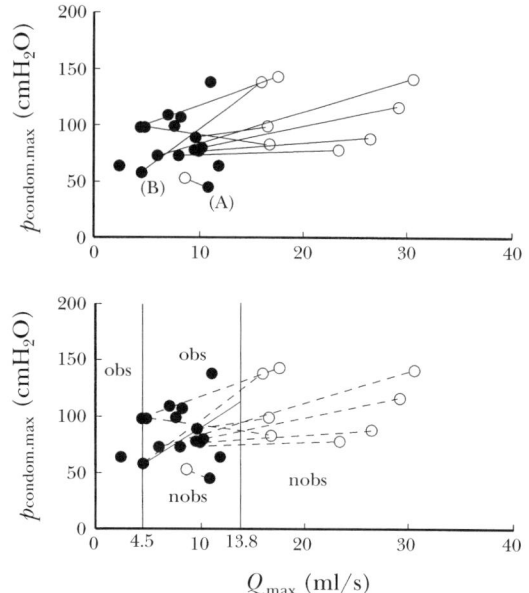

Figure 9 Maximum condom pressure, $p_{condom.max}$, is plotted versus maximum free flow rate, Q_{max}, in patients before (closed circles) and after (open circles) transurethral resection of the prostate, in the top panel. Lines connect measurements made in the same patient. In the lower panel, the data set is plotted in classification areas derived in a different group of patients (see Figure 8, lowest panel)

remained the same after the operation, implying that this patient probably voided with a weakly contracting bladder. A second patient (labelled (B)) voided intermittently before the operation. After the operation, not only the flow rate but also the condom pressure had increased enormously. This example illustrates that a condom pressure measurement is not reliable in a patient who voids intermittently. In the remaining patients, the maximum flow rate increased, on average, 160%. The condom pressures were (on average) increased by 20% after TURP. We did not expect to find this small increase, because the detrusor was unaltered. We think that, owing to the increased flow rate, a better pressure transmission between bladder and condom existed, resulting in a higher condom pressure after the operation.

In Figure 9, lower panel, the non-invasive classification areas were added to the condom pressure–flow rate plot. Eight of the nine post-operative evaluations fell in the non-obstructed areas (nobs), and only ten of the 16 successful preoperative evaluations fell in the obstructed areas (obs). The line separating the 'obs' from the 'nobs' seems to be defined too high, since six of the 16 patients before the TURP fell in the non-obstructed areas. However, four of these six patients were near the obstructed area border and showed improvement after the operation. As the non-invasive evaluation is based on the ICS nomogram, our preliminary finding suggests that some patients diagnosed (invasively) as non-obstructed on the basis of the ICS-nomogram might still benefit from surgical relief of the prostate. The non-invasive nomogram as proposed was derived from a small population studied in one center. For general application, a larger multicenter study is necessary to establish more definite borderlines.

Scientific application

The condom method to measure bladder pressure non-invasively is well tolerated by both volunteers and patients. For large-scale application of this method, an integrated measurement set-up was developed. It is based on the use of reusable domes that are attached to a reusable pressure transducer. Each dome has an inflow port to which a modified incontinence condom is attached, and three outflow ports with different resistance values. The disposable tubes attached to the outflow resistances can be closed by pneumatic valves. The valves and transducer are fixed on a standard rotating-disc flow transducer. Recently, the medical ethics boards of two academic centers approved two population-based studies using this patient-friendly measurement technique. The first study is being carried out by the Sector Furore, Erasmus MC. A large group of 825 healthy male volunteers aged 38–77 will be studied three times in 5 years to evaluate changes in urinary bladder contractility secondary to age-related prostatic enlargement. To date, a first evaluation of two pressure measurements in 191 volunteers has been completed. As the second measurement was not systematically different from the first, there was no bias. The reproducibility was good, and comparable to that of invasive pressure flow studies. Unexpected adverse events were mild and inherent to the subject's sensibility and vulnerability. It can be concluded that the condom-type catheter for measuring bladder pressure non-invasively is suitable for this epidemiological study.

The second study is being carried out at the Department of General Practice, University of Maastricht. In a randomized controlled trial, the effects of an increased water intake (1.5 l daily) in 160 patients aged 55–75 years with a moderate symptom score (International Prostate Symptom Score, IPSS 8–19) on bladder contractility is being tested. The rationale behind this intervention is the animal study observation that increasing urine output may improve bladder function. On this basis it is hypothesized that increasing the workload on the human bladder will also lead to an increase in bladder contractility. Changes in bladder contractility will be monitored using the condom-type catheter. In addition, it will be tested whether improving bladder contractility will lead to relief of LUTS.

End of classical urodynamics?

The results of measurements made in healthy volunteers and patients with LUTS show that, if the free flow rate of the subject exceeds 5.4 ml/s, straining is avoided and the flow of urine is continuous, a reliable bladder pressure measurement can be carried out using the condom method. The question may therefore be asked: can the condom method replace the classical, invasive urodynamics? It has been shown that isovolumetric bladder pressure measured with the condom method can be used to classify BOO by combining it with a free flow rate. Therefore, in patients with a not too weak flow rate (mild voiding symptoms), this method can replace classical urodynamics to classify BOO. If the voiding symptoms are more severe, i.e. voiding with a very poor flow rate or straining, invasive urodynamics is still the only tool to be used. Also, for the assessment of bladder

stability, compliance or dys-synergia, invasive urodynamics is currently the only choice. In addition to replacing classical urodynamics in a subgroup of patients, the non-invasive method may also widen the clinical application of urodynamics. An example is formed by patients treated for BOO, for instance, by TURP. Nowadays, an invasive pressure–flow study is not always done in these patients because of its morbidity. However, a poor flow rate could be the result of a weakly contracting bladder as well as BOO. Many patients undergo surgery without a urodynamic diagnosis to differentiate between the causes of voiding complaints. The condom method provides a patient-friendly alternative for investigating this group of patients. Moreover, the test could be repeated in almost all patients after the operation. Such a post-treatment evaluation is rare, but essential for a clinical evaluation of alternative therapies.

Finally, the condom method opens up a unique opportunity for population-based research. At present, the condom method is being applied in two epidemiological studies. The recruited male volunteers are free of voiding symptoms or have only mild voiding complaints.

Future research

Neither the condom method nor the classical pressure–flow test pinpoint the exact location of an infravesical obstruction. For example, in patients with BOO, the outcome of the test does not discriminate between prostatic obstruction or meatus stenosis. An alternative measurement method to diagnose BOO non-invasively and possibly to detect the location of the obstruction is based on the recording of noise produced in the urethra during voiding. We have demonstrated that this urethral noise can be measured using a microphone pressed against the perineum[8]. The noise recorded is related to the flow rate through the urethra (Figure 10). However, the origin of the noise and its relation to urethral resistance is as yet undefined. It has been suggested that the recorded noise may be caused by turbulence resulting from narrowing

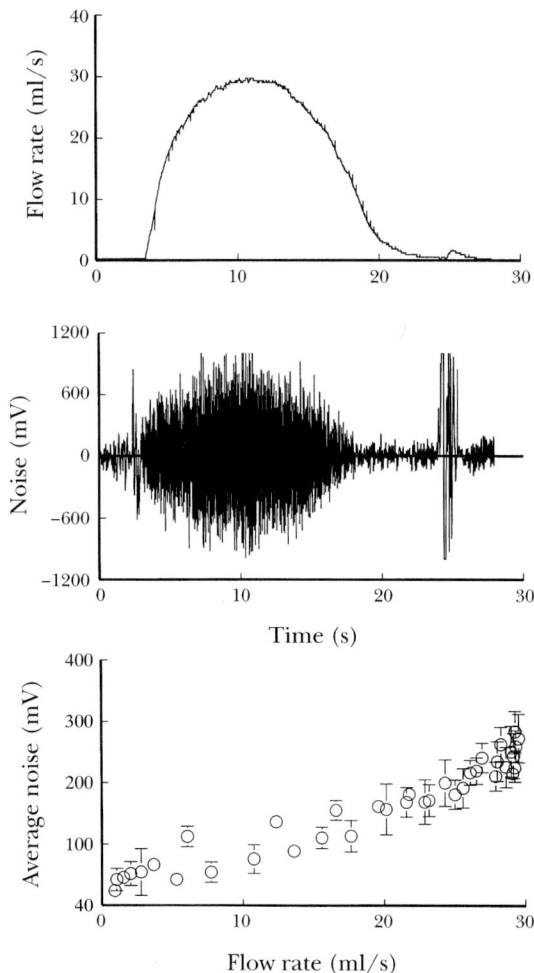

of the urethra through the enlarged prostate. The aim of our current project is to develop a biophysical model of the urethra to study noise production in relation to urethral resistance. The modelling results will be verified by measurements in healthy volunteers and in patients with LUTS. In this way, we hope to establish the recording of urethral noise as a clinical, non-invasive classification tool.

Acknowledgement

This research was supported by the Technology Foundation STW, applied division of The Netherlands Organization for Scientific Research (NWO) and the technology program of the Ministry of Economic Affairs.

Figure 10 Simultaneous measurement of flow rate (top panel) and urethral noise (middle panel) using a perineal microphone. Average noise is plotted against flow rate (lowest panel) to illustrate the dependency

References

1. van Mastrigt R, Kranse M. Accuracy of non-invasive urodynamics in diagnosing infravesical obstruction. *Neurourol Urodynam* 1995;14:451–2
2. Pel JJM, van Mastrigt R. Non-invasive measurement of bladder pressure using an external condom catheter. *Neurourol Urodynam* 1999;18:455–75
3. Rikken B, Pel JJM, van Mastrigt R. Repeated non-invasive bladder pressure measurements with an external catheter. *J Urol* 1999;162:474–9

4. Griffths DJ, Hofner K, van Mastrigt R, *et al.* Standardization of terminology of lower urinary tract function: pressure–flow studies of voiding, urethral resistance and urethral obstruction. *Neurourol Urodynam* 1997;16:1–18

5. Pel JJM, van Mastrigt R. The variable outflow resistance catheter: a new method to measure the bladder pressure noninvasively. *J Urol* 2001;165: 647–52

6. Pel JJM, Spigt MG, Knottnerus JA, *et al.* A modified procedure to non-invasively measure the bladder pressure: preloading the condom. *Neurourol Urodynam* 2001;20:386–8

7. Pel JJM, Bosch JLHR, Blom JHM, *et al.* Development of a non-invasive strategy to classify bladder outlet obstruction in male patients with LUTS. *Neurourol Urodynam* 2002;21:117–25

8. van Koeveringe AJ, van Mastrigt R. A relation between the sound produced by the urethral turbulence in patients and objectively assessed subvesical obstruction. *Neurourol Urodynam* 1991; 10:442–3

Screening for prostate cancer within the benign prostatic hypertrophy population: current evidence and future directions

12

M. R. Cooperberg and P. R. Carroll

Epidemiology

Benign prostatic hypertrophy (BPH) and prostate cancer are the most common benign and malignant neoplasias, respectively, in aging men in the USA[1]. An estimated 189 000 new cases of prostate cancer are expected in 2002; this figure represents a relative levelling of annual incidence, following a sharp peak and subsequent decline in the early 1990s with the introduction of prostate-specific antigen (PSA) screening in a previously unscreened population[2]. The histological prevalence is higher: autopsy studies have found prostate cancer with volume > 0.5 ml or extracapsular spread in 6.0% and 15.6% of men in their 50s and 70s, respectively[3].

An accurate epidemiological description of BPH is less straightforward, as the disease may be defined alternatively by histology, symptomatology and/or urodynamic parameters. The terms 'lower urinary tract symptoms (LUTS)' and 'prostatism' are often used synonymously with BPH, although they may define somewhat distinct patient populations. Autopsy studies have found histological BPH in over 40% of men in their 50s, and in nearly 90% of men in their 80s[4]. Population-based studies of older men with no documented history of prostate pathology have found prevalence rates of LUTS varying from 35% among a cohort of Michigan men over age 60, to 80% of French men 50–80 years old. The prevalence of relatively severe symptoms in each of these cohorts was 15% and 13%, respectively[5].

A number of recent studies have sought to characterize the prevalence of prostate cancer among patients with BPH. Among a referral population of 224 patients with LUTS, Lepor and colleagues reported a 6.7% rate of prostate cancer detection[6]. Fowler and associates performed sextant biopsies on 128 patients with LUTS, negative digital rectal examination (DRE), PSA > 4.0 ng/ml and prostate volume > 75 ml. They found malignancy in 13%; of the 57 patients who underwent open prostatectomy, 11 and 4% were found to have pT1a and pT1b prostate cancer, respectively[7].

Other investigators have specifically analyzed the effects of PSA screening on prostate cancer detection among BPH patients. Mai and co-workers reviewed 533 transurethral resection of the prostate (TURP) specimens from 1989–90 and 449 specimens from 1997–99, finding cancer in 12.9% of the former and 8.0% of the latter; the trend was explained by a decrease in T1b rather than T1a tumors, suggesting a downward stage migration[8]. Tombal and colleagues likewise reviewed 1648 BPH prostatectomy specimens over a 13-year period. They reported an 11% incidence of prostate cancer, decreasing from 23 to 7% over the study period; like Mai and co-workers, they found the decrease to be explained by T1b tumors (15–2%), while the rate of T1a tumors remained nearly constant[9]. Finally, Simons and colleagues compared prostate cancer mortality among Rhode Island men treated surgically for BPH with the population-based expected rate, and found no significant increased risk (relative risk 1.14, confidence interval 0.96–1.33)[10]. The conclusion of a recent systematic review of the literature was that available data do not indicate a significantly elevated risk of prostate cancer among patients with BPH[11].

No epidemiological study to date has established an etiological role for BPH in the development of prostate cancer[3], although the two conditions share endocrine characteristics such as androgen dependence, as well as some common oncological features. The oncoprotein ErbB-2/Neu has been identified in both BPH and prostate cancer tissue[12]; on the other hand, transforming growth factor-β1 exerts a mitogenic effect in prostate cancer but is pro-apoptotic in BPH[13]. Other recent work on prostatic epithelial–stromal interactions has demonstrated that fibroblasts isolated from prostate cancer specimens can induce malignant transformation in epithelial cells derived from BPH tissue, but not from normal prostate glands[14].

Screening: general concerns

No clear consensus exists across medical specialties with respect to the benefits of PSA screening in the general population. The American Urological Association[15] and the American Cancer Society[16] recommend annual PSA and DRE screening for men starting at 50 years old (40 or 45 in high-risk patients); the American College of Preventive Medicine[17] and the American College of Physicians–American Society of Internal Medicine[18], on the other hand, do not. Survey data across three US states of practices by generalists and internists suggest that only 67% of family physicians and 40% of internists routinely screen men over 50[19].

The presence of LUTS does not predict prostate cancer incidence[3], but it does increase the likelihood of PSA testing, as do a diagnosis of BPH and/or prior history of prostate surgery[20]. BPH patients are also, of course, more likely to be seen by a urologist; a 1997 Gallup survey found that 92% of urologists employed routine PSA testing among their BPH patients[21]. The

Agency for Health Care Policy and Research[22] and the International Consultation on BPH[23] both recommend PSA measurement in those BPH patients for whom an incidental diagnosis of prostate cancer would spur a change in management (generally referring to patients with at least a 10-year life expectancy).

Prostate cancer detected incidentally during work-up or surgery for BPH may not necessarily be clinically significant. In the series of Tombal and colleagues, 8% of T1a patients opting for surveillance progressed at a mean of 73 months, whereas 29% of T1b patients progressed at a mean of 17 months[9]. Kearse and associates followed 304 TURP patients for a minimum of 8 years, concluding that the risk of progression and death among T1a prostate cancer patients was not significantly elevated over those confirmed to have only BPH on pathological examination[24]. Epstein and co-workers found, conversely, that even low-volume T1a tumors may progress and cause mortality with extended follow-up[25]. Fowler and colleagues also point out that, with the decline in surgical management for BPH, men with T1a/b prostate cancer are increasingly likely to be undiagnosed[26].

A fundamental caveat with respect to interpretation of studies of diagnostic tests' predictive ability is raised periodically in reviews of the prostate cancer screening literature (see, for example, reference 27) and should be reiterated here: most studies report sensitivity (i.e. the proportion of cancers that will be diagnosed) and specificity (i.e. the proportion of unnecessary biopsies that may be avoided) of a test in a given population, and frequently present receiver operating characteristic (ROC) curve areas as a means of comparing competing tests. The calculation of these measures, however, is highly dependent on the prevalence among the study population of the disease in question. Thus, if a test's threshold value is calculated to yield high sensitivity among a referral population in whom prostate cancer is relatively common, in a general screening population the same test would retain high sensitivity but may have very low specificity. For this reason, the positive and negative predictive values (PPV and NPV) of a test, reported less frequently, are more relevant to most clinical decision-making. For ROC comparisons among unfractionated PSA and other assays between prostate cancer and BPH patients, Jung and colleagues have suggested matching patients by unfractionated PSA, to compensate for unequal distribution of PSA values between the two groups[28], but such adjustments are not usually performed.

Prostate-specific antigen

Unfractionated

Serum PSA measurement has revolutionized the detection of prostate cancer in the general population, and has produced a significant downward stage migration in the epidemiology of the disease[29]. Benign disease, however, can also elevate the PSA: 28% of men with histologically proven BPH have a PSA over 4.0 ng/ml[22]. In fact, the similarity in the epidemiology of the two conditions and their frequent coexistence constitutes one of the greatest impediments to the specificity of PSA testing for prostate cancer. BPH confounds PSA screening via a number of mechanisms. Unfractionated PSA correlates with prostate volume in a log-linear fashion; the relationship between the two variables becomes stronger with advancing patient age[30]. Conversely, finasteride, a common treatment for BPH, reduces PSA levels by roughly 50% after 6 months of therapy. While 'correcting' the PSA by doubling the reported value has been suggested for men taking finasteride[31], the actual percentage change may range from −81 to +20%[32]. (Of note, alpha blockers and saw palmetto[33], two other commonly used medications among BPH patients, do not significantly affect PSA.) Urinary retention, a frequent complication of BPH, can produce further increases in PSA of up to six-fold; levels have been reported to drop by 50% within 48 h of relief of obstruction[34].

In the general screening population, unfractionated PSA has a sensitivity of 67.5–80% and specificity of 60–70%, given a threshold for normal of 4.0 ng/ml[35]. PSA levels above 4.0 ng/ml are found in approximately 8–13% of men with neither BPH nor prostate cancer, and in more than 30% of men with BPH but not prostate cancer[3]. Among patients with PSA 4–10 ng/ml, only about 25% with normal DRE results in fact have prostate cancer[36]. The specificity of PSA in men with PSA 4–10 ng/ml falls to as low as 50%, owing to the broad overlap in PSA levels between men with BPH and prostate cancer in this range[37]. In particular, Monda and colleagues found that PSA could not reliably differentiate BPH from T1a prostate cancer[38]. In the series of BPH patients of Lepor and colleagues, PSA and DRE screening had a sensitivity of 86.7 and 80.0%, specificity of 80.9 and 86.3%, and PPV of 25 and 30%, respectively[6].

Digital rectal examination still detects up to 25% of prostate cancers that present in the setting of PSA less than 4 ng/ml[39], and therefore remains an essential part of prostate cancer screening, in the context of BPH or otherwise. Certainly, however, the PPV of DRE goes up with increasing PSA, ranging from 4 to 11% in men with PSA 0–2.9 ng/ml, and from 33 to 83% in those with PSA 3–9.9 ng/ml[40]. Owing to the inability of unfractionated PSA to discriminate reliably between prostate cancer and BPH, a number of modifications and refinements have been proposed over the past decade, and currently stand at various levels of development. This review focuses on those that have been specifically evaluated in the context of differentiating BPH from prostate cancer in a screening population. It should be noted that none of these tests has yet shown consistent enough benefit to win the endorsement of the American Urological Association's PSA best practices policy[35].

PSA density

Prostate-specific antigen density (PSAD), described by Benson and colleagues in 1992[41], refers to the serum PSA divided by the prostate volume as calculated from transrectal ultrasound (TRUS) measurements using the prolate ellipsoid formula. This measurement attempts to improve the specificity of PSA testing for prostate cancer by accounting for the PSA changes produced by BPH. The ratio of PSA-producing epithelium to stroma is relatively preserved in BPH, and the serum PSA is thought to rise at a relatively constant rate of roughly 0.3 ng/ml per gram of hyperplastic tissue. In prostate cancer, however, the concentration of epithelial cells in a given volume of prostate tissue increases; moreover, the 'leaky' nature of the neoplastic endothelium allows a greater amount of PSA to enter the bloodstream, producing an increase in PSA as great as 3.5 ng/ml per gram of tumor[42]. A study by Furuya and co-workers of patients undergoing open or transurethral prostatectomy for BPH found that each gram of BPH tissue removed reduced the PSA by an average of 0.18 ng/ml, and that after surgical treatment for BPH, PSA should return to normal levels in a patient without concurrent prostate cancer[43].

Benson and colleagues analyzed a cohort of 595 men with PSA levels between 4.1 and 10 ng/ml, and found mean PSAD values of 0.297 and 0.208 among men with and without prostate cancer, respectively ($p < 0.0001$). They constructed a PSAD-based nomogram that calculated prostate cancer risk estimates ranging from 3 to 100%[41]. An updated analysis of 733 patients found mean PSAD values of 0.285 and 0.199 among biopsy-positive and -negative patients, and 0.165 among those with no indication for biopsy. They concluded that a PSAD > 0.15 corresponded to an 18% positive biopsy probability among those with an abnormal DRE or TRUS, and a 6% probability among those with no abnormality[44].

A Japanese study of 63 men with histologically confirmed BPH and 234 men with prostate cancer found PSA levels between 4 and 10 ng/ml in 36 and 25 men, respectively. The BPH patients had a mean prostate volume (determined by transabdominal ultrasound) and PSA of 17.1 ± 8.2 ml and 6.42 ± 1.82 ng/ml, respectively, for a mean PSAD of 0.218 ± 0.085. The prostate cancer patients, by contrast, had a mean volume and PSA of 33.4 ± 14.1 ml and 7.8 ± 2.15 ng/ml, for a PSAD of 0.572 ± 0.363. The authors found that PSAD measurement yielded > 90% sensitivity and 56% specificity for distinguishing BPH from prostate cancer. Other PSAD studies have been reviewed previously by Beduschi and Oesterling[45].

Drawbacks to PSAD measurement include the need to perform TRUS to obtain the measurement, the operator-dependent nature of TRUS estimation of prostate volume and the variable stromal–epithelial ratio among individuals. In a large, prospective, multicenter study of nearly 5000 men screened for prostate cancer with PSA and PSAD, Catalona and associates found that TRUS-measured volume correlated poorly ($r = 0.61$) with pathological prostate weight, and that employing a PSAD cut-off of 0.15 to guide biopsy decisions would miss 47% of cancers among patients with PSA levels between 4 and 10 ng/ml[36].

Transition zone-adjusted PSA

BPH is almost exclusively restricted to the transition zone of the prostate, whereas prostate cancer most often affects the peripheral zone. Kalish and colleagues therefore proposed that adjusting the PSA for the transition zone volume rather than the total prostate volume would better reflect the relative contribution to PSA from BPH tissue, particularly in the PSA 'gray zone' of 4–10 ng/ml[46]. The transition zone-adjusted PSA (PSAT) does in fact appear to distinguish BPH from prostate cancer more accurately than PSAD. Kurita and associates performed TRUS-guided biopsies on 164 consecutive patients with elevated PSA and/or abnormal DRE. They found cancer in 27.2%, and calculated ROC areas of 0.667 for PSA, 0.663 for PSAD (not significant) and 0.826 for PSAT ($p < 0.01$)[47].

Zlotta and co-workers evaluated PSA density parameters for histologically proven BPH ($n = 74$) and prostate cancer ($n = 88$) patients, finding mean PSAD values of 0.12 ± 0.07 and 0.22 ± 0.12, respectively, and PSAT values of 0.21 ± 0.13 and 1.02 ± 0.70. They estimated that using PSAT with a threshold of 0.35 would miss 10% of cancers, versus 34% using PSAD with a threshold of 0.15. Again using a threshold of 0.35, they calculated sensitivity and specificity for PSAT of 90 and 93% for patients with total

PSA 0.25–10 ng/ml, and 94 and 89% for patients with PSA 4–10 ng/ml[48]. In a separate study, Zlotta and co-workers also found that assessment of prostate volume by TRUS was more accurate for the transition zone (correlation with pathological weight $r = 0.95$, variability −17 to +18%) than for the whole prostate ($r = 0.78$, variability −21 to +30%)[49], further supporting the concept of PSAT rather than PSAD measurement.

PSA free fraction

Another area in which improvements to PSA screening have been emerging over the past decade is the assessment of molecular fractions of PSA. PSA in the serum complexes primarily with α_1-antichymotrypsin (ACT) and α_2-macroglobulin (A2M). Standard PSA immunoassays detect free PSA (fPSA, 5–30% of the detectable fraction) and PSA complexed to ACT (cPSA, 60–95% of the detectable fraction); PSA complexed to A2M, which represents up to 40% of the true total serum PSA, is not detected in standard assays[50]. Stenman and colleagues noted that the ratio of the PSA–ACT complex to the total detectable PSA (tPSA) tends to be elevated in prostate cancer[51]; shortly thereafter, Christensson and associates found that the cPSA : tPSA ratio is higher in prostate cancer patients than in BPH patients, and conversely that the fPSA is lower (18% in prostate cancer vs. 28% in BPH, $p < 0.0001$). They calculated a specificity for prostate cancer of 73% for a fPSA fraction < 18%, compared with 55% for tPSA > 4 ng/ml[52]. Another advantage of fPSA in the context of BPH is that it does not appear to be affected by finasteride[53].

Catalona and associates calculated median free/total PSA (f/tPSA) ratios of 9.2% in men with prostate cancer, 15.9% in those with prostate cancer and BPH, and 18.8% in those with BPH only. They proposed a cut-off of 23.4%, for a sensitivity of 90% and specificity of 31.3%[54]. In a prospective study of 773 men, 379 with prostate cancer and 394 with BPH, with tPSA 4–10 ng/ml, they used a f/tPSA cut-off of 25%, yielding a sensitivity of 95% and specificity of 20%. Significantly, they reported that the cancers detected in men with f/tPSA > 25% tended to occur in older patients, and were more likely to be of lower grade and volume[55]. Performance of f/tPSA was found to be comparable in White and Black men[56]. Horninger and colleagues simultaneously measured f/tPSA and PSAT, finding that among 308 screened volunteers, a PSAT threshold of 0.22 could eliminate 24.4% of unnecessary biopsies, while an f/tPSA ratio of < 20% could eliminate 45.5%. Combining the two tests, they reported, could reduce the unnecessary biopsy rate by 54.2%[57]. Other studies of f/tPSA have recently been reviewed[58,59]. Of the various PSA adjuncts, f/tPSA is currently the most frequently used in practice for patients with PSA 4–10 ng/ml.

α_1-Antichymotrypsin-complexed PSA

With the introduction of a new immunoassay for cPSA[60], interest has grown in the possibility of replacing the f/tPSA ratio – which requires two biochemical measures – with the cPSA alone, an approach that would lower both costs and variability owing to the multiplicity of tPSA and fPSA assays available and their attendant range of specificities[61]. If its clinical utility were comparable to that of the f/tPSA ratio, the cPSA would also offer the advantage of better longevity in stored serum[62]; instability of fPSA may have compromised retrospective studies of its predictive ability[63].

Brawer and colleagues recently published an updated analysis of PSA fractions using the new assay among 272 patients with and 385 patients without prostate cancer. At a set sensitivity of 95%, they calculated specificity for cPSA > 2.75 ng/ml of 24%, compared with 18% for tPSA > 3.06 ng/ml, and 23% for the f/tPSA ratio. For patients with tPSA 4–10 ng/ml, 95% sensitivity of tPSA is achieved with a tPSA cut-off of > 4.24 ng/ml, for a specificity of 7%; in this range, a cPSA cut-off of 3.70 ng/ml yields a specificity of 18%, while that of a 23% f/tPSA ratio threshold is 17%. The performance of cPSA over f/tPSA was particularly evident in the lower range of tPSA levels between 4 and 6 ng/ml[64]. Okegawa and associates conducted a similar analysis in the range of tPSA 4–10, reporting that a cPSA threshold of 3.9 ng/ml yielded 96% sensitivity and 18% specificity. However, in this series, while the ratio of f/cPSA outperformed all other PSA-based measures in ROC analysis, cPSA alone was not significantly better than tPSA[65].

If cPSA does in fact perform better than f/tPSA, or even if it is merely comparable, the new assay may offer significant economic advantages. A recent cost–benefit analysis for primary screening compared tPSA > 4.0 ng/ml, f/tPSA ratio < 25% (performed when tPSA is 4–10 ng/ml) and cPSA at various thresholds. This study found cPSA with a cut-off of 3.8 ng/ml to be the dominant strategy, increasing the PPV of the screening test from 31.0% for tPSA to 32.8%, and preventing 17% of unnecessary biopsies. However, at this threshold, the sensitivity fell to 81%, compared with 92.4% for tPSA; to raise the sensitivity of cPSA above 90%, a threshold of 3.0 ng/ml would have to be used, which would reduce the specificity to the point at which tPSA would become more cost-effective[66].

A significant caveat is offered, by one study by Jung and colleagues, which looked explicitly at cPSA performance in distinguishing BPH from prostate cancer. These investigators analyzed 91 men with no prostate disease, 144 men with untreated prostate cancer and 89 men with BPH. They found that the ratio of c/tPSA was similar to that of f/tPSA in its ability to distinguish BPH and prostate cancer (ROC area 0.851 vs. 0.838), but that cPSA alone was not significantly different from tPSA (ROC area 0.632 vs. 0.568). In this analysis, the specificity of cPSA at 90% sensitivity was only 25%, compared with 55% for f/tPSA and 18% for tPSA[67]. Stamey and Yemoto, likewise, found that the f/tPSA and f/cPSA ratios had ROC values over 0.80, but that cPSA alone was only marginally more specific than tPSA[68]. A final study of the f/cPSA ratio from Filella and colleagues in 178 BPH and 44 prostate cancer patients found, similarly, that f/cPSA (ROC area 0.887, specificity 72% at 90% sensitivity) was more accurate than f/tPSA (ROC area 0.872, specificity 59% at 90% sensitivity)[69].

Human kallikrein 2

PSA is a member of the human kallikrein gene family, designated hK3. A closely related molecule, hK2, shares roughly 80% amino acid homology with PSA. hK2 is also highly prostate-specific, and may be more prostate cancer-specific than PSA[70]. hK2 levels are significantly different among healthy volunteers, men with BPH, men with localized prostate cancer and men with advanced prostate cancer[71]. Kwiatkowski and colleagues analyzed 90 consecutive patients with LUTS and tPSA between 4 and 10 ng/ml. They diagnosed 20 prostate cancer and 70 BPH patients, and compared hK2, f/tPSA, the hK2/tPSA ratio and the hK2/fPSA ratio. While hK2 alone and hK2/tPSA did not distinguish significantly between prostate cancer and BPH, hK2/fPSA had better accuracy (94.4% sensitivity and 60.3% specificity with an ROC area of 0.86) than f/tPSA (25.2% cut-off for 94.4% sensitivity and 27.6% specificity, ROC area 0.76)[72].

Magklara and colleagues likewise studied 106 prostate cancer and 100 histologically confirmed patients with BPH and tPSA 2.5–10 ng/ml. Again, hK2/fPSA performed better than f/tPSA, although the ROC areas were both lower and closer (0.69 vs. 0.64) in this data set. With 95% specificity, the hK2/fPSA ratio identified 25% of patients with cancer who had tPSA in the range 2.5–4.5 ng/ml[73]. Finally, Ylikoski and co-workers recently reported a novel method of assessing the presence of both PSA and hK2 mRNAs in the serum by simultaneous reverse transcriptase-polymerase chain reaction, a method that in early reports appears to be highly accurate in distinguishing benign from malignant prostate disease[74].

Comparisons

A number of investigators have recently undertaken direct comparisons among the various combinations of assays described above in defined populations of prostate cancer and BPH patients. A study by Moon and colleagues of 67 Korean patients (22 prostate cancer and

45 BPH) with PSA 4–10 ng/ml calculated higher accuracy for PSAT with a cut-off of 0.35 (86% sensitivity and 89% specificity) than for f/tPSA, PSAD or tPSA[75]. In contrast, Matsuyama and associates found that among 97 Japanese men (24 prostate cancer and 73 BPH), f/tPSA (cut-off 17%) had equal sensitivity (92%) and higher specificity (56 vs. 40%) than PSAT (cut-off 0.3); in a logistic regression analysis of the 65 men with tPSA 4–10 ng/ml, only f/tPSA significantly predicted disease status[76].

Kurita and co-workers introduced a new degree of subtlety to the comparison literature, comparing PSAD, PSAT and f/tPSA among 297 patients with tPSA 4–10 ng/ml, of whom 21% were found to have prostate cancer on biopsy. The ROC areas for the overall cohort were 0.680 for tPSA, 0.684 for PSAD, 0.764 for PSAT and 0.748 for f/tPSA. However, on subgroup analysis they found that the best test depended on the prostate volume: among those with prostate volume < 40 ml, the ROC area for f/tPSA increased to 0.885, yielding sensitivity and specificity of 87 and 75%, respectively, at a threshold of 40%. For those with volume ≥ 40 ml, however, the highest ROC area was achieved with PSAT (0.817), for a sensitivity and specificity of 88 and 56% at a threshold of 0.17[77]. Another study by Djavan and colleagues confirmed these findings, concluding once again that f/tPSA and PSAT demonstrated the best performance in distinguishing BPH from prostate cancer in a cohort of 974 patients, but that PSAT was significantly affected by smaller prostate volume (< 30 ml) and/or transition zone (< 20 ml)[78].

Taneja and co-workers further explored the variability in reported specificities for PSAT, analyzing a cohort of 235 men biopsied for PSAs of 4–10 ng/ml. They determined PSAD and PSAT specificities at threshold levels calculated to yield 95% sensitivity, using the whole cohort and subsets defined by prostate volume < 30, 30–40 and 40–60 ml. For the whole cohort, 95% sensitivity was realized at cut-offs of 0.20 for PSAT and 0.13 for PSAD. At these thresholds, the specificity of PSAT was only 37.5% vs. 29.6% for PSAD, and was 0 and 2%, respectively, among glands under 30 g in size. On the other hand, if 95% sensitivity thresholds were calculated for each volume group, specificity could be increased to as high as 45.7% for a PSAT threshold of 0.193 for glands 40–60 ml in size (vs. 30.8% for PSAD > 0.126), while for glands under 30 ml, PSAT > 0.280 was 28.2% specific, vs. 5.6% specificity for PSAD > 0.159[79]. Stamey and Yemoto likewise found that adjustment for transition zone volume improved the performance of any molecular fraction of PSA[68].

Finally, a recent study by Horinaga and associates was the first to combine molecular fractionation and volume adjustment, calculating the cPSA/ transition zone volume ratio (cPSAT) among 144 patients undergoing repeat biopsy (a subset of 86 had PSA 4–10 ng/ml). Prostate cancer was detected in 39 patients (19 of the subset), and tPSA did not differ significantly between those with and without cancer. The cPSAT had the highest ROC areas of a number of tests analyzed (0.756, 0.768 for the subset), and was the only one with significant discriminatory power in a logistic regression analysis[80].

These insightful studies appear to confirm an intuitive hypothesis, that adjustment of PSA for volume would add the most discriminatory information among BPH patients with large prostate volumes, whereas for those with smaller prostates, PSAD would not vary significantly and measures of molecular fractions of PSA would be more helpful. They also once again underscore the critical importance of considering the denominator – i.e. the characteristics of the study group relative to the target population to be screened – when interpreting reported sensitivity and specificity values.

PSA 2–4 ng/ml

Most of the studies discussed have focused on patients in the 'gray zone' of tPSA 4–10 ng/ml. PSA levels above 10 are generally felt to warrant biopsy regardless of other parameters. The definition of 4 as the threshold of 'normal', however, has always been arbitrary. Oesterling and colleagues defined age-specific cut-offs for tPSA ranging from 2.5 for men aged 40–49 to

6.5 for those aged 70–79[81]. Other groups have published ranges for African–American[82] and Asian men[83]. Such age-specific reference ranges offer the promise of improving sensitivity among younger men, who are less likely to have concurrent BPH and would benefit most from aggressive treatment of localized disease, while decreasing the rates of biopsies and potentially unnecessarily invasive interventions in older patients. In other large series[84,85], however, age did not significantly affect the performance of PSA with a threshold of 4.0, and age-specific ranges have not won universal endorsement, nor are they recommended by the manufacturers of PSA assays[58].

Recent studies have suggested that the prevalence of prostate cancer in the PSA 2.5–4 ng/ml range is actually comparable to the rate in the 4–10 ng/ml range, and moreover that cancers detected in this range are clinically significant in 80% of cases and have Gleason scores of 7 or greater in up to 50%[86]. Haese and associates recently reported that, among 1602 screened patients, 756 had negative DRE and PSA 4–10 ng/ml, while an additional 219 had negative DRE and PSA 2–4 ng/ml. They found that varying f/tPSA cut-offs of 18–25% yielded sensitivities of 63.7–92.5% and specificities of 57.5–18.7% for the 4–10-ng/ml group, and sensitivities of 46.3–75.6% and specificities of 73.6–37.6% for the 2–4-ng/ml group. On average, 3–5 biopsies were required to detect each cancer in the lower-PSA group; 35 of the 41 cancers detected had Gleason scores of 7 or greater[87].

Roehl and co-workers reported a series of 965 screened volunteers with PSA 2.6–4 ng/ml. Of these, 25% had prostate cancer detected on biopsy. A 25% f/tPSA cut-off had an 85% sensitivity and 19% specificity, while sensitivity and specificity for a 30% cut-off were 93 and 9%, respectively. Of the 241 patients in this cohort who underwent radical prostatectomy, 95% had clinically significant tumors, of which 80% were organ-confined on pathological examination[88]. Recker and colleagues have reported diagnosis of prostate cancer using a screening f/tPSA ratio of < 20% in patients with tPSA as low as 1 ng/ml[89].

These are the largest studies to date, but do not specifically address the differentiation of BPH from prostate cancer. A prospective study by Djavan and associates found that f/tPSA (threshold 41%) and PSAT (threshold 0.095) had the best performance among 273 men with PSA 2.5–4 ng/ml, of whom 207 had BPH on histology and 66 had prostate cancer. The ROC areas were 0.749 and 0.701, respectively, with specificities of 29.3% and 17.2%[90].

New directions

A number of novel approaches to distinguishing prostate cancer from BPH have recently been reported and are currently under development. Charrier and colleagues, for example, have found via two-dimensional gel electrophoresis that BPH sera contain higher percentages of low-molecular-weight fPSA elements than prostate cancer sera; they reported that the ratio of these elements to a standard fPSA measurement could correctly diagnose 100% of 40 BPH cases and 82.5% of 52 prostate cancer cases, compared with 73 and 42.5% correctly diagnosed via a standard f/tPSA assay[91]. Mikolajczyk and associates have demonstrated that a significant fraction of fPSA is actually composed of inactive precursor forms of PSA (pPSA)[92]. Various isoforms of pPSA with truncated leader sequences have been shown to distinguish very reliably between BPH and prostate cancer in tissue extracts[93–95], but have yet to be tested in serum assays.

Yet another variation on PSA testing is the ratio of serum PSA to urinary PSA, which Hillenbrand and colleagues found could distinguish BPH from prostate cancer in a set of 105 patients[96]. An early report by Dobrowolski and associates suggested that measurement of the vascular/stromal coefficient via TRUS incorporating power Doppler may be able to distinguish normal, BPH and prostate cancer tissue[97]. Xiao and co-workers have developed an assay for serum prostate-specific membrane antigen (sPSMA), a specific and highly conserved marker of prostate cancer. In preliminary tests, the mean sPSMA level was 623.1 ng/ml in prostate cancer patients and

117.1 ng/ml in BPH patients, this nearly six-fold difference indicating a very promising result[98]. On the other hand, transforming growth factor-β1, known to be markedly elevated in prostate cancer, in another study did not discriminate significantly among 32 prostate cancer and ten BPH patients[99].

Rather than focusing on single markers, Adam and colleagues published a proteomic approach, analyzing serum protein fingerprints obtained by surface-enhanced laser desorption/ionization (SELDI) mass spectrometry. They identified a pattern of nine proteins whose expression could distinguish 167 prostate cancer patients from 77 BPH patients and 82 age-matched healthy men with 96% accuracy. In a prospective, blinded test set, the pattern had a sensitivity of 83%, a specificity of 97% and a PPV of 96% (91% for the whole study population)[100]. Although very labor-intensive, this approach holds great promise for future refinement and automation.

Other investigators have combined known and novel markers with interesting preliminary results. While serum insulin-like growth factor I (IGF-I) has not consistently been able to distinguish BPH from prostate cancer, Koliakos and colleagues found in a group of 34 prostate cancer and 131 BPH patients that IGF-I correlates with PSA and fPSA levels only in prostate cancer patients; the ratio of PSA/IGF-I in fact had better ROC characteristics than f/tPSA in this group[101]. Finally, the ProstAsure Index is an artificial neural network model that incorporates PSA and several other preclinical variables, which, in early trials, has demon-strated better performance than the f/tPSA ratio in distinguishing BPH from prostate cancer in patients with PSA 4–10 ng/ml and 2.5–4 ng/ml[58].

Conclusions and future directions

Although screening for prostate cancer in any population remains controversial, and is the subject of ongoing randomized trials, patients with signs or symptoms of BPH should be offered early detection efforts, as discovery of clinically significant prostate cancer may alter treatment recommendations. In addition, certain treatments for BPH, such as trans-urethral resection, may exclude patients from receiving some treatment options for their prostate cancer, or make such procedures more morbid.

The best method of early detection in this patient population remains unclear. It appears likely that even if cPSA cannot match the f/tPSA ratio in terms of accuracy, it may, if borne out in prospective trials, prove a better initial screening test than tPSA. Future studies of volume-depending parameters such as PSAT should probably focus on patients with prostate volumes over 30 or 40 ml; in any event, studies should account for volume in comparing patient cohorts. Certainly the coming years will see the availability of better clinical tools to identify occult prostate cancer among BPH patients, tools that should increase the acceptance of prostate cancer screening in the general medical community.

References

1. Hall MC, Roehrborn CG, McConnell JD. Is screening for prostate cancer necessary in men with symptoms of benign prostatic hyperplasia? *Semin Urol Oncol* 1996;14:122–33
2. Jemal A, Thomas A, Murray T, Thun M. Cancer statistics, 2002. *CA Cancer J Clin* 2002;52:23–47
3. Guess HA. Benign prostatic hyperplasia and prostate cancer. *Epidemiol Rev* 2001;23:152–8
4. Berry SJ, Coffey DS, Walsh PC, Ewing LL. The development of human benign prostatic hyperplasia with age. *J Urol* 1984;132:474–9

5. Guess HA. Epidemiology and natural history of benign prostatic hyperplasia. *Urol Clin North Am* 1995;22:247–61

6. Lepor H, Owens RS, Rogenes V, Kuhn E. Detection of prostate cancer in males with prostatism. *Prostate* 1994;25:132–40

7. Fowler JE Jr, Bigler SA, Kolski JM. Prostate cancer detection in candidates for open prostatectomy. *J Urol* 1998;160:2107–10

8. Mai KT, Isotalo PA, Green J, Perkins DG, Morash C, Collins JP. Incidental prostatic adenocarcinomas and putative premalignant lesions in TURP specimens collected before and after the introduction of prostate-specific antigen screening. *Arch Pathol Lab Med* 2000; 124:1454–6

9. Tombal B, De Visccher L, Cosyns JP, *et al.* Assessing the risk of unsuspected prostate cancer in patients with benign prostatic hypertrophy: a 13-year retrospective study of the incidence and natural history of T1a–T1b prostate cancers. *BJU Int* 1999;84:1015–20

10. Simons BD, Morrison AS, Young RH, Verhoek-Oftedahl W. The relation of surgery for prostatic hypertrophy to carcinoma of the prostate. *Am J Epidemiol* 1993;138:294–300

11. Young JM, Muscatello DJ, Ward JE. Are men with lower urinary tract symptoms at increased risk of prostate cancer? A systematic review and critique of the available evidence. *BJU Int* 2000;85:1037–48

12. Giri DK, Wadhwa SN, Upadhaya SN, Talwar GP. Expression of NEU/HER-2 oncoprotein (p185neu) in prostate tumors: an immunohistochemical study. *Prostate* 1993;23:329–36

13. Lee C, Sintich SM, Mathews EP, *et al.* Transforming growth factor-β in benign and malignant prostate. *Prostate* 1999;39:285–90

14. Olumi AF, Grossfeld GD, Hayward SW, Carroll PR, Tlsty TD, Cunha GR. Carcinoma-associated fibroblasts direct tumor progression of initiated human prostatic epithelium. *Cancer Res* 1999; 59:5002–11

15. American Urological Association Prostate Cancer Clinical Guidelines Panel. *Report on the management of clinically localized prostate cancer.* Baltimore, MD: AUA, 1995

16. Smith RA, von Eschenbach AC, Wender R, *et al.* American Cancer Society guidelines for the early detection of cancer: update of early detection guidelines for prostate, colorectal, and endometrial cancers. *CA Cancer J Clin* 2001;51:38–75, quiz 77–80

17. Ferrini R, Woolf SH. American College of Preventive Medicine practice policy. Screening for prostate cancer in American men. *Am J Prev Med* 1998;15:81–4

18. American College of Physicians. Screening for prostate cancer. *Ann Intern Med* 1997;126: 480–4

19. Kim HL, Benson DA, Stern SD, Gerber GS. Practice trends in the management of prostate disease by family practice physicians and general internists: an internet-based survey. *Urology* 2002;59:266–71

20. Meigs JB, Barry MJ, Giovannucci E, Rimm EB, Stampfer MJ, Kawachi I. High rates of prostate-specific antigen testing in men with evidence of benign prostatic hyperplasia. *Am J Med* 1998; 104:517–25

21. Gee WF, Holtgrewe HL, Blute ML, *et al.* 1997 American Urological Association Gallup survey: changes in diagnosis and management of prostate cancer and benign prostatic hyperplasia, and other practice trends from 1994 to 1997. *J Urol* 1998;160:1804–7

22. McConnell JD, Barry MJ, Bruskewitz RC. *Benign prostatic hyperplasia: diagnosis and treatment.* Clinical practice guideline no. 8 (pub 94–0582). Rockville, MD: Agency for Health Care Policy and Research, 1994

23. Denis L, Griffiths K, Khoury S, *et al.* eds. *Proceedings of the 4th International Consultation on BPH.* Plymouth, UK: Health Publication, 1998

24. Kearse WS Jr, Seay TM, Thompson IM. The long-term risk of development of prostate cancer in patients with benign prostatic hyperplasia: correlation with stage A1 disease. *J Urol* 1993;150:1746–8

25. Epstein JI, Paull G, Eggleston JC, Walsh PC. Prognosis of untreated stage A1 prostatic carcinoma: a study of 94 cases with extended followup. *J Urol* 1986;136:837–9

26. Fowler JE Jr, Pandey P, Bigler SA, Yee DT, Kolski JM. Trends in diagnosis of stage T1a–b prostate cancer. *J Urol* 1997;158:1849–52

27. Presti JC Jr, Carroll PR. Use of prostate-specific antigen (PSA) and PSA density in the detection of stage T1 carcinoma of the prostate. *Semin Urol Oncol* 1996;14:134–8

28. Jung K, Stephan C, Lein M, *et al.* Receiver-operating characteristic as a tool for evaluating the diagnostic performance of prostate-specific antigen and its molecular forms – what has to be considered? *Prostate* 2001;46:307–10

29. Catalona WJ, Smith DS, Ratliff TL, Basler JW. Detection of organ-confined prostate cancer is increased through prostate-specific antigen-based screening. *J Am Med Assoc* 1993;270: 948–54

30. Roehrborn CG, Boyle P, Gould AL, Waldstreicher J. Serum prostate-specific antigen as a predictor of prostate volume in men with benign prostatic hyperplasia. *Urology* 1999; 53:581–9

31. Gormley GJ, Ng J, Cook T, Stoner E, Guess H, Walsh P. Effect of finasteride on prostate-specific antigen density. *Urology* 1994;43:53–8, discussion 58–9

32. Guess HA, Heyse JF, Gormley GJ, Stoner E, Oesterling JE. Effect of finasteride on serum PSA concentration in men with benign prostatic hyperplasia. Results from the North American phase III clinical trial. *Urol Clin North Am* 1993;20:627–36

33. Gerber GS, Zagaja GP, Bales GT, Chodak GW, Contreras BA. Saw palmetto (*Serenoa repens*) in men with lower urinary tract symptoms: effects on urodynamic parameters and voiding symptoms. *Urology* 1998;51:1003–7

34. Semjonow A, Roth S, Hamm M. Re: non-traumatic elevation of prostate-specific antigen following cardiac surgery and extracorporeal cardiopulmonary bypass. *J Urol* 1995;155:295

35. Carroll P, Coley C, McLeod D, *et al*. Prostate-specific antigen best practice policy – part I: early detection and diagnosis of prostate cancer. *Urology* 2001;57:217–24

36. Catalona WJ, Richie JP, deKernion JB, *et al*. Comparison of prostate specific antigen concentration versus prostate specific antigen density in the early detection of prostate cancer: receiver operating characteristic curves. *J Urol* 1994;152:2031–6

37. Shershon PD, Barry MJ, Osterling JE. Serum prostate-specific antigen discriminates weakly between men with benign prostatic hyperplasia and patients with organ-confined prostate cancer. *Eur Urol* 1994;25:1994

38. Monda JM, Barry MJ, Oesterling JE. Prostate specific antigen cannot distinguish stage T1a (A1) prostate cancer from benign prostatic hyperplasia. *J Urol* 1994;151:1291–5

39. Basler JW, Thompson IM. Lest we abandon digital rectal examination as a screening test for prostate cancer. *J Natl Cancer Inst* 1998; 90:1761–3

40. Schroder FH, van der Maas P, Beemsterboer P, *et al*. Evaluation of the digital rectal examination as a screening test for prostate cancer. Rotterdam section of the European Randomized Study of Screening for Prostate Cancer. *J Natl Cancer Inst* 1998;90:1817–23

41. Benson MC, Whang IS, Olsson CA, McMahon DJ, Cooner WH. The use of prostate specific antigen density to enhance the predictive value of intermediate levels of serum prostate specific antigen. *J Urol* 1992;147:817–21

42. Babaian RJ, Fritsche HA, Evans RB. Prostate specific antigen and the prostate gland volume: correlation and clinical application. *J Clin Lab Anal* 1990;4:135

43. Furuya Y, Akakura K, Tobe T, Ichikawa T, Igarashi T, Ito H. Changes in serum prostate-specific antigen following prostatectomy in patients with benign prostate hyperplasia. *Int J Urol* 2000;7:447–51

44. Seaman E, Whang M, Olsson CA, Katz A, Cooner WH, Benson MC. PSA density (PSAD). Role in patient evaluation and management. *Urol Clin North Am* 1993;20:653–63

45. Beduschi MC, Oesterling JE. Prostate-specific antigen density. *Urol Clin North Am* 1997;24: 323–32

46. Kalish J, Cooner WH, Graham SD Jr. Serum PSA adjusted for volume of transition zone (PSAT) is more accurate than PSA adjusted for total gland volume (PSAD) in detecting adeno-carcinoma of the prostate. *Urology* 1994;43: 601–6

47. Kurita Y, Ushiyama T, Suzuki K, Fujita K, Kawabe K. PSA value adjusted for the transition zone volume in the diagnosis of prostate cancer. *Int J Urol* 1996;3:367–72

48. Zlotta AR, Djavan B, Marberger M, Schulman CC. Prostate specific antigen density of the transition zone: a new effective parameter for prostate cancer prediction. *J Urol* 1997;157: 1315–21

49. Zlotta AR, Djavan B, Damoun M, *et al*. The importance of measuring the prostatic transition zone: an anatomical and radiological study. *BJU Int* 1999;84:661–6

50. McCormack RT, Rittenhouse HG, Finlay JA, *et al*. Molecular forms of prostate-specific antigen and the human kallikrein gene family: a new era. *Urology* 1995;45:729–44

51. Stenman UH, Leinonen J, Alfthan H, Rannikko S, Tuhkanen K, Alfthan O. A complex between prostate-specific antigen and α_1-antichymotrypsin is the major form of prostate-specific antigen in serum of patients with prostatic cancer: assay of the complex improves clinical sensitivity for cancer. *Cancer Res* 1991;51:222–6

52. Christensson A, Bjork T, Nilsson O, *et al*. Serum prostate specific antigen complexed to α_1-antichymotrypsin as an indicator of prostate cancer. *J Urol* 1993;150:100–5

53. Pannek J, Marks LS, Pearson JD, *et al*. Influence of finasteride on free and total serum prostate specific antigen levels in men with benign prostatic hyperplasia. *J Urol* 1998;159:449–53

54. Catalona WJ, Smith DS, Wolfert RL, *et al*. Evaluation of percentage of free serum prostate-specific antigen to improve specificity of prostate cancer screening. *J Am Med Assoc* 1995;274:1214–20

55. Catalona WJ, Partin AW, Slawin KM, *et al*. Use of the percentage of free prostate-specific antigen to enhance differentiation of prostate cancer from benign prostatic disease: a prospective multicenter clinical trial. *J Am Med Assoc* 1998; 279:1542–7

56. Catalona WJ, Partin AW, Slawin KM, *et al.* Percentage of free PSA in black versus white men for detection and staging of prostate cancer: a prospective multicenter clinical trial. *Urology* 2000;55:372–6

57. Horninger W, Reissigl A, Klocker H, *et al.* Improvement of specificity in PSA-based screening by using PSA-transition zone density and percent free PSA in addition to total PSA levels. *Prostate* 1998;37:133–7, discussion 138–9

58. Polascik TJ, Oesterling JE, Partin AW. Prostate specific antigen: a decade of discovery – what we have learned and where we are going. *J Urol* 1999;162:293–306

59. Woodrum DL, Brawer MK, Partin AW, Catalona WJ, Southwick PC. Interpretation of free prostate specific antigen clinical research studies for the detection of prostate cancer. *J Urol* 1998;159:5–12

60. Allard WJ, Zhou Z, Yeung KK. Novel immunoassay for the measurement of complexed prostate-specific antigen in serum. *Clin Chem* 1998;44:1216–23

61. Brawer MK. Clinical usefulness of assays for complexed prostate-specific antigen. *Urol Clin North Am* 2002;29:193–203, xi

62. Ferreri L, Bankson D, Brawer MKL. Long-term stability of complex prostate specific antigen (PSA) in frozen serum. *J Urol* 1999;161:318A

63. Woodrum D, French C, Shamel LB. Stability of free prostate-specific antigen in serum samples under a variety of sample collection and sample storage conditions. *Urology* 1996;48:33–9

64. Brawer MK, Cheli CD, Neaman IE, *et al.* Complexed prostate specific antigen provides significant enhancement of specificity compared with total prostate specific antigen for detecting prostate cancer. *J Urol* 2000;163:1476–80

65. Okegawa T, Kinjo M, Watanabe K, *et al.* The significance of the free-to-complexed prostate-specific antigen (PSA) ratio in prostate cancer detection in patients with a PSA level of 4.1–10.0 ng/ml. *BJU Int* 2000;85:708–14

66. Ellison L, Bright S, Cheli C, Partin A. Cost–benefit analysis of total PSA, free/total PSA and complexed PSA for prostate cancer screening [Abstract]. *J Urol* 2002;167:45A

67. Jung K, Elgeti U, Lein M, *et al.* Ratio of free or complexed prostate-specific antigen (PSA) to total PSA: which ratio improves differentiation between benign prostatic hyperplasia and prostate cancer? *Clin Chem* 2000;46:55–62

68. Stamey TA, Yemoto CE. Examination of the three molecular forms of serum prostate specific antigen for distinguishing negative from positive biopsy: relationship to transition zone volume. *J Urol* 2000;163:119–26

69. Filella X, Alcover J, Corral JM, Molina R, Beardo P, Ballesta AM. Free to complexed PSA ratio in differentiating benign prostate hyperplasia from prostate cancer. *Anticancer Res* 2001;21:3717–20

70. Darson MF, Pacelli A, Roche P, *et al.* Human glandular kallikrein 2 (hK2) expression in prostatic intraepithelial neoplasia and adenocarcinoma: a novel prostate cancer marker. *Urology* 1997;49:857–62

71. Becker C, Piironen T, Pettersson K, *et al.* Discrimination of men with prostate cancer from those with benign disease by measurements of human glandular kallikrein 2 (hK2) in serum. *J Urol* 2000;163:311–16

72. Kwiatkowski MK, Recker F, Piironen T, *et al.* In prostatism patients the ratio of human glandular kallikrein to free PSA improves the discrimination between prostate cancer and benign hyperplasia within the diagnostic 'gray zone' of total PSA 4 to 10 ng/ml. *Urology* 1998;52:360–5

73. Magklara A, Scorilas A, Catalona WJ, Diamandis EP. The combination of human glandular kallikrein and free prostate-specific antigen (PSA) enhances discrimination between prostate cancer and benign prostatic hyperplasia in patients with moderately increased total PSA. *Clin Chem* 1999;45:1960–6

74. Ylikoski A, Pettersson K, Nurmi J, *et al.* Simultaneous quantification of prostate-specific antigen and human glandular kallikrein 2 mRNA in blood samples from patients with prostate cancer and benign disease. *Clin Chem* 2002;48:1265–71

75. Moon DG, Cheon J, Kim JJ, Yoon DK, Koh SK. Prostate-specific antigen adjusted for the transition zone volume versus free-to-total prostate-specific antigen ratio in predicting prostate cancer. *Int J Urol* 1999;6:455–62

76. Matsuyama H, Baba Y, Yamakawa G, Yamamoto N, Naito K. Diagnostic value of prostate-specific antigen-related parameters in discriminating prostate cancer. *Int J Urol* 2000;7:409–14

77. Kurita Y, Terada H, Masuda H, Suzuki K, Fujita K. Prostate specific antigen (PSA) value adjusted for transition zone volume and free PSA (γ-seminoprotein)/PSA ratio in the diagnosis of prostate cancer in patients with intermediate PSA levels. *Br J Urol* 1998;82:224–30

78. Djavan B, Zlotta AR, Remzi M, *et al.* Total and transition zone prostate volume and age: how do they affect the utility of PSA-based diagnostic parameters for early prostate cancer detection? *Urology* 1999;54:846–52

79. Taneja SS, Tran K, Lepor H. Volume-specific cutoffs are necessary for reproducible application of prostate-specific antigen density of the

transition zone in prostate cancer detection. *Urology* 2001;58:222–7

80. Horinaga M, Nakashima J, Ishibashi M, *et al.* Clinical value of prostate specific antigen based parameters for the detection of prostate cancer on repeat biopsy: the usefulness of complexed prostate specific antigen adjusted for transition zone volume. *J Urol* 2002;168:986–90

81. Oesterling JE, Jacobsen SJ, Chute CG, *et al.* Serum prostate-specific antigen in a community-based population of healthy men. Establishment of age-specific reference ranges. *J Am Med Assoc* 1993;270:860–4

82. Morgan TO, Jacobson SJ, McCarthy WF, *et al.* Age-specific reference ranges for serum prostate specific antigen in black men. *N Engl J Med* 1996;335:304

83. Oesterling JE, Kumamoto Y, Tsukamoto T, *et al.* Serum prostate-specific antigen in a community-based population of healthy Japanese men: lower values than for similarly aged white men. *Br J Urol* 1995;75:347–53

84. Catalona WJ, Richie JP, Ahmann FR, *et al.* Comparison of digital rectal examination and serum prostate specific antigen in the early detection of prostate cancer: results of a multicenter clinical trial of 6630 men. *J Urol* 1994;151:1283–90

85. Littrup PJ, Kane RA, Mettlin CJ, *et al.* Cost-effective prostate cancer detection. Reduction of low-yield biopsies. Investigators of the American Cancer Society National Prostate Cancer Detection Project. *Cancer* 1994;74:3146–58

86. Catalona WJ, Smith DS, Ornstein DK. Prostate cancer detection in men with serum PSA concentrations of 2.6 to 4.0 ng/ml and benign prostate examination. Enhancement of specificity with free PSA measurements. *J Am Med Assoc* 1997;277:1452–5

87. Haese A, Dworschack RT, Partin AW. Percent free prostate specific antigen in the total prostate specific antigen 2 to 4 ng/ml range does not substantially increase the number of biopsies needed to detect clinically significant prostate cancer compared to the 4 to 10 ng/ml range. *J Urol* 2002;168:504–8

88. Roehl KA, Antenor JA, Catalona WJ. Robustness of free prostate specific antigen measurements to reduce unnecessary biopsies in the 2.6 to 4.0 ng/ml range. *J Urol* 2002;168:922–5

89. Recker F, Kwiatkowski MK, Huber A, *et al.* Prospective detection of clinically relevant prostate cancer in the prostate specific antigen range 1 to 3 ng/ml combined with free-to-total ratio 20% or less: the Aarau experience. *J Urol* 2001;166:851–5

90. Djavan B, Zlotta A, Kratzik C, *et al.* PSA, PSA density, PSA density of transition zone, free/total PSA ratio, and PSA velocity for early detection of prostate cancer in men with serum PSA 2.5 to 4.0 ng/ml. *Urology* 1999;54:517–22

91. Charrier JP, Tournel C, Michel S, *et al.* Differential diagnosis of prostate cancer and benign prostate hyperplasia using two-dimensional electrophoresis. *Electrophoresis* 2001;22:1861–6

92. Mikolajczyk SD, Grauer LS, Millar LS, *et al.* A precursor form of PSA (pPSA) is a component of the free PSA in prostate cancer serum. *Urology* 1997;50:710–14

93. Mikolajczyk SD, Marker KM, Millar LS, *et al.* A truncated precursor form of prostate-specific antigen is a more specific serum marker of prostate cancer. *Cancer Res* 2001;61:6958–63

94. Mikolajczyk SD, Millar LS, Wang TJ, *et al.* A precursor form of prostate-specific antigen is more highly elevated in prostate cancer compared with benign transition zone prostate tissue. *Cancer Res* 2000;60:756–9

95. Mikolajczyk SD, Millar LS, Wang TJ, *et al.* 'BPSA', a specific molecular form of free prostate-specific antigen, is found predominantly in the transition zone of patients with nodular benign prostatic hyperplasia. *Urology* 2000;55:41–5

96. Hillenbrand M, Bastian M, Steiner M, *et al.* Serum-to-urinary prostate-specific antigen ratio in patients with benign prostatic hyperplasia and prostate cancer. *Anticancer Res* 2000;20:4995–6

97. Dobrowolski Z, Jaszczynski J, Drewniak T, Habrat W. Assessing the vascular–stromal coefficient in patients with benign prostatic hyperplasia or prostate cancer using transrectal ultrasonography and power Doppler analysis. *BJU Int* 2002;89:601–3

98. Xiao Z, Adam BL, Cazares LH, *et al.* Quantitation of serum prostate-specific membrane antigen by a novel protein biochip immunoassay discriminates benign from malignant prostate disease. *Cancer Res* 2001;61:6029–33

99. Wolff JM, Fandel T, Borchers H, Brehmer B Jr, Jakse G. Transforming growth factor-β1 serum concentration in patients with prostatic cancer and benign prostatic hyperplasia. *Br J Urol* 1998;81:403–5

100. Adam BL, Qu Y, Davis JW, *et al.* Serum protein fingerprinting coupled with a pattern-matching algorithm distinguishes prostate cancer from benign prostate hyperplasia and healthy men. *Cancer Res* 2002;62:3609–14

101. Koliakos G, Chatzivasiliou D, Dimopoulos T, *et al.* The significance of PSA/IGF-1 ratio in differentiating benign prostate hyperplasia from prostate cancer. *Dis Markers* 2000;16:143–6

Androgen supplementation in older men: what is the impact on prostate-specific antigen, prostate growth and lower urinary tract symptoms?

13

L. Gooren and M. Bunck

Introduction

The prostate is a hormone-dependent organ. Its growth is stimulated and its size and secretory function are maintained by the continued presence of serum testosterone at approximately eugonadal male levels. Testosterone in the circulation is largely bound to proteins. Approximately 60% is bound to sex hormone-binding globulin (SHBG) and around 38% more loosely to albumin. Only 2–3% of circulating testosterone is unbound and diffuses into organs. Thereafter, it is subjected to a variety of steroid metabolic steps that regulate activity, and finally the inactivation of the steroid hormone. Over 95% of testosterone that enters the prostate is converted to 5α-dihydrotestosterone (DHT)[1]. DHT binds to the same hormone receptor as testosterone, but its biopotency is considerably higher. There is an abundance of androgen receptors in the prostate, probably more than in any other tissue[2]. The result is that the prostate is capable of accumulating testosterone, and local concentrations of androgens are approximately ten times higher than in the circulation. In the adult prostate, androgens continuously play a role in the maintenance of the gland in the mature and differentiated state by homeostatic mechanisms that are androgen-dependent. Prostate size and plasma levels of prostate-specific antigen (PSA) are decreased in androgen-deficient men, and increase again with androgen replacement, but not

significantly exceeding the size and PSA levels in age-matched controls[3–5].

In a recent study, Bhasin and colleagues[6] showed that, in healthy (18–35 years old) men whose endogenous testosterone production was almost totally suppressed by administration of a luteinizing hormone-releasing hormone (LHRH) agonist, PSA levels could be restored to normal by administration of 25 mg testosterone weekly, resulting in plasma testosterone levels of 125 ng/dl (4.3 nmol/l), while the reference range of testosterone is in the order of 8–24 nmol/l. Higher doses of testosterone replacement had no additional effect on plasma PSA levels. Prostate volumes were not measured in this study. So, on the basis of androgen replacement studies and the study by Bhasin and colleagues[6], there is reason to believe that there is no linear relationship between prostate volume and PSA levels on the one hand and plasma testosterone levels on the other. In men chronically abusing anabolic-androgen steroids (body-builders), the total prostate volume was not larger whereas the central prostate volume was approximately 20% larger, compared with age-matched controls; PSA levels were not different between the two groups[7]. Above a threshold value of plasma testosterone there seems to be no additional effect on PSA values, while only supraphysiological doses increase the central prostate volume but not the total prostate volume. In summary, the prostate is an exquisitely androgen-dependent organ, capable of accumulating testosterone through its high androgen receptor content and amplifying the action of testosterone through reduction to DHT. Via these mechanisms the prostate is capable of maintaining its function with relatively low-to-normal peripheral testosterone levels, higher levels not adding substantially to its size or to PSA production.

The following addresses the potential risks of administration of testosterone to androgen-deficient aging men, in particular the risks for benign prostatic hyperplasia and lower urinary tract symptoms (LUTS), and associated PSA levels, but first the rationale for androgen administration to a subgroup of aging men is discussed.

Decline of androgens in old age

Initially cross-sectional studies[8,9], but later also longitudinal studies[10], documented a statistical decline of plasma testosterone by approximately 30% in healthy men between the ages of 25 and 75 years. The pathophysiological mechanism behind the age-related decline of testosterone production lies mainly at the level of the testis[10], but also the hypothalamic–pituitary stimulation of testicular steroidogenesis wanes with aging[11]. Plasma levels of SHBG[9] increase with aging, resulting in lower unbound levels of plasma testosterone. As a result, plasma testosterone levels not bound to SHBG (which are critical for its biological action) may decrease by even 50% over that period. Also, systemic diseases (cardiac, pulmonary, gastrointestinal or rheumatic) that occur increasingly with aging are a cause of declining plasma levels of testosterone[11]. The fall of testosterone levels in (a subgroup of) aging men suggests a parallel with the female menopause, but in men the decline of testosterone levels is more gradual and less precipitous, in comparison with the decline of estrogen production in the female menopause. While it has been shown that plasma testosterone, in particular free testosterone, declines with aging, it remains uncertain what percentage of men

become truly testosterone-deficient with aging, warranting androgen replacement. Stringent criteria for testosterone deficiency have not been formulated. In a study of 300 healthy men between the ages of 20 and 100 years, Kaufman and Vermeulen[9], defining their reference range of testosterone between 11 and 40 nmol/l, found subnormal testosterone levels in more than 20% above the age of 60 years and 35% above the age of 70 years, but 15% of men above the age of 80 years still had testosterone values above 20 nmol/l! Men who have lower-than-normal testosterone values in old age are difficult to identify using clinical criteria. Many signs of aging, such as loss of bone and muscle mass, and loss of sexual functions and mental capacity, closely resemble symptoms of androgen deficiency. It is difficult, if not impossible, to determine whether these signs of aging are related to the decline of androgens with aging, or whether they can be ascribed to the aging process *per se*. Only intervention studies provide a clue to this question. In view of the increasing number of aged persons world-wide and the increasing demand for quality of life, and not simply longevity, the phenomenon of declining androgen levels with aging commands our attention.

Clinical relevance of declining androgen levels with aging

Bone mass

Similar to the situation in women, men show a progressive loss of bone with an exponential increase in the incidence of bone fractures with aging[12,13], albeit that the exponential increase in men starts at a later age (6–8 years later) than in women. Both androgen levels and bone mass decline with age. The actions of androgens on bone might be indirect. A recent study found evidence that bioavailable testosterone levels are positively associated with insulin-like growth factors; the latter correlated again with bone mineral density of the femur and the calcaneus[14]. The available studies in hypogonadal men receiving androgen replacement treatment show that their bone mass increases but does not become normal[15]. Some studies have found a beneficial effect of androgen supplementation in old age on bone density[16–18] or on biochemical indices of bone turnover. A recent well-designed study demonstrated that elevation of testosterone values in men over 65 years to mid-normal levels for young men did not increase lumbar spine density overall, but did increase it in those men with low pre-treatment serum testosterone levels[19]. The last finding validates the assumption that lower-than-normal androgen levels in aging men are a factor in the development of osteoporosis. A role for estrogens, aromatization products of androgens, in the health of male bones is becoming clear. Two cases of men with an impairment of the biological effects of estrogens, presenting with delayed epiphyseal closure and osteopenia, have stirred up interest in the role of estrogens in acquiring and maintaining bone mineral density in men. It could be shown in another man with aromatase deficiency that estrogen administration had a significant beneficial effect on skeletal growth and bone maturation (for review see reference 20). Androgen receptors are present at low densities in osteoblasts, which express 5α-reductase activity. So, there is evidence that androgens *per se* exert effects on (peak) bone mass in men, but part of the effects may be ascribed to aromatization to estrogens, which may occur locally in bone and may therefore not be fully evident from plasma levels of estrogens. The currently available evidence supports a role of estrogens in the bone loss of aging men[13,21]. Thus, with the present state of knowledge it would therefore seem desirable that, for induction and maintenance of bone mass, the type of androgens administered should be aromatizable.

Lean body mass and muscle strength

Androgens have an anabolic effect on muscles, especially the muscles of the upper body. With aging there is a decrease in muscle mass, most of the time associated with an increase in adipose tissue, predominantly in the abdominal and also upper body regions[22]. The interesting question of whether the decline of muscle mass and that of androgen levels with aging are causally inter-related has not been resolved[23]. In a cross-sectional study in aging men, 65–97 years of age, muscle mass was significantly associated with serum free testosterone, physical activity, cardiovascular disease and insulin-like growth factor-I (IGF-I). However, grip strength, probably more relevant, was associated with age independent of muscle mass[24]. Three studies that investigated the effect of testosterone supplementation in small groups of aging men found an increase of lean body mass and an improvement in handgrip strength[24] or lower-limb muscle function, although the magnitude of the improvement was not reported[25]. Tenover[18] found an improvement in lean body mass but no clear increase in muscle strength. A recent study established that administration of testosterone to men over 65 years of age, achieving serum levels in the mid-normal range, decreased fat mass and increased lean body mass but did not increase the strength of knee extension and flexion[26]. Another recent study of parenteral testosterone administration over 12 weeks found neither an increase in lean body mass nor in muscle strength. This study focused on lower-extremity muscles, being probably more relevant for stair climbing, chair rising and walking[27]. Strength of the quadriceps and triceps surae is much more significant in old age, since they determine gait speed, balance, rising from a seated position and stair climbing, and are most impaired in old age. A very positive effect of resistance training has been observed in aging subjects (for review see reference 28). In conclusion, the causal role of declining androgen levels with aging in loss of muscle mass/strength awaits further corroboration. Androgen therapy may have an effect on lean body mass, but the effects on muscle strength are much less certain. Declining growth hormone levels might be significant as well.

Androgens and sexual/psychological functions

Reliable studies on the relationships between androgens and psychological functions are of rather recent date. There is now solid evidence that androgens stimulate sexual appetite. With regard to erectile function the situation is somewhat less clear. It has become clear, however, that in males between 20 and 50 years approximately 60–80% of the normal physiological levels suffice to maintain sexual functions, and that increasing testosterone levels above that threshold adds little to sexual functioning. Whether this holds true for aging men remains to be established. Most aging men complain of erectile failure rather than of loss of libido; therefore, it is not certain that their sexual functioning will improve much upon androgen supplementation.

There is some evidence to suggest that testosterone may influence performance in cognitive tasks[29,30], which is supported by the finding that testosterone administration to older men enhances performance in measures of spatial cognition. Testosterone has also been associated with general mood-elevating effects, and some studies have found associations between lowered testosterone levels and depressive symptoms[30,31]. Depression is not rare in aging men, and impairs their quality of life[32]. So, the effects that declining levels of androgens may have on mood and on specific aspects of cognitive functioning in aging are worthy of research.

Significance of estrogens in male (patho)physiology

Of late, estrogens, largely a product of peripheral aromatization of androgens, have received great attention. Traditionally conceptualized as 'female hormones', estrogens appear to have unexpected but important effects on the male reproductive system (for review see reference 33). Estrogen receptor knock-out mice show abnormalities of the testis and accessory sex organs[33]. With regard to the aging male, estrogen effects on bone, the cardiovascular system and adipogenesis are significant. It becomes increasingly clear that estrogens have important effects on the final phases of skeletal maturation and bone mineralization, and some studies in aging men show that estrogen levels correlate better with bone mineral density than androgen levels (for review see reference 34). Impaired estrogen action in men leads to dyslipidemia and to impaired flow-dependent vasodilatation in peripheral arteries, in response to an ischemic stimulus[35] probably resulting from endothelial dysfunctioning. Also, the effects of estrogens on the brain are increasingly recognized[36]. Actions include effects on cognitive function, co-ordination of movement, pain and affective state. An intriguing possibility is the putative neuroprotective effect of estrogens preventing or retarding Alzheimer's disease. A better understanding of estrogen receptor physiology with its two subtypes may open up possibilities for selective effects of estrogens in men. This may also be significant for the potentially negative effect of estrogens on prostate disease in old age (see below). Several studies of Vermeulen's group[9] have indicated that plasma estrogen levels do not change with aging in men, resulting in an increased estrogen/androgen ratio in the aging male. Plasma estrogens show a strong correlation with body fat. Severely testosterone-deficient men, however, also have low plasma estrogen levels.

Benefits and risks of androgen supplementation in old age

The phenomena described above might suggest that some signs and symptoms of aging are related to the (statistically reliably demonstrated) decline of androgen levels with old age. However, it is likely that aging itself is the most prominent determinant of this process. The question arises whether androgen supplementation for (selected) aging men might benefit their health. Naturally, before an informed decision can be made, the potential benefits and the disadvantages have to be weighed carefully. On balance, androgens enjoy a dubious medical reputation. They have been implicated in some typically age-related medical conditions of men, such as cardiovascular and prostate disease. Although there is certainly truth in these assumptions, some views need to be modified.

Androgens in cardiovascular disease

Traditionally, it has been thought that the relationship between sex steroids and cardiovascular disease is predominantly determined by the relatively detrimental effects of androgens on lipid profiles. It is then paradoxical that, in cross-sectional studies of men, low levels of testosterone[37–39] appear to be associated with coronary disease and myocardial infarction. Recent research indeed shows that the effects of androgens are much broader than on lipids alone, and that there are effects on other biological systems such as fat distribution, endocrine/paracrine factors produced by the vascular wall (such as endothelins, nitric oxide), blood platelets and coagulation. These studies suggest the intriguing possibility that, in spite of the overall negative effects of androgens on lipid profiles, a lower-than-normal androgen level in aging men is associated with an increase of atherosclerotic disease. It is now commonly accepted that preferential accumulation of fat in the abdominal region is associated with an increased risk of non-insulin-dependent diabetes mellitus (NIDDM) and cardiovascular disease, not only in obese subjects but also even in non-obese subjects[40]. A large number of cross-sectional studies have established a relationship between abdominal obesity and cardiovascular risk factors such as hypertension, dyslipidemia (elevated levels of cholesterol, triglycerides and low-density lipoproteins and low levels of high-density lipoproteins) and impaired glucose tolerance with hyperinsulinemia, a cluster known as the 'insulin resistance syndrome' or 'metabolic syndrome'[41,42]. A number of studies have documented that visceral obesity is associated with low plasma total testosterone levels[43–46]. It remains to be determined whether testosterone administration to men with visceral obesity and low testosterone levels will improve their cardiovascular risk profile.

The above information is relevant to the subject of prostate disease, since obesity and hyperinsulinism and high leptin levels (an index of obesity) seem to be associated with prostate disease in old age (see below).

Prostate disease and androgen supplementation in old age

An immediate concern of androgen supplementation in old age is the development and/or progression of prostate diseases such as benign prostatic hyperplasia (BPH) and prostate carcinoma. Although the etiology of BPH is unknown, it is widely accepted that both conditions do not develop without testosterone exposure early in life up to early adulthood. The present position of experts in the field is that androgens do not truly cause BPH or prostate carcinoma, but that they have a 'permissive' role, also evidenced by the beneficial effects of treatment aiming to reduce the biological effects of androgens on both conditions[47]. This contribution does not address the risks of development of prostate cancer, but focuses on the risks of BPH and LUTS potentially associated with androgen administration to aging men. In this regard, two kinds of information seem pertinent. First, is there a relationship between sex steroid levels and the development and severity of BPH? Second, what are the findings in men receiving androgen administration, usually hypogonadal men, particularly when they are of advanced age?

Epidemiological findings show that, as is common knowledge, the risk of BPH increases sharply with aging. In a 9-year follow-up of 1019 men in the Massachusetts Male Aging Study, no relationship between the development of BPH and serum levels of androgens and estrogens could be detected[48]. An intriguing finding reported by Jin and colleagues[49] studying the effects of androgen deficiency and replacement on prostate zonal volumes was that, even in testosterone-deficient men, the volume of the prostate increases with aging from mid-life on. Apparently, prostate volume shows an age-related increase even in the presence of lower-than-normal testosterone levels. A study in Austrian men provided no evidence that plasma testosterone correlated with prostate volume in elderly men with LUTS[50]. In a series of studies in monozygotic and dizygotic twin pairs, Meikle and co-workers[51] could establish the significance of age and genetic and hereditary factors in the development of prostate enlargement, while testosterone, dihydrotestosterone and testosterone bound to SHBG were not significant factors in prostate size. In summary, the available epidemiological evidence does not provide strong clues that serum levels of androgens or estrogens predict the development of BPH later in life.

With regard to BPH, there is no evidence that androgen administration to hypogonadal[3,51-53] or to eugonadal men[54] increases the incidence of BPH over that observed in control eugonadal men. In the study of Jin and colleagues[49], testosterone replacement in hypogonadal men was unable to restore prostate volume to the size of that in eugonadal men. In hypogonadal men receiving parenteral testosterone preparations, some of the time plasma testosterone levels exceeded the normal range, but apparently this was without consequence for prostate safety[3,49]. A number of studies of androgen supplementation in elderly men who were not hypogonadal have shown that, in the short term, there is only a modest increase in prostate size and in levels of PSA[3,54,55]. In men who had low plasma testosterone for their age and who received testosterone administration, there was no or almost no increase in prostate size or PSA over the placebo groups. When PSA levels increased, then this occurred after 4 weeks of androgen administration until 6 months, whereafter no further increase was observed for as long as 2.5 years. Neither were there changes in urine flow or prostate symptom scores[17-19,25-27,55,56].

So, in conclusion, on the basis of epidemiological and testosterone replacement studies (sometimes resulting in supraphysiological levels), peripheral levels of testosterone (over and above a critical minimal value) are not significant determinants of prostate size and serum PSA. With regard to these insights, restoring plasma testosterone levels to within the normal range seems a defensible treatment option in androgen-deficient men in view of the potential benefits of androgens on bone, muscle, brain and maybe also the cardiovascular system.

Estrogens in prostate disease

It is argued above that estrogens in men of all ages are very relevant for their beneficial effects on bone, the cardiovascular system and maybe the brain. So, it seems pertinent that, in old age, not only androgens but also estrogens remain within normal limits. The counterpart is that not only androgens but also estrogens play an important role in prostate development[57]. Recent knowledge indicates that prostate development depends on the synergistic effect between androgens and estrogens[58,59]. Furthermore, this synergistic effect characterizes the different stages of prostate development in human life.

It is highly remarkable that androgen-related prostate diseases such as BPH and prostate carcinoma develop in a period of life when serum androgen levels are declining in most men, so androgens cannot serve as the only causative factor. However, it is of note that finasteride, a 5α-reductase inhibitor, is capable of reducing prostate volume in patients with BPH by reducing DHT levels[60]. Similarly, LHRH agonists and flutamide, lowering, respectively, androgen production and androgen biological action, are capable of reducing prostate volume in men with BPH. Plasma DHT levels in elderly men are either unchanged or slightly decreased[8], but a slightly elevated DHT level has been found in men with BPH[61]. There is evidence that the development of BPH is correlated to serum estradiol levels[62]. It has been controversial whether, similar to androgens, serum estrogen levels fall with increasing age. Testicular and adrenal androgens are the precursors of estrogens in men, and since both show a decline with aging, it seems reasonable to expect that serum estrogen levels would fall, too. But an important determinant of serum estrogen in old age is subcutaneous fat, and since most men gain weight with aging, there are a significant number of aging men whose serum estrogen levels do not decline. Apart from these considerations it is questionable whether the androgen/estrogen (patho) physiology of the prostate can be judged by the levels of circulating sex steroids. Through its high androgen receptor content, the prostate is capable of accumulating androgens in concentrations considerably higher than in the circulation. Part of the testosterone is locally converted to estradiol, thus allowing local interactions of estrogens and androgens. So, it follows that serum levels of testosterone, DHT and estradiol provide an incomplete picture of the hormonal action within the prostate itself. Since BPH occurs typically in the aging male, the resultant increase in the estradiol/testosterone ratio has been implicated in its pathogenesis, mainly on the basis of observations in dogs.

Histologically, BPH is more of a stromal disease than an epithelial disease. For example, one study found that concentrations of estradiol and estrone increased in the stroma but not in the epithelium, as a function of age[63]. In the normal situation, as opposed to BPH, the concentrations of estradiol and estrone are higher in the epithelium of the prostate than in the stroma. The stromal DHT level shows no correlation with age[63]. One hypothesized mechanism for the effects of estrogens on the prostate is that estrogens can induce transcriptional activity of the androgen receptor[64]. From this, it would seem that inhibition of the biological effects of estradiol might have a beneficial effect on stromal hyperplasia, but studies using the aromatase inhibitor atamestane show that a reduction in estrogen level has no consistently beneficial effect on clinically established BPH[65,66]. Interruption of the negative feedback of estrogens on the hypothalamopituitary axis, however, caused an increase in the level of circulating androgens, which may be an undesired effect. The relationship between estrogens and prostate cancer has received less attention. A recent study indicates that estradiol levels were lower while cortisol levels were higher in men with prostate cancer, compared with age-matched men with LUTS[50]. In summary, while studies in laboratory animals and in vitro show a convincing role for estrogens in prostate pathology of old age, reduction of estrogen action has not yet resulted in successful therapeutic interventions in prostate disease.

Other factors in prostate (patho)physiology

It is increasingly recognized that not only sex hormones but also other hormones and growth factors influence prostate growth, development and disease. Several of these hormonal factors and growth factors interact with androgens and estrogens for their biological expression.

Growth hormone

Growth hormone is a major anabolic hormone, promoting body growth and numerous metabolic processes. Growth hormone binds to the epithelial and stromal cells of the prostate. There is evidence that, in cases of growth hormone excess, prostate enlargement occurs. Growth hormone levels have been found to be higher in men with prostate carcinoma[67]. The overall trend in aging men is, however, a decline of growth hormone, which is more profound than the decline of testosterone when serum levels in the fifth to eighth decades are compared with levels in the second and third decades of life.

The insulin-like growth factor (IGF) axis is a multicomponent network of molecules involved in the regulation of cell growth. The axis includes IGFs, receptors, IGF-binding proteins (IGFBPs) and a group of IGFBP proteases. IGF-I and -II are regarded as two protein growth factors. IGFs are produced in the liver, and enter the circulation and act like hormones, but they may also be produced locally in the tissues. A functional IGF system has been demonstrated in the prostate[68]. Prostate epithelial cells contain IGF-I receptors, and prostatic stromal cells produce and secrete IGF-II. Meanwhile, it is likely that, owing to their mitogenic effects, the IGFs are involved in prostatic disease[69]. Also, nerve growth factor has been postulated to be involved in the etiology of BPH through a mechanism of stromal–epithelial interaction[70].

Insulin has a major function in glucose storage and metabolism. Insulin receptors have been found in rat prostatic epithelial cells but not in stromal cells.

Meanwhile, a relationship between prostate disease and overweight has been found. Since being overweight is associated with hyperinsulinemia, insulin may be one of the links between overweight and prostate pathology[71–74].

Sex hormone-binding globulin

SHBG is a plasma protein synthesized and secreted by the liver. SHBG is best known as a carrier protein for sex steroids. Its initial description stemmed from its ability to bind estrogens and androgens, and its capacity to regulate the free concentration of the steroids that bind to it. However, not only is it a binding protein in the circulation, but it also binds to a specific receptor on the cell membranes. In plasma, SHBG is divided into liganded (bound to a sex steroid) and unliganded forms. Liganded SHBG has no physiological effect on the target cells of the sex steroids because the complex of steroid + SHBG cannot be bound to the sex steroid receptor. Additionally, it participates in signal transduction for certain steroid hormones at the cell membrane. It binds with high affinity to a specific membrane receptor (RSHBG) in prostate stromal and epithelial cells, wherein the SHBG–RSHBG complex forms. An appropriate steroid binds to this complex and results in increases of intracellular cyclic adenosine monophosphate (cAMP)[75,76].

Suitable testosterone preparations

While the evidence that some aging men with proven testosterone deficiency will benefit from androgen supplements is growing, the question becomes whether we have suitable testosterone preparations[77]. The androgen deficiency of the aging male is only partial and, consequently, only partial substitution will be required; it should, preferably, not suppress the hypothalamopituitary hormone secretion, and it should leave the residual testicular androgen production intact. The conventional parenteral testosterone preparations do not meet this requirement; even for young hypogonadal men

they are less than ideal, if not obsolete, on grounds of the strongly fluctuating plasma testosterone level following administration. Oral or transdermal testosterone may be better candidates, although both preparations are associated with high plasma DHT levels following resorption. Whether the elevation of plasma DHT with oral or transdermal administration should be a matter of concern is not known. The target organs of testosterone, in as far as they convert testosterone to DHT, have high local concentrations of DHT, and plasma levels of DHT might rather be a reflection of conversions in these target organs from which the products leak into the circulation. It is currently unknown whether elevated plasma levels of DHT would be of pathophysiological significance. Two recent studies administering DHT to aging men for androgen replacement did not notice any adverse effect on the prostate in the short term[78,79]. In view of the potential role of estrogens in prostate disease in old age, the question has been raised whether administration of DHT might even be advantageous, since DHT cannot be aromatized to estradiol. In cases of hormone deficiencies, traditional endocrinology aims to replace the missing hormone with a substitute hormone, ideally mimicking the natural hormone in molecular structure as closely as possible. Increasing insight into how hormones exert their biological effects has paved the way for rethinking this traditional aim. There may be clinical situations in which the full spectrum is redundant, or may even be harmful by carrying a (long-term) health risk. So, there might be a need for androgens intentionally designed not to render the full spectrum of androgenic actions of the normal testosterone molecule[80]. 7α-Methyl-19-nortestosterone, which is aromatized to estradiol but not 5α-reduced to DHT, and has a very potent anabolic effect but a less potent effect on the prostate, is such a compound. Its biopotency is approximately ten times more than that of normal testosterone with regard to its antigonadotropic and anabolic actions, while the effects on prostate volume are only twice as potent, thereby providing evidence of its potential prostate-sparing effect. How far this type of androgen signifies progress, with regard to safety for the prostate, remains to be determined[81].

The androgen receptor is a transcription factor and a member of the extended family of nuclear receptors, and insights into nuclear receptor activation and function have provided the molecular underpinnings for tissue-selective molecules targeting steroid and other nuclear receptors. Recently, a novel family of non-steroidal molecules has been identified, with selectivity and specificity for the androgen receptor. These compounds possess partial antagonist and partial agonist activity[82]. The availability of these molecules with their diversity of ligands provides the opportunity to explore the utility and activities of so-called selective androgen receptor modulators (SARMs)[80].

Conclusions

There is now convincing evidence that, in a subset of aging men, plasma testosterone levels fall below a critical level, resulting in hypogonadism. This state of testosterone deficiency has an impact on bone, muscle and brain function, and is possibly a factor in the accumulation of visceral fat, which, in turn, has a significant impact on the cardiovascular risk profile. From the above it follows that androgen replacement in selected men with proven androgen deficiency will have beneficial effects. The almost immediate reaction is to question androgen administration in aging men, in view of its potential harmful effects on prostate disease. BPH is typically a disease of the aging male, its incidence increasing sharply with age. This automatic response needs rethinking. Epidemiological studies provide no clues that the levels of circulating androgens are correlated with or predict prostate disease. Similarly, androgen replacement studies in men do not suggest that these men suffer to a higher degree from prostate disease than control

subjects. This is despite the observation that treatment with parenteral testosterone is, part of the time, associated with strongly supraphysiological testosterone levels. Studies providing a definitive answer to whether testosterone replacement in aging men is safe, with regard to the initiation or progression of prostate disease, would require inclusion of several thousand men, and the finances and logistics for such studies are lacking.

The fact that prostate diseases occur in men at a time when most men show an age-related decline of androgens has prompted research into factors other than androgens to explain the age-related increase in prostate disease. On the basis of animal models of BPH, the role of estrogens has received serious attention, although this has not resulted in substantial therapeutically successful interventions aiming at reducing estrogen effects on the prostate. Such interventions would conflict with the recent evidence that estrogens are significant in men for the health of their bones, brain and cardiovascular function. In epidemiological studies, elements of the so-called metabolic syndrome have been found to correlate with prostate disease (obesity, hyperinsulinism, hyperleptinemia). It is remarkable that the metabolic syndrome is associated with lowered testosterone levels, and might theoretically be improved with androgen administration!

On the basis of the above information, it seems a defensible practice to treat aging men with androgens if and when they are testosterone-deficient. Follow-up with regard to side-effects is needed. Before androgens are prescribed, a digital rectal examination of the prostate, a prostate symptom score and determination of PSA level should be undertaken. A re-evaluation after 3 months should take place, whereafter the patient can be checked after longer intervals. Naturally, the patient should be forewarned that prostate symptoms may occur during androgen administration, which may or may not be related to the administration of androgens.

References

1. Frick J, Aulitzky W. Physiology of the prostate. *Infection* 1991;19(Suppl 3):S115–18
2. Leav I, McNeal JE, Kwan PW, *et al.* Androgen receptor expression in prostatic dysplasia (prostatic intraepithelial neoplasia) in the human prostate: an immunohistochemical and *in situ* hybridization study. *Prostate* 1996;29: 137–45
3. Behre HM, Bohmeyer J, Nieschlag E. Prostate volume in testosterone-treated and untreated hypogonadal men in comparison to age-matched normal controls. *Clin Endocrinol (Oxf)* 1994;40:341–9
4. Meikle AW, Arver S, Dobs AS, *et al.* Prostate size in hypogonadal men treated with a nonscrotal permeation-enhanced testosterone transdermal system. *Urology* 1997;49:191–6
5. Cooper CS, Perry PJ, Sparks AE, *et al.* Effect of exogenous testosterone on prostate volume, serum and semen prostate specific antigen levels in healthy young men. *J Urol* 1998;159:441–3
6. Bhasin S, Woodhouse L, Casaburi R, *et al.* Testosterone dose–response relationships in healthy young men. *Am J Physiol Endocrinol Metab* 2001;281:E1172–81
7. Jin B, Turner L, Walters WA, *et al.* The effects of chronic high dose androgen or estrogen treatment on the human prostate [Corrected]. *J Clin Endocrinol Metab* 1996;81:4290–5
8. Gray A, Feldman HA, McKinlay JB, *et al.* Age, disease, and changing sex hormone levels in middle-aged men: results of the Massachusetts Male Aging Study. *J Clin Endocrinol Metab* 1991;73:1016–25
9. Kaufman JM, Vermeulen A. Declining gonadal function in elderly men. *Baillière's Clin Endocrinol Metab* 1997;11:289–309
10. Morley JE, Kaiser FE, Perry HM III, *et al.* Longitudinal changes in testosterone, luteinizing hormone, and follicle-stimulating hormone in healthy older men. *Metabolism* 1997;46:410–13
11. Handelsman DJ. Testicular dysfunction in systemic disease. *Endocrinol Metab Clin North Am* 1994;23:839–56
12. Orwoll ES, Klein RF. Osteoporosis in men. *Endocr Rev* 1995;16:87–116
13. Jones G, Nguyen T, Sambrook P, *et al.* Progressive loss of bone in the femoral neck in elderly people: longitudinal findings from the Dubbo osteoporosis epidemiology study. *Br Med J* 1994; 309:691–5
14. Pfeilschifter J, Scheidt-Nave C, Leidig-Bruckner G, *et al.* Relationship between circulating insulin-like growth factor components and sex hormones in a population-based sample of 50- to 80-year-old men and women. *J Clin Endocrinol Metab* 1996;81:2534–40
15. Finkelstein JS, Neer RM, Biller BM, *et al.* Osteopenia in men with a history of delayed puberty. *N Engl J Med* 1992;326:600–4
16. Katznelson L, Finkelstein JS, Schoenfeld DA, *et al.* Increase in bone density and lean body mass during testosterone administration in men with acquired hypogonadism. *J Clin Endocrinol Metab* 1996;81:4358–65
17. Morley JE, Perry HM III, Kaiser FE, *et al.* Effects of testosterone replacement therapy in old hypogonadal males: a preliminary study. *J Am Geriatr Soc* 1993;41:149–52
18. Tenover JS. Effects of testosterone supplementation in the aging male. *J Clin Endocrinol Metab* 1992;75:1092–8
19. Snyder PJ, Peachey H, Hannoush P, *et al.* Effect of testosterone treatment on bone mineral density in men over 65 years of age. *J Clin Endocrinol Metab* 1999;84:1966–72
20. Faustini-Fustini M, Rochira V, Carani C. Oestrogen deficiency in men: where are we today? *Eur J Endocrinol* 1999;140:111–29
21. Rudman D, Drinka PJ, Wilson CR, *et al.* Relations of endogenous anabolic hormones and physical activity to bone mineral density and lean body mass in elderly men. *Clin Endocrinol (Oxf)* 1994;40:653–61
22. Bross R, Javanbakht M, Bhasin S. Anabolic interventions for aging-associated sarcopenia. *J Clin Endocrinol Metab* 1999;84:3420–30
23. Nair KS. Muscle protein turnover: methodological issues and the effect of aging. *J Gerontol A Biol Sci Med Sci* 1995;50:107–12
24. Baumgartner RN, Waters DL, Gallagher D, *et al.* Predictors of skeletal muscle mass in elderly men and women. *Mech Ageing Dev* 1999;107: 123–36
25. Sih R, Morley JE, Kaiser FE, *et al.* Testosterone replacement in older hypogonadal men: a 12-month randomized controlled trial. *J Clin Endocrinol Metab* 1997;82:1661–7
26. Urban RJ, Bodenburg YH, Gilkison, C, *et al.* Testosterone administration to elderly men increases skeletal muscle strength and protein synthesis. *Am J Physiol* 1995;269:E820–6
27. Snyder PJ, Peachey H, Hannoush P, *et al.* Effect of testosterone treatment on body composition and muscle strength in men over 65 years of age. *J Clin Endocrinol Metab* 1999;84:2647–53
28. Clague JE, Wu FC, Horan MA. Difficulties in measuring the effect of testosterone replacement therapy on muscle function in older men. *Int J Androl* 1999;22:261–5

29. Janowsky JS, Oviatt SK, Orwoll ES. Testosterone influences spatial cognition in older men. *Behav Neurosci* 1994;108:325–32

30. Barrett-Connor E, Goodman-Gruen D, Patay B. Endogenous sex hormones and cognitive function in older men. *J Clin Endocrinol Metab* 1999;84:3681–5

31. Seidman SN, Walsh BT. Testosterone and depression in aging men. *Am J Geriatr Psychiatry* 1999;7:18–33

32. Araujo AB, Durante R, Feldman HA, *et al.* The relationship between depressive symptoms and male erectile dysfunction: cross-sectional results from the Massachusetts Male Aging Study. *Psychosom Med* 1998;60:458–65

33. Couse JF, Korach KS. Estrogen receptor null mice: what have we learned and where will they lead us? *Endocr Rev* 1999;20:358–417

34. Riggs BL, Khosla S, Melton LJ III. A unitary model for involutional osteoporosis: estrogen deficiency causes both type I and type II osteoporosis in postmenopausal women and contributes to bone loss in aging men. *J Bone Miner Res* 1998;13:763–73

35. Sudhir K, Komesaroff PA. Clinical review 110: cardiovascular actions of estrogens in men. *J Clin Endocrinol Metab* 1999;84:3411–15

36. McEwen BS, Alves SE. Estrogen actions in the central nervous system. *Endocr Rev* 1999;20:279–307

37. Barrett-Connor E. Lower endogenous androgen levels and dyslipidemia in men with non-insulin-dependent diabetes mellitus. *Ann Intern Med* 1992;117:807–11

38. Swartz CM, Young MA. Low serum testosterone and myocardial infarction in geriatric male inpatients. *J Am Geriatr Soc* 1987;35:39–44

39. Vermeulen A, Kaufman JM. Androgens and cardiovascular disease in men and women. *Aging Male* 1998;1:35–50

40. Kannel WB, Cupples LA, Ramaswami R, *et al.* Regional obesity and risk of cardiovascular disease; the Framingham Study. *J Clin Epidemiol* 1991;44:183–90

41. Despres JP, Marette A. Relation of components of insulin resistance syndrome to coronary disease risk. *Curr Opin Lipidol* 1994;5:274–89

42. Bjorntorp P. Visceral obesity: a civilization syndrome. *Obesity Res* 1993;1:206–22

43. Marin P, Arver S. Androgens and abdominal obesity. *Baillière's Clin Endocrinol Metab* 1998;12:441–51

44. Seidell JC, Bjorntorp P, Sjostrom L, *et al.* Visceral fat accumulation in men is positively associated with insulin, glucose, and C-peptide levels, but negatively with testosterone levels. *Metabolism* 1990;39:897–901

45. Tchernof A, Labrie F, Belanger A, *et al.* Relationships between endogenous steroid hormone, sex hormone-binding globulin and lipoprotein levels in men: contribution of visceral obesity, insulin levels and other metabolic variables. *Atherosclerosis* 1997;133:235–44

46. Simon D, Charles MA, Nahoul K, *et al.* Association between plasma total testosterone and cardiovascular risk factors in healthy adult men: the Telecom Study. *J Clin Endocrinol Metab* 1997;82:682–5

47. Marcelli M, Cunningham GR. Hormonal signaling in prostatic hyperplasia and neoplasia. *J Clin Endocrinol Metab* 1999;84:3463–8

48. Meigs JB, Mohr B, Barry MJ, *et al.* Risk factors for clinical benign prostatic hyperplasia in a community-based population of healthy aging men. *J Clin Epidemiol* 2001;54:935–44

49. Jin B, Conway AJ, Handelsman DJ. Effects of androgen deficiency and replacement on prostate zonal volumes. *Clin Endocrinol (Oxf)* 2001;54:437–45

50. Schatzl G, Reiter WJ, Thurridl T, *et al.* Endocrine patterns in patients with benign and malignant prostatic diseases. *Prostate* 2000;44:219–24

51. Meikle AW, Stephenson RA, Lewis CM, *et al.* Effects of age and sex hormones on transition and peripheral zone volumes of prostate and benign prostatic hyperplasia in twins. *J Clin Endocrinol Metab* 1997;82:571–5

52. Sasagawa I, Nakada T, Kazama T, *et al.* Volume change of the prostate and seminal vesicles in male hypogonadism after androgen replacement therapy. *Int Urol Nephrol* 1990;22:279–84

53. Behre HM, von Eckardstein S, Kliesch S, *et al.* Long-term substitution therapy of hypogonadal men with transscrotal testosterone over 7–10 years. *Clin Endocrinol (Oxf)* 1999;50:629–35

54. Wallace EM, Pye SD, Wild SR, *et al.* Prostate-specific antigen and prostate gland size in men receiving exogenous testosterone for male contraception. *Int J Androl* 1993;16:35–40

55. Holmang S, Marin P, Lindstedt G, *et al.* Effect of long-term oral testosterone undecanoate treatment on prostate volume and serum prostate-specific antigen concentration in eugonadal middle-aged men. *Prostate* 1993;23:99–106

56. de Lignieres B. Transdermal dihydrotestosterone treatment of 'andropause'. *Ann Med* 1993;25:235–41

57. Thomas JA, Keenan EJ. Effects of estrogens on the prostate. *J Androl* 1994;15:97–9

58. Suzuki K, Takezawa Y, Suzuki T, *et al.* Synergistic effects of estrogen with androgen on the prostate – effects of estrogen on the prostate of androgen-administered rats and 5α-reductase activity. *Prostate* 1994;25:169–76

59. Suzuki K, Ito K, Suzuki T, *et al.* Synergistic effects of estrogen and androgen on the prostate: effects of estrogen on androgen- and estrogen-receptors, BrdU uptake, immunohistochemical

study of AR, and responses to antiandrogens. *Prostate* 1995;26:151–63

60. Gormley GJ, Stoner E, Bruskewitz RC, *et al.* The effect of finasteride in men with benign prostatic hyperplasia. The Finasteride Study Group. *N Engl J Med* 1992;327:1185–91

61. Hammond GL, Kontturi M, Vihko P, *et al.* Serum steroids in normal males and patients with prostatic diseases. *Clin Endocrinol (Oxf)* 1978;9:113–21

62. Gann PH, Hennekens CH, Longcope C, *et al.* A prospective study of plasma hormone levels, nonhormonal factors, and development of benign prostatic hyperplasia. *Prostate* 1995;26:40–9

63. Krieg M, Nass R, Tunn S. Effect of aging on endogenous level of 5α-dihydrotestosterone, testosterone, estradiol, and estrone in epithelium and stroma of normal and hyperplastic human prostate. *J Clin Endocrinol Metab* 1993;77:375–81

64. Yeh S, Miyamoto H, Shima H, *et al.* From estrogen to androgen receptor: a new pathway for sex hormones in prostate. *Proc Natl Acad Sci USA* 1998;95:5527–32

65. Schweikert HU, Tunn UW, Habenicht UF, *et al.* Effects of estrogen deprivation on human benign prostatic hyperplasia. *J Steroid Biochem Mol Biol* 1993;44:573–6

66. Radlmaier A, Eickenberg HU, Fletcher MS, *et al.* Estrogen reduction by aromatase inhibition for benign prostatic hyperplasia: results of a double-blind, placebo-controlled, randomized clinical trial using two doses of the aromatase-inhibitor atamestane. Atamestane Study Group. *Prostate* 1996;29:199–208

67. Colao A, Marzullo P, Spiezia S, *et al.* Effect of two years of growth hormone and insulin-like growth factor-I suppression on prostate diseases in acromegalic patients. *J Clin Endocrinol Metab* 2000;85:3754–61

68. Cohen P, Peehl DM, Rosenfeld RG. The IGF axis in the prostate. *Horm Metab Res* 1994;26:81–4

69. Shi R, Berkel HJ, Yu H. Insulin-like growth factor-I and prostate cancer: a meta-analysis. *Br J Cancer* 2001;85:991–6

70. Graham CW, Lynch JH, Djakiew D. Distribution of nerve growth factor-like protein and nerve growth factor receptor in human benign prostatic hyperplasia and prostatic adenocarcinoma. *J Urol* 1992;147:1444–7

71. Hsing AW, Chua S Jr, Gao YT, *et al.* Prostate cancer risk and serum levels of insulin and leptin: a population-based study. *J Natl Cancer Inst* 2001;93:783–9

72. Stattin P, Soderberg S, Hallmans G, *et al.* Leptin is associated with increased prostate cancer risk: a nested case–referent study. *J Clin Endocrinol Metab* 2001;86:1341–5

73. Hammarsten J, Hogstedt B. Hyperinsulinaemia as a risk factor for developing benign prostatic hyperplasia. *Eur Urol* 2001;39:151–8

74. Lehrer S, Diamond EJ, Stagger S, *et al.* Increased serum insulin associated with increased risk of prostate cancer recurrence. *Prostate* 2002;50:1–3

75. Ding VD, Moller DE, Feeney WP, *et al.* Sex hormone-binding globulin mediates prostate androgen receptor action via a novel signaling pathway. *Endocrinology* 1998;139:213–18

76. Hryb DJ, Nakhla AM, Kahn SM, *et al.* Sex hormone-binding globulin in the human prostate is locally synthesized and may act as an autocrine/paracrine effector. *J Biol Chem* 2002;277:26618–22

77. Bhasin S, Bagatell CJ, Bremner WJ, *et al.* Issues in testosterone replacement in older men. *J Clin Endocrinol Metab* 1998;83:3435–48

78. Ly LP, Jimenez M, Zhuang TN, *et al.* A double-blind, placebo-controlled, randomized clinical trial of transdermal dihydrotestosterone gel on muscular strength, mobility, and quality of life in older men with partial androgen deficiency. *J Clin Endocrinol Metab* 2001;86:4078–88

79. Kunelius P, Lukkarinen O, Hannuksela ML, *et al.* The effects of transdermal dihydrotestosterone in the aging male: a prospective, randomized, double blind study. *J Clin Endocrinol Metab* 2002;87:1467–72

80. Negro-Vilar A. Selective androgen receptor modulators (SARMs): a novel approach to androgen therapy for the new millennium. *J Clin Endocrinol Metab* 1999;84:3459–62

81. Cummings DE, Kumar N, Bardin CW, *et al.* Prostate-sparing effects in primates of the potent androgen 7α-methyl-19-nortestosterone: a potential alternative to testosterone for androgen replacement and male contraception. *J Clin Endocrinol Metab* 1998;83:4212–19

82. Zhi L, Tegley CM, Marschke KB, *et al.* Switching androgen receptor antagonists to agonists by modifying C-ring substituents on piperidino [3,2-g]quinolinone. *Bioorg Med Chem Lett* 1999;9:1009–12

Diagnosis, classification and therapy development for human prostate cancer using biochip technologies and post-genomic era molecular medicine

14

O.-P. Kallioniemi, M. Wolf, L. Bubendorf and S. Mousses

Introduction

Prostate cancer has remained a mysterious disease in terms of its etiology, biological and genetic basis, natural history, clinical presentation and progression. Substantial controversies exist about issues such as screening, diagnosis and treatment. Research into the molecular basis of prostate cancer has revealed numerous clues to the disease process, but definitive solutions to clinical dilemmas are few in number, and no effective therapies exist for advanced prostate cancer. We are now becoming more aware of the enormous complexity that underlies the molecular 'wiring diagram' of the cancer cells. In the light of this extreme complexity, it is hardly surprising that the few genes, such as the androgen receptor, that have so far been used as targets for therapy development have not yielded a cure. New tools, technologies and resources will be needed to unravel the mysteries of prostate cancer. Such technologies have now started to emerge with the launch of the post-genomics era and biochip technologies.

Now that the human genome sequence is published[1], we have at our disposal the building blocks of human life. Knowledge of our genes also forms the basis for a rational understanding of the cancer development process. Advances in translational genomics could profoundly impact upon prostate cancer research, early diagnosis, molecular classification and therapy development, and lead us towards personalized medicine. Genome sequence, however, is only the first frontier, and much additional research will be needed to turn this basic research breakthrough into a deeper understanding of cancer development, and particularly into clinical benefits. The possibilities of basic science do not change medical practice overnight. More likely, this will take a decade for the progress to flow to the clinical arena, and will require active participation of both clinicians and basic scientists. Also, we will need to develop better tools to analyze not only the genome (DNA), but also the transcriptome (RNA) and proteome (proteins). These data will have to be integrated to develop a comprehensive, global view of the cancer development process and to identify weak points as targets for drug development.

In this chapter we review some of the possibilities and challenges that lie ahead as we move from genome sequence to research on functional genomics and proteomics and to molecular diagnostics and treatment tailored against the biological properties of the cancer cells. The focus of this review is describing technologies that may facilitate applied genomics research and clinical implementation.

Genomics: now we know it all, or do we?

A conservative estimate of the number of genes in the human genome is ~35 000[1]. This is only slightly more than the number of genes in lower organisms, such as fly (*Drosophila*) or worm (*Caenorhabditis elegans*). The relatively low number of human genes highlights a number of important features of human cell biology. First, non-coding regulatory sites in the genome are likely to be critical in directing the complex gene expression patterns of human cells. Second, the process of RNA splicing determines how many proteins will be made from a given gene sequence. A single gene sequence may be transcribed and spliced into multiple different mRNA species, each of which encodes a different protein variant. Third, each protein may then undergo multiple, highly complex post-translational modifications, such as glycosylation, phosphorylation, etc. Therefore, a single gene may encode dozens, if not hundreds, of different proteins, often with differing or even opposing effects. Fourth, several genes are not encoding proteins, but produce RNA molecules that have a regulatory role. Methods that would enable us comprehensively to survey all this complexity of the transcriptome and proteome do not even exist yet. However, substantial advances in exploring functional genomics of prostate cancer have taken place using cDNA microarray technologies.

Functional genomics: the 'living genome'

Functional genomics refers to the analysis of gene expression changes throughout the genome using microarrays and other high-throughput tools. The expression levels of all human genes can be quantified simultaneously by hybridizing labelled cDNAs from a tumor sample against a microarray of oligos or cDNA clones representing all human genes. Such gene expression profiles are highly useful for diagnostic efforts. For example, two or more different tumor types can be objectively identified, and subclasses of tumors with a similar histological appearance, but different biological or clinical properties, can be distinguished.

Several applications of the technology in prostate cancer research have already been published. Luo and co-workers studied the differences in gene expression profiles between benign prostatic hyperplasia and prostate cancer[2]. They reported that the patterns of gene expression in these samples were significantly different, facilitating diagnostic classification and understanding of the molecular basis of these diseases, as well as identifying markers for clinical diagnosis and therapy. We identified characteristic gene expression patterns in human prostate cancer before, during and after androgen-deprivation therapy[3]. Characteristic gene expression patterns could be defined for all these states. Two distinct gene expression programs contributed to hormone therapy failure: first, reactivation of androgen-responsive genes, and second, activation of other, progression-associated genes. Finally, gene expression profiling can be used to identify critical target genes for therapy. For example, activation of the EZH2 gene, a polycomb group protein involved in transcriptional repression, was shown to be causally involved in prostate cancer growth and metastatic progression[4].

Comparative genomic hybridization microarrays: identifying primary gene targets that may drive cancer progression

The vast amount of data collected by cDNA microarrays raises the question whether these gene expression changes reflect primary genetic alterations driving tumor progression or secondary downstream changes. In leukemias and lymphomas, cytogenetic clues have played a major role in pinpointing critical primary cancer genes and therapeutic targets, whereas only limited progress in similar studies of solid tumors has so far been achieved. Integration of the 'functional genomic view' of the cancer genome with the 'genetic or chromosomal view' could lead to the identification of primary genes playing a critical role in the development and progression of solid tumors.

New array-based comparative genomic hybridization (CGH) technologies enable the study of gene copy number changes (amplifications and deletions) throughout the genome virtually at a single gene resolution[5].

Furthermore, consequences that gene copy number changes have on gene expression patterns can be readily studied. This makes it possible directly to identify genes that are activated by DNA amplifications. As demonstrated for the HER-2 oncogene, which is amplified and overexpressed in breast cancer, such amplification target genes may provide invaluable starting points for anticancer drug development.

We hybridized differentially labelled genomic DNA from prostate cancer cell lines and normal reference to a microarray of cDNA clones (Wolf and colleagues, unpublished data). This made it possible to measure copy number changes of 15 000 genes throughout the genome at a time. Prostate cancer cells often have amplifications of the 10q22 chromosomal region, indicating that this region may harbor genes that play a role in prostate cancer progression. High-resolution CGH microarray analysis indicated that there are several regions of amplification at 10q, and pinpointed the critical regions of involvement with virtually single gene precision. Furthermore, analysis of gene expression changes of all genes along chromosome 10 indicated that the amplifications lead to the activation of numerous genes, some of which could possibly serve as candidate targets for therapy development. CGH microarray analysis may significantly help to narrow down the focus in the search of therapeutically important genes in the genome.

Cell-based microarrays: functional studies of cancer cells

Cell microarrays or cell chips enable the analysis of consequences of gene up-regulation or down-regulation on cell functions, phenotypes or signalling pathways. Compared with the descriptive molecular profiling methods of genomics and proteomics, cell-based microarrays provide information on cause and effect relationships, and are therefore ideally applicable to the validation of targets for novel anticancer therapies.

Cell-based arrays can be constructed using a number of methods. An ingenious method for this purpose was described by the Sabatini group at the Whitehead Institute[6]. Genes in expression vectors are printed as a microarray on a glass slide. Instead of using the array in a hybridization experiment, the microarray slide is placed in a cell culture flask, and living cells are plated to grow on top of the microarray. In a process called reverse transfection, the cDNA clones enter cells and are being translated to a protein, which may in turn have a measurable phenotypic or molecular effect on the cells. The process of reverse transfection can be substantially scaled up to analyze hundreds, if not thousands, of genes.

Similarly, using antisense oligonucleotides or small interfering RNAs[4], one could specifically turn down the expression of specific genes in the cells and explore the consequences on cell phenotypes. Modulating the expression levels of genes in living cells in a microarray format has powerful implications for exploring the cell signalling pathways, identifying drug targets and facilitating a 'systems biology' approach to the studies of the 'wiring diagrams' of cancer cells. Cell microarrays and other functional assay systems are fundamentally different from regular genomics and proteomics technologies that only enable analyses of gene and protein expression changes as well as correlations and patterns among these molecules. In contrast, cell-based microarrays make it possible to infer cause and effect associations and consequences of gene expression alterations.

Tissue microarrays: clinical translation of genomics and proteomics

Often the molecular targets of interest need to be studied in the context of cancer or normal tissues, integrating morphological information with the molecular level data and expanding the studies to large cohorts of patients, perhaps hundreds or thousands of cases. For such analyses, assay costs may become prohibitively expensive when dozens of targets need to be explored. Furthermore, sufficient quantities of fresh–frozen tissues are often not available for molecular analyses.

Tissue microarray (TMA) technology is based on the arraying of hundreds of tissue specimens at high density on microscope slides[7]. TMA technology enables rapid visualization of molecular targets in thousands of arrayed tissue specimens at a time, at the DNA, RNA or protein level. This facilitates rapid translation of molecular discoveries to clinical applications, particularly when large cohorts of patient samples from retrospective tissue archives, tissue banks or clinical trial materials need to be investigated. By revealing the cellular localization, prevalence and clinical significance of candidate target molecules in tissues, TMAs are ideally suitable for genomics-based diagnostic and drug target discovery, validation and prioritization.

TMAs have a number of advantages compared with conventional techniques of analyzing tissue samples. The speed of molecular analysis is increased by up to 100-fold, precious tissues are not destroyed and a large number of different molecular targets can be analyzed from consecutive TMA sections. The ability to study archival tissue specimens is an important advantage, as such specimens are usually more readily available in existing tumor banks in large quantities, often with associated demographic, pathological, clinical, treatment and follow-up data. Furthermore, such tissues are not at all applicable to other high-throughput genomic and proteomic surveys. Construction and analysis of TMAs can be automated, increasing the throughput further.

There are many applications of TMA technology in cancer research, including:

(1) Identification of the inter- and intracellular molecular target distribution in tumor samples;

(2) Analysis of the frequency of molecular alterations in large tumor materials;

(3) Exploration of tumor progression by including samples from normal tissues, hyperplasia, invasion, metastasis and therapy failure;

(4) Identification of predictive or prognostic factors and validation of newly discovered genes as diagnostic and therapeutic targets.

TMAs provide a high-throughput methodology for microscopic examination of tissue specimens in the post-genome era.

Using TMA technology, we showed how amplification of the androgen receptor (AR) gene and overexpression of the insulin-like growth factor-binding protein-2 (IGFBP-2) were common in hormone-refractory end-stage prostate cancers, but infrequent in untreated primary tumors[8,9]. These kinds of clinical associations could be rapidly ascertained by constructing a prostate cancer 'progression TMA' that included dozens of tissue samples from all stages of prostate cancer development, starting from normal prostate, and progressing through benign prostatic hyperplasia, prostatic intraepithelial neoplasia and localized clinical cancer to metastatic and hormone-refractory end-stage cancer. Perrone and co-workers[10] reported differences in tumor proliferation rates between matched prostate cancer cases from Caucasians and African–Americans using TMA technology. This indicates how demographic, genetic or other etiological risk factors can be rapidly associated with molecular or phenotypic characteristics of cancers. Dhanasekaran and co-workers identified and validated prognostic biomarkers in prostate cancer (hepsin transmembrane protease and a serine–threonine kinase PIM-1[11] as well as the EZH2 gene[4]).

Conclusions

Progress in genome sequencing has initiated a new wave of research based on the comprehensive molecular profiling of prostate cancers. Genome sequence-based research has led to 'functional genomic' and, most recently, 'proteomic' research strategies that all produce an overview of the molecular fingerprint of the cancer genome. The challenge for the future is how to turn the enormous quantities of research data obtained using these tools into knowledge of the signalling cascades and molecular wiring diagrams. This should be highly useful to identify 'weak links' in the cellular signal processing network that could be targeted therapeutically. The second enormous challenge is how to translate these data to the clinical setting. The tools, technologies and strategies described in this review of translational cancer genomics research may facilitate this goal. All the various technologies will need to be integrated with sample acquisition and pathological and clinical characterization of the tumors and patients, as well as with the process of clinical trials, to identify the role that this new post-genomic era 'molecular medicine' could have on the management of prostate cancer patients in the future.

References

1. http://genome.cse.ucsc.edu/, http://www.ncbi.nlm.nih.gov/, http://www.ensembl.org/
2. Luo J, Duggan DJ, Chen Y, et al. Human prostate cancer and benign prostatic hyperplasia: molecular dissection by gene expression profiling. Cancer Res 2001;61:4683–8
3. Mousses S, Wagner U, Chen Y, et al. Failure of hormone therapy in prostate cancer involves restoration of an androgen dependent gene expression program and activation of rapamycin sensitive signaling. Oncogene 2001;20:6718–23
4. Varambally S, Dhanasekaran SM, Zhou M, et al. The polycomb protein EZH2 is involved in progression of prostate cancer. Nature (London) 2002;419:624–9
5. Pollack JR, Perou CM, Alizadeh AA, et al. Genome-wide analysis of DNA copy-number changes using cDNA microarrays. Nature Genet 1999;23:41–6
6. Ziauddin J, Sabatini DM. Microarrays of cells expressing defined cDNAs. Nature (London) 2001;411:107–10
7. Kononen J, Bubendorf L, Kallioniemi A, et al. Tissue microarrays for high-throughput molecular profiling of tumor specimens. Nature Med 1998;4:844–7
8. Bubendorf L, Kononen J, Koivisto P, et al. Survey of gene amplifications during prostate cancer progression by high-throughout fluorescence in situ hybridization on tissue microarrays. Cancer Res 1999;59:803–6
9. Bubendorf L, Kolmer M, Kononen J, et al. Hormone therapy failure in human prostate cancer: analysis by complementary DNA and tissue microarrays. J Natl Cancer Inst 1999;91:1758–64
10. Perrone EE, Theoharis C, Mucci NR, et al. Tissue microarray assessment of prostate cancer tumor proliferation in African–American and white men. J Natl Cancer Inst 2000;92:937–9
11. Dhanasekaran SM, Barrette TR, Ghosh D, et al. Delineation of prognostic biomarkers in prostate cancer. Nature (London) 2001;412:822–6

Candidate genetic markers and therapeutic targets in hereditary and sporadic prostate cancer

15

P. Berthon

Introduction

Improvements in screening and treatment have led to a steady decline in mortality from prostate cancer over the past 10 years. Yet prostate cancer remains a leading cause of death among European and North American men over 50[1]. Localized tumors can be removed by radical surgery or destroyed by radiotherapy, but almost 40% of patients already have occult metastases that necessitate second-line therapy. Since the work of Huggins and colleagues in the 1940s[2], androgen withdrawal, aimed at triggering hormone-dependent apoptosis of the prostatic epithelium, has been the cornerstone of treatment for advanced, metastatic prostate adenocarcinomas. However, patients who relapse during hormone withdrawal therapy have no curative treatment options. The search for genetic, epigenetic and environmental factors involved in this malignancy really started in the early 1990s, when the first genetic map was released[3], and was boosted by publication of the human genome in 2001[4].

Genetic factors involved in prostate carcinogenesis can be divided into three categories according to their origin and penetrance (i.e. the frequency of individuals with a given genotype who develop prostate cancer), namely inherited predisposition, inherited susceptibility and acquired events.

Inherited predisposition to prostate cancer

Epidemiological studies conducted over the past 50 years have identified familial clusters of prostate cancer, pointing to an inherited form of the disease. Hereditary prostate cancer is generally diagnosed in families in which at least three first-degree relatives have the disease, or in which two relatives are diagnosed before age 55 years[5]. Carter's model suggests the transmission of a rare autosomal dominant gene (allele frequency 0.003) with high age-dependent penetrance (88% at 85 years). The cumulative proportions of affected subjects with this gene have been estimated at 43%, 34% and 9%, respectively, before 55, 70 and 85 years of age[6,7]. The very steep increase in the frequency of prostate cancer with age in elderly men, and improvements in early detection (in terms of both age and stage), have demonstrated familial clustering in elderly men with no evidence of inherited factors (high age-dependent phenocopy rate).

To identify this predisposing gene, several genome-wide screening studies have been performed in familial prostate cancer. At least six predisposing genes have so far been identified (Figure 1), namely *HPC1* in chromosome region 1q24–25, *PCaP* on 1q42.2–43, *CaPB* on 1p36, *Elac2* on 17p11.2, *HPC20* on 20q13 and *HPCX* on Xq27–28, the last being X-recessive[8]. The genetic heterogeneity of prostate cancer has hindered attempts to confirm these findings. Moreover, precise genetic mapping remains problematic despite the availability of most of the human genome sequence. To identify a culprit gene, it is necessary to analyze the full sequences of up to 150 genes present in the target region, and to compare linked and non-linked family members. In addition, the candidate genetic alteration may lie within

Inherited predisposing event

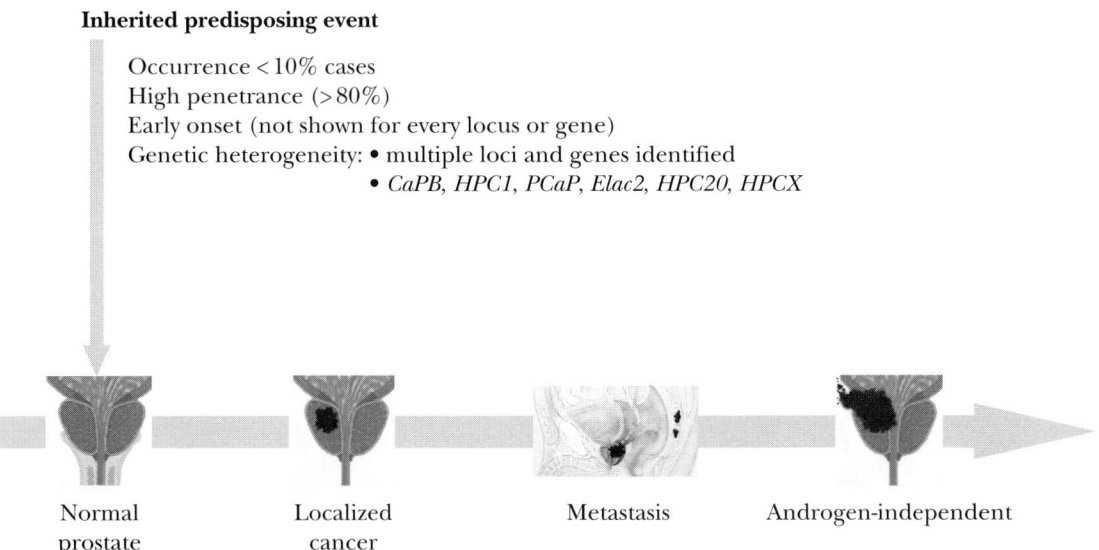

Occurrence < 10% cases
High penetrance (>80%)
Early onset (not shown for every locus or gene)
Genetic heterogeneity: • multiple loci and genes identified
• *CaPB, HPC1, PCaP, Elac2, HPC20, HPCX*

Normal prostate   Localized cancer   Metastasis   Androgen-independent

Figure 1   Main criteria of inherited predisposition to prostate cancer

the coding sequence, the splicing regions or the promoter. This may explain why only one gene – *Elac2* on 17p11.2 – has so far been cloned. Attempts to confirm *Elac2* as a prostate cancer-predisposing gene remain inconclusive.

Associations between clinical parameters and inheritance have been studied. Hereditary prostate cancer is diagnosed, on average, 6–7 years earlier than sporadic prostate cancer[9,10]. On the other hand, the relationship between inherited predisposing genes and prostate cancer progression based on standard clinical parameters is controversial[11].

Available microsatellite markers cannot be used to estimate the individual risk of developing prostate cancer. Regular prostate-specific antigen (PSA) assay should be started before age 50 years in members of high-risk families, who should also be offered basic genetic counselling[9].

Inherited susceptibility to prostate cancer

Apart from a positive family history, the only recognized risk factors for prostate cancer are age and ethnicity. Melanoderms have a higher risk of developing prostate cancer than Caucasians and flavoderms. Both genetic and environmental factors are thought to underlie these ethnic differences. Polymorphisms of the genes encoding the androgen receptor, 5α-reductase type II (*SRD5A2*), p450c17 (*CYP17*), aromatase (*CYP19*) and the vitamin D receptor, leading to variations in endogenous factors such as circulating levels of sex steroids, have been linked to the risk of prostate cancer (Figure 2). These polymorphisms may explain risk variations among ethnic groups and geographic areas[12].

These observations have prompted population-based association studies to determine the role of genetic polymorphisms, single nucleotide polymorphisms (SNPs) and microsatellite instabilities. For example, several studies of North American populations have revealed links between shorter CAG repeats (< 22 or < 18) of the androgen receptor exon 1 and the incidence, age of onset or stage of prostate cancer. No such link was found in a French–German Caucasian population, pointing to the importance of the ethnic mix of the North American population. Polymorphisms of the vitamin D receptor gene have been linked to prostate cancer susceptibility in both Europe and North America[13]. Association studies between the 171-bp allele of *CYP19* and the risk of prostate carcinoma suggested that aromatase

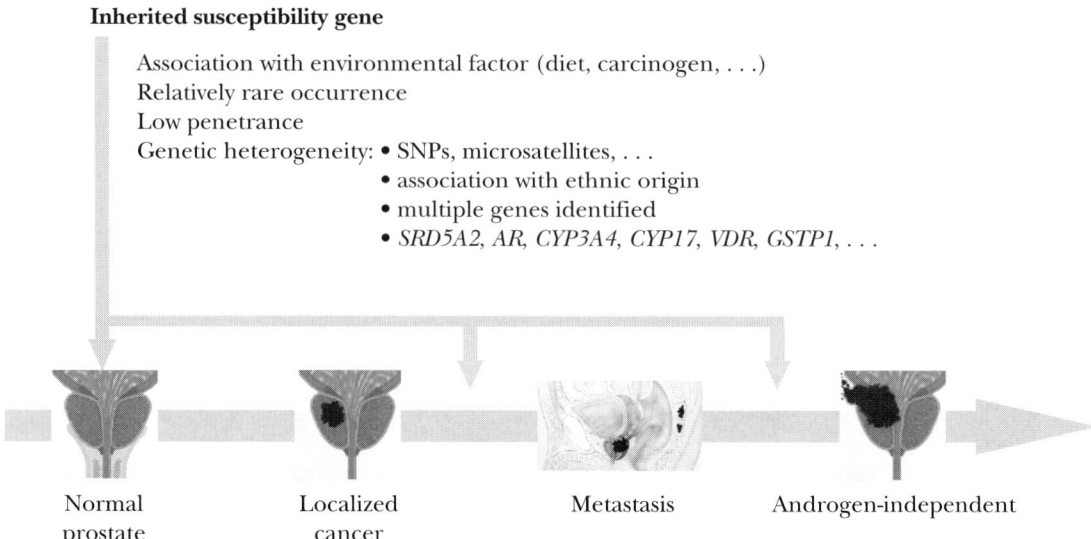

Inherited susceptibility gene

Association with environmental factor (diet, carcinogen, . . .)
Relatively rare occurrence
Low penetrance
Genetic heterogeneity: • SNPs, microsatellites, . . .
                   • association with ethnic origin
                   • multiple genes identified
                   • *SRD5A2, AR, CYP3A4, CYP17, VDR, GSTP1*, . . .

| Normal prostate | Localized cancer | Metastasis | Androgen-independent |

Figure 2 Main criteria of inherited susceptibility to prostate cancer. These subtle genetic alterations could be associated with both disease onset and tumor aggressiveness. SNP, single nucleotide polymorphism

could be used as a new indicator for prostate carcinoma prevention, at least in Western Europe[14]. Some individuals may carry both high- and low-risk markers (e.g. *CYP17*A2 allele and V89L in *SRD5A2*), resulting in no overall difference in risk across the population. The observed discrepancies might also be due to difficulties in obtaining well-defined populations, documenting environmental factors and developing appropriate statistical models to analyze this complex multitrait disease. A polygenic model incorporating multiple loci of individual genes might thus maximize the chances of identifying individuals with high-risk genotypes.

A large proportion of familial prostate cancers may be due not to segregation of a few major gene mutations with monogenic inheritance but rather to familial sharing of alleles at many loci, each leading to a small increase in risk.

Sporadic genetic alterations in prostate cancer

Maintaining genomic integrity is of primary importance for the cell. If this integrity is altered, leading to proliferation, the daughter cells may contain clonal alterations such as subtle mutations, microdeletions or amplifications, losses or gains of chromosomes, and chromosomal rearrangements. Gross cytogenetic modifications have been observed in prostate cancer, but most results point to a role of loss of heterozygosity (LOH) and subtle mutations (Figure 3). These alterations may affect genomic stability by inactivating 'mutator' genes (DNA mismatch repair activity), or by stimulating telomerase activity. Also, these alterations may involve gain (oncogene activation) or loss of function (tumor suppressor gene inactivation) of genes involved in specific signalling pathways or complex physiological processes such as angiogenesis and apoptosis.

The most consistent losses of heterozygosity in prostate adenocarcinoma affect regions of chromosome arms 7q, 8p, 10q, 13q, 16q, 17q and 18q[15] (Figure 4). These regions have recently been studied by using regularly spaced polymorphic probes (microsatellite markers). Several deleted regions have thus been identified on a given chromosome arm, further complicating the identification of relevant tumor-suppressor genes. For example, at least three deleted regions have been found on chromosome arm 8p, and most are common to

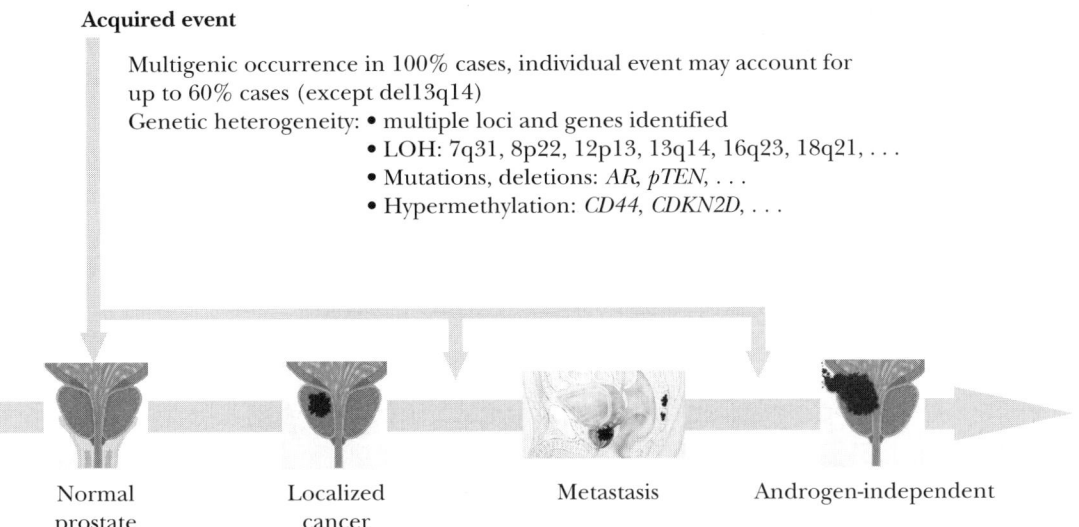

Acquired event

Multigenic occurrence in 100% cases, individual event may account for up to 60% cases (except del13q14)

Genetic heterogeneity: • multiple loci and genes identified
  • LOH: 7q31, 8p22, 12p13, 13q14, 16q23, 18q21, . . .
  • Mutations, deletions: *AR, pTEN,* . . .
  • Hypermethylation: *CD44, CDKN2D,* . . .

Normal prostate	Localized cancer	Metastasis	Androgen-independent

Figure 3 Main criteria of lifetime-acquired genetic events involved in the initiation and progression of prostate cancer. LOH, loss of heterozygosity

prostate carcinoma and other malignancies[16]. This suggests that a single suppressor gene may play a part in the genesis of several cancers or, alternatively, that each of several genes in a given region has a particular function in one type of cancer.

Loss of heterozygosity (LOH) on chromosome arm 13q14 is one of the most recurrent anomalies in sporadic prostate tumors (Figure 5). This LOH is believed to unmask recessive mutations that inactivate one or more tumor-suppressor genes that normally regulate normal cell growth and suppress abnormal cell proliferation. While 13q14 LOH was initially suspected to affect *RB1*, a key cell-cycle regulator, the main target that is deleted or down-regulated as a result of 13q14 LOH remains to be identified. One gene, *CHC1-L* (chromosome condensation 1-like), has been mapped to the smallest common deleted region. *CHC1-L* expression is significantly reduced in prostate tumors compared with normal prostate tissues, as measured by real-time quantitative reverse transcriptase-polymerase chain reaction (RT-PCR). Although *CHC1-L* is not an obvious candidate, given its known homology to *RCC1* (a guanine nucleotide exchange factor for the *Ras*-related guanosine triphosphatase (GTPase)

Ran), the frequent and marked decrease in its expression in prostate cancer, together with the different frequency of *CHC1-L* variant isoforms between normal and neoplastic prostate tissues, suggests either that it plays a pivotal role in prostate cancer or that it is adjacent to a gene with such a role[17]. Several other candidate genes have been mapped since the *Human Genome Working Draft* was published[4], and are currently being evaluated for correlations between LOH status, individual gene expression and second allele alterations.

LOH and target genes lying in these regions are good candidates for molecular diagnosis and prognostication. Genetic alterations in prostatic cells collected in urinary sediments show promise in this respect[18]. Some such alterations are potential prognostic factors, such as deletion of chromosome region 8p22 (prediction of disease progression)[19] and deletions at 12p12–13 and 13q (tumor aggressiveness)[20–22] (Figure 6). Chromosome regions 7q31, 8p22, 12p13, 13q14, 16q23.2 and 18q21 have been analyzed in prostatic cells collected in urinary sediments after prostatic massage, with the aim of determining the diagnostic value of genetic alterations in conjunction with PSA assay. One major objective is to reduce the rate

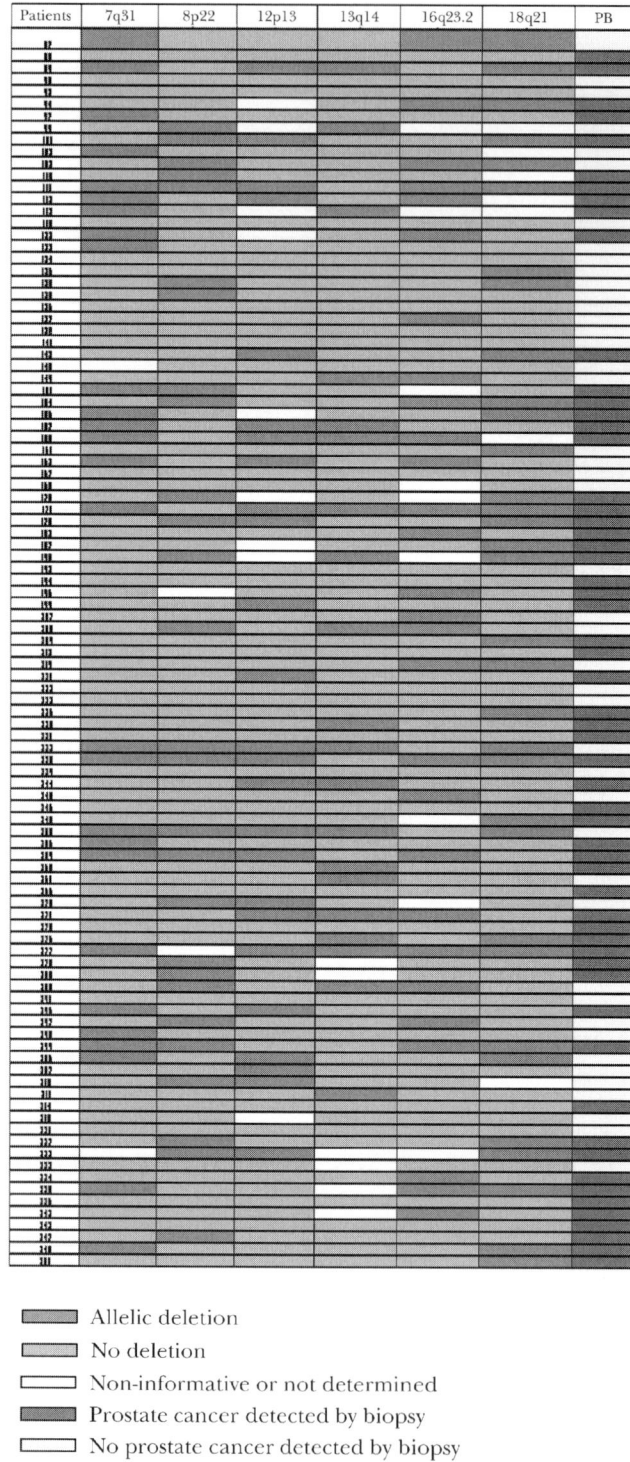

Figure 4 Results of loss of heterozygosity (LOH) analysis of six chromosome regions in 103 patients with total prostate-specific antigen (tPSA) values ranging from 2.5 to 10 ng/ml. Note the high frequency of loss of heterozygosity even in early-stage prostate cancer

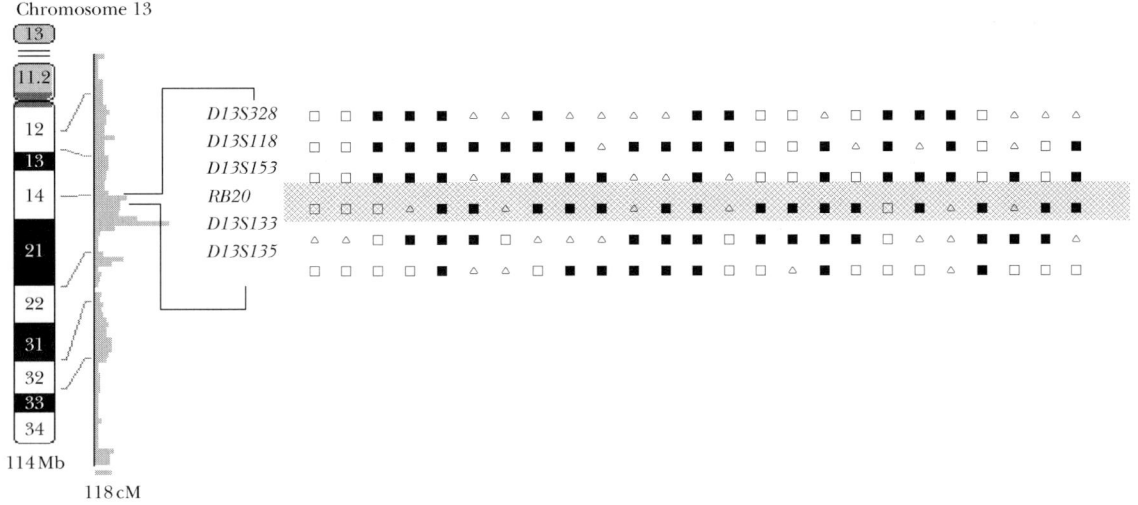

Figure 5 Loss of heterozygosity on chromosome arm 13q14 in prostate cancer patients, defining a minimal commonly deleted region around the *RB1* locus (shaded zone). Filled squares, microsatellite instability; open squares, no deletion (informative); open triangles, homozygotes (non-informative)

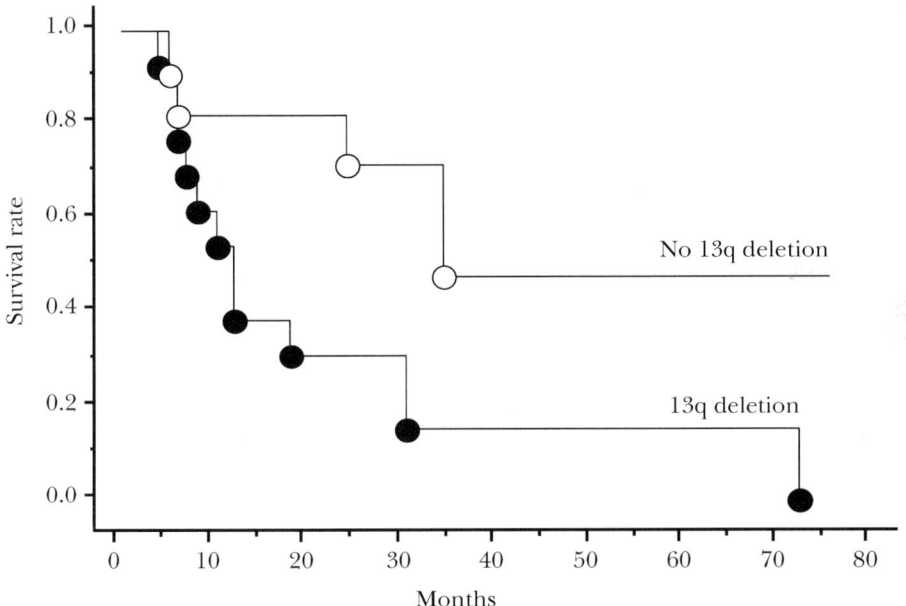

Figure 6 Survival of prostate cancer patients with and without deletions in chromosome arm 13q14

of unnecessary prostate biopsies. The LOH–free/total PSA combination reportedly has 91.9% diagnostic sensitivity, a value far higher than that obtained for telomerase activity[23] or *GSTP1* hypermethylation (27%)[24]. However, some 'false-negative' patients have

non-informative loci (because of marker homozygosity), reducing the sensitivity and specificity of the test.

LOH should lead to down-regulation of tumor suppressor genes. These genes and their protein products are considered as negative regulators of cell growth, DNA repair, etc. These underexpressed genes are not currently very promising as therapeutic targets, as most treatments are designed to antagonize a biological function rather than to mimic a missing function. However, we are confident that careful analysis of gene functions, their localization at the cellular level and their signalling pathways should rapidly lead to therapeutic advances.

Conclusions

Identification of genetic events involved in prostate cancer onset and progression should eventually improve the diagnosis, prognostication and treatment of this very frequent disease. As in other complex diseases such as schizophrenia, diabetes and breast cancer, the hunt for inherited predisposing and susceptibility genes, and for acquired genetic alterations, will require much time and energy. Statistical power and combined analysis, including the stratification of genetic information according to clinical and environmental factors, are required to determine the precise contribution of genetic events to prostate cancer, at both the individual and the population level. Original diagnostic and therapeutic approaches based on specific genetic defects should soon become available.

References

1. http:/www.dep.iarc.fr
2. Huggins C, Stevens RE, Hodges CV. Studies on prostatic cancer: II. The effects of castration on advanced carcinoma of the prostate gland. *Arch Surg* 1991;43:209–23
3. Weissenbach J, Gyapay G, Dib C, *et al.* A second-generation linkage map of the human genome. *Nature (London)* 1992;359:794–801
4. Human genome, public and private. *Nature* 2001;409:745–964
5. Cussenot O, Valeri A, Berthon P, *et al.* Hereditary prostate cancer and other genetic predisposition to prostate cancer. *Urol Int* 1998;5:30–4
6. Carter BS, Beaty TH, Steinberg GD, *et al.* Mendelian inheritance of familial prostate cancer. *Proc Natl Acad Sci USA* 1992;89:3367–71
7. Carter BS, Bova GS, Beaty TH, *et al.* Hereditary prostate cancer: epidemiologic and clinical features. *J Urol* 1993;150:797–802
8. Ostrander EA, Stanford J. Genetics of prostate cancer: too many loci, too few genes. *Am J Hum Genet* 2000;67:1367–75
9. Valeri A, Cormier L, Moineau MP, *et al.* Targeted screening for prostate cancer in high risk families: early onset is a significant risk factor for disease in first degree relatives. *J Urol* 2002;168:483–7
10. Bratt O. Hereditary prostate cancer: clinical aspects. *J Urol* 2002;168:906–13
11. Valeri A, Azzouzi R, Drelon E, *et al.* Early-onset hereditary prostate cancer is not associated with specific clinical and biological features. *Prostate* 2000;45:66–71
12. Cussenot O, Valeri A. Heterogeneity in genetic susceptibility to prostate cancer. *Eur J Intern Med* 2001;12:11–16
13. Correa-Cerro L, Berthon P, Haussler J, *et al.* Vitamin D receptor polymorphisms as markers in prostate cancer. *Hum Genet* 1999;105:281–7
14. Latil AG, Azzouzi R, Cancel GS, *et al.* Prostate carcinoma risk and allelic variants of genes involved in androgen biosynthesis and metabolism pathways. *Cancer* 2001;92:1130–7
15. Latil A, Lidereau R. Genetic aspects of prostate cancer. *Virchow's Arch* 1998;432:389–406
16. Rodriguez E, Sreekantaiah C, Chaganti RSK. Genetic changes in epithelial solid neoplasia. *Cancer Res* 1994;54:3398–406
17. Latil A, Morant P, Fournier G, *et al. CHC1-L*, a candidate gene for prostate carcinogenesis at 13q14.2, is frequently affected by loss of heterozygosity and underexpressed in human prostate cancer. *Int J Cancer* 2002;99:689–96
18. Cussenot O, Teillac P, Berthon P, *et al.* Noninvasive detection of genetic instability in cells from prostatic secretion as a marker of prostate cancer. *Eur J Intern Med* 2001;12:17–19
19. Matsuyama H, Pan Y, Oba K, *et al.* Deletions on chromosome 8p22 may predict disease

progression as well as pathological staging in prostate cancer. *Clin Cancer Res* 2001;7:3139–43

20. Latil A, Bieche I, Pesche S, *et al.* Loss of heterozygosity at chromosome arm 13q and *RB1* status in human prostate cancer. *Hum Pathol* 1999; 30:809–15

21. Dong JT, Chen C, Stultz BG, *et al.* Deletion at 13q21 is associated with aggressive prostate cancers. *Cancer Res* 2000;60:3880–3

22. Kibel AS, Faith DA, Bova GS, *et al.* Loss of heterozygosity at 12P12–13 in primary and metastatic prostate adenocarcinoma. *J Urol* 2000; 164:192–6

23. Meid FH, Gygi CM, Leisinger HJ, *et al.* The use of telomerase activity for the detection of prostatic cancer cells after prostatic massage. *J Urol* 2001;165:1802–5

24. Cairns P, Esteller M, Herman JG, *et al.* Molecular detection of prostate cancer in urine by *GSTP1* hypermethylation. *Clin Cancer Res* 2001;7:2727

Basic research on prostate cancer: signal transduction

16

Z. Culig

Introduction

Prostate cancer remains the most frequently diagnosed tumor in the Western world, and its incidence is increasing also in Asian countries in parallel with ongoing changes in life-style. There are encouraging developments owing to the improved possibility of the early diagnosis of prostate cancer. Therapeutic approaches for non-organ-confined disease remain limited, however. Endocrine therapy is based on the pioneering work by Huggins and Hodges, who first demonstrated that withdrawal of androgens leads to retardation of prostate cancer growth[1]. Considerable efforts in prostate cancer research are being undertaken to improve the understanding of signal transduction pathways of steroid and peptide hormones, growth factors, cytokines and neurotransmitters. Signal transduction research is focused either on mechanisms underlying tumor progression to therapy resistance or on identification of early changes, which are a characteristic feature of clinically significant prostate tumors. Results obtained in these studies could also improve prostate cancer chemoprevention in the future. The development of resistance towards endocrine therapy is associated with multiple molecular alterations and the disregulation of expression of growth-regulatory molecules or their receptors. In some cases, growth factors or cytokines exhibit pleiotropic effects on prostate cancer cells. Activation of different signalling pathways by the same molecules in diverse cell lines could result in either growth stimulation or inhibition.

New technologies are increasingly utilized in prostate cancer signal research. The use of laser capture microdissection allows analyses in selected subpopulations of prostate cancer cells. Tissue microarrays make possible investigations of a large number of genes of interest. Although new targets for therapy could be identified in this way, it should be emphasized that there is a need for evaluation of the functional significance of genes overexpressed in prostate cancer specimens.

Owing to increased interest in prostate cancer in the scientific community, clinical trials with signal transduction inhibitors have been initiated. For example, the epidermal growth factor receptor (EGFR) has been targeted by monoclonal antibodies cetuximab and trastuzumab, and low-molecular-weight inhibitors of the EGFR tyrosine kinase.

The focus of the present chapter is the signalling of selected regulators of prostate growth – steroid and peptide hormones and cytokines – and their involvement in the development and progression of prostate cancer (Table 1).

Androgen signalling in prostate cancer

Both epithelial and stromal cells of the prostate respond to androgen stimulation and express the androgen receptor (AR). The AR protein is a transcription factor composed of 919 amino acids, and consists of the three main regions: well-conserved ligand- and DNA-binding domains and the N-terminal region, which contains a variable number of polyglutamine (CAG) and polyglycine (GGN) stretches. In general, a shorter number of polyglutamine repeats is associated with an increased transcriptional activity of the AR. Differences in the number of polyglutamine repeats between races have been reported[2]. African–American males are at greater risk of developing prostate cancer, and they also have the highest frequency

Table 1 Steroid and peptide regulators of prostate cancer growth

Hormone	Receptor	Effect	Alterations
Androgen	androgen receptor	proliferation, differentiation	receptor up-regulation, receptor mutations
Estrogen	estrogen receptors α and β	proliferation	down-regulation of β receptor
EGF	EGF receptor	proliferation	
TGF-α	EGF receptor	proliferation	up-regulation
TGF-β	TGF-β receptors	inhibition of proliferation, angiogenesis, immunosuppression	loss of receptors
bFGF	FGF receptors	angiogenesis	up-regulation
IGF-I	IGF receptor I	anti-apoptotic	altered binding-protein expression
IL-6	IL-6 receptor	pleiotropic	up-regulation

EGF, epidermal growth factor; TGF, transforming growth factor; bFGF, basic fibroblast growth factor; IGF, insulin-like growth factor; IL-6, interleukin-6

of short CAG repeats. The length of that polymorphic repeat has been correlated with prediction of prognosis[3], prostate cancer progression[4] or survival[5], although definitive consensus on some of these issues has not been reached.

The AR is expressed in the vast majority of human prostate cancers, including tumors derived from patients who have failed endocrine therapy[6,7]. Quantitative analyses of AR expression based on binding assays with radiolabelled ligands are not routinely used in diagnostic procedures in prostate carcinoma. Several prostate cancer cell lines are AR-negative, and therefore do not reflect the clinical situation. In human prostate cancer specimens, there is no evidence for gross deletions in the AR molecule. Point mutations have been discovered by several investigators, and the majority of these alterations are located in the conserved domains of the AR. The controversy as to the frequency of AR mutations in various stages of the disease has been solved, since a recent study has provided clear evidence that mutations frequently occur in advanced stages of prostate cancer[8]. AR transcriptional activity is measured either in cells that express endogenous AR or in heterologous cells that are transfected with AR cDNA. It is induced by androgens and, to a lesser extent, by other steroid hormones. AR transcriptional activity is strictly concentration-dependent, and does not parallel regulation of cellular proliferation of

LNCaP (lymph node cancer of the prostate) cells, which express a mutated AR. These cells show a typical biphasic regulation of proliferation in response to androgenic hormones; low doses of androgen enhance proliferation, whereas higher concentrations cause a progressive decline in cell growth[9]. The effect of androgens on proliferation is associated with the up-regulation of cyclin-dependent kinases 2 and 4[10]. In contrast, the inhibitory action of high doses of androgenic hormones on prostate cancer cells is associated with induction of the cell cycle inhibitor p27[11,12]. Importantly, low doses of androgens promote phosphorylation of the retinoblastoma gene[12]. Retinoblastoma binds to the transcription factor E2F, and prevents unrestricted cellular proliferation when its hypophosphorylated form is predominant. Thus, changes in phosphorylation of retinoblastoma protein are regulated by androgens.

Functional characterization of several mutated receptors in prostate cancer has revealed increased activation by non-androgenic steroids and antiandrogens, and it is believed that this activation is important for tumor progression. Two non-steroidal antiandrogens are used for prostate cancer endocrine therapy, hydroxyflutamide and bicalutamide. They both bind to the AR with low affinity, but they do not allow acquisition of a transcriptionally active conformation of the receptor. Another important difference between agonists and antagonists of the AR is that only agonists enhance interactions between the N-terminal region and the C terminal. In many aspects, there are similarities between AR, glucocorticoid receptor and progesterone receptor interactions with target DNA sequences. For example, it has been reported that not only androgens, but also the glucocorticoid hormone dexamethasone, induce expression of the AR-regulated prostate-specific antigen (PSA) gene[13].

The first AR mutation detected in prostate cancer was one in LNCaP cells, in which the two antiandrogens act in different manners[14]. Whereas hydroxyflutamide enhances cellular proliferation, promotes dissociation of heat shock proteins from the receptor and increases functional activity of the AR, bicalutamide acts as an AR antagonist in the LNCaP cell line[15]. However, it has been observed that after long-term androgen ablation there is an up-regulation of AR activity also after stimulation by bicalutamide[16]. In studies of ARs using patient material, it has been shown that hydroxyflutamide but not bicalutamide frequently activates mutated receptors[17]. For a practicing urologist, it is interesting to note that some patients whose ARs are stimulated by hydroxyflutamide respond to second-line therapy with bicalutamide.

AR mutations with a broadened activation spectrum have also been detected in the xenograft CWR22 and in the cell line MDA PCa 2a[18,19]. AR mutations might be one of the underlying mechanisms for the antiandrogen withdrawal syndrome, which has been reported for many drugs used in prostate cancer endocrine therapy[20]. Growth of some prostate cancers might be stimulated by a complex formed between the AR and estrogen receptor β, which leads to activation of the mitogen-activated protein kinase (MAPK) signalling pathway[21]. In contrast to estrogen receptor β, estrogen receptor α is predominantly expressed in prostate stroma.

For a clinician, it is important to distinguish between beneficial short-term effects of endocrine therapy and effects of long-term treatment, which include adaptation mechanisms. A potential problem with endocrine therapy is up-regulation of AR expression, which could occur because of amplification of the AR gene, increased mRNA expression or increased protein stability[22–24]. Amplification of the AR gene is a typical feature of a subset of recurrent prostate cancers. Thus, one can speculate that, after long-term treatment with an anti-androgen, the doses are not sufficient to prevent signalling through the AR. Other studies with long-term androgen-deprived cells showed that they become resistant to various inducers of apoptosis, and in this context mimic the situation in prostate cancer patients[25,26].

Importantly, the AR has a role in maintenance of the differentiated function of the prostate. This is particularly evident in the case of ligand-independent activation of the receptor by interleukin-6 (IL-6) and butyrate (Figure 1)[27,28]. These compounds cause inhibition of proliferation of LNCaP cells but stimulate PSA gene expression through activation of the AR. Stable expression of AR cDNA in PC-3 cells also generates sublines with a less malignant phenotype[29,30]. Because of situations in which the AR mediates growth-inhibitory and prodifferentiation effects, it is not easy to assess all possible consequences of therapeutic down-regulation of AR expression. The AR was down-regulated in short-term experiments by antisense oligonucleotides[31], interleukin-1β[32] or anti-inflammatory drugs[33]. In those reports, there was a clear inhibition of LNCaP proliferation and PSA expression.

However, in many cases, activation of the AR in the absence of androgens is observed with compounds that show a growth-stimulatory effect. These substances are growth factors, growth factor-related molecules and neuropeptides[34–36]. This mechanism might be of crucial importance in advanced carcinoma of the prostate in conditions with low androgen supply. It is notable that the ability of anti-androgens to inhibit non-androgenic activation of the AR might be greatly reduced[37,38]. This is, however, not surprising, because several non-steroidal compounds activate signalling pathways of MAPK, which phosphorylate the AR in

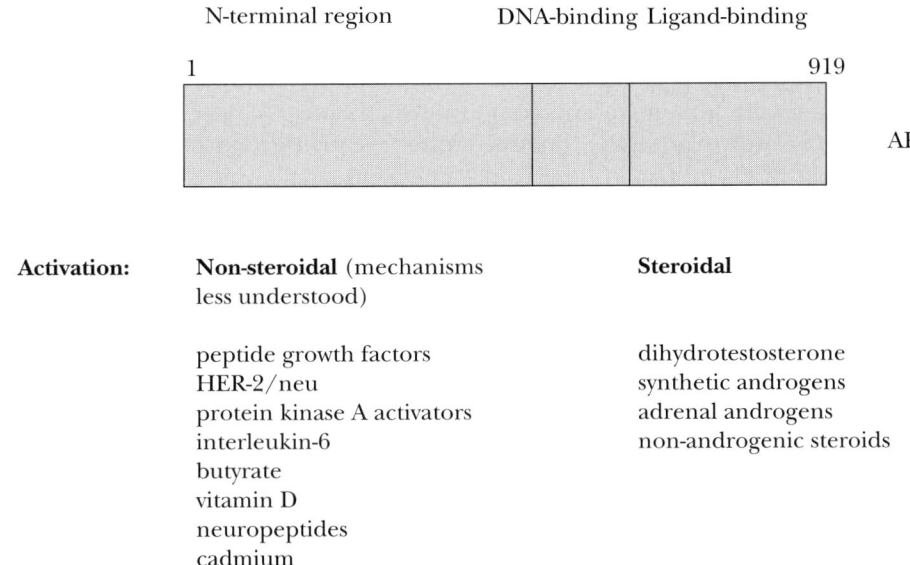

Figure 1 Activation of the androgen receptor (AR) by androgens and non-steroidal activators. AR ligand-independent activation could result either in stimulation of cellular proliferation or in secretion of prostate-specific proteins, such as prostate-specific antigen (PSA) which is up-regulated in response to interleukin-6 (IL-6) and butyrate

the N-terminal region[37]. Enhancement of AR activity by MAPK has obvious clinical importance. MAPK phosphorylation increases with high Gleason grades and after androgen ablation[39].

In addition, changes in expression or function of AR-associated proteins might contribute to prostate cancer progression. These proteins, coactivators or corepressors, modulate AR activity by interaction with the transcriptional machinery. There are an increasing number of coactivators detected, and it is difficult to identify those which have a predominant role in cancer tissue. A role for the AR-associated protein ARA70 in different AR-mediated regulations has been suggested[40,41]. However, research from other laboratories does not support specific coactivation of the AR by ARA70[42,43]. According to two recent reports, the expression of AR-associated proteins SRC-1, TIF2 and RAC3 increases with progression towards therapy resistance[44,45]. For many other coregulatory proteins, it is known that they enhance AR activity to a similar extent, and studies of their functional significance have to be performed.

Disregulation of growth factor signal transduction in prostate cancer

The MAPK signalling pathway links signal transduction of growth factors and the AR in carcinoma of the prostate. Besides activating MAPK, these peptides act through other signalling pathways, for example the pathway of phosphatidylinositol 3-kinase. There is evidence for overexpression of some growth factors in carcinoma of the prostate. Epidermal growth factor (EGF) and transforming growth factor-α (TGF-α), both of which bind to the EGFR, are differentially expressed in benign and malignant prostate tissue[46]. In benign prostate tissue, there is predominant expression of EGF, whereas prostate cancer metastases stain predominantly for TGF-α. There is ongoing controversy whether EGF-related molecule HER-2/neu expression is elevated in prostate cancer. HER-2 is an important activator of the AR, and its overexpression is frequently associated with malignant transformation.

TGF-β is a pleiotropic regulator of prostate growth that exhibits different effects on cell growth *in vitro* and *in vivo*. It is considered an important growth-inhibitory factor for prostate cells in culture, where it antagonizes stimulatory effects of EGF[47]. Inhibitory action, however, depends on duration of treatment and percentage of serum in individual experiments. Prostate cancer cells PC-3 and DU-145 respond to TGF-β by reducing their proliferation, whereas growth of LNCaP cells cannot be retarded by the growth factor. In earlier studies, it was suggested that this is due to absence of the TGF-β receptor type I[48]. However, studies carried out by others have revealed that there is missing expression of the receptor type II[49]. Overexpression of that receptor in LNCaP cells results in restoration of TGF-β responsiveness. In clinical specimens, either receptor could be lost in advanced carcinoma of the prostate[50]. In addition, TGF-β intermediary effectors caspase-1 and caspase-3 also decrease in human prostate cancer[51]. *In vivo*, TGF-β influences angiogenesis and suppresses immune response. Therefore, it is not surprising that prostate cancer cells stably transfected with TGF-β cDNA confer a growth advantage *in vivo*. Elevated levels of TGF-β were measured in some studies in sera from prostate cancer patients[52].

Similar elevation of growth factor serum levels have been reported for basic fibroblast growth factor (bFGF, FGF-2), which is involved in promotion of metastasis by regulation of matrix metalloproteinases and angiogenesis[53,54]. bFGF is expressed in prostate cancer cell lines PC-3 and DU-145 but not in LNCaP cells, and is capable of down-regulating AR expression[55,56]. It is mainly contained in the extracellular matrix, and only a very small percentage is secreted. The presence of bFGF in prostate tissues was initially reported in stromal cells[57]. In more recent publications, it was recognized that some tumor cells also show bFGF immunoreactivity[54]. Keratinocyte growth factor (KGF), which belongs to the same family of peptides, is implicated in mediation of androgenic effects between the stromal and epithelial compartments of the prostate[58], as evidenced in studies with coculture of prostatic cells. However, *in vivo* experiments did not confirm that role of KGF[59]. KGF binds to the variant IIIb isoform of the FGF receptor-2,

whereas bFGF binds to the isoform IIIc, whose expression is up-regulated in prostate cancer[60]. Therapeutic approaches to down-regulate bFGF in cancer may be based on an antagonistic effect of interferons-α and -β[61]. Transfection of cells with a recombinant adenovirus expressing dominant-negative FGF receptor-1 led to G_2 growth arrest[62]. Little is known about signalling pathways by which FGF enhances growth of prostate cancer cells and down-regulates AR expression.

Recent studies have focused on the other member of the FGF family of growth factors, FGF-8, which is expressed in high-grade prostate intraepithelial neoplasia lesions and in prostate cancer[63]; administration of neutralizing anti-FGF-8 antibodies abolished the effect of androgens on cell growth[64]. LNCaP cells generated to overexpress FGF-8b proliferated at a high rate and increased invasive potential[65].

Insulin-like growth factor-I (IGF-I) has been suggested to be associated with increased prostate cancer risk[66]. IGF-I action is determined by its association with several binding proteins, and the growth factor is implicated in regulation of apoptosis, mitogenic responses and AR activity.

Interleukin-6: a pleiotropic regulator of prostate cancer growth

Interleukin-6 (IL-6) binds to the membrane receptor, which is composed of the ligand-binding subunit gp 80 and signal-transducing subunit gp 130. IL-6 signalling leads to activation of pathways of signal transducers and activators of transcription (STAT) and MAPK. Twillie and associates were the first to report increased levels of IL-6 in sera from patients with metastatic prostate cancer[67]. These results were confirmed by other researchers and extended by Giri and associates[68]. The most interesting observation from their work is that IL-6 expression is elevated in tissue extracts obtained from patients with organ-confined carcinoma of the prostate. In addition, IL-6 receptor expression also increases in prostate cancer. Taken together with results from immunohistochemical studies[69], these findings indicate the presence of IL-6 autocrine and paracrine loops in carcinoma of the prostate. Stimulation of growth of prostate cells by IL-6 has been reported for primary epithelial cultures, a cell line established from high-grade prostate intraepithelial neoplasia and PC-3 cells[68,70,71]. In the case of PC-3 cells, IL-6 acts as a survival factor mainly by activating the phosphatidylinositol-3 kinase pathway[71]. For regulation of growth of LNCaP cells, divergent results have been reported[72,73]. The discrepancy might occur because of the use of different LNCaP passages and sera in various laboratories. The mechanism responsible for inhibition of LNCaP cell proliferation involves down-regulation of cyclin-dependent kinases and induction of the cell cycle inhibitor p27[74]. It is, however, well established that IL-6 is a potent activator of the AR[27,75,76]. This activation results in stimulation of PSA protein expression. Signalling pathways of several protein kinases and STAT are required for AR activation by IL-6. The AR is also activated by the IL-6-related cytokine oncostatin M, which is a paracrine regulator of prostate cancer cell growth[38]. In studies of IL-6 signalling, it is particularly interesting that LNCaP cells initially inhibited by IL-6 change their response after prolonged treatment with the cytokine[77]. They acquire a growth advantage *in vitro*, do not respond to IL-6 by growth inhibition and express endogenous IL-6. The subline developed after long-term treatment with IL-6, LNCaP–IL-6+, may represent a useful model for studies of IL-6 signalling in prostate cancer progression.

As well as effects on cellular proliferation, apoptosis and AR activation, IL-6 is also implicated in regulation of neuroendocrine differentiation in prostate cancer cells[78]. Because of the pleiotropic nature of its effects, IL-6 should be considered a target in the development of novel therapies for carcinoma of the prostate.

In conclusion, it has become clear that prostate cancer cell growth is associated with multiple alterations in signalling pathways. It is therefore unlikely that a single therapeutic approach will substantially reduce prostate cancer mortality. Therefore, research should be directed towards establishing reasonable combined therapies in the future.

References

1. Huggins C, Hodges CV. Studies on prostatic cancer: the effects of castration, of estrogen and of androgen injection on serum phosphatases in metastatic carcinoma of the prostate. *Cancer Res* 1941;1:293–7
2. Nelson KA, Witte JS. Androgen receptor CAG repeats and prostate cancer. *Am J Epidemiol* 2002;155:883–90
3. Suzuki H, Akakura K, Komiya A, *et al.* CAG polymorphic repeat lengths in androgen receptor gene among Japanese prostate cancer patients: potential predictor of prognosis after endocrine therapy. *Prostate* 2002;51:219–24
4. Nam RK, Elhaji Y, Krahn MD, *et al.* Significance of the CAG repeat polymorphism of the androgen receptor gene in prostate cancer progression. *J Urol* 2000;164:567–72
5. Edwards SM, Badzioch MD, Minter R, *et al.* Androgen receptor polymorphisms: association with prostate cancer risk, relapse and overall survival. *Int J Cancer* 1999;84:458–65
6. Van der Kwast TH, Schalken J, Ruizeveld de Winter JA, *et al.* Androgen receptors in endocrine-therapy-resistant human prostate cancer. *Int J Cancer* 1991;48:189–93
7. Hobisch A, Culig Z, Radmayr C, *et al.* Distant metastases from prostatic carcinoma express androgen receptor protein. *Cancer Res* 1995; 55:3068–72
8. Marcelli M, Ittmann M, Mariani S, *et al.* Androgen receptor mutations in prostate cancer. *Cancer Res* 2000;60:944–9
9. Lee C, Sutkowski DM, Sensibar JA, *et al.* Regulation of proliferation and production of

prostate-specific antigen in androgen-sensitive prostatic cancer cells, LNCaP, by dihydrotestosterone. *Endocrinology* 1995;136:796–805

10. Lu S, Tsai SY, Tsai MJ. Regulation of androgen-dependent prostatic cancer cell growth: androgen regulation of CDK2, CDK4, and CKI p16 genes. *Cancer Res* 1997;57:4511–16

11. Tsihlias J, Zhang W, Bhattacharya N, *et al.* Involvement of p27 (Kip1) in G_1 arrest by high dose 5α-dihydrotestosterone in LNCaP human prostate cancer cells. *Oncogene* 2000;19:670–9

12. Hofman K, Svinnen JV, Verhoeven G, *et al.* E2F activity is biphasically regulated by androgens in LNCaP cells. *Biochem Biophys Res Commun* 2001; 283:97–101

13. Cleutjens CB, Steketee K, van Eekelen CC, *et al.* Both androgen receptor and glucocorticoid receptor are able to induce prostate-specific antigen expression, but differ in their growth-stimulating properties of LNCaP cells. *Endocrinology* 1997;138:5293–300

14. Veldscholte J, Ris-Stalpers C, Kuiper GGJM, *et al.* A mutation in the ligand binding domain of the androgen receptor of human LNCaP cells affects steroid binding characteristics and response to anti-androgens. *Biochem Biophys Res Commun* 1990;17:534–40

15. Veldscholte J, Berrevoets CA, Zegers ND, *et al.* Hormone-induced dissociation of the androgen receptor–heat-shock protein complex: use of a new monoclonal antibody to distinguish transformed from nontransformed receptors. *Biochemistry* 1992;31:7422–30

16. Culig Z, Hoffman J, Erdel M, *et al.* Switch from antagonist to agonist of the androgen receptor blocker bicalutamide is associated with prostate tumour progression in a new model system. *Br J Cancer* 1999;81:242–51

17. Taplin ME, Bubley GJ, Ko YJ, *et al.* Selection for androgen receptor mutations in prostate cancers treated with androgen antagonist. *Cancer Res* 1999;59:2511–15

18. Tan J, Sharief Y, Hamil KG, *et al.* Dehydroepiandrosterone activates mutant androgen receptors expressed in the androgen-dependent human prostate cancer xenograft CWR22 and LNCaP cells. *Mol Endocrinol* 1997;11:450–9

19. Zhao XY, Boyle B, Krishman AV, *et al.* Two mutations identified in the androgen receptor of the new human prostate cancer cell line MDA PCa 2a. *J Urol* 1999;162:2192–9

20. Culig Z, Klocker H, Bartsch G, *et al.* Mutations of androgen receptor in carcinoma of the prostate – significance for endocrine therapy. *Am J Pharmacogenomics* 2001;1:241–9

21. Migliaccio A, Castoria G, Di Domenico M, *et al.* Steroid-induced androgen receptor–oestradiol receptor β–Src complex triggers prostate cancer cell proliferation. *EMBO J* 2000;19:5406–17

22. Visakorpi T, Hyytinen E, Koivisto P, *et al. In vivo* amplification of the androgen receptor gene and progression of human prostate cancer. *Nature Genet* 1995;9:401–6

23. Kokontis J, Takakura K, Hay N, *et al.* Increased androgen receptor activity and altered c-*myc* expression in prostate cancer cells after long-term androgen deprivation. *Cancer Res* 1994;54: 1566–73

24. Gregory CW, Johnson RT Jr, Mohler JL, *et al.* Androgen receptor stabilization in recurrent prostate cancer is associated with hypersensitivity to low androgen. *Cancer Res* 2001;61:2892–8

25. Gao M, Ossowski L, Ferrari AC. Activation of Rb and decline in androgen receptor protein precede retinoic acid-induced apoptosis in androgen-dependent LNCaP cells and their androgen-independent derivative. *J Cell Physiol* 1999;179:336–46

26. Murillo H, Huang H, Schmidt LJ, *et al.* Role of PI3K signaling in survival and progression of LNCaP prostate cancer cells to the androgen refractory state. *Endocrinology* 2001;142:4795–805

27. Hobisch A, Eder IE, Putz T, *et al.* Interleukin-6 regulates prostate-specific protein expression in prostate carcinoma cells by activation of the androgen receptor. *Cancer Res* 1998;58:4640–5

28. Sadar MD, Gleave ME. Ligand-independent activation of the androgen receptor by the differentiation agent butyrate in human prostate cancer cells. *Cancer Res* 2000;60:5825–31

29. Yuan S, Trachtenberg J, Mills GB, *et al.* Androgen-induced inhibition of cell proliferation in an androgen-insensitive prostate cancer cell line (PC-3) transfected with a human androgen receptor complementary DNA. *Cancer Res* 1993;53:1304–11

30. Bonaccorsi L, Carloni V, Muratori M, *et al.* Androgen receptor expression in prostate carcinoma cells suppresses α6β4 integrin-mediated invasive phenotype. *Endocrinology* 2000;141:3172–82

31. Eder IE, Culig Z, Ramoner R, *et al.* Inhibition of LNCaP prostate cancer cells by means of androgen receptor antisense oligonucleotides. *Cancer Gene Ther* 2000;7:997–1007

32. Culig Z, Hobisch A, Herold M, *et al.* Interleukin-1β mediates the modulatory effects of monocytes on LNCaP human prostate cancer cells. *Br J Cancer* 1998;78:1004–11

33. Zhu W, Smith A, Young CY. A nonsteroidal anti-inflammatory drug, flufenamic acid, inhibits the expression of androgen receptor in LNCaP cells. *Endocrinology* 1999;140:5451–4

34. Culig Z, Hobisch A, Cronauer MV, *et al.* Androgen receptor activation in prostatic tumor cell lines by insulin-like growth factor-I, keratinocyte growth factor, and epidermal growth factor. *Cancer Res* 1994;54:5474–8

35. Craft N, Shostak Y, Carey M, *et al.* A mechanism for hormone-independent prostate cancer through modulation of androgen receptor signaling by the HER-2/neu tyrosine kinase. *Nature Med* 1999;5:280–5

36. Lee LF, Guan J, Qiu Y, *et al.* Neuropeptide-induced androgen independence in prostate cancer cells: roles of nonreceptor tyrosine kinases Etk/Bmx, Src, and focal adhesion kinase. *Mol Cell Biol* 2001;21:8385–97

37. Yeh S, Lin HK, Kang HY, *et al.* From HER2/Neu signal cascade to androgen receptor and its coactivators: a novel pathway by induction of androgen target genes through MAP kinase in prostate cancer cells. *Proc Natl Acad Sci USA* 1999;96:5458–63

38. Godoy-Tundidor S, Hobisch A, Pfeil K, *et al.* Acquisition of agonistic properties of non-steroidal antiandrogens after treatment with oncostatin M in prostate cancer cells. *Clin Cancer Res* 2002;8:2356–61

39. Gioeli D, Mandell JW, Petroni GR, *et al.* Activation of mitogen-activated protein kinase associated with prostate cancer progression. *Cancer Res* 1999;59:279–84

40. Yeh S, Miyamoto H, Shima H, *et al.* From estrogen to androgen receptors: a new pathway for sex hormones in prostate. *Proc Natl Acad Sci USA* 1998;95:5527–32

41. Miyamoto H, Yeh S, Wilding G, *et al.* Promotion of agonist activity of antiandrogens by the androgen receptor coactivator, ARA70, in human prostate cancer DU145 cells. *Proc Natl Acad Sci USA* 1998;95:7379–84

42. Alen P, Claessens F, Schoenemakers E, *et al.* Interaction of the putative androgen receptor-specific coactivator ARA70/ELE1α with multiple steroid receptors and identification of an internally deleted ELE1β isoform. *Mol Endocrinol* 1999;13:117–28

43. Gao T, Brantley K, Bolu E, *et al.* RFG (ARA70, ELE1) interacts with the human androgen receptor in a ligand-dependent fashion, but functions only weakly as a coactivator in co-transfection assays. *Mol Endocrinol* 1999;13: 1645–56

44. Gregory CW, He B, Johnson RT Jr, *et al.* A mechanism for androgen receptor-mediated prostate cancer recurrence after androgen deprivation therapy. *Cancer Res* 2001;61:4315–19

45. Gnanapragasam VJ, Leung HY, Pulimood AS, *et al.* Expression of RAC3, a steroid hormone receptor co-activator in prostate cancer. *Br J Cancer* 2001;85:1928–36

46. Scher HI, Sarkis A, Reuter V, *et al.* Changing pattern of expression of the epidermal growth factor receptor and transforming growth factor α in the progression of prostatic neoplasms. *Clin Cancer Res* 1995;1:545–50

47. Sutkowski DM, Fong CJ, Sensibar JA, *et al.* Interaction of epidermal growth factor and transforming growth factor β in human prostatic epithelial cells in culture. *Prostate* 1992;21:133–43

48. Kim IY, Ahn HJ, Zelner DJ, *et al.* Genetic change in transforming growth factor β (TGF-β) receptor type I gene correlates with insensitivity to TGF-β1 in human prostate cancer cells. *Cancer Res* 1996;56:44–8

49. Guo Y, Kyprianou N. Overexpression of transforming growth factor-βI receptor type II restores transforming growth factor-βI sensitivity and signaling in human prostate cancer cells. *Cell Growth Differ* 1998;9:185–93

50. Kim IY, Ahn HJ, Zelner DJ, *et al.* Loss of expression of transforming growth factor β type I and II receptors correlates with tumor grade in human prostate cancer tissues. *Clin Cancer Res* 1996;2:1255–61

51. Winter RN, Kramer A, Borowski A, *et al.* Loss of caspase-1 and caspase-3 protein expression in human prostate cancer. *Cancer Res* 2001;61: 1227–32

52. Adler HI, McCurdy MA, Kattan MW, *et al.* Elevated levels of circulating interleukin-6 and transforming growth factor-β1 in patients with metastatic prostatic carcinoma. *J Urol* 1999; 161:182–7

53. Meyer GE, Yu E, Siegal JA, *et al.* Serum basic fibroblast growth factor in men with and without prostate carcinoma. *Cancer* 1995;76:2304–11

54. Cronauer MV, Hittmair A, Eder IE, *et al.* Basic fibroblast growth factor levels in cancer cells and in sera of patients suffering from proliferative disorders of the prostate. *Prostate* 1997;31:223–33

55. Nakamoto T, Chang CS, Li AK, *et al.* Basic fibroblast growth factor in human prostate cancer cells. *Cancer Res* 1992;52:571–7

56. Cronauer MV, Nessler-Menardi C, Klocker H, *et al.* Androgen receptor protein is down-regulated by basic fibroblast growth factor in prostate cancer cells. *Br J Cancer* 2000;82:39–45

57. Sherwood E, Lee C, Kozlowsky JM. Basic fibroblast growth factor: a potential mediator of stromal growth in the human prostate. *Endocrinology* 1992;130:2955–63

58. Yan G, Fukabori Y, Nikolaropoulos S, *et al.* Heparin-binding keratinocyte growth factor is a candidate stromal-to-epithelial-cell andromedin. *Mol Endocrinol* 1992;6:2123–8

59. Nemeth JA, Zelner DJ, Lang S, *et al.* Keratinocyte growth factor in the rat ventral prostate: androgen-independent expression. *J Endocrinol* 1998;156:115–25

60. Yan G, Fukabori Y, MacBride G, *et al.* Exon switching and activation of stromal and embryonic fibroblast growth factor (FGF)–FGF receptor genes in prostate epithelial cells accompany

stromal independence and malignancy. *Mol Cell Biol* 1993;13:4513–22

61. Singh RK, Gutman M, Bucana CD, *et al.* Interferons α and β down-regulate the expression of basic fibroblast growth factor in human carcinomas. *Proc Natl Acad Sci USA* 1995;92:4562–6

62. Ozen M, Giri D, Ropiquet F, *et al.* Role of fibroblast growth factor receptor signaling in prostate cancer cell survival. *J Natl Cancer Inst* 2001;93:1783–90

63. Valve EM, Nevalainen MT, Nurmi MJ, *et al.* Increased expression of FGF-8 isoforms and FGF receptors in human premalignant prostatic intraepithelial neoplasia lesions and prostate cancer. *Lab Invest* 2001;81:815–26

64. Tanaka A, Furuya A, Yamasaki M, *et al.* High frequency of fibroblast growth factor (FGF) 8 expression in clinical prostate cancers and breast tissues, immunohistochemically demonstrated by a newly established neutralizing monoclonal antibody against FGF 8. *Cancer Res* 1998;58:2052–6

65. Song Z, Powell WC, Kasahara N, *et al.* The effect of fibroblast growth factor 8, isoform b, on the biology of prostate carcinoma cells and their interaction with stromal cells. *Cancer Res* 2000;60:6730–6

66. Chan JM, Stampfer MJ, Giovanucci E, *et al.* Plasma insulin-like growth factor-I and prostate cancer risk: a prospective study. *Science* 1998;279:563–6

67. Twillie DA, Eisenberger MA, Carducci MA, *et al.* Interleukin-6: a candidate mediator of human prostate cancer morbidity. *Urology* 1995;45:542–9

68. Giri D, Ozen M, Ittmann M. Interleukin-6 is an autocrine growth factor in human prostate cancer. *Am J Pathol* 2001;159:159–65

69. Hobisch A, Rogatsch H, Hittmair A, *et al.* Immunohistochemical localization of interleukin-6 and its receptor in benign, premalignant and malignant prostate tissue. *J Pathol* 2000;191:239–44

70. Liu XH, Kirschenbaum A, Lu M, *et al.* Prostaglandin E(2) stimulates prostatic intraepithelial neoplasia cell growth through activation of the interleukin-6/GP130/STAT-3 signaling pathway. *Biochem Biophys Res Commun* 2002;290:249–55

71. Chung TD, Yu JJ, Kong TA, *et al.* Interleukin-6 activates phosphatidylinositol-3 kinase, which inhibits apoptosis in human prostate cancer cell lines. *Prostate* 2000;42:1–7

72. Degeorges A, Tatoud R, Fauvel Lafeve F, *et al.* Stromal cells from human benign prostate hyperplasia produce a growth-inhibitory factor for LNCaP prostate cancer cells, identified as interleukin-6. *Int J Cancer* 1996;68:207–14

73. Okamoto M, Lee C, Oyasu R. Interleukin-6 as a paracrine and autocrine growth factor in human prostatic carcinoma cells *in vitro. Cancer Res* 1997;57:141–6

74. Mori S, Murakami-Mori K, Bonavida B. Interleukin-6 induces G$_1$ arrest through induction of p27 (Kip1), a cyclin-dependent kinase inhibitor, and neuron-like morphology in LNCaP prostate tumor cells. *Biochem Biophys Res Commun* 1999;257:609–14

75. Chen T, Wang LH, Farrar WL. Interleukin 6 activates androgen receptor-mediated gene expression through a signal transducer and activator of transcription 3-dependent pathway in LNCaP prostate cancer cells. *Cancer Res* 2000;60:2132–5

76. Lin DL, Whitney MC, Yao Z, *et al.* Interleukin-6 induces androgen responsiveness in prostate cancer cells through up-regulation of androgen receptor expression. *Clin Cancer Res* 2001;7:1773–81

77. Hobisch A, Ramoner R, Fuchs D, *et al.* Prostate cancer cells (LNCaP) generated after long-term interleukin-6 treatment express interleukin-6 and acquire an interleukin-6-partially resistant phenotype. *Clin Cancer Res* 2001;7:2941–8

78. Zelivianski S, Verni M, Moore C, *et al.* Multipathways for transdifferentiation of human prostate cancer cells into neuroendocrine-like phenotype. *Biochim Biophys Acta* 2001;1539:28–43

Stem cells and differentiation in human prostate cancer

17

J. R. Masters, T. N. Alam, C. L. Foley, I. Laczkó and D. L. Hudson

Introduction

Human prostate epithelium consists of two cell layers within which three cell types are recognized: basal, luminal and neuroendocrine cells, each of which has many phenotypic variants. Prostate cancers contain cells with similar phenotypes, but the patterns of growth and differentiation are altered to varying extents within each cancer.

An important concept is that the degree of differentiation is inversely proportional to the capacity for cell division. In normal prostate epithelial cells, there is a relatively strict division of labor, and cells that produce prostate-specific antigen (PSA) are unlikely to be proliferative. In contrast, one of the characteristics of prostate cancer is the blurring of this distinction.

In order to understand prostate cancer cell differentiation, it is first necessary to understand normal prostate epithelial cell growth and differentiation. Many studies of normal and abnormal prostate tissue derived from fetuses, boys, young men and older men have been published. However, few definitive conclusions have been reached.

The aim of this review is to summarize the literature describing the patterns of differentiation seen in human normal prostate epithelium and consider how these are altered in prostate cancer.

Prostate normal epithelial cell lineages

In the normal prostate epithelium, a nearly complete layer of basal, relatively undifferentiated cells is the progenitor of the luminal layer of columnar PSA-secreting cells[1-3]. Interspersed amongst these cells are scattered individual or small groups of neuroendocrine cells. It is thought that the stem cells reside in the basal layer, where the majority of cell division occurs.

A number of interrelated questions arise, including:

(1) What is the sequence of phenotypes during prostate epithelial cell differentiation?

(2) Is there, in some areas, a cell layer between the basal cells and the secretory cells?

(3) What is the phenotype of the cells transiting between the basal and luminal layers?

(4) Does prostate epithelium contain some cells with characteristics of both basal and luminal cells?

(5) What is the origin of the neuroendocrine cells?

(6) Is stem cell division monodirectional or can the prostate epithelial stem cell give rise to two populations of transit amplifying cells, one of which divides to give basal cells and one to luminal cells?

(7) What are the differences in the patterns of differentiation between the transition, central and peripheral zones of the human prostate?

(8) Which cell type(s) give rise to prostate cancer?

Study of these questions has been facilitated by the use of a number of markers, particularly cytokeratins (CKs). The classical lineage markers are CK5/14 (and p63) for basal cells, CK8/18 (and PSA, nuclear androgen receptor (AR), prostate-specific membrane antigen

(PSMA) and prostatic acid phosphatase (PSAP)) for luminal cells and chromogranin A or CD56 for neuroendocrine cells. However, extending the range of markers studied has demonstrated that there are many other phenotypes present in both the basal and luminal layers.

Stem cell theory and prostate epithelial cell differentiation

Most of the theories concerning prostate epithelial cell differentiation are based on stem cell theory. Stem cell theory suggests that within each tissue there is a small population of long-lived cells that has two properties, multipotency and self-renewal. Prostate epithelial stem cells not only give rise to all the other cell types within the prostate epithelium, but also have the capacity for self-renewal (every time they divide at least one of the daughter cells is a stem cell). The stem cells divide infrequently, but give rise to a population of rapidly dividing cells called transit amplifying cells that, in turn, produce the differentiated cells of the prostate (Figure 1).

If stem cell theory is correct, the most important cells within the prostate epithelium are the stem cells. Many discussion articles have been written concerning prostate epithelial stem cells and their role in normal development, benign prostatic hyperplasia (BPH) and cancer[1,2,5–8].

In cell culture, the ability of single cells to develop colonies is equated with stem and transit amplifying cells[4]. The colony-forming ability of human prostate epithelium was first described by Peehl and colleagues[9,10]. They showed that, at low plating densities (100 cells per 5-cm Petri dish), about 5% of the epithelial cells formed colonies, and that some of these were very large.

Similar findings were made by Hudson and co-workers[11], who extended Peehl's work by distinguishing colonies derived from stem and transit amplifying cells. Prostate epithelial cells were cloned in a serum-free medium (PrEGM; BioWhittaker, Wokingham, UK). A small population of cells (about 0.5% of the cells plated)

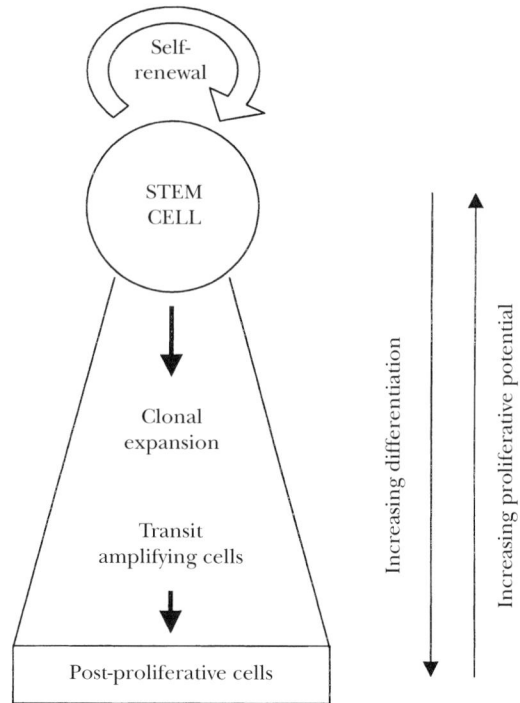

Figure 1 Schematic representation of stem cell differentiation hierarchy. As cells move down the hierarchy, they progressively lose proliferative potential and gain differentiated characteristics. The resultant post-proliferative cell population is differentiated but non-dividing. From reference 4

was able to form very large colonies comprising mainly small tightly packed cells. The majority of the colonies (about 4.5% of cells plated) were smaller, and contained a mixture of small tightly packed undifferentiated and larger differentiated cells. The large colonies differentiated into basal and intermediate cells in Matrigel (Becton Dickinson, Oxford, UK), and when grown as xenografts in the subrenal capsule assay formed glandular prostate tissue. It was suggested that the large colonies were the product of prostate epithelial stem cells and the smaller colonies of transit amplifying cells[11].

Two types of colony were also obtained by cloning human prostate epithelial cells, by Collins and associates[12]. The morphology of the colonies differed somewhat from those described by Peehl[10] and Hudson[11], perhaps owing to the inclusion of serum in the growth medium. By preselecting for CD44-positive cells, Collins and associates isolated basal epithelial cells and showed that the colony-forming cells express high levels of α2 integrin on their surface. Frozen section studies indicated that about 15% of the basal cells express high levels of α2 integrin on their surface[12].

A further issue is whether any of these studies of stem cells provide information that is relevant to questions concerning the lineage of the prostate epithelial cells discussed in the next section. Interestingly, Collins and associates[12] found that 5% of the clonogenic cells express CK18, compared with 50% of the basal cells in an unselected population. It was suggested that CK18 expression is a marker of basal cells committed to differentiation[12].

The studies of Peehl and colleagues[10] and subsequent workers indicate that prostate epithelial stem cells can be isolated *in vitro*. Some clues to the properties of these stem cells have been gleaned from recent studies, but it is not yet possible to identify and isolate pure single prostate epithelial stem cells. Until definitive cell surface markers are identified,

analogous to those used to isolate hematopoietic stem cells, the isolation and characteristics of individual human prostate epithelial stem cells will remain elusive.

Models of prostate epithelial cell differentiation

Bonkhoff and Remberger[2] suggested that all the epithelial cell types within the prostate epithelium are derived from a common stem cell in the basal layer (Figure 2). Rather than concentrating on the basal and luminal layers, the primary distinction is between stem, proliferative and non-proliferative cells[2]. Some of the cells in the basal layer were found to express AR protein and/or mRNA, and it is suggested that these are the precursors of the luminal layer of columnar PSA-secreting cells.

By increasing the range of cytokeratin markers, Nagle and colleagues[13] demonstrated that basal cells can variably express CKs 5, 6, 8, 10, 13, 14, 18 and 19, and luminal cells can variably express CKs 5, 7, 8, 13, 18 and 19. Cytokeratin 15 staining was also described by Sherwood and associates[14], and Hudson and

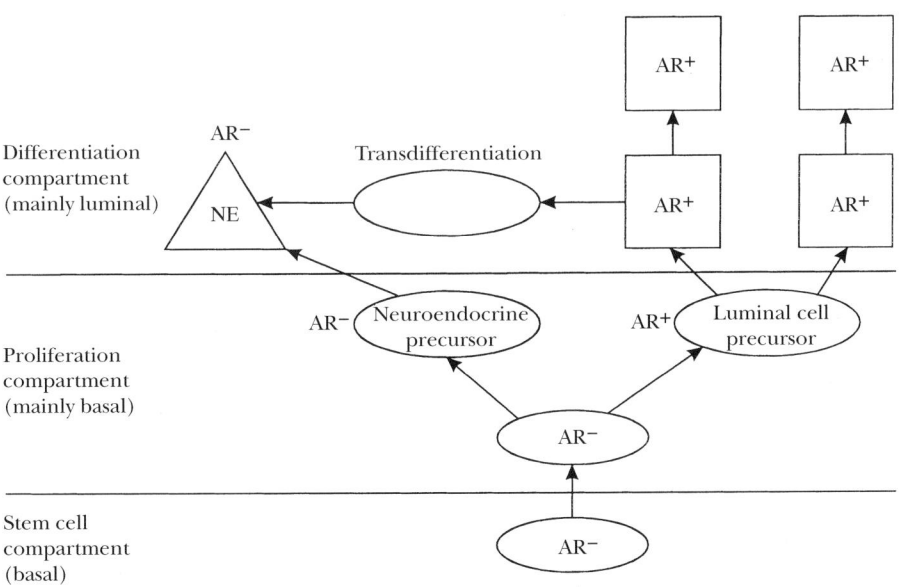

Figure 2 Simplified diagrammatic representation of the model of prostate epithelial cell differentiation described by Bonkhoff and Remberger[2]. NE, neuroendocrine

colleagues[15] saw CK15 and CK17 staining in BPH tissue. Hudson and colleagues[15] also saw CK19 in some luminal cells, as well as many basal cells (Figure 3), confirming the finding of Peehl and co-workers[16]. It was suggested that the CK19-positive population may represent the cells transiting from the basal to the luminal layer[15].

The clear distinction between basal and luminal markers has been questioned by Xue and co-workers[17], and van Leenders and associates[18]. It is suggested that a stem cell fraction expresses high levels of CK5/14 in conjunction with low levels of CK18. A transit amplifying or intermediate population loses K14 expression and, as the cells differentiate, K18 is up-

regulated and K5 down-regulated, leading to terminally differentiated cells expressing K18 only (Figure 4). Interestingly, both Bonkhoff and associates[19] and Xue and co-workers[17] have observed occasional PSA expression in the basal layer, also suggesting that there may not be an absolute distinction between the phenotypes of the basal and luminal layers.

A third cell layer between the basal and luminal layers was described by de Marzo and colleagues[6], identified by a low level of p27[kip1] expression. This protein is expressed at high levels in resting cells, but is down-regulated in proliferating cells. The basal layer was found to be heterogeneous for p27[kip1] expression, and a layer of p27[kip1] negative cells was present in

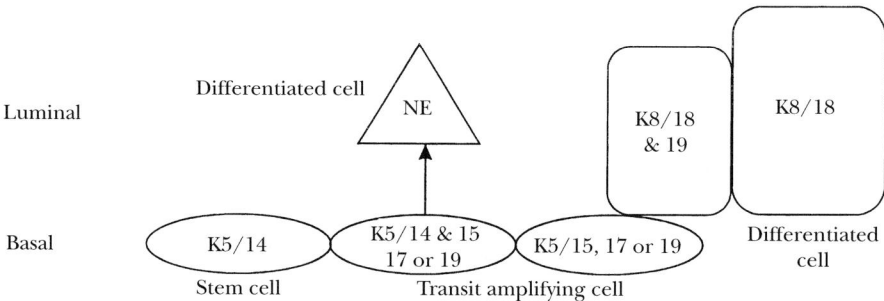

Figure 3 Simplified diagrammatic representation of the model of prostate epithelial cell differentiation described by Hudson and colleagues[15]. NE, neuroendocrine

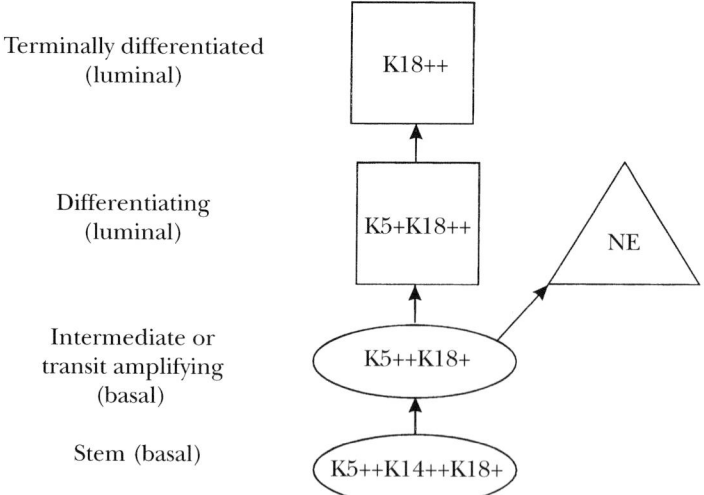

Figure 4 Simplified diagrammatic representation of the model of prostate epithelial cell differentiation described by van Leenders and colleagues[18]. NE, neuroendocrine; +, degree of expression

some areas between the basal and luminal layers[6].

The concept of a bidirectional stem cell was described by Wang and associates[20], based on studies of fetal prostate. The human prostate begins to develop at about the tenth week of gestation, as a series of outbuddings from the urogenital sinus epithelium into the surrounding mesenchyme. By the 16th week of gestation, basal, secretory PSA-producing and neuroendocrine cells are all present[20]. Fetal urogenital sinus epithelium was studied before and during the development of prostatic buds and ducts and from adult prostate of mice, rats and humans, with similar results in all three species (Figure 5).

The key finding of Wang and associates[20] was that almost all the epithelial cells of the urogenital sinus express a full complement of basal and luminal markers, including CK5/14 and CK8/18, as well as glutathione-S-transferase pi (GSTpi), CK19 and p63. As prostate development proceeds, luminal and basal cell populations are delineated, but at all stages a proportion of the basal cells continue to express all these markers, and these cells are found in

the adult at a low frequency (about 0.6% of basal cells). A strong argument was made that these are the stem cells of the adult prostate[20]. It was suggested that this theory can be tested by studying the potential of clonal cells to give rise to other prostate epithelial cell types[20].

Prostatic intraepithelial neoplasia

Prostatic intraepithelial neoplasia (PIN) is generally accepted to be a precursor of prostate cancer[21], and consequently provides clues to changes that occur in the differentiation pathway during the development of prostate cancer.

Three grades of PIN are recognized: 1, 2 and 3, with the highest grade representing carcinoma *in situ*. In ducts and acini containing PIN, there is disruption of the basal layer seen in 0.7% of grade 1, 15% of grade 2 and 56% of grade 3 PIN. Early evidence of invasion was frequently observed in association with grade 3 PIN[21].

Patterns of cell proliferation are altered in PIN. In normal prostate tissue and BPH, 70–80% of the proliferative cells are seen in the basal layer[15,19]. In low-grade (1) PIN nearly 70%

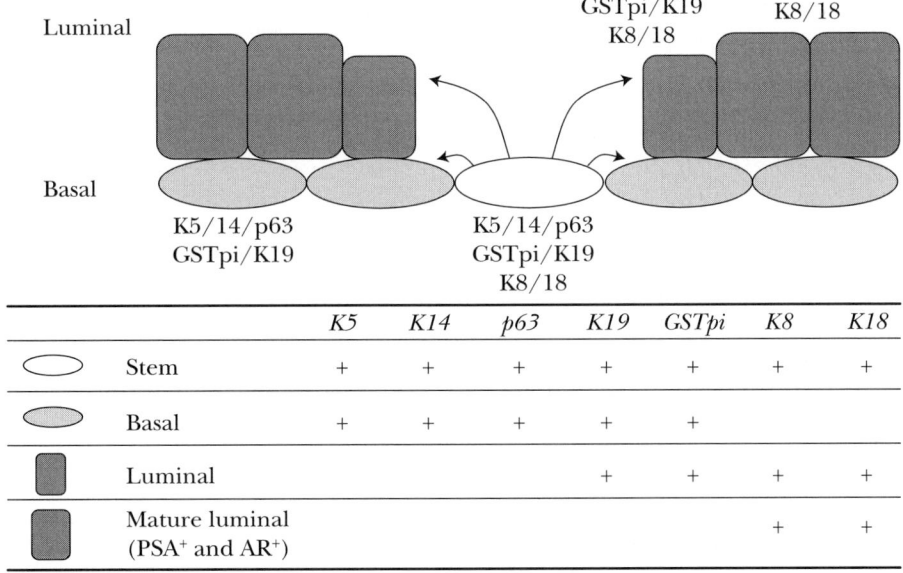

		K5	K14	p63	K19	GSTpi	K8	K18
⬭	Stem	+	+	+	+	+	+	+
⬭	Basal	+	+	+	+	+		
▮	Luminal				+	+	+	+
▮	Mature luminal (PSA+ and AR+)						+	+

Figure 5 Simplified diagrammatic representation of the model of prostate epithelial cell differentiation described by Wang and colleagues[20]. GSTpi, glutathione-S-transferase pi; PSA, prostate-specific antigen; AR, androgen receptor

of the proliferative cells are in the luminal layer, and this increases to over 90% in high-grade (2 and 3) PIN[19].

In terms of differentiation, an increased proportion of the luminal cells are positive for CK19 in PIN[13]. Overexpression of Bcl-2 (an antiapoptotic protein) and the *RET* oncogene[22] is observed in high-grade PIN[23], together with changes in the distribution of metalloproteinases[24].

Prostate cancer cell differentiation

In prostate cancer, the predominant cell type has a phenotype with characteristics of the luminal layer[25–29]. The majority of the cancer cells express CK8/18 and PSA and have nuclei that stain strongly for AR protein. Another basal cell marker, p63, is absent in prostate cancer[30]. At least 95% of both primary and metastatic prostate cancers stain for PSA[31], but higher-grade cancers stain less intensively than lower-grade cancers[32].

Most cancers also contain a few neuro-endocrine cells, and in a small minority this is the predominant cell type. Occasional cancer cells are positive for both PSA and chromogranin A[9].

While the majority of prostate cancer cells have a luminal phenotype, cells with inter-mediate characteristics can also be observed in many cancers, perhaps reflecting the origin of these cancers. Antibodies to the luminal and basal cell markers CD57 and CD44[33] were used to sort single cells isolated from primary and metastatic prostate cancers by Liu and colleagues[34]. Most primary tumors and one lymph node metastasis contained a predomi-nance of cells with the luminal marker CD57, while two other metastases contained cells with a mainly basal CD44-positive phenotype[34].

In order to study the expression of basal cell markers, 14 cases of prostate cancer (Gleason scores 6–9) with metastases to lymph nodes were stained with the antibody 34βE12, which recognizes CKs 1, 5, 10 and 14[35]. Staining was observed in 7/13 (54%) primary tumors and 6/14 (43%) metastases.

An earlier study had also clearly shown that some prostate cancers express basal cyto-keratins[36]. In low-grade cancers (Gleason grades 1–3), 35% (range 0–90%) of the cancer cells stained positive, compared with 25% and 0% of Gleason grade 4 and 5 cancers, respectively[36]. Cells that coexpress the basal cytokeratin and CK18 may represent a transit amplifying population in prostate cancer[36].

A comparison of CK5 and CK18 staining was undertaken by de Medina and colleagues[37], using prostate cancer tissue from 24 untreated, 15 hormone-deprived and ten hormone-relapsed patients. It was confirmed that prostate cancer can coexpress CK5 and CK18. The percentage of cancer cells staining with the basal marker CK5 increased from 14% in the untreated group to 47% and 38% in the hormone-treated and hormone-relapsed groups, respectively. Similar figures were obtained for another basal cell marker, epidermal growth factor (EGF) receptor[37].

In order to determine whether the prostate cancer cells expressing a basal cell phenotype were early (CK5/14-expressing) or inter-mediate (CK14-negative), antibodies specific for CK5, CK14 and CK18 labelled with different fluorescent dyes were used to stain 56 prostate cancer metastases[8]. All the cancers were CK18-positive and CK14-negative. CK5 staining was observed in 29% of the untreated cancers, 75% of the cancers undergoing androgen deprivation and 57% of hormone-relapsed prostate cancers. Approximately half the tumors contained neuroendocrine cells, regardless of hormone treatment[8].

Stem cell theory and prostate cancer cell differentiation

A stem cell model has been proposed for cancer, corresponding to the stem cell model in normal tissue. Three tumor cell populations are pre-dicted: stem, transit amplifying and terminally differentiated[38]. If prostate cancer conforms to the stem cell model, then it is derived from a single cell that expands clonally to give rise to further stem cells as well as transit amplifying and differentiated cells.

The direct evidence for cancer stem cells is the observation that most cancers have a monoclonal origin. Clonal markers, such as the Philadelphia chromosome, can be found in every cancer cell. A second line of evidence for a stem cell model for cancer is derived from clonogenic assays. Colony-forming assays of prostate and other types of cancer indicate that the proportion of clonogenic cells is low (usually less than 1%). This observation could have two explanations. It is possible that all the cells in the cancer have an equally low probability of proliferating *in vitro* or that there is a small stem cell fraction delineated by the clonogenic assays. These possibilities have been distinguished in human acute myeloid leukemia (AML). It was shown that, in most cases, only a small fraction of the leukemic cells (CD34[+]CD38[−], corresponding to the phenotype of the normal progenitor stem cells) can be xenografted in NOD/SCID (non-obese diabetic/severe combined immunodeficiency disorder) mice. Thus, proliferative capacity differs among AML cells, and only a small subpopulation (leukemia stem cells) can proliferate and transfer the disease[39].

Markers of basal, luminal and neuro-endocrine cells can be found in prostate cancers, in part corresponding to the pattern of differentiation in normal prostate epithelium. This observation suggests that cancer cells undergo processes that are analogous to the self-renewal and differentiation of normal stem cells, and provides circumstantial evidence that prostate cancer conforms to stem cell theory.

Prostate cancer stem cells

If it is correct that prostate cancer conforms to stem cell theory, then the question is, in which type of cell does prostate cancer arise? Theoretically, a cancer stem cell could be derived from a cell at any stage of differentiation. One concept is that a differentiated cell can gain proliferative capacity and 'de-differentiate' as the cancer progresses[4]. At the other end of the spectrum, cancer may arise in a stem cell[4,40].

It has been proposed that prostate cancer originates in a normal stem cell[5]. During progression to an invasive stage, the cells lose their basal phenotype and acquire luminal cell characteristics. An intermediate stage can be seen in PIN, in which the proliferative compartment is inverted and shifts to the luminal cell layer.

Alternatively, it has been proposed that prostate cancer originates in an intermediate transit amplifying cell[8,36], perhaps in the luminal layer[6]. Following androgen withdrawal, the proportion of cancers containing a basal cell phenotype increases[7,8,37], suggesting a basal cell origin from either stem or transit amplifying cells.

A luminal cell origin of prostate cancer has also been proposed[25,26,29,34], based on the luminal cell phenotype of most prostate cancers.

Most of the evidence concerning the origin of malignant stem cells comes from studies of hematopoietic cancers. The advantage of studying leukemias and lymphomas is that stem cell and lineage markers are available for the hematopoietic system, in contrast to prostate and most other epithelial tissues.

Evidence for a normal stem cell origin comes from human AML. Most of the cells capable of forming human AML xenografts in NOD/SCID mice have a CD34[+]CD38[−] phenotype, as do the hematopoietic stem cells. In contrast, CD34[+]CD38[+] AML cells are incapable of forming xenografts[39]. Thus, the cells capable of initiating human AML in the mice possess the differentiative and proliferative capacities and the potential for self-renewal expected of a leukemic stem cell[39]. As with AML, both chronic myelogenous leukemia and acute lymphoblastic leukemia contain characteristic genetic changes in cells that have the same cell surface phenotype as the normal hematopoietic precursors[41,42].

A second line of evidence also comes from human AML. An 8;21 translocation is common in AML, producing a fusion gene. In AML patients in remission, cells containing transcripts from this fusion gene can be isolated from the bone marrow. However, these cells are not leukemic and produce normal

151

myeloerythroid cells *in vitro*[43]. It was also shown that, whereas the leukemic blasts were CD34+CD38−Thy-1−, normal stem cells were CD34+CD38−Thy-1+. Therefore, the initiating event must have occurred in normal hematopoietic stem cells, with the subsequent genetic changes occurring in either downstream Thy-1 progenitors or in hematopoietic stem cells that lost Thy-1 expression[43].

There seems little doubt that many leukemias arise in normal stem cells. However, the evidence also suggests that leukemias progress as a result of further genetic changes. These further genetic changes do not necessarily occur in the cancer stem cells, and could occur either in transit amplifying or more differentiated cancer cells. Prostate cancer may develop and progress in a similar manner.

In cases where inherited mutations are present, then it is more likely that a cancer stem cell could be derived from a transit amplifying cell: for example, in individuals born with mutations in tumor suppressor genes such as the retinoblastoma gene, or transgenic mice whose cells constitutively express viral genes such as SV40 large T antigen or other genes that influence cell survival (for examples see reference 40).

In prostate cancer, it is believed that up to 20 years may elapse before a cancer is clinically detectable, and that a cancer is two-thirds to three-quarters through its proliferative life span before it can be detected. If it is necessary for the prostate cancer stem cell to acquire 5–10 mutations before clinically apparent disease develops, it seems probable that in most cases the cancer arises in the only cell type that can survive for a sufficiently long period, the normal prostate epithelial stem cell.

Once a stem cell has acquired one or two mutations, it will then pass these mutations to all its progeny, including the transit amplifying cells with their much greater proliferative potential. These mutations may confer self-renewal capacity and extended life span on the transit amplifying cells. Therefore, while the initiating events probably occur in a normal prostate epithelial stem cell, it is possible that the expansion and progression of the cancer occurs in the genetically modified highly proliferative transit amplifying cells as a result of further genetic changes.

The pattern of differentiation seen in prostate cancer may therefore depend how far down the pathway of differentiation the subsequent genetic events occur. Further progression, for example to metastatic and hormone-independent disease, could occur as a result of additional clonal expansions[44,45].

References

1. Isaacs JT, Coffey DS. Etiology and disease process of benign prostatic hyperplasia. *Prostate* 1989;2 (Suppl):33–50
2. Bonkhoff H, Remberger K. Differentiation pathways and histogenetic aspects of normal and abnormal prostatic growth: a stem cell model. *Prostate* 1996;28:98–106
3. Robinson EJ, Neal DE, Collins AT. Basal cells are progenitors of luminal cells in primary cultures of differentiating human prostatic epithelium. *Prostate* 1998;37:149–60
4. Buick RN, Pollak MN. Perspectives on clonogenic tumor cells, stem cells, and oncogenes. *Cancer Res* 1984;44:4909–18
5. Bonkhoff H. Role of the basal cells in premalignant changes of the human prostate: a stem cell concept for the development of prostate cancer. *Eur Urol* 1996;30:201–5
6. de Marzo AM, Meeker AK, Epstein JI, Coffey DS. Prostate stem cell compartments: expression of the cell cycle inhibitor p27Kip1 in normal, hyperplastic, and neoplastic cells. *Am J Pathol* 1998;153:911–19

7. Bui M, Reiter RE. Stem cell genes in androgen-independent prostate cancer. *Cancer Metastasis Rev* 1998–99;17:391–9

8. van-Leenders GJ, Schalken JA. Stem cell differentiation within the human prostate epithelium: implications for prostate carcinogenesis. *BJU Int* 2001;88(Suppl 2):35–42

9. Peehl DM, Stamey TA. Serum-free growth of adult human prostatic epithelial cells. *In Vitro Cell Dev Biol* 1986;22:82–90

10. Peehl DM, Wong ST, Stamey TA. Clonal growth characteristics of adult human prostatic epithelial cells. *In Vitro Cell Dev Biol* 1988;24: 530–6

11. Hudson DL, O'Hare M, Watt FM, Masters JR. Proliferative heterogeneity in the human prostate: evidence for epithelial stem cells. *Lab Invest* 2000;80:1243–50

12. Collins AT, Habib FK, Maitland NJ, Neal DE. Identification and isolation of human prostate epithelial stem cells based on alpha(2)beta(1)-integrin expression. *J Cell Sci* 2001;114:3865–72

13. Nagle RB, Brawer MK, Kittelson J, Clark V. Phenotypic relationships of prostatic intra-epithelial neoplasia to invasive prostatic carcinoma. *Am J Pathol* 1991;138:119–28

14. Sherwood ER, Berg LA, Mitchell NJ, McNeal JE, Kozlowski JM, Lee C. Differential cytokeratin expression in normal, hyperplastic and malignant epithelial cells from human prostate. *J Urol* 1990;143:167–71

15. Hudson DL, Guy AT, Fry P, O'Hare MJ, Watt FM, Masters JR. Epithelial cell differentiation pathways in the human prostate: identification of intermediate phenotypes by keratin expression. *J Histochem Cytochem* 2001;49:271–8

16. Peehl DM, Sellers RG, McNeal JE. Keratin 19 in the adult human prostate: tissue and cell culture studies. *Cell Tissue Res* 1996;285:171–6

17. Xue Y, Smedts F, Debruyne FM, de-la-Rosette JJ, Schalken JA. Identification of intermediate cell types by keratin expression in the developing human prostate. *Prostate* 1998;34:292–301

18. van-Leenders G, Dijkman H, Hulsbergen-van-de-Kaa C, Ruiter D, Schalken J. Demonstration of intermediate cells during human prostate epithelial differentiation *in situ* and *in vitro* using triple-staining confocal scanning microscopy. *Lab Invest* 2000;80:1251–8

19. Bonkhoff H, Stein U, Remberger K. Multi-directional differentiation in the normal, hyperplastic, and neoplastic human prostate: simultaneous demonstration of cell-specific epithelial markers. *Hum Pathol* 1994;25:42–6

20. Wang Y, Hayward S, Cao M, Thayer K, Cunha G. Cell differentiation lineage in the prostate. *Differentiation* 2001;68:270–9

21. Bostwick DG, Brawer MK. Prostatic intra-epithelial neoplasia and early invasion in prostate cancer. *Cancer* 1987;59:788–94

22. Dawson DM, Lawrence EG, MacLennan GT, *et al.* Altered expression of *RET* proto-oncogene product in prostatic intraepithelial neoplasia and prostate cancer. *J Natl Cancer Inst* 1998;90: 519–23

23. Johnson MI, Robinson MC, Marsh C, Robson CN, Neal DE, Hamdy FC. Expression of Bcl-2, Bax, and p53 in high-grade prostatic intra-epithelial neoplasia and localized prostate cancer: relationship with apoptosis and proliferation. *Prostate* 1998;37:223–9

24. Upadhyay J, Shekarriz B, Nemeth JA, *et al.* Membrane type 1-matrix metalloproteinase (MT1-MMP) and MMP-2 immunolocalization in human prostate: change in cellular localization associated with high-grade prostatic intra-epithelial neoplasia. *Clin Cancer Res* 1999;5: 4105–10

25. Brawer MK, Peehl DM, Stamey TA, Bostwick DG. Keratin immunoreactivity in the benign and neoplastic human prostate. *Cancer Res* 1985;45: 3663–7

26. Nagle RB, Ahmann FR, McDaniel KM, Paquin ML, Clark VA, Celniker A. Cytokeratin characterization of human prostatic carcinoma and its derived cell lines. *Cancer Res* 1987;47:281–6

27. O'Malley FP, Grignon DJ, Shum DT. Usefulness of immunoperoxidase staining with high-molecular-weight cytokeratin in the differential diagnosis of small-acinar lesions of the prostate gland. *Virchow's Arch A Pathol Anat Histopathol* 1990;417:191–6

28. Sherwood ER, Theyer G, Steiner G, Berg LA, Kozlowski JM, Lee C. Differential expression of specific cytokeratin polypeptides in the basal and luminal epithelia of the human prostate. *Prostate* 1991;18:303–14

29. Okada H, Tsubura A, Okamura A, *et al.* Keratin profiles in normal/hyperplastic prostates and prostate carcinoma. *Virchow's Arch A Pathol Anat Histopathol* 1992;421:157–61

30. Signoretti S, Waltregny D, Dilks J, *et al.* p63 is a prostate basal cell marker and is required for prostate development. *Am J Pathol* 2000;157: 1769–75

31. Ford TF, Butcher DN, Masters JR, Parkinson MC. Immunocytochemical localisation of prostate-specific antigen: specificity and application to clinical practice. *Br J Urol* 1985;57:50–5

32. Ellis DW, Leffers S, Davies JS, Ng AB. Multiple immunoperoxidase markers in benign hyperplasia and adenocarcinoma of the prostate. *Am J Clin Pathol* 1984;81:279–84

33. Liu AY, True LD, LaTray L, *et al.* Cell–cell interaction in prostate gene regulation and

cytodifferentiation. *Proc Natl Acad Sci USA* 1997;94:10705–10

34. Liu AY, True LD, LaTray L, *et al.* Analysis and sorting of prostate cancer cell types by flow cytometry. *Prostate* 1999;40:192–9

35. Googe PB, McGinley KM, Fitzgibbon JF. Anticytokeratin antibody 34 beta E12 staining in prostate carcinoma. *Am J Clin Pathol* 1997;107: 219–23

36. Verhagen AP, Ramaekers FC, Aalders TW, Schaafsma HE, Debruyne FM, Schalken JA. Colocalization of basal and luminal cell-type cytokeratins in human prostate cancer. *Cancer Res* 1992;52:6182–7

37. de Medina S, Salomon L, Colombel M, *et al.* Modulation of cytokeratin subtype, EGF receptor, and androgen receptor expression during progression of prostate cancer. *Hum Pathol* 1998;29:1005–12

38. Mackillop WJ, Ciampi A, Till JE, Buick RN. A stem cell model of human tumor growth: implications for tumor cell clonogenic assays. *J Natl Cancer Inst* 1983;70:9–16

39. Bonnet D, Dick JE. Human acute myeloid leukemia is organized as a hierarchy that originates from a primitive hematopoietic cell. *Nature Med* 1997;3:730–7

40. Reya T, Morrison SJ, Clarke MF, Weissman IL. Stem cells, cancer, and cancer stem cells. *Nature (London)* 2001;414:105–11

41. George AA, Franklin J, Kerkof K, *et al.* Detection of leukemic cells in the CD34(+)CD38(−) bone marrow progenitor population in children with acute lymphoblastic leukemia. *Blood* 2001;97: 3925–30

42. Mauro MJ, Druker BJ. Chronic myelogenous leukemia. *Curr Opin Oncol* 2001;13:3–7

43. Miyamoto T, Weissman IL, Akashi, K. AML1/ ETO-expressing nonleukemic stem cells in acute myelogenous leukemia with 8;21 chromosomal translocation. *Proc Natl Acad Sci USA* 2000; 97:7521–6

44. Foulds L. Tumor progression. *Cancer Res* 1957;17:355–6

45. Nowell PC. Tumor progression: a brief historical perspective. *Semin Cancer Biol* 2002;12:261–6

Role of the stromal microenvironment in carcinogenesis of the prostate

18

G. R. Cunha, S. W. Hayward, Y. Z. Wang and W. A. Ricke

Introduction

Prostatic development occurs as a result of an epithelial–mesenchymal interaction, which is the basic developmental mechanism employed by all organs and organ systems composed of an epithelial parenchyma, e.g. male and female urogenital tracts, the gastrointestinal system and the integument. For hormone target organs of the reproductive tract, an additional layer of developmental regulation occurs via the hormonal milieu. Thus, development of the prostate is dependent upon fetal testicular androgens, whose effects are mediated via androgen receptors expressed in fetal urogenital sinus mesenchyme.

Reciprocal mesenchymal–epithelial interactions in prostatic development

The prostate develops from the embryonic urogenital sinus via interactions between the endodermal epithelium of the urogenital sinus (UGE) and the mesoderm-derived urogenital sinus mesenchyme (UGM). UGM–UGE interactions are obligatory for prostatic development. When UGE and UGM are grown by themselves, prostatic development does not occur. However, when UGM and UGE are reassociated, prostatic development proceeds provided that androgens are present. During prostatic development, androgen-dependent inductive signals from UGM direct the developmental process[1]. Prostate-inducing signals arise from spatially distinct areas within the UGM[2,3], which elicit development of the well-defined lobar subdivisions of the rodent prostate[2–4]. UGM specifies prostatic identity in the undifferentiated

UGE, induces prostatic bud formation, elicits prostatic bud growth and branching morphogenesis, promotes prostatic epithelial differentiation into secretory epithelial cells and determines the types of secretory proteins expressed. These conclusions have been derived from mesenchymal–epithelial recombination experiments in which UGM has been grown in association with a variety of heterotypic epithelia. The tissue recombinant composed of embryonic UGM plus epithelium of the urinary bladder (BLE) has been the most informative experiment. When UGM + BLE tissue recombinants were grown under the renal capsule of male hosts (and thus exposed to endogenous androgens), the bladder epithelium differentiated into prostatic epithelium. Unexpectedly, UGM induced prostatic development from either embryonic bladder epithelium or fully differentiated adult bladder epithelium[5,6]. Adult bladder epithelium is a highly specialized non-glandular androgen receptor-negative epithelium that lines the bladder. In UGM + BLE tissue recombinants, inductive influences from the UGM re-specify epithelial identity from bladder to prostate. Three to four days after transplantation of UGM + adult BLE tissue recombinants, prostatic buds emerge from the basal aspect of the bladder epithelium[5]. These solid epithelial buds elongate and undergo branching morphogenesis and canalize into ducts in a fashion similar to that of developing prostate. The UGM-induced adult bladder epithelium differentiates into tall columnar secretory luminal cells, interspersed by non-secretory basal cells located on the basement membrane. These two cell types express the correct range of differentiation markers distinctive of mature prostatic epithelium. The induced bladder epithelium resembles prostatic epithelium both at the light and electron microscopic levels. Androgen receptors develop in the originally androgen receptor-negative bladder epithelium of UGM + BLE tissue recombinants, and prostate-specific secretory proteins are expressed[5,7–9]. Thus, embryonic UGM induces prostatic identity, formation and elongation of prostatic buds, ductal branching morphogenesis and functional prostatic histodifferentiation in bladder epithelium. The fact that an adult bladder epithelium can be induced to undergo this remarkable change in histodifferentiation implies a continued importance of epithelial–stromal interactions into adulthood, presumably for the maintenance of adult epithelial differentiation. A likely interpretation of these data is that adult bladder epithelium contains a pleuripotent population, which is capable of responding to inductive mesenchyma. Such pleuripotent epithelial cells, which might represent a stem cell population, have the capacity to give rise to entirely new phenotypes when induced by heterotypic UGM.

While UGM induces prostatic epithelial differentiation, prostatic epithelium in a reciprocal fashion induces UGM to differentiate into smooth muscle. Evidence supporting a role of prostatic epithelium as the inducer of smooth muscle is based upon studies in which undifferentiated embryonic mouse or rat UGM was grown beneath the renal capsule of male hosts for 4 weeks. Such UGM grafts formed only small amounts of smooth muscle. In contrast, when rat or mouse UGM was grafted with epithelium of adult prostate, bladder or embryonic urogenital sinus derived from rat or mouse, prostatic ducts developed that were surrounded by α-actin-positive smooth muscle cells organized into thin sheaths, as is appropriate for rodent prostate[10]. Significantly, rat UGM formed thick sheets of smooth muscle in tissue recombinants composed of rat UGM plus human prostatic epithelium[11,12], which is the pattern of smooth muscle characteristic of

human prostate. This demonstrates that human prostatic epithelium both induced the rat UGM to undergo smooth muscle differentiation and determined the spatial patterning of the smooth muscle. Thus, the prostate develops as a result of reciprocal cell–cell interactions in which UGM induces prostatic epithelial differentiation, and developing prostatic epithelium induces smooth muscle differentiation in the UGM. The ultimate result of these reciprocal epithelial–mesenchymal interactions is the development of mature prostatic tissue in which the epithelium expresses a highly differentiated secretory phenotype and specific secretory proteins, and the mesenchyme develops into a mature prostatic stroma predominantly composed of smooth muscle cells.

Paracrine influences of androgens and estrogens on prostatic development

As discussed above, mesenchymal–epithelial interactions play critical roles in development of the prostate. Moreover, prostatic development is absolutely dependent upon androgens, which act via androgen receptors. During prostatic development, androgens acting via mesenchymal–epithelial interactions induce prostatic buds, ductal growth and branching and epithelial proliferation. Thus, the field of prostatic development lies at the boundary between developmental biology and endocrinology. In this regard, the ontogeny of androgen receptors in the prostate is particularly informative. Several investigators have confirmed that prior to and during prostatic development, the UGM expresses high levels of androgen receptors, while androgen receptors are initially undetectable in the epithelium[13,14]. Indeed, when prostatic buds emerge from the urogenital sinus epithelium, androgen receptors are undetectable even in the induced epithelial buds. This finding suggests that mesenchymal androgen receptors (and not epithelial androgen receptors) are implicated in the early phases of prostatic development. Androgen receptors are at first detected in developing prostatic epithelium in the neonatal mouse and rat, as the solid epithelial buds begin to canalize[15–17]. Thus, the appearance of epithelial androgen receptors coincides with postnatal aspects of prostatic development. To elucidate the respective roles of epithelial versus mesenchymal androgen receptors in prostatic development, tissue recombinants were analyzed that had been prepared with mesenchyme and epithelium from wild-type (wt) and androgen receptor-negative testicular feminization (Tfm) mice (Figure 1). Epithelium from wt and Tfm mice undergo prostatic development when combined with wt–UGM. The common feature of these two tissue recombinants is the expression of androgen receptors in the UGM. The other two tissue recombinants, Tfm–UGM + Tfm–epithelium and Tfm–UGM + wt–epithelium, do not

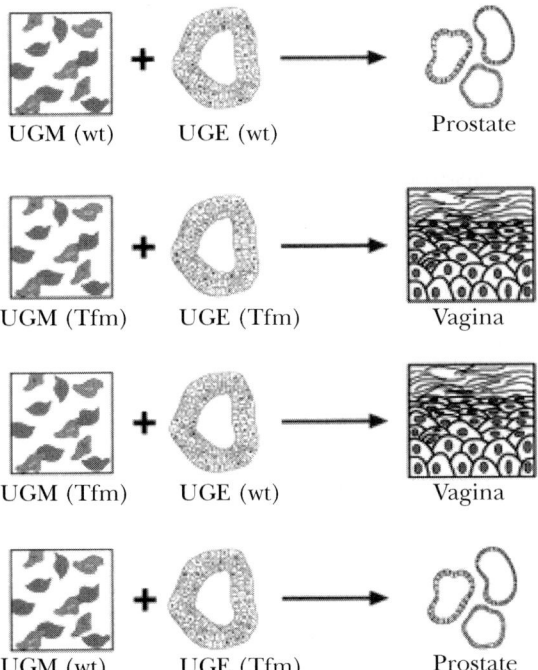

Figure 1 A summary of tissue recombination experiments between urogenital sinus mesenchyme (UGM) and epithelium (UGE) from testicular feminization (Tfm) and wild-type (wt) embryos. A positive androgenic response (prostatic morphogenesis) occurs when wt mesenchyme is grown in association with either wt or Tfm epithelium. Conversely, vagina-like differentiation occurs when either wt or Tfm epithelium is grown in association with Tfm mesenchyme

undergo prostatic development in the presence of androgens (Figure 1). The lack of prostatic development in these two tissue recombinants prepared with androgen receptor-negative Tfm–UGM suggested a critical role for mesenchymal androgen receptors in prostatic development, an idea that was confirmed through analysis of tissue recombinants composed of wt–UGM + Tfm– epithelium. In wt–UGM + Tfm–epithelium tissue recombinants, the androgen receptor-deficient Tfm epithelium underwent androgen-dependent ductal morphogenesis, epithelial proliferation and columnar cytodifferentiation, thus forming glandular epithelium resembling prostate[18]. This demonstrates that certain 'androgenic effects' on epithelium do not require epithelial androgen receptors. Instead, many epithelial androgenic effects are elicited by paracrine factors produced by androgen receptor-positive mesenchyme.

To investigate the function of epithelial androgen receptors, tissue recombinants composed of androgen receptor-positive wt–UGM + androgen receptor-positive wt– epithelium have been compared with tissue recombinants composed of androgen receptor-positive wt–UGM + androgen receptor-negative–Tfm epithelium. Such tissue recombinants differ only in the presence or absence of epithelial androgen receptors. These experiments demonstrated that, while the Tfm epithelium was induced to undergo prostatic differentiation, prostatic secretory proteins were not expressed[9,19]. Thus, epithelial androgen receptors are required for expression of androgen receptor-dependent secretory proteins.

While the prostate is primarily considered to be an androgen target, it is also responsive to estrogens. One well-known effect of estrogen on the prostate is squamous metaplasia[20]. Estrogenic effects are mediated via estrogen receptors expressed in the developing and adult prostate[21,22]. Given the paracrine action of androgen on the prostate mediated via stromal androgen receptors, we considered the possibility that prostatic squamous metaplasia may be similarly induced via stromal estrogen receptors (ERs). Experiments using ERα- and

ERβ-null mice demonstrated that ERα, and not ERβ, is essential for induction of prostatic squamous metaplasia by diethylstilbestrol (DES)[20,23]. To determine the respective roles of epithelial versus stromal ERα in induction of prostatic squamous metaplasia, the following tissue recombinants were prepared with prostatic epithelium (PRE) and stroma (S) from wt and ERα knock-out (αERKO) mice: wt–S + wt–PRE, αERKO–S + αERKO–PRE, wt–S + αERKO–PRE and αERKO–S + wt–PRE. DES induced squamous metaplasia only in wt–S + wt–PRE tissue recombinants. Tissue recombinants containing αERKO–PRE and/or αERKO–S (αERKO–S + αERKO–PRE, wt–S + αERKO–PRE and αERKO–S + wt–PRE) were not induced by DES to become metaplastic. Thus, estrogenic induction of prostatic squamous metaplasia appeared to require the action of estrogen via stromal ERα (paracrine mechanism) as well as the direct action of estrogen via epithelial ERα. The significance of paracrine action of estrogen on the prostate has also been suggested in studies of neo-natal imprinting of the prostate[24,25]. Studies have demonstrated ERα and ERβ in both prostatic epithelial and stromal cells during various stages of development [21,25–28], and the tissue recombinant studies point formally to the importance of both stromal and epithelial ERα in estrogenic response in the prostate.

In a broader perspective, it is known that estrogens and progesterone regulate epithelial proliferation in hormone target organs of the male and female genital tracts. Comparable wild-type/steroid receptor-null tissue recombinants have been constructed with epithelium and mesenchyme from wild-type, ERα-null or progesterone receptor-null mice. Such experiments demonstrated that for all three classes of steroids (androgens, estrogens and progesterone) epithelial proliferation is regulated *in vivo* via the appropriate hormone receptors in the stromal cells in organs such as the prostate, uterus, vagina and mammary gland[29–32]. Thus, regulation of proliferation of normal epithelia by sex steroids occurs via paracrine mechanisms. In contrast, hormonal regulation of epithelial differentiation and

function requires direct hormone action mediated by epithelial hormone receptors[33,34]. It should be emphasized that these ideas are applicable to normal epithelia and probably not to neoplastic epithelia. For example, andro-genic regulation of epithelial proliferation during prostatic carcinogenesis appears to involve conversion from a paracrine to an autocrine mechanism of androgen-stimulated growth[35].

Role of stroma in hormonal carcinogenesis of the prostate

Epidemiological studies suggest a vital role of steroid hormones in prostate carcinogenesis[36], and, because the prostate is a target for both androgens and estrogens, both of these hormones have been implicated in prostatic carcinogenesis. The role of androgens and estrogens in prostatic carcinogenesis is suggested by several observations:

(1) Prostate cancer does not occur in eunuchs castrated early in life;

(2) In men and dogs, which are both suscept-ible to prostatic carcinogenesis, testos-terone secretion and plasma testosterone levels decline with age, while plasma free estrogen levels remain unchanged or increase during aging when prostate cancer develops and is diagnosed. Thus, elevation in the ratio of estrogen to testosterone is temporally related with the development of benign prostatic hyperplasia and pros-tate cancer[37,38];

(3) American Blacks, who have the highest incidence of prostatic cancer in the world, exhibit elevations in both plasma free testosterone and estradiol levels[39];

(4) Testosterone in combination with 17β-estradiol induces prostatic hyperplasia and dysplasia in mice, and induces prostate cancer in rats and in rUGM + Rb–/–PRE tissue recombinants[40–46].

Hormonal induction of prostate cancer is thought to require signalling through androgen and estrogen receptors, which are expressed in the prostate. The respective roles of androgen receptor, ERα and ERβ in prostatic carcinogenesis are currently under investigation through:

(1) Use of knock-out mice lacking ERα (αERKO mice) or ERβ (βERKO mice);

(2) Use of BPH-1 cells null for androgen receptor and estrogen receptors;

(3) Use of tissue recombinants that allow dissection of androgen receptor, ERα and ERβ signalling pathways.

Hormonal carcinogenesis in the prostate is independent of epithelial androgen receptors

As discussed above, certain androgenic responses in normal prostatic epithelial cells are mediated through stromal versus epithelial androgen receptors, such as epithelial proliferation, ductal branching morphogenesis, ductal canalization and cytodifferentiation into basal and luminal cells[29,47,48]. Likewise, in adulthood, androgens act via stromal androgen receptors (predominantly localized in the prostatic smooth muscle cells[17,49–51]) to maintain a fully differentiated growth-quiescent gland. Epithelial androgen receptors are required for secretory function in adulthood[9,19].

To elucidate the role of androgen receptors in prostate carcinogenesis, tissue recombinants were prepared by combining rat embryonic UGM (rUGM) plus BPH-1 cells (a clonally derived immortalized, non-tumorigenic human prostatic epithelial cell line)[52]. Androgen receptors are undetectable in BPH-1 prostatic epithelial cells by immunocytochemical and reverse transcriptase-polymerase chain reaction (RT-PCR) techniques[53]. ERα and ERβ are also not demonstrable in BPH-1 cells by immunocytochemical techniques. BPH-1 cells grafted by themselves under the renal capsule of untreated or testosterone + estradiol-treated (T + E2-treated) male hosts survive, but do not undergo tumorigenesis. This lack of a tumorigenic response in grafts of BPH-1 cells coincides with the apparent lack of androgen

and estrogen receptors. When BPH-1 cells are combined with rUGM (rUGM + BPH-1 recombinants) and grown in untreated male mice, relatively normal prostatic development occurs, with the formation of branched solid and canalized ductal structures. On the other hand, when rUGM + BPH-1 tissue recombinants are grown in T + E2-treated mice, BPH-1 cells undergo malignant transformation. As described above, androgen and estrogen receptors are undetectable in BPH-1 cells[52,53], while androgen and estrogen receptors are expressed in rUGM (Figure 2). Thus, the only androgen and estrogen receptors in rUGM + BPH-1 recombinants reside in the stroma. This suggests a critical role of stroma and stromal hormone receptors in mediating hormonal carcinogenesis of the prostate. Thus, hormonal carcinogenesis appears to involve paracrine mechanisms, as is the case for certain hormonal effects during normal prostatic growth and development. It is important to recognize that the carcinogenic effect of T + E2 in rUGM + BPH-1 tissue recombinants involves malignant progression of an epithelium harboring pre-existing genetic lesions, as the parental BPH-1 epithelial cells, while non-tumorigenic, are immortal and aneuploid[53,54]. Thus, this model differs from the induction of tumors in genetically normal prostatic epithelium, and instead may well mimic in some way the promotion of spontaneously occurring human prostate tumors.

ERα, but not ERβ, mediates hormonal carcinogenesis in the prostate

Estrogen plays an important role in the pathobiology of prostatic epithelium. Estrogens act through two specific estrogen receptors, ERα and ERβ[55,56]. While estrogen receptors in the prostate are difficult to detect by immunocytochemical methods, ERα has been consistently detected in prostatic stroma[26,57], and is also expressed in prostatic squamous metaplasia[58] (Wang and Cunha, unpublished data). ERβ is expressed at high levels in both prostatic epithelium and stroma in the developing prostate, but in adulthood ERβ is restricted

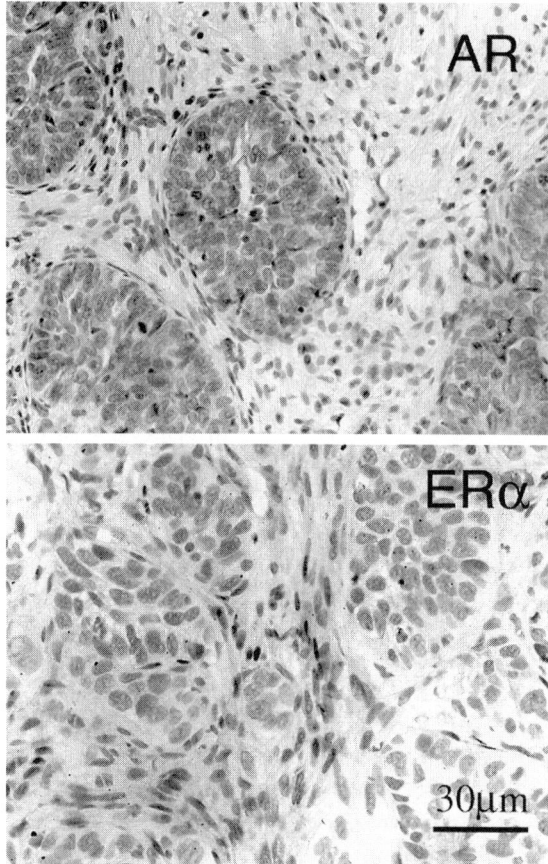

Figure 2 Rat embryonic urogenital sinus mesenchyme plus BPH-1 cells (clonally derived immortalized, non-tumorigenic human prostatic epithelial; cell line) (UGM + BPH-1) tissue recombinants stained for androgen receptor (top) and estrogen receptor α (bottom). Note androgen receptor (AR)- and estrogen receptor α (ERα)-positive cells in the stroma and the absence of these receptors in the epithelial structures formed by the BPH-1 cells

primarily to prostatic epithelial cells[58]. As described above, induction of prostatic squamous metaplasia is dependent upon ERα (and not ERβ), and ERα appears to be required simultaneously in both the epithelium and stroma[23]. The role of epithelial versus stromal ERα and ERβ in prostatic carcinogenesis is unknown and is currently under investigation.

Testosterone (T) in combination with estradiol (E_2) is an effective method of inducing prostatic cancer in adult Noble rats[40–44]. Likewise, mice treated with T + E_2 develop prostatic

hyperplasia and dysplasia[45]. Induction of hormonal carcinogenesis by T + E_2 in mice means that the power of mouse genetics can be used to elucidate the underlying molecular mechanisms. In this regard, treatment of αERKO mice with T + E_2 does not elicit prostatic hyperplasia or dysplasia[45], suggesting a key role of ERα in hormonal carcinogenesis. In support of this concept, ERβ knock-out mice (which express ERα) developed prostatic hyperplasia and dysplasia comparable to that seen in wild-type mice when treated with T + E_2 (Wang and Cunha, unpublished data). This emphasizes the importance of signalling through ERα in the induction of prostatic carcinogenesis. To determine the respective roles of epithelial versus stromal ERα in prostatic carcinogenesis, tissue recombinant experiments are under way in which prostatic epithelium (PRE) and stroma (S) are derived from wt and αERKO mice as follows: wt–S + wt–PRE,   αERKO–S + αERKO–PRE, wt–S + αERKO–PRE and αERKO–S + wt–PRE. Grafts of these tissue recombinants will be treated with T + E_2 to assess the effects of estrogen in hormonal carcinogenesis of the prostate. In support of this experimental approach are the recent findings that wild-type mouse UGM can be substituted for rat UGM in hormonal carcinogenesis studies. When wt–mouse UGM + BPH-1 tissue recombinants are grown for 6 months in untreated hosts, growth is modest, and benign epithelial structures develop. However, wt–mouse UGM + BPH-1 tissue recombinants grown for 6 months in T + E_2-treated hosts develop large tumors (Figure 3).

Reciprocal homeostatic interactions between prostatic stroma and epithelium in adulthood

The normal adult prostate is composed of two tissue compartments: an epithelial compartment and a fibromuscular stroma. The stroma of the adult prostate contains primarily smooth muscle cells and fibroblasts, both derived from embryonic UGM. Normal adult prostate contains highly differentiated functional

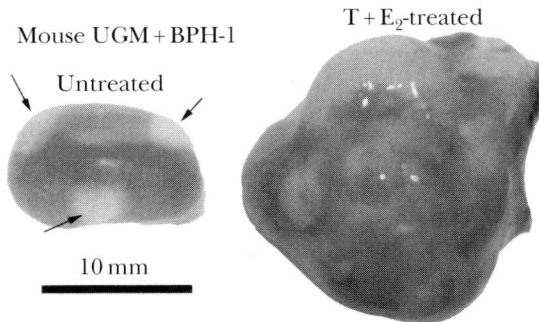

Mouse UGM + BPH-1

Untreated

T + E₂-treated

10 mm

Figure 3 Gross appearance of mouse embryonic urogenital sinus mesenchyme plus BPH-1 cells (UGM + BPH-1) tissue recombinants harvested after 6 months of growth in untreated and testosterone + estradiol-treated (T + E$_2$-treated) male nude mouse hosts. In untreated hosts the mouse UGM + BPH-1 tissue recombinants give rise to small benign growths (arrows), whereas in T + E$_2$-treated hosts the mouse UGM + BPH-1 tissue recombinants form large tumors that completely overgrow the host's kidney. Each kidney received three identical grafts

epithelial and stromal cells. Under steady state androgenic conditions of the adult male, the prostate contains differentiated smooth muscle cells in intimate relationship with highly differentiated and functional prostatic epithelium. Both cell types are growth-quiescent, with levels of proliferation and cell death extremely low and in balance. It should be emphasized that the growth-quiescent, homeostatic state in adulthood occurs in the presence of high levels of systemic androgens, which at earlier stages (fetal, neonatal and pubertal) were profoundly growth stimulatory. This adult homeostatic growth-quiescent state appears to be dependent upon maintenance of the normal architectural associations between adult prostatic epithelium and stroma, because proliferation occurs when epithelial and stromal cultures are established from growth-quiescent adult prostate. Proliferative activity in cultures of adult prostatic epithelial and stromal cells is related to marked de-differentiation of both cell types. Thus, perturbation or elimination of normal stromal–epithelial interactions is associated with de-differentiation and elicits proliferation of both adult prostatic stromal and epithelial cells.

Cell–cell interactions in the adult prostate can also be altered by associating adult growth-quiescent epithelium (PRE) with embryonic prostatic inductive mesenchyme. For this purpose, an approximately 300-μm segment of an adult mouse prostatic duct is associated with embryonic rat UGM (rUGM + mPRE). Such 300-μm fragments of adult prostatic ducts contain about 5000 epithelial cells. When grown in male hosts, rUGM + mPRE recombinants form about 30–50 mg wet weight of prostatic tissue in 1 month, which contains 20×10^6–30×10^6 mouse prostatic epithelial cells[59,60]. Surprisingly, if the adult prostatic duct is derived from the ventral prostate, UGM or neonatal seminal vesicle mesenchyme (SVM, also a prostatic inducer) elicits the development of prostatic epithelium, expressing secretory proteins specific to the dorsal–lateral and anterior prostatic lobes[59,60]. This observation on mesenchymal respecification of lobar identity in adult prostatic epithelium in combination with the ability of UGM and SVM to induce prostatic differentiation in adult bladder epithelium[61] provides yet another example of the responsiveness of adult epithelia to the stromal microenvironment. Thus, the adult stromal microenvironment plays a fundamental role in regulating adult epithelial proliferation and differentiation. The corollary to this idea is that alterations in normal homeostatic stromal–epithelial interactions in adulthood may play a role in prostatic pathogenesis.

Role of stroma in carcinogenesis: a historical perspective

The concept that stroma may play a role in initiation and promotion of cancer has been considered for many years, and is based upon the pathological literature demonstrating that 'tumor stroma' is commonly different from normal stroma[62,63]. Indeed, 'peritumoral dermis' has been shown to be mitogenic on embryonic epidermis[64]. Studies of neoplastic transformation of embryonic mouse submandibular gland epithelium by polyoma virus showed that malignant transformation occurred when salivary gland epithelium was grown in association with embryonic salivary gland mesenchyme, but not when isolated epithelium was grown by itself[65]. A key milestone in the field of microenvironmental influences in cancer was the book, *Tissue Interactions in Carcinogenesis* published in 1972[66]. This collection of reviews emphasized that deregulation of stromal– epithelial interactions may contribute to both early and late stages of cancer formation, and that the prolonged interaction of the carcinoma cell with its abnormal stromal microenvironment played an important role in the carcinogenic process.

Once a carcinoma develops, the neoplastic epithelial cells may be responsive to stromal influences that may either exacerbate the malignancy or have possible therapeutic significance. In this latter regard, De Cosse and colleagues reported that mammary carcinoma cells exhibit a more orderly histodifferentiation and a lower proliferative rate when grown in association with embryonic mammary mesenchyme[67,68]. When basal cell carcinomas were grown in association with normal stroma, the malignant epidermal cells differentiated with an apparent loss of their former malignant properties[69]. Transitional cell carcinomas of the bladder grown in association with UGM were induced to differentiate into adenocarcinomatous structures resembling prostatic neoplasms (presumably associated with a change in the biology of the neoplasm)[70]. Similarly, human colon carcinoma cells differentiated in response to embryonic rat intestinal mesenchyme[71,72].

The idea that interactions between embryonic prostatic mesenchyme and malignant prostatic epithelial cells could possibly be used as a therapeutic strategy to inhibit tumorigenic growth was examined by combining rat Dunning prostatic adenocarcinoma R3327 epithelium (DTE) with UGM or SVM. It is worth noting that, while the Dunning tumor is considered an adenocarcinoma, an immortal stroma of uncertain origin has been passaged along with the malignant epithelial cells through countless generations of serial transplantation. This Dunning tumor stroma (DTS) is abnormal, being composed of fibroblastic

cells with an almost complete absence of smooth muscle. In addition, the basement membrane between the malignant epithelium and the stroma is frequently discontinuous or excessively reduplicated[73]. Thus, the stromal–epithelial interactions in the parental Dunning tumor are clearly abnormal. To determine whether malignant DTE cells might be modified by a more 'normal' stromal environment, DTE cells were grown for 1 month either alone or in combination with embryonic UGM or neonatal SVM, both known to be prostatic inductors[23,74]. Grafts of Dunning tumor containing DTE plus DTS demonstrated the characteristic histopathology of the Dunning tumor, forming tumors containing small ducts lined by one or more layers of undifferentiated epithelial cells. In contrast, DTE cells combined with UGM or SVM differentiated into tall columnar epithelial cells arranged in large cystic ducts[75–78]. These changes in histodifferentiation of the DTE induced by UGM or SVM were associated with a marked decrease in tumorigenesis and a significantly lower proliferation rate, in comparison with the parental Dunning tumor[76]. Upon harvest of SVM + DTE recombinants, the highly differentiated ducts on the recombinants were grafted directly into new male hosts or were combined with fresh SVM to form secondary SVM + DTE tissue recombinants. Ducts previously induced by SVM and secondary SVM + DTE tissue recombinants exhibited minimal growth during a 3-month period, and maintained a highly differentiated state. Conversely, control grafts composed of Dunning tumor alone (DTS + DTE) formed large (5–7 g) tumors during the same time period. The highly differentiated state of the SVM-induced DTE cells and apparent loss or reduction in tumorigenesis were associated with a dramatic decrease in epithelial [^{3}H]thymidine labelling index[76]. Significantly, smooth muscle cells, which were apparently derived from the SVM, were found in close apposition to the highly differentiated, relatively growth-quiescent DTE in these secondary SVM + DTE tissue recombinants[73].

Taken together, the above examples serve to underscore the continued importance of stromal–epithelial interactions in carcinomas. Continued responsiveness of carcinoma cells such as the DTE cells to their stromal microenvironment may provide the biological means of regulating both differentiation and proliferation of a carcinoma, perhaps to therapeutic benefit.

The biological effects of normal and 'tumor stroma' on carcinomas reviewed above imply an alteration in the cellular and extracellular matrix (ECM) of the stroma immediately adjacent to carcinoma cells. Such stromal changes have been documented in several tumors[79–83]. For example, in mammary tumors, the histology and growth characteristics of carcinoma-associated fibroblasts are different from that of fibroblasts associated with normal breast epithelial cells, in that abnormal myofibroblasts are associated with invasive breast carcinoma cells[84]. Other phenotypic changes attributed to carcinoma-associated fibroblasts include abnormal migratory behavior in vitro[85], alterations in cell surface molecules[86,87], altered expression of a variety of growth factors (platelet-derived growth factor, insulin-like growth factor-I and -II, transforming growth factor-β1, hepatocyte growth factor/epithelial scatter factor and keratinocyte growth factor[83,88–92]), expression of prostaglandin-synthesizing enzymes[93,94] and alterations in ECM[95,96]. While these phenotypic changes have been documented in carcinoma-associated fibroblasts from a variety of tumors, their significance or contribution to tumor growth, progression and differentiation are poorly understood. Recently, we have tested the hypothesis that carcinoma-associated fibroblasts (CAF) may affect tumor progression.

Role of carcinoma-associated fibroblasts in progression of human prostate cancer

Adult human prostatic stroma normally comprises a fibromuscular matrix, predominantly composed of smooth muscle cells. These stromal cells express androgen receptors, and respond to androgens by restricting prostatic epithelial proliferation via homeostatic stromal–epithelial interactions[97]. In contrast, stromal cells surrounding prostatic carcinoma cells are more typically fibroblastic or myofibroblastic[11,50,98–100]. In the prostate, we have used the term carcinoma-associated fibroblasts (CAF) to describe the stromal cells within and surrounding a tumor[101]. Others, notably Rowley and co-authors, have described the same stromal phenotype as 'reactive stroma'[99,100].

As reviewed above, stromal–epithelial interactions play a critical role in normal development and adult function[18]. We hypothesized (as summarized in Figure 4) that prostatic carcinogenesis is coupled with changes in local interactions between the stromal microenvironment and genetically initiated incipient tumor cells[11,50,102]. Thus, altered stromal–epithelial interactions are suggested to promote malignant progression and tumorigenesis[11,50,102,103].

One of the initial experiments to test the idea that stromal cells may facilitate prostatic carcinogenesis involved a tissue recombination system developed by Thompson and colleagues[104]. In these experiments, the urogenital sinus (prostatic anlagen) or its individual mesenchymal (UGM) or epithelial (UGE) components were transfected with a virus carrying the myc and ras oncogenes. Tissue recombinants containing uninfected UGM + infected UGE developed epithelial hyperplasias. Tissue recombinants containing infected UGM + uninfected UGE developed stromal desmoplasias. Tissue recombinants containing infected UGM + infected UGE developed carcinomas[104]. These findings demonstrated that changes in both the epithelium and stroma were required for prostatic carcinogenesis to occur.

We have shown that human prostatic CAF can promote carcinogenesis in immortal but non-tumorigenic human prostatic epithelial cells[101]. CAF isolated from human prostate tumors and recombined with the SV40T immortalized human prostatic epithelial cells, BPH-1 cells[53], promoted carcinogenesis, while normal prostatic fibroblasts did not (Figure 5 Table 1). CAF + BPH-1 tissue recombinants formed large poorly differentiated tumors[101], while growth was meager in tissue recombinants

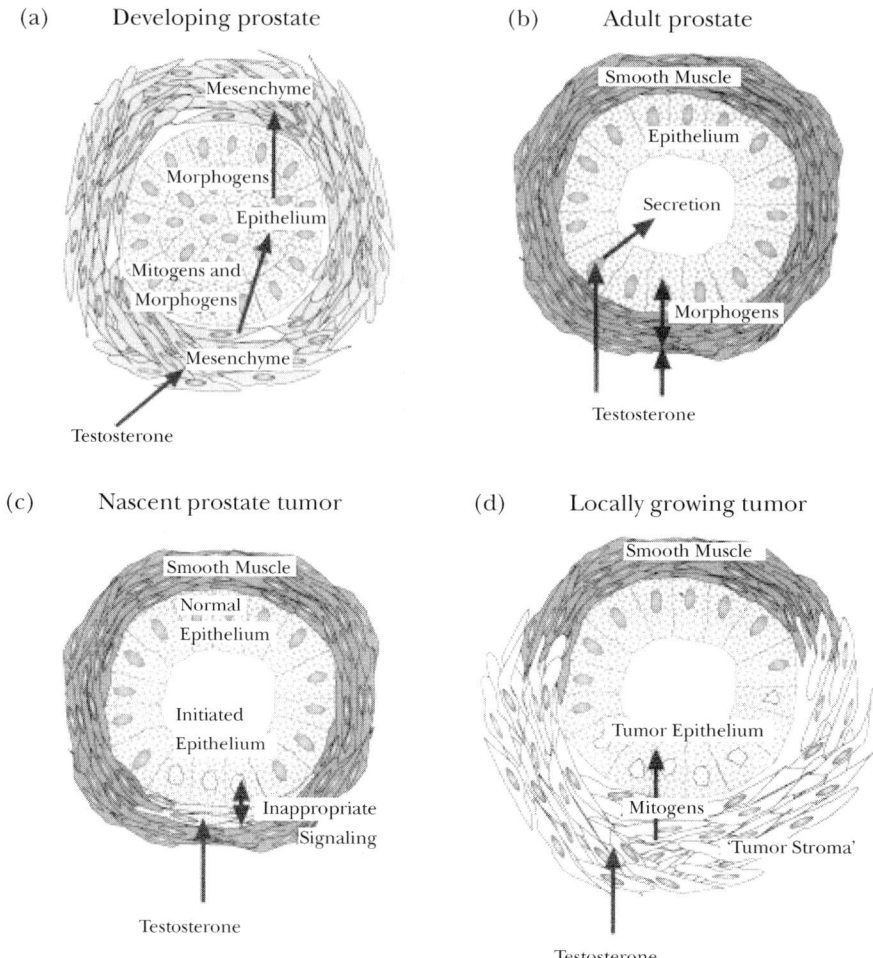

Figure 4 Interactions between the epithelial and the stromal/mesenchymal components of the prostate during development and adulthood. During prostatic development (a) low levels of androgens, acting through the mesenchymal androgen receptor, stimulate proliferation and differentiation of prostatic epithelium. Concurrently the epithelium induces differentiation of the mesenchyme into smooth muscle. In the normal adult (b) high levels of circulating androgens, acting through androgen receptors located in the smooth muscle, maintain the morphology of growth-quiescent adult epithelium. Secretory function is elicited by direct androgenic stimulation of androgen receptors in the differentiated columnar epithelium. Epithelial and smooth muscle differentiation is maintained by reciprocal paracrine-acting homeostatic factors. In early tumors we have hypothesized that following genetic insult to the epithelium (c) signalling between the epithelium and the adjacent smooth muscle begins to become abnormal, leading (d) to the formation of a fibroblastic 'tumor stroma', which responds to androgenic stimulation by producing paracrine-acting mitogens, fuelling a cycle of tumor proliferation and epithelial and stromal de-differentiation

composed of normal prostatic fibroblasts plus BPH-1 cells. Thus, unlike normal adult prostatic stroma, CAF did not respond to androgens by restricting epithelial proliferation, but instead stimulated epithelial proliferation and carcinogenesis. In experimental models in which BPH-1 cells were combined with normal stroma derived from fetal UGM, epithelial growth was also stimulated, but tumorigenesis did not occur, suggesting that simple stimulation of epithelial proliferation is not the single determinant in CAF-induced promotion of

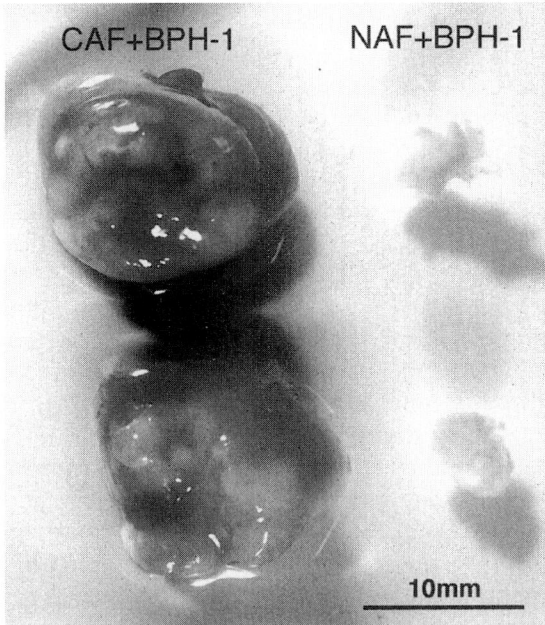

CAF+BPH-1   NAF+BPH-1

10mm

Figure 5 Gross appearance of tissue recombinants prepared with BPH-1 cells associated with either carcinoma-associated fibroblasts (CAF) or normal-associated fibroblasts (NAF) harvested after 85 days of growth in male nude mouse hosts. CAF + BPH-1 tissue recombinants weighed ~ 1300 mg and NAF + BPH-1 tissue recombinants weighed ~ 10 mg

Table 1 Summary of the results of recombining human prostatic fibroblasts from normal human prostate (NPF) or from prostate cancer (CAF) with either normal human prostatic epithelium or with the SV40T immortalized (and thus genetically initiated) human prostatic epithelial cell line BPH-1. Recombinants were grafted to athymic mouse hosts and allowed to grow for 41 days. Tumors developed only when the initiated epithelium (BPH-1) was associated with CAF

Cell recombination	Result (epithelial differentiation and graft wet weight)
NPF + normal epithelium	normal differentiation, wet weight > 10 mg
CAF + initiated epithelium	squamous differentiation, wet weight > 10 mg
NPF + normal epithelium	solid epithelial cords, no tumor, wet weight > 10 mg
CAF + initiated epithelium	tumor, median wet weight 132 mg

tumorigenesis[52]. The inference is that stromal cells surrounding a human prostate carcinoma stimulate proliferation and promote carcinogenesis, while normal stroma does not.

The tumorigenic process promoted by CAF in the parental non-tumorigenic BPH-1 cells involved alteration in gene expression and further genetic alterations, suggesting that CAF play an active, dynamic role in tumor progression. Specifically, CAF from human prostatic carcinomas induced tumorigenesis and elicited a characteristic pattern of genetic change associated with malignant progression[54,105]. A comparison of BPH-1 epithelial cells, induced to become tumorigenic by exposure to CAF (BPH-1[CAFTD]), and BPH-1 cells, induced to become tumorigenic as a result of hormonal carcinogenesis (BPH-1[TETD])[52], revealed many common changes as well as changes unique to the mode of cancer induction. BPH-1[CAFTD] and the BPH-1[TETD] cells share amplification of chromosomes 11q and 20q and loss of chromosomes 3q, 8p and 10p. Conversely, the cells induced by CAF contained multiple non-reciprocal translocations and a series of complex harlequin chromosomes based on chromosome 7, while BPH-1[TETD] cells that underwent hormonal carcinogenesis were much more likely to contain reciprocal translocations and show harlequin chromosomes based on chromosome 5[54,105]. These data support the contention that interactions between the stromal and epithelial cells within a tumor influence genetic changes across tissue layer boundaries.

Others have previously examined fibroblast–epithelial interactions in tumor growth and development, using immortalized fibroblasts or tumorigenic fibroblastic cell lines[92,106–111] rather than the mortal fibroblasts (CAF) used in our study[101]. On the whole, studies using immortalized fibroblasts or tumorigenic fibroblastic cell lines have reported that such fibroblasts accelerate tumorigenesis when co-inoculated with carcinoma cells of proven tumorigenicity. These studies[106,108,109] are fundamentally different from our study[101], which used an immortalized epithelial cell line shown to be non-tumorigenic by rigorous criteria. The report of carcino-sarcomatous development in combinations of sarcoma cells plus non-tumorigenic immortalized prostatic epithelial cells[107] likewise differs from our study, in that sarcoma cells (as opposed to CAF) were used. More important, evidence that the non-tumorigenic immortalized prostatic epithelial cells had actually become carcinomatous was not assessed directly, in that tumorigenic growth of the epithelial cells themselves was not demonstrated. More comparable to our CAF + BPH-1 studies are the reports by Thompson and colleagues that carcinoma development occurs following introduction of the *myc* and *ras* oncogenes into both UGM and UGE used to prepare prostatic reconstructions[112,113]. Likewise, induction of bladder carcinogenesis in tissue recombinants composed of carcinogen-treated epithelium plus carcinogen-treated bladder stroma[114,115] are relevant to our studies, even though strictly speaking the stromal cells used in these later studies cannot be considered CAF. However, the CAF + BPH-1 model firmly establishes the idea that carcinoma-associated fibroblasts can play a central role in progression to full malignancy of initiated but non-tumorigenic cells.

The mechanisms by which 'tumor stroma' influences the process of tumorigenesis are not known, even though it is clear that carcinomatous changes in the epithelium are frequently associated with concomitant alterations in the stroma. Thus, altered stromal– epithelial interactions foster progression to malignancy. Differential regulation of growth factors and proteases, which can modulate the local microenvironment, have been reported during carcinogenesis in several model systems (see December 2002 issue of *Differentiation*). It is also possible, indeed likely, that prostatic tumor stromal cells respond to androgens by producing growth factors that induce epithelial proliferation[12,97,116,117]. Stromal cells associated with carcinomas are known to produce a variety of matrix metalloproteinases that profoundly affect stromal–epithelial signalling and thus may affect tumor initiation, growth, migration, angiogenesis, apoptosis, invasion and metastasis[118]. Future work on the cellular and molecular mechanisms of interactions between stromal microenvironment and carcinoma cells may provide new therapeutic strategies for regulating carcinoma growth and/or apoptosis, to the benefit of patients suffering from cancer. For further information, see reviews in the December 2002 issue of *Differentiation*.

Acknowledgements

This work was supported in part by National Institutes of Health (NIH) grants CN–15114–MAO, CA 89520, CA 84294, CA 59831, DK 52708, DK 47517, DK 45861 and CA 64872, Department of Defense Prostate Cancer Research Program Grant DAMD 17–02–1–0151 and a grant from the Prostate Cancer Research Foundation of Canada.

References

1. Cunha GR, Donjacour AA, Cooke PS, *et al.* The endocrinology and developmental biology of the prostate. *Endocr Rev* 1987;8:338–62
2. Sugimura Y, Norman JT, Cunha GR, *et al.* Regional differences in the inductive activity of the mesenchyme of the embryonic mouse urogenital sinus. *Prostate* 1985;7:253–60
3. Timms B, Lee C, Aumuller G, *et al.* Instructive induction of prostate growth and differentiation by a defined urogenital sinus mesenchyme. *Microsc Res Tech* 1995;30:319–32

4. Takeda H, Suematsu N, Mizuno T. Transcription of prostatic steroid binding protein (PSBP) gene is induced by epithelial–mesenchymal interaction. *Development* 1990; 110:273–82

5. Cunha GR, Fujii H, Neubauer BL, *et al.* Epithelial–mesenchymal interactions in prostatic development. I. Morphological observations of prostatic induction by urogenital sinus mesenchyme in epithelium of the adult rodent urinary bladder. *J Cell Biol* 1983;96:1662–70

6. Cunha GR, Sekkingstad M, Meloy BA. Heterospecific induction of prostatic development in tissue recombinants prepared with mouse, rat, rabbit, and human tissues. *Differentiation* 1983; 24:174–80

7. Cunha GR, Reese BA, Sekkingstad M. Induction of nuclear androgen-binding sites in epithelium of the embryonic urinary bladder by mesenchyme of the urogenital sinus of embryonic mice. *Endocrinology* 1980;107: 1767–70

8. Cunha GR. Androgenic effects upon prostatic epithelium are mediated via trophic influences from stroma. In Kimball FA, Buhl AE, Carter DB, eds. *New Approaches to the Study of Benign Prostatic Hyperplasia.* New York: AR Liss, 1984:81–102

9. Cunha GR, Young P. Inability of Tfm (testicular feminization) epithelial cells to express androgen-dependent seminal vesicle secretory proteins in chimeric tissue recombinants. *Endocrinology* 1991;128:3293–8

10. Cunha GR, Battle E, Young P, *et al.* Role of epithelial–mesenchymal interactions in the differentiation and spatial organization of visceral smooth muscle. *Epithelial Cell Biol* 1992;1:76–83

11. Hayward SW, Cunha GR, Dahiya R. Normal development and carcinogenesis of the prostate: a unifying hypothesis. *Ann NY Acad Sci* 1996;784:50–62

12. Hayward SW, Haughney PC, Rosen MA, *et al.* Interactions between adult human prostatic epithelium and rat urogenital sinus mesenchyme in a tissue recombination model. *Differentiation* 1998;63:131–40

13. Cooke PS, Young P, Cunha GR. Androgen receptor expression in developing male reproductive organs. *Endocrinology* 1991;128:2867–73

14. Takeda H, Chang C. Immunohistochemical and *in situ* hybridization analysis of androgen receptor expression during the development of the mouse prostate gland. *J Endocrinol* 1991;129:83–9

15. Moeller H, Blank B, Lander K, *et al.* Ontogeny of the androgen receptor in rat ventral prostate during sexual development. *Res Exp Med* 1987;187:287–94

16. Prins GS, Jung MH, Vellanoweth RL, *et al.* Age-dependent expression of the androgen receptor gene in the prostate and its implication in glandular differentiation and hyperplasia. *Dev Genet* 1996;18:99–106

17. Prins GS, Birch L. The developmental pattern of androgen receptor expression in rat prostate lobes is altered after neonatal exposure to estrogen. *Endocrinology* 1995;136:1303–14

18. Cunha GR, Alarid ET, Turner T, *et al.* Normal and abnormal development of the male urogenital tract: role of androgens, mesenchymal–epithelial interactions and growth factors. *J Androl* 1992;13:465–75

19. Donjacour AA, Cunha GR. Assessment of prostatic protein secretion in tissue recombinants made of urogenital sinus mesenchyme and urothelium from normal or androgen–insensitive mice. *Endocrinology* 1993;131: 2342–50

20. Risbridger G, Wang H, Frydenberg M, *et al.* The metaplastic effects of estrogen on prostate epithelium: proliferation of cells with basal cell phenotype. *Endocrinology* 2001;142:2443–50

21. Cooke PS, Young P, Hess RA, *et al.* Estrogen receptor expression in developing epididymis, efferent ductules and other male reproductive organs. *Endocrinology* 1991;128:2874–79

22. Jung-Testas I, Groyer MT, Bruner-Lorand J, *et al.* Androgen and estrogen receptors in rat ventral prostate epithelium and stroma. *Endocrinology* 1981;109:1287–9

23. Risbridger G, Wang H, Young P, *et al.* Evidence that epithelial and mesenchymal estrogen receptor-α mediates effects of estrogen on prostatic epithelium. *Dev Biol* 2001;229:432–42

24. Chang WY, Wilson MJ, Birch L, *et al.* Neonatal estrogen stimulates proliferation of periductal fibroblasts and alters the extracellular matrix composition in the rat prostate. *Endocrinology* 1999;140:405–15

25. Prins GS, Birch L, Couse JF, *et al.* Estrogen imprinting of the developing prostate gland is mediated through stromal estrogen receptor α: studies with α-ERKO and β-ERKO mice. *Cancer Res* 2001;61:6089–97

26. Prins GS, Birch L. Neonatal estrogen exposure up-regulates estrogen receptor expression in the developing and adult rat prostate lobes. *Endocrinology* 1997;138:1801–9

27. Prins GS, Marmer M, Woodham C, *et al.* Estrogen receptor-β messenger ribonucleic acid ontogeny in the prostate of normal and neonatally estrogenized rats. *Endocrinology* 1998;139:874–83

28. Weihua Z, Makela S, Andersson LC, *et al.* A role for estrogen receptor β in the regulation of growth of the ventral prostate. *Proc Natl Acad Sci USA* 2001;98:6330–5

29. Sugimura Y, Cunha GR, Bigsby RM. Andro-genic induction of deoxyribonucleic acid synthesis in prostatic glands induced in the urothelium of testicular feminized (Tfm/Y) mice. *Prostate* 1986;9:217–25

30. Cooke P, Buchanan D, Young P, *et al.* Stromal estrogen receptors (ER) mediate mitogenic effects of estradiol on uterine epithelium. *Proc Natl Acad Sci USA* 1997;94:6535–40

31. Kurita T, Young P, Brody J, *et al.* Stromal progesterone receptors mediate the inhibitory effects of progesterone on estrogen-induced uterine epithelial cell (UtE) proliferation. *Endocrinology* 1998;139:4708–13

32. Cunha GR, Young P, Hom YK, *et al.* Elucidation of a role of stromal steroid hormone receptors in mammary gland growth and development by tissue recombination experiments. *J Mammary Gland Biol Neoplasia* 1997;2:393–402

33. Buchanan DL, Setiawan T, Lubahn DL, *et al.* Tissue compartment-specific estrogen receptor participation in the mouse uterine epithelial secretory response. *Endocrinology* 1998;140:484–91

34. Buchanan DL, Kurita T, Taylor JA, *et al.* Role of stromal and epithelial estrogen receptors in vaginal epithelial proliferation, stratification and cornification. *Endocrinology* 1998;139:4345–52

35. Gao J, Arnold JT, Isaacs JT. Conversion from a paracrine to an autocrine mechanism of androgen-stimulated growth during malignant transformation of prostatic epithelial cells. *Cancer Res* 2001;61:5038–44

36. Montie JE, Pienta KJ. Review of the role of androgenic hormones in the epidemiology of benign prostatic hyperplasia and prostate cancer. *Urology* 1994;43:892–9

37. Brendler CB, Berry SJ, Ewing LL, *et al.* Spontaneous benign prostatic hyperplasia in the beagle. Age-associated changes in serum hormone levels, and the morphology and secretory function of the canine prostate. *J Clin Invest* 1983;71:1114–23

38. Hayes RB, de Jong FH, Raatgever J, *et al.* Physical characteristics and factors related to sexual development and behaviour and the risk for prostatic cancer. *Eur J Cancer Prev* 1992;1:239–45

39. Ross R, Bernstein L, Judd H, *et al.* Serum testosterone levels in healthy young black and white men. *J Natl Cancer Inst* 1986;76:45–8

40. Ho SM, Yu M. Selective increase in type II estrogen-binding sites in the dysplastic dorso-lateral prostates of noble rats. *Cancer Res* 1993;53:528–32

41. Leav I, Ho SM, Ofner P, *et al.* Biochemical alterations in sex hormone-induced hyper-plasia and dysplasia of the dorsolateral prostates of Noble rats. *J Natl Cancer Inst* 1988;80:1045–53

42. Noble RL. The development of prostatic adenocarcinoma in Nb rats following pro-longed sex hormone administration. *Cancer Res* 1977;37:1929–33

43. Yu M, Leav BA, Leav I, *et al.* Early alterations in *ras* protooncogene mRNA expression in testos-terone and estradiol-17β induced prostatic dysplasia of Noble rats. *Lab Invest* 1993;68:33–44

44. Wang YZ, Wong YC. Sex hormone-induced prostatic carcinogenesis in the Noble rat: the role of insulin-like growth factor-I (IGF-I) and vascular endothelial growth factor (VEGF) in the development of prostate cancer. *Prostate* 1998;35:165–77

45. Wang YZ, Hayward SW, Cao M, *et al.* Role of estrogen signaling in prostatic hormonal carcinogenesis. *J Urol* 2001;165:1320

46. Wang Y, Hayward SW, Donjacour AA, *et al.* Hormonal carcinogenesis of the Rb-knockout mouse prostate. *Cancer Res* 2000;60:6008–17

47. Cunha GR, Chung LWK. Stromal–epithelial interactions: I. Induction of prostatic pheno-type in urothelium of testicular feminized (Tfm/Y) mice. *J Steroid Biochem* 1981;14:1317–21

48. Shannon JM, Cunha GR. Characterization of androgen binding and deoxyribonucleic acid synthesis in prostate-like structures induced in testicular feminized (Tfm/Y) mice. *Biol Reprod* 1984;31:175–83

49. Cunha GR. Role of mesenchymal–epithelial interactions in normal and abnormal develop-ment of the mammary gland and prostate. *Cancer* 1994;74:1030–44

50. Hayward SW, Rosen MA, Cunha GR. Stromal–epithelial interactions in normal and neoplastic prostate. *Br J Urol* 1997;79(Suppl 2):18–26

51. Prins G, Birch L, Greene G. Androgen receptor localization in different cell types of the adult rat prostate. *Endocrinology* 1991;129:3187–99

52. Wang Y, Sudilovsky D, Zhang B, *et al.* A human prostatic epithelial model of hormonal carcino-genesis. *Cancer Res* 2001;61:6064–72

53. Hayward SW, Dahiya R, Cunha GR, *et al.* Establishment and characterization of an immortalized but non-tumorigenic human prostate epithelial cell line: BPH-1. *In Vitro* 1995;31A:14–24

54. Phillips J, Hayward S, Wang Y, *et al.* The con-sequences of chromosomal aneuploidy on gene expression profiles in a cell line model for pros-tate carcinogenesis. *Cancer Res* 2001;61:8143–9

55. Couse JF, Korach KS. Estrogen receptor null mice: what have we learned and where will they lead us? *Endocr Rev* 1999;20:358–417

56. Kuiper GG, Enmark E, Pelto-Huikko M, *et al.* Cloning of a novel receptor expressed in rat

prostate and ovary. *Proc Natl Acad Sci USA* 1996;93:5925–30

57. Lau KM, Leav I, Ho SM. Rat estrogen receptor-α and -β, and progesterone receptor mRNA expression in various prostatic lobes and microdissected normal and dysplastic epithelial tissues of the Noble rats. *Endocrinology* 1998;139:424–7

58. Adams JY, Leav I, Lau KM, *et al.* Expression of estrogen receptor β in the fetal, neonatal, and prepubertal human prostate. *Prostate* 2002;52: 69–81

59. Hayashi N, Cunha GR, Parker M. Permissive and instructive induction of adult rodent prostatic epithelium by heterotypic urogenital sinus mesenchyme. *Epithelial Cell Biol* 1993;2: 66–78

60. Norman JT, Cunha GR, Sugimura Y. The induction of new ductal growth in adult prostatic epithelium in response to an embryonic prostatic inductor. *Prostate* 1986;8:209–20

61. Donjacour AA, Cunha GR. Seminal vesicle mesenchyme induces prostatic morphology and secretion in urinary bladder epithelium. *J Cell Biol* 1988;107:609a

62. Bosman FT, de Bruine A, Flohil C, *et al.* Epithelial–stromal interactions in colon cancer. *Int J Dev Biol* 1993;37:203–11

63. Seljelid R, Jozefowski S, Sveinbjornsson B. Tumor stroma. *Anticancer Res* 1999;19:4809–22

64. Redler P, Lustig ES. Differences in the growth-promoting effect of normal and peritumoral dermis on epidermis *in vitro. Dev Biol* 1968; 17:679–91

65. Dawe CJ. Epithelial–mesenchymal interactions in relation to the genesis of polyoma virus-induced tumours of mouse salivary gland. In Tarin D, ed. *Tissue Interactions in Carcinogenesis.* London: Academic Press, 1972:305–58

66. Tarin D, ed. *Tissue Interactions in Carcinogenesis.* London: Academic Press, 1972

67. De Cosse J, Gossens CL, Kuzma JF. Breast cancer: induction of differentiation by embryonic tissue. *Science* 1973;181:1057–8

68. De Cosse JJ, Gossens CL, Kuzma JF, *et al.* Embryonic inductive tissues that cause histological differentiation of murine mammary carcinoma *in vitro. J Natl Cancer Inst* 1975; 54:913–21

69. Cooper M, Pinkus H. Intrauterine transplantation of rat basal cell carcinoma: a model for reconversion of malignant to benign growth. *Cancer Res* 1977;37:2544–52

70. Fujii H, Cunha GR, Norman JT. The induction of adenocarcinomatous differentiation in neoplastic bladder epithelium by an embryonic prostatic inductor. *J Urol* 1982;128:858–61

71. Fukamachi H, Mizuno T, Kim YS. Morphogenesis of human colon cancer cells with fetal rat mesenchymes in organ culture. *Experientia* 1986;42:312–15

72. Fukamachi H, Mizuno T, Kim YS. Gland formation of human colon cancer cells combined with foetal rat mesenchyme in organ culture: an ultrastructural study. *J Cell Sci* 1987;87:615–21

73. Wong YC, Cunha GR, Hayashi N. Effects of mesenchyme of embryonic urogenital sinus and neonatal seminal vesicle on the cyto-differentiation of the Dunning tumor: ultra-structural study. *Acta Anat* 1992;143:139–50

74. Cunha GR. Epithelio-mesenchymal interactions in primordial gland structures which become responsive to androgenic stimulation. *Anat Rec* 1972;172:179–96

75. Hayashi N, Cunha GR, Wong YC. Influence of male genital tract mesenchymes on differentiation of Dunning prostatic adenocarcinoma. *Cancer Res* 1990;50:4747–54

76. Hayashi N, Cunha GR. Mesenchyme-induced changes in neoplastic characteristics of the Dunning prostatic adenocarcinoma. *Cancer Res* 1991;51:4924–30

77. Tam NNC, Phil M, Wang YZ, *et al.* The influence of mesenchyme of neonatal seminal vesicle and embryonic urogenital sinus on the morphologic and functional cytodifferentiation of Dunning prostatic adenocarcinoma: roles of growth factors and proto-oncogenes. *Urol Oncol* 1997;3:85–93

78. Hayashi N, Tsuji M, Sugimura Y, *et al.* Change in the morphological and functional cyto-differentiation induced by seminal vesicle mesenchyme in cell suspensions of rat Dunning prostatic adenocarcinoma cells. *Int J Cancer* 1996;68:788–94

79. Basset P, Wolf C, Chambon P. Expression of the stromelysin-3 gene in fibroblastic cells of invasive carcinomas of the breast and other human tissues: a review. *Breast Cancer Res Treat* 1993;24:185–93

80. Chiquet-Ehrismann R, Mackie EJ, Pearson CA, *et al.* Tenascin: an extracellular matrix protein involved in tissue interactions during fetal development and oncogenesis. *Cell* 1986;47: 131–9

81. Singer C, Rasmussen A, Smith HS, *et al.* Malignant breast epithelium selects for insulin-like growth factor II expression in breast stroma: evidence for paracrine function. *Cancer Res* 1995;55:2448–54

82. Wright JH, McDonnell S, Portella G, *et al.* A switch from stromal to tumor cell expression of stromelysin-1 mRNA associated with the conversion of squamous to spindle carcinomas during mouse skin tumor progression. *Mol Carcinog* 1994;10:207–15

83. Yee D, Paik S, Lebovic GS, *et al.* Analysis of insulin-like growth factor I gene expression in malignancy: evidence for a paracrine role in human breast cancer. *Mol Endocrinol* 1989; 3:509–17

84. Ronnov-Jessen L, Petersen OW, Bissell MJ. Cellular changes involved in conversion of normal to malignant breast: importance of the stromal reaction. *Physiol Rev* 1996;76:69–125

85. Schor SL, Schor AM, Rushton G. Fibroblasts from cancer patients display a mixture of both foetal and adult-like phenotypic characteristics. *J Cell Sci* 1988;90:401–7

86. Chaudhuri S, Koprowska I, Rowinski J. Different agglutinability of fibroblasts underlying various precursor lesions of human uterine cervical carcinoma. *Cancer Res* 1975; 35:2350–4

87. Oishi K, Romijn JC, Schroeder FH. The surface character of separated prostatic cells and cultured fibroblasts of prostatic tissue as determined by concanavalin-a hemadsorption. *Prostate* 1981;2:11–21

88. Ellis MJ, Singer C, Hornby A, *et al.* Insulin-like growth factor mediated stromal–epithelial interactions in human breast cancer. *Breast Cancer Res Treat* 1994;31:249–61

89. Frazier KS, Grotendorst GR. Expression of connective tissue growth factor mRNA in the fibrous stroma of mammary tumors. *Int J Biochem Cell Biol* 1997;29:153–61

90. Nakamura T, Matsumoto K, Kiritoshi A, *et al.* Induction of hepatocyte growth factor in fibroblasts by tumor-derived factors affects invasive growth of tumor cells: *in vitro* analysis of tumor–stromal interactions. *Cancer Res* 1997; 57:3305–13

91. Ponten F, Ren Z, Nister M, *et al.* Epithelial–stromal interactions in basal cell cancer: the PDGF system. *J Invest Dermatol* 1994;102:304–9

92. Yan G, Fukabori Y, McBride G, *et al.* Exon switching and activation of stromal and embryonic FGF/FGF receptor genes in prostate epithelial cells accompanies stromal independence and malignancy. *Mol Cell Biol* 1993;13: 4513–22

93. Shattuck-Brandt RL, Lamps LW, Heppner Goss KJ, *et al.* Differential expression of matrilysin and cyclooxygenase-2 in intestinal and colorectal neoplasms. *Mol Carcinog* 1999;24:177–87

94. Shattuck-Brandt RL, Varilek GW, Radhika A, *et al.* Cyclooxygenase 2 expression is increased in the stroma of colon carcinomas from IL-10(−/−) mice. *Gastroenterology* 2000;118: 337–45

95. Pupa SM, Menard S, Forti S, *et al.* New insights into the role of extracellular matrix during

tumor onset and progression. *J Cell Physiol* 2002;192:259–67

96. Werb Z, Ashkenas J, MacAuley A, *et al.* Extracellular matrix remodeling as a regulator of stromal–epithelial interactions during mammary gland development, involution and carcinogenesis. *Braz J Med Biol Res* 1996; 29:1087–97

97. Hayward SW, Cunha GR. The prostate: development and physiology. *Radiol Clin North Am* 2000;38:1–14

98. Arnold JT, Isaacs JT. Mechanisms involved in the progression of androgen-independent prostate cancers: it is not only the cancer cell's fault. *Endocr Relat Cancer* 2002;9:61–73

99. Rowley DR. What might a stromal response mean to prostate cancer progression? *Cancer Metastasis Rev* 1998;17:411–19

100. Tuxhorn JA, Ayala GE, Rowley DR. Reactive stroma in prostate cancer progression. *J Urol* 2001;166:2472–83

101. Olumi AF, Grossfeld GD, Hayward SW, *et al.* Carcinoma-associated fibroblasts direct tumor progression of initiated human prostatic epithelium. *Cancer Res* 1999;59:5002–11

102. Hayward SW, Grossfeld GD, Tlsty TD, *et al.* Genetic and epigenetic influences in prostatic carcinogenesis. *Int J Oncol* 1998;13:35–47

103. Grossfeld G, Hayward S, Tlsty T, *et al.* The role of stroma in prostatic carcinogenesis. *Endocr Relat Cancer* 1998;5:253–70

104. Thompson TC, Timme TL, Kadmon D, *et al.* Genetic predisposition and mesenchymal–epithelial interactions in *ras* + *myc*-induced carcinogenesis in reconstituted mouse prostate. *Mol Carcinog* 1993;7:165–79

105. Hayward S, Wang Y, Cao M, *et al.* Malignant transformation in a non-tumorigenic human prostatic epithelial cell line. *Cancer Res* 2001; 61:8135–42

106. Camps JL, Chang SM, Hsu TC, *et al.* Fibroblast-mediated acceleration of human epithelial tumor growth *in vivo*. *Proc Natl Acad Sci USA* 1990;87:75–9

107. Chung LW, Chang SM, Bell C, *et al.* Co-inoculation of tumorigenic rat prostate mesenchymal cells with non-tumorigenic epithelial cells results in the development of carcinosarcoma in syngeneic and athymic animals. *Int J Cancer* 1989;43:1179–87

108. Gleave M, Hsieh JT, Gao CA, *et al.* Acceleration of human prostate cancer growth *in vivo* by factors produced by prostate and bone fibroblasts. *Cancer Res* 1991;51:3753–61

109. Gleave ME, Hsieh JT, von Eschenbach AC, *et al.* Prostate and bone fibroblasts induce human prostate cancer growth *in vivo*: implications for bidirectional tumor–stromal cell interaction

in prostate carcinoma growth and metastasis. *J Urol* 1992;147:1151–9

110. Noel A, Munaut C, Nusgens B, *et al.* The stimulation of fibroblasts' collagen synthesis by neoplastic cells is modulated by the extracellular matrix. *Matrix* 1992;12:213–20

111. Picard O, Rolland Y, Poupon MF. Fibroblast-dependent tumorigenicity of cells in nude mice: implication for implantation of metastases. *Cancer Res* 1986;46:3290–4

112. Thompson TC, Kadmon D, Timme TL, *et al.* Experimental oncogene induced prostate cancer. In Isaacs JT, ed. *Prostate Cancer: Cell and Molecular Mechanisms in Diagnosis and Treatment.* Cold Spring Harbor: Cold Spring Harbor Laboratory Press, 1991:55–72

113. Thompson TC, Southgate J, Kitchener G, *et al.* Multistage carcinogenesis induced by *ras* and *myc* oncogenes in a reconstituted organ. *Cell* 1989;56:917–30

114. Momose H, Uchida K, Kakinuma H, *et al.* Involvement of urine in epithelial–stromal interactions in urinary bladder carcinogenesis. *Cancer Lett* 1990;53:91–6

115. Uchida K, Samma S, Momose H, *et al.* Stimulation of urinary bladder tumorigenesis by carcinogen-exposed stroma. *J Urol* 1990; 143:618–21

116. Haughney PC, Hayward SW, Dahiya R, *et al.* Species-specific detection of growth factor gene expression in developing prostatic tissue. *Biol Reprod* 1998;59:93–9

117. Wong YC, Wang YZ. Growth factors and epithelial–stromal interactions in prostate cancer development. *Int Rev Cytol* 2000;199: 65–116

118. Lynch CC, Matrisian LM. MMPs in tumor–host cell communication. *Differentiation* 2002; 70:561–73

Prostate cancer xenograft models 19

J. C. Romijn

Introduction

Despite intensive research efforts, the biological processes contributing to the development and progression of prostate cancer are still incompletely understood. For a long time, the scarcity of experimental models for prostate cancer has been a major obstacle to the rapid advancement of our knowledge about important issues such as the mechanisms of prostate cancer progression. The generation of suitable models is therefore of critical importance to achieve further progress in the elucidation of such fundamental processes.

It is difficult to explain why so few model systems could be established for such a common type of cancer, which is now one of the most frequently diagnosed cancers in males in the Western world. A possible reason for the limited existence of prostate cancer models of animal origin is that only few species (dogs and rats) develop prostate cancer spontaneously. One of the first and certainly the most widely used animal model system for prostate cancer is the Dunning rat model[1]. Over the years, a variety of sublines with different biological properties (including metastatic ability) have been isolated from the parental Dunning R3327 cell line and extensively characterized[2]. Studies using these cell lines have contributed much to the current understanding of prostate tumor cell biology. Nevertheless, owing to the possible occurrence of species-specific differences there is a preference for using models of human rather than animal origin for studying (human) prostate cancer. Unfortunately, a common experience is that it is extremely difficult to establish human prostatic cancer cell lines in culture. Only a few cell lines have been reported in the literature[3–6] and, in fact, some of the more recently described cell lines are considered to be cross-contaminants of already existing cell lines[7]. Moreover, most of the recognized prostate cancer cell lines do not exhibit features that are characteristic of prostatic cells, such as expression of prostate-specific antigen (PSA) and androgen receptors and/or responsiveness to androgens. As an exception, the LNCaP (lymph node cancer of the prostate) model has retained the ability to produce PSA and respond to androgens, but this cell line appears to have a mutation in the steroid-binding domain of the androgen receptor[8]. Alternatively, *in vivo* models might be generated by heterotransplantation of human prostate cancer tissue in immune-deficient animals. In this review, the establishment of such models is described and their characteristics summarized.

The nude mouse model

A hairless mutant mouse, which appeared to be homozygous for an autosomal recessive gene (symbol: *nu*), was reported for the first time in 1962[9] and its phenotype was described in more detail a few years later[10]. It was found that this mouse not only was hairless but also lacked a normally developed thymus, and therefore was deficient in its cell-mediated immune response[11]. Other defects include reduced fertility[12]. Taking advantage of the immune-deficient status, the athymic nude mouse has been used as a host for human tissues, and tumor tissues in particular, since the 1970s[13]. Schröder and co-workers were probably the first to use this approach for maintenance and growth of human prostate tissues[14].

Human prostate cancer xenografts in nude mice (Erasmus PC series)

Under the inspiring leadership of Fritz H. Schröder, the Experimental Urology Research Group of the Erasmus University Rotterdam started with a series of heterotransplantations of human prostate cancer tissues in 1977, with the purpose of generating new experimental model systems for prostate cancer. The animals used were initially obtained from their own nude mouse breeding colony of a BALB/c mouse background. Tumor fragments were implanted subcutaneously near the shoulders in male mice. Already in 1977 this strategy appeared to be very successful, and led to the establishment of the PC-82 xenograft cell line[14] (discussed more extensively below). Over the subsequent period of 10 years, more than 150 prostate cancer tissues were transplanted, but with relatively little success. Only two new xenograft lines were established during that period, PC-133 in 1981 and PC-135 in 1982. This discouraging low success rate has not yet been explained, but the observation that prostate cancer tissue is notoriously difficult to grow *in vivo* as well as *in vitro* has also been experienced by other investigators. In a concurrent series of renal carcinomas transplanted in nude mice in our laboratory the success rate was 35%, indicating that low take rate is a problem inherent to the nature of prostate tissues. World-wide, only one other new xenograft cell line, PC-EW[15], was reported to be established during that period.

In the years 1988–91 another series of transplantations was undertaken in our laboratory. Surprisingly, this resulted in the establishment of seven new xenograft models[16], extending our panel to ten different models. The characteristics of these models are summarized in Table 1. One of the most important features of this panel is that it represents various stages of clinical prostate cancer with corresponding different biological behaviors[17]. It includes models such as PC-82, PC-295, PC-329 and PC-310 that are strictly androgen-dependent for their growth, as demonstrated by the lack of tumor development upon implantation into castrated male mice. The responsiveness of established tumors from these four models to androgen withdrawal is quantitatively different, however. While PC-295 tumors regress rapidly and almost completely within a few weeks[18], long-term androgen depletion induces partial regression of PC-82 tumors that can be restimulated by androgen even after a 79-day period[19]. In models PC-295 and PC-310, androgen depletion induces the appearance of neuroendocrine-differentiated cells[18,20]; these models have therefore been applied to study the role of neuroendocrine differentiation in prostate cancer progression. On the other side of the spectrum, the models PC-133, PC-135, PC-324 and PC-339 should be considered truly androgen-independent. These xenografts grow

Table 1 Human prostate cancer xenografts (Erasmus PC series)

Tumor model	Year	Tissue of origin	Androgen response	AR	PSA
PC-82	1977	prostate	dependent	+	+
PC-133	1981	bone	independent	−	−
PC-135	1982	prostate	independent	−	−
PC-295	1990	lymph node	dependent	+	+
PC-310	1990	prostate	dependent	+	+
PC-324	1991	prostate (TURP)	independent	−	−
PC-329	1991	prostate	dependent	+	+
PC-339	1991	prostate (TURP)	independent	−	−
PC-346*	1991	prostate (TURP)	responsive	+	+
PC-374	1991	scrotal skin	responsive	+	+

*Several sublines are available; TURP, transurethral resection of the prostate; AR, androgen receptor; PSA, prostate-specific antigen; +, expresses or secretes; −, does not express or secrete

equally well in intact or castrated male mice, and their growth rate cannot be influenced by hormonal manipulation. The PC-346 and PC-374 xenografts are very interesting because they have an intermediate position. PC-374 is androgen-responsive but not -dependent, since tumors grow in castrated males although at a slower rate than in intact or androgen-supplemented male mice. Similarly, the PC-346 model, which was originally considered androgen-dependent, is in fact an androgen-responsive tumor model. In the mean time, a number of sublines have been derived from the original PC-346 model as well as from a second model, PC-346B, which originates from the same patient. This subpanel of related PC-346 sublines (see below) will be extremely valuable for studying the mechanisms of prostate cancer progression to androgen-independent autonomous growth[21]. All androgen-dependent or -responsive xenografts listed in Table 1 contained (wild-type) androgen receptor (AR). PSA was detected at tumor model- and tumor load-dependent levels in the serum of mice carrying androgen-dependent or -responsive xenografts.

The PC-82 model

PC-82 was the first permanent *in vivo* human prostate cancer model described[14]. This model had several characteristics that appeared to be much more representative for clinical prostate cancer than those of any other experimental model system at that time. These properties included:

(1) Relatively slow growth rate (tumor doubling time approximately 15 days)[22];

(2) Cribriform growth pattern, similar to the original tumor histology[14];

(3) Production of prostate-specific factors: prostatic acid phosphatase[23] and PSA in later years; at the time of PC-82 establishments, PSA was not yet known;

(4) Presence of androgen receptors[24];

(5) Strict dependence on androgen for growth[22,25].

These tumor characteristics appeared to be well preserved over a large number of subsequent mouse passages.

Its strict androgen dependence is probably the most conspicuous property of PC-82, and has made this model an important tool for studies of the hormonal regulation of tumor growth. To ensure adequate and reproducible PC-82 tumor growth in nude mice, the animals are routinely supplemented with testosterone encapsulated in Silastic® tubing implants[26]. The PC-82 model does *not* progress to androgen independence, even after long-term androgen deprivation, and is *non*-metastatic.

The PC-346 model system

One of the most interesting newer xenograft model systems is, without doubt, the PC-346 model. This model was obtained after implantation of tissue from a transurethral resection of the prostate (TURP) of a non-progressed prostate cancer patient. From this material two xenograft lines were established, PC-346 and PC-346B, that had slightly different characteristics, e.g. with respect to growth rate[21]. Both were androgen-responsive, expressed a normal (wild-type) AR and secreted PSA. The PC-346 xenograft was originally considered to be androgen-dependent, since tumors did not generally develop in female mice or in castrated males. Established PC-346 tumors, however, did show the clinically relevant feature of progression towards androgen-independent growth following androgen ablation. Castration of mice with PC-346 tumors resulted in a variable tumor response[21], ranging from clear-cut regression to relatively minor reduction in growth rate. All tumors remained androgen-responsive and could be restimulated to restore their normal growth rate by androgen supplementation or by retransplantation in intact male mice. This indicates that regrowth after castration was not caused by a selection mechanism (with preferential outgrowth of pre-existing hormone-insensitive cells), but rather should be attributed to adaptation of the tumor to the androgen-depleted environment. Occasionally, tumor regrowth after androgen ablation resulted in the generation of truly androgen-independent cells. One of these events resulted in the establishment of the subline PC-346I, that grows equally well in intact and castrated males or even in female mice. Molecular analyses have shown that the AR in PC-346I cells is mutated in the same way as the AR of LNCaP cells[21]. Other, 'spontaneously' developed androgen-independent sublines of PC-346 have been isolated in the mean time (PC-346SI). These tumor cells appeared to have a non-mutated AR. Interestingly, androgen-independent sublines were generated also from PC-346B xenografts. The AR found in these sublines (PC-346BI, PC-346SBI) was not mutated.

The subpanel of PC-346 xenografts and its derivatives constitutes a unique set of related cell lines that should be extremely valuable for studying the processes associated with progression to autonomous androgen-independent prostate cancer growth.

Other prostate cancer xenograft models

In recent years, prostate cancer xenografts have also been developed in several other laboratories. An overview is given in Table 2.

Four serially transplantable xenografts, CWR21, CWR22, CWR31 and CWR91, were obtained after subcutaneous injection of minced tissue from 22 primary prostatic carcinomas in testosterone-supplemented nude mice[27]. With the aim of improving tumor development, tissue fragments were suspended in Matrigel. Characteristics of these xenografts have not been further described, except for CWR22. The latter xenograft cell line contains AR, produces PSA and is androgen-responsive for growth[28]. Androgen withdrawal generally led to a marked tumor regression, sometimes followed by tumor relapse[35]. Relapsed tumors (CWR22R) frequently had increased metastatic ability to the lungs[35].

Mixing with Matrigel was also applied for the generation of LAPC xenografts[29]. Two successful attempts (from an initial series of eight) resulted in the establishment of LAPC-3 and -4, which both express AR and PSA. LAPC-3 tumors grow androgen-independently, and LAPC-4 tumors are androgen-sensitive and regress after castration but commonly then progress to androgen-independence. A third xenograft, LAPC-9, was established later[30]. Similar to LAPC-4, this xenograft stops growing in response to castration, and remains in a dormant but viable and androgen-responsive state until an androgen-independent population starts to grow out.

Table 2 Other human prostate cancer xenograft models

Tumor model	Tissue of origin	Androgen sensitive	AR	PSA	Reference
CWR21	prostate	?	?	?	27
CWR22	prostate	+	+*	+	27, 28
CWR31	prostate	?	?	?	27
CWR91	prostate	?	?	?	27
LAPC-3	prostate	−	+	+	29
LAPC-4	lymph node	+	+	+	29
LAPC-9	bone	+	+	+	30
LuCaP23.1	lymph node	+	+	+	31
LuCaP23.8	lymph node	+	+	+	31
LuCaP23.12	liver	+	+	+	31
LuCaP49	prostate	−	−	−	32
MDA PCa-31	liver	?	+	+	33
MDA PCa-40	liver	?	−	−	33
MDA PCa-43	adrenal	?	+	+	33
MDA PCa-44	skin	?	−	−	33
PAC120	prostate	+	?	+	34

*Mutated androgen receptor (AR); PSA, prostate-specific antigen; +, expresses or secretes (AR or PSA); −, does not express or secrete (AR or PSA)

Transplantation of metastatic prostate cancer tissue (from lymph nodes and liver) in BALB/c nude mice resulted in the establishment of three xenograft lines of the LuCaP23 series[31], which were reported to be androgen-sensitive and to express AR and PSA. Their response to androgen ablation is variable, ranging from minimal and short-lasting to prolonged responses, more or less similar to our observations with PC-346 xenografts. Recently, the establishment of an androgen-insensitive xenograft, LuCaP49, was reported by the same investigators[32]. This xenograft, propagated in severe combined immune deficient (SCID) mice, has a neuroendocrine phenotype.

Establishment of four different xenografts from metastatic prostate cancer tissue in liver, adrenals and skin was reported recently[33]. These xenografts also express AR and PSA, but detailed characterization studies have not been published.

Very recently, another research group described the establishment and characterizaton of the androgen-responsive xenograft PAC120[34].

Possible determinants of xenograft establishment

As described in this review, efforts to generate new human prostate cancer xenograft models have resulted in the establishment of a panel of models that adequately covers a whole spectrum of prostate cancer types. Nevertheless, it should be mentioned that the success rate for establishing such models is disappointingly low. The reasons why the great majority of attempts have failed are not at all clear. Factors relating to the condition of the transplanted tissue, as well as host-associated properties making up the tumor cell microenvironment, might be involved. Clearly, viability of the original tumor tissue fragments will play an important role. Unfortunately, there is no experimental evidence, nor general consensus, about the optimal preimplantation conditions with regard to time, temperature, storage/transport conditions, tissue fragment size, etc.

In any case, even within a very viable population of tumor cells, the survival rate after *in vivo* implantation will be poor. We earlier showed that only 10% of (radio-labelled, viable) PC-3 tumor cells survived for a period of 24 h after implantation[36]. Active immunological mechanisms, which are still residual in nude mice (macrophages, natural killer cells), are not likely to play a major role in this process. In our hands, but also reported by others[27], there was no clear beneficial effect of the use of SCID mice instead of conventional nudes. Nevertheless, the type of animal used could well influence the results. It is a striking observation that, in our laboratory, the success rate for establishing serially transplantable lines went up from less than 2% (3/> 150) in the years 1977–87 to 14% (7/51) in the years 1988–91[17]. When the latter period was split up further, it was noticed that only one of the first 35 transplants was successful (3%), but six out of the last 16 (38%). This enhancement coincided with the change in the nude mouse strain used: NMRI *nu/nu* instead of BALB/c *nu/nu*. Other differences (tissue origin, etc.) were not identified. Comparative studies to demonstrate that the superior results should indeed be ascribed to the use of NMRI mice have not been performed, however. In line with our findings, it has also been noticed that endogenous malignancies (sarcomas, lymphomas) are relatively frequently formed in NMRI nude mice[37], which is in fact a potential disadvantage of the use of these animals.

The possible mechanisms of strain-dependence of transplantability are completely unknown. Angiogenic activity and/or recruitment of suitable stromal matrices might play a role. It is known that the stromal compartment (including blood vessels) of xenograft tumors is of mouse origin. Formation of reactive stroma is an important aspect of (prostate) cancer growth and progression[38]. It cannot be excluded that species effects influence the exchange of original (human) stroma for the murine counterpart. Once xenografts have been established, no differences in growth behavior are seen upon retransplantation in either NMRI or BALB/c nude mice.

Further developments

Further extension of the xenograft model system can be achieved by using implantation routes other than the subcutaneous inoculation site. Orthotopic (intraprostatic) implantation will be the most realistic model, since it provides the most natural environment for prostate cells and allows organ-specific interactions to occur. From the technical point of view, orthotopic implantation is now a procedure that can be performed routinely[39,40]. The orthotopic model also has some disadvantages, however. First, the tumor sample has to be inoculated in a reproducible but small volume. The most suitable material for this, single-cell tumor suspension, is not readily available from most xenograft lines. A favorable exception, however, is PC-346 from which a permanent *in vitro* cell line, PC-346C, has been developed in our laboratory. A second problem is the difficulty of adequately monitoring tumor growth, since orthotopic tumors are not as readily accessible as subcutaneous tumors. This problem also has now been solved, using the technique of transrectal ultrasonography (TRUS)[41]. This method, employing tiny ultrasound probes, has been fully validated by demonstrating the excellent correlation between TRUS values and actual tumor weights and/or plasma PSA levels in mice with orthotopic PC-346C tumors[42].

One aspect that is still insufficiently covered by the current panel of xenograft models is the metastatic process. Subcutaneous tumors only rarely metastasize. Metastatic spread of orthotopic tumors is more likely to occur, but will still be dependent on the specific characteristics of the implanted tumor cells. Using the orthotopic PC-346C model we were able to detect the presence of prostatic mRNA in liver, lungs and lymph nodes (Van Weerden and colleagues, unpublished data), but overt metastatic deposits were generally not seen. The clinical importance of the metastatic process demands the development of additional experimental models with the propensity to metastasize, preferably to the bones.

Concluding remarks

Prostate cancer xenograft models have contributed and will continue to contribute to the elucidation of many important questions concerning the biology of prostate cancer. Xenograft models will be valuable tools for finding an answer to a number of still open fundamental questions with regard to the biological behavior of prostate cancer cells. Moreover, xenograft models are extremely useful, reproducible sources of well-characterized tumor material that will be needed for molecular studies. Finally, representative xenograft models are crucial for reliable testing of new treatment modalities. Further extension of the current panel of xenograft models is still needed, however, and should preferably be focused on the inclusion of models with enhanced metastatic ability.

References

1. Smolev J, Heston WDW, Scott WW, *et al.* Characterization of the Dunning R-3327-H prostatic carcinoma: an appropriate model for prostatic cancer. *Cancer Treat Rep* 1977;61: 273–87
2. Isaacs JT, Isaacs WB, Feitz WFJ, *et al.* Establishment and characterization of seven Dunning rat prostatic cancer cell lines and their use in developing methods for predicting metastatic abilities of prostatic cancers. *Prostate* 1986;9: 261–81
3. Stone KR, Mickey DD, Wunderli H, *et al.* Isolation of a human prostate carcinoma cell line (DU145). *Int J Cancer* 1978;21:274–81
4. Kaighn ME, Narayan KS, Ohnuki Y, *et al.* Establishment and characterization of a human

prostatic carcinoma cell line (PC-3). *Invest Urol* 1979;17:16–23

5. Horoszewicz JS, Leong SS, Kawinsky E, *et al.* LNCaP model of human prostatic carcinoma. *Cancer Res* 1983;43:1809–18

6. Weijerman PC, König JJ, Wong ST, *et al.* Lipofection-mediated immortalization of human prostatic epithelial cells of normal and malignant origin using human papillomavirus type 18 DNA. *Cancer Res* 1984;54:5579–83

7. Van Bokhoven A, Varella-Garcia M, Korch C, *et al.* Widely used prostate carcinoma cell lines share common origins. *Prostate* 2001;47:36–51

8. Veldscholte J, Ris-Stalpers C, Kuiper GGJM, *et al.* A mutation in the ligand binding domain of the androgen receptor of human LNCaP cells affects steroid binding characteristics and response to antiandrogens. *Biochem Biophys Res Commun* 1990;173:534–40

9. Isaacson JH, Cattanach BM. [Report.] *Mouse News Letter* 1962;27:31

10. Flanagen SP. Nude, a hairless gene with pleiotropic effects in the mouse. *Genet Res* 1966;8:295–309

11. Pantelouris EM. Absence of thymus in a mouse mutant. *Nature (London)* 1968;217:370–1

12. Rebar RW, Morandini IC, Petze JE, *et al.* Hormonal basis of reproductive defects in athymic mice: reduced gonadotropins and testosterone in males. *Biol Reprod* 1982;27:1267–76

13. Rygaard J, Povlsen CO. Heterotransplantation of a human malignant tumor to 'nude' mice. *Acta Pathol Microbiol Scand* 1969;77:758–60

14. Hoehn W, Schröder FH, Riemann JF, *et al.* Human prostatic adenocarcinoma: some characteristics of a serially transplantable line in nude mice (PC82). *Prostate* 1980;1:95–104

15. Hoehn W, Wagner M, Riemann JF, *et al.* Prostatic adenocarcinoma PC-EW, a new human tumor line transplantable in nude mice. *Prostate* 1984;5:445–52

16. Van Weerden WM, de Ridder CMA, Verdaasdonk CL, *et al.* Development of seven new human prostate tumor xenograft models and their histopathological characterization. *Am J Pathol* 1996;149:1055–62

17. Van Weerden WM, Romijn JC. Use of nude mouse xenograft models in prostate cancer research. *Prostate* 2000;43:263–71

18. Jongsma J, Oomen MH, Noordzij MA, *et al.* Kinetics of neuroendocrine differentiation in an androgen dependent human prostate xenograft model. *Am J Pathol* 1999;154:543–51

19. Van Steenbrugge GJ, Groen M, Romijn JC, *et al.* Biological effects of hormonal treatment regimens on a transplantable human prostatic tumor line (PC-82). *J Urol* 1984;131:812–17

20. Jongsma J, Oomen MH, Noordzij MA, *et al.* Androgen deprivation of the PC-310 human prostate cancer model system induces neuro-endocrine differentiation. *Cancer Res* 2000;60:741–8

21. Van Weerden WM, de Ridder CMA, Erkens S, *et al.* Tumor progression of the androgen-responsive human prostate tumor xenograft PC-346. *Contrib Oncol* 1999;54:325–30

22. Van Steenbrugge GJ, van Dongen JJW, Reuvers PJ, *et al.* Transplantable human prostatic carcinoma (PC-82) in athymic nude mice: I. Hormone dependence and the concentration of androgens in plasma and tumor tissue. *Prostate* 1987;11:195–210

23. Van Steenbrugge GJ, Bolt-de Vries J, Blankenstein MA, *et al.* Effect of hormone treatment on prostatic acid phosphatase in a serially transplantable human prostatic adeno-carcinoma (PC-82). *J Urol* 1983;129:630–3

24. Van Steenbrugge GJ, Blankenstein MA, Bolt-de Vries J, *et al.* Transplantable human prostatic carcinoma (PC-82) in athymic nude mice: II. Tumor growth and androgen receptors. *Prostate* 1988;12:145–56

25. Van Weerden WM, van Steenbrugge GJ, van Kreuningen A, *et al.* Assessment of the critical level of androgen for growth response of trans-plantable human prostatic carcinoma (PC-82) in nude mice. *J Urol* 1991;145:631–4

26. Van Steenbrugge GJ, Groen M, de Jong FH, *et al.* The use of steroid-containing Silastic implants in male nude mice: plasma hormone levels and the effect of implantation on the weights of the ventral prostate and seminal vesicles. *Prostate* 1984;5:639–47

27. Pretlow TG, Wolman SR, Micale MA, *et al.* Xenografts of primary human prostatic carcinoma. *J Natl Cancer Inst* 1993;85:394–8

28. Wainstein MA, He F, Robinson D, *et al.* CWR 22: androgen dependent xenograft model derived from a primary human prostatic carcinoma. *Cancer Res* 1994;54:6049–52

29. Klein KA, Reiter RE, Redula J, *et al.* Progression of metastatic human prostate cancer to androgen-independence in immunodeficient SCID mice. *Nat Med* 1997;3:402–8

30. Craft N, Chhor C, Tran C, *et al.* Evidence for clonal outgrowth of androgen-independent prostate cancer cells from androgen-dependent tumors through a two-step process. *Cancer Res* 1999;59:5030–6

31. Ellis WJ, Vessella RL, Buhler KR, *et al.* Character-ization of a novel androgen-sensitive, prostate-specific antigen-producing prostatic carcinoma xenograft: LuCaP23. *Clin Cancer Res* 1996;2:1039–48

32. True LD, Buhler K, Quinn J, *et al.* A neuroendocrine/small cell prostate carcinoma

xenograft – LuCaP49. *Am J Pathol* 2002;161: 705–15

33. Navone NM, Logothetis CJ, von Eschenbach AC, *et al.* Model systems of prostate cancer: uses and limitations. *Cancer Metastasis Rev* 1999;17:361–71

34. De Pinieux G, Legrier ME, Poirson-Bichat F, *et al.* Clinical and experimental progression of a new model of human prostate cancer and therapeutic approach. *Am J Pathol* 2001;159:753–64

35. Nagabhushan M, Milller CM, Pretlow TP, *et al.* CWR22: the first human prostate cancer xenograft with strongly androgen-dependent and relapsed strains both *in vivo* and in soft agar. *Cancer Res* 1996;56:3042–6

36. Romijn JC, Verkoelen CF, Schroeder FH. Measurement of the survival of human tumor cells after implantation in athymic nude mice. *Int J Cancer* 1986;38:97–101

37. Van Weerden WM, Romijn JC, de Ridder CMA, *et al.* Frequent occurrence of spontaneous tumors in NMRI athymic nude mice. *Contrib Oncol* 1996;51:41–4

38. Tuxhorn JA, Ayala GE, Rowley DR. Reactive stroma in prostate cancer progression. *J Urol* 2001;166:2472–83

39. Rembrink K, Romijn JC, Ruizeveld de Winter JA, *et al.* Orthotopic implantation of human prostate cancer cell lines: a clinically relevant animal model for metastatic prostate cancer. *Prostate* 1997;31:168–74

40. Fu X, Herrera H, Hoffman RM. Orthotopic growth and metastasis of human prostate carcinoma in nude mice after transplantation of histological intact tissue. *Int J Cancer* 1992;52: 987–90

41. Kusaka N, Nasu Y, Arata R, *et al.* Transrectal ultrasound for monitoring murine orthotopic prostate tumor. *Prostate* 2001;47:118–24

42. Kraaij R, van Weerden WM, de Ridder CMA, *et al.* Validation of transrectal ultrasonographic volumetry for orthotopic prostate tumours in mice. *Lab Anim* 2002;36:165–72

Hormonal regulation of prostate cancer

20

C. A. Berrevoets, A. Umar and A. O. Brinkmann

Introduction

Androgens are important steroid hormones for expression of the male phenotype. They have characteristic roles during male sexual differentiation, during the development and maintenance of secondary male characteristics, and during the initiation and maintenance of spermatogenesis[1]. The two most important androgens in this respect are testosterone and 5α-dihydrotestosterone. Each androgen has its own specific role during male sexual differentiation: testosterone is directly involved in the development and differentiation of Wolffian duct-derived structures, whereas 5α-dihydrotestosterone, a metabolite of testosterone, is the active ligand in a number of other androgen target tissues (e.g. urogenital sinus, prostate, urogenital tubercle, penis, hair follicle).

Mechanism of androgen action

The actions of androgens are mediated by the androgen receptor. This ligand-dependent transcription factor belongs to the superfamily of nuclear receptors. In this respect, testosterone and 5α-dihydrotestosterone can be considered to act as tissue-selective androgen receptor modulators during fetal sexual differentiation and during development and maintenance of the male phenotype. In Figure 1, a simplified model of androgen action in a typical androgen target cell is depicted.

Despite the two different ligands, only one androgen receptor cDNA has been identified and cloned[2–5]. The concept of two hormones acting via one receptor is generally accepted to explain the different actions of androgens.

In the present overview, some aspects of androgen action are presented, with particular emphasis on structural and functional properties of the androgen receptor protein after binding androgens, and a specific group of androgen receptor modulators, the anti-androgens. In addition, a model for selective androgen receptor modulation by anti-androgens is proposed, in which the role of the nuclear receptor corepressor (N-CoR) is highlighted.

Structural aspects of the androgen receptor

The androgen receptor protein displays a large homology in the DNA-binding domain and in the ligand-binding domain with the other members of the steroid hormone receptor subfamily[6]. Recently, the crystal structures of the human androgen receptor ligand-binding domain in complex with the synthetic ligand methyltrienolone (R1881) and 5α-dihydrotestosterone, respectively, have been determined[7,8]. The crystallographic data predict a three-dimensional structure, with typical nuclear receptor ligand-binding domain folding. Interestingly, in the ligand-binding pocket, 20 amino acid residues have been identified that interact more or less directly with the bound ligand[7]. Crystallographic data on the ligand-binding domain complexed with an agonist predict 11 helices (no helix 2), with two anti-parallel β-sheets arranged in a so-called helical sandwich pattern. In the agonist-bound conformation, the carboxy-terminal helix 12 is positioned in an orientation allowing closure of

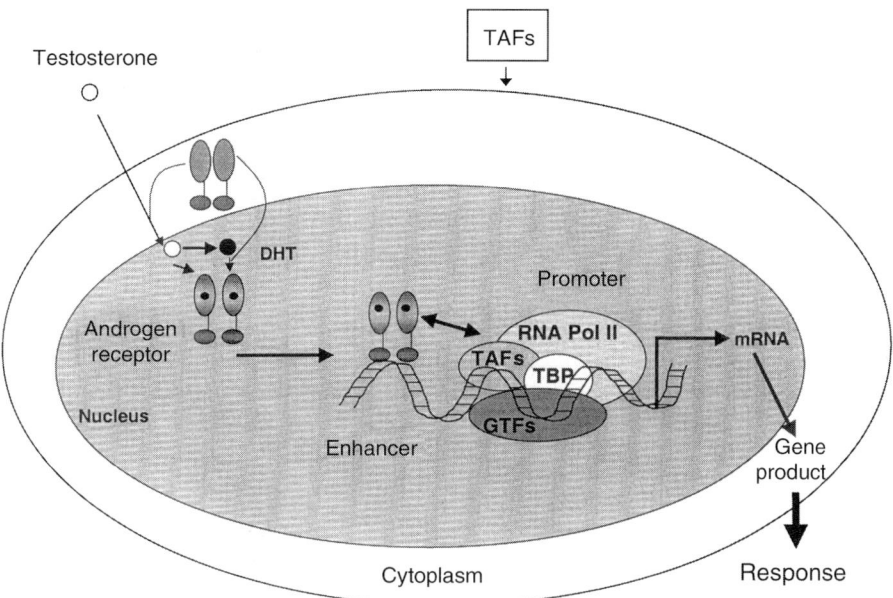

Figure 1 Simplified model of androgen action in an androgen target cell. The key protein is the androgen receptor, which binds testosterone directly or its active metabolite 5α-dihydrotestosterone (DHT). The receptor enters the nucleus via an intrinsic nuclear localization signal. Upon steroid hormone binding, which may occur either in the cytoplasm or in the nucleus, the androgen receptor binds as dimer to specific DNA elements present as enhancers in upstream promoter sequences of androgen target genes. Important is the direct and indirect communication of the androgen receptor complex with several components of the transcription machinery (e.g. RNA polymerase II (RNA Pol II), TATA box binding protein (TBP), TBP associating factors (TAFs), general transcription factors (GTFs)). This communication via so-called coactivators triggers mRNA synthesis and, consequently, protein synthesis, which finally results in an androgen response

the ligand-binding pocket. The folding of the ligand-binding domain upon hormone binding results in a globular structure, with an interaction surface for binding of interacting proteins such as coactivators. In this way, the androgen receptor recruits selectively a number of proteins, and can communicate with other partners of the transcription initiation complex (Figure 1). Crystal structure data of the androgen receptor ligand-binding domain complexed with an antagonist are currently lacking, but would be very valuable for understanding the recruitment of possible corepressors.

Antiandrogen binding to the androgen receptor: structural consequences

Androgen receptor antagonists are compounds that interfere in some way in the biological effects of androgens, and are therefore frequently used in the treatment of androgen-based pathologies (e.g. prostate cancer, hirsutism).

The steroidal antiandrogens cyproterone acetate (CPA) and RU38486 (RU486; mifepristone) have partial agonist and antagonistic actions. Interestingly, both compounds also display partial progestational and glucocorticoid action, and are therefore considered not to be pure antiandrogens. The nonsteroidal antiandrogens hydroxyflutamide, nilutamide and bicalutamide are pure antiandrogens[9–11].

In contrast to the full antagonists hydroxyflutamide and bicalutamide, CPA and RU486 can partially activate the androgen receptor with respect to transcription activation (Figure 2)[12,13]. As determined by proteolytic

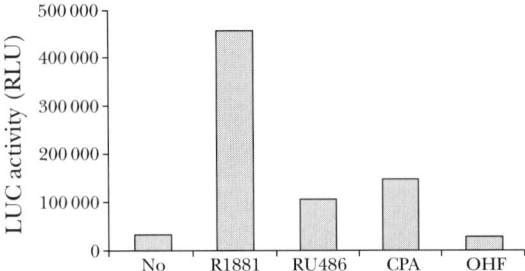

Figure 2 Comparison of transcription activation of the androgen receptor by different ligands (androgen (R1881), 1 nmol/l; RU486, cyproterone acetate (CPA), hydroxyflutamide (OHF), all 1 μmol/l). Transcriptional activation of an androgen-responsive promoter was measured in Chinese hamster ovary (CHO) cells after transfection of androgen receptor cDNA and the reporter plasmid MMTV-LUC (mouse mammary tumor virus luciferase), and was expressed in relative light units (RLU)

degradation studies, binding of androgens by the androgen receptor results in two consecutive conformational changes of the receptor molecule. Initially, a fragment of 35 kDa, spanning the complete ligand-binding domain and part of the hinge region, is protected by the ligand. After prolonged incubation times, a second conformational change occurs, resulting in protection of a smaller fragment of 29 kDa[12,13]. In the presence of several anti-androgens (e.g. CPA, hydroxyflutamide and bicalutamide), only the 35-kDa fragment is protected, and no smaller fragments are detectable upon longer incubations. Obviously, the 35-kDa fragment is correlated with an inactive conformation, whereas the second conformational change, only inducible by agonists and considered the necessary step for transcription activation, is lacking upon binding of anti-androgens. Further analyses with specific antibodies against different epitopes in the 35-kDa and 29-kDa fragments reveal that only the most COOH-terminal end of the androgen receptor protein is represented by the 29-kDa fragment[12,13].

Antiandrogens and a special androgen receptor mutant in prostate cancer

In prostate cancer, initial tumor growth depends on the presence of an activated androgen receptor. In general, prostate cancer patients benefit temporarily from androgen-ablation therapies. However, growth of the majority of prostate tumors changes during tumor development from androgen-dependent to androgen-independent. In these apparently hormone-independent tumors, high nuclear androgen receptor expression levels exist. In some hormone-refractory prostate cancers, androgen receptor gene amplification occurs or androgen receptor mutations are found, which can modify the ligand specificity[14–16].

The androgen receptor (AR) gene in the LNCaP (lymph node) prostate cancer cell line contains a point mutation at codon 877 (ACT to GCT), which leads to a threonine to alanine substitution[15]. This substitution has a dramatic effect on the ligand specificity and trans-activating function of the AR. It renders the receptor, and as a consequence the growth of LNCaP cells, responsive to most antiandrogens (e.g. CPA, hydroxyflutamide; but not bicalutamide) and to the natural low-affinity ligands estradiol, progesterone and adrenal gland androgens[17–19]. The Thr877Ala substitution has not only been found in the LNCaP cell line, but has also been detected in prostate cancer patients. This mutation has preferentially been found in hormone-refractory tumors, underscoring its functional importance[16]. In contrast to other antagonists such as hydroxyflutamide and CPA, the binding of RU486 to the mutated AR from LNCaP cells is not different from that to the wild-type receptor. This suggests that RU486 is interacting in a different way with the AR ligand-binding domain. This is supported by proteolytic degradation studies, in which RU486 protects different AR fragments (30 kDa and 25 kDa), compared with normal agonists (35 kDa and 29 kDa), indicating that RU486 induces different conformational changes in the ligand-binding domain of the AR[12,13]. It seems that proper folding of the

COOH-terminal part of the AR (helices 11 and 12) is not essential for the optimal binding and partial agonistic action of RU486.

Mechanism of action of antiandrogens

It has been known for some time that interaction of nuclear receptors with basal transcription factors is necessary for the control of hormone-dependent transcription activation (see Figure 1). However, more recently it has become clear that additional protein factors, called coactivators, are also involved. Most of these proteins have a broad specificity, and appear to interact with the ligand-binding domain of nuclear receptors, leading to an increase in nuclear receptor activity. For some nuclear receptors, proteins that inhibit the receptor activity, so-called corepressors (N-CoR, and silencing mediator for retinoid and thyroid hormone receptors (SMRT)), have been described[20,21]. These corepressors associate with the receptor in the absence of ligand (e.g. retinoid acid receptor and thyroid hormone receptor), or in the presence of an anti-hormone (progesterone receptor (PR), estrogen receptor (ER))[22,23]. In the latter case, binding of an antagonist (RU486 or tamoxifen), and not of an agonist, results in a conformational change of the ligand-binding domain (LBD) appropriate for interaction with a corepressor and inappropriate for interaction with coactivators. For the AR, several coactivators have been described to increase its activity (e.g. TIF2, SRC1, ARA70)[24–26]. Also, several protein factors have been identified that interact with the AR and repress transcriptional activity of agonist-bound AR (e.g. cyclin D1, tumor susceptibility gene 101, p21-activated kinase, SRY, HBO1, AES, TR-4)[27–33].

Recently, studies have been published in which it was unequivocally demonstrated that the AR can interact with the corepressors N-CoR and SMRT, in the presence of an antiandrogen and also in the presence of agonists[34–37].

As described above, RU486 is a partial AR agonist, and induces a conformational change of the AR-LBD different from that induced by other antiandrogens and androgens. Since it

was described that N-CoR interacts with the RU486-occupied PR, we investigated the effect of N-CoR on the activity of RU486-occupied AR in Chinese hamster ovary (CHO) cells. Co-transfection of N-CoR led to a decrease in AR activity (75% reduction) after incubation with RU486. Furthermore, when an AR–VP16 fusion protein was used instead of the AR protein, the effect of N-CoR was even more pronounced (Figure 3). The RU486-induced partial activity was almost completely abolished after co-transfection with N-CoR. As determined by Western immunoblotting, AR expression in CHO cells was not reduced by N-CoR cotransfection, excluding the possibility that repression of AR activity by N-CoR was due to a decrease of AR protein levels. In contrast, when the synthetic androgen R1881 was used, only a slight decrease in AR activity was observed upon transfection with N-CoR. Similar results were obtained with another partial agonist, CPA. The repression of AR activity by N-CoR was not dependent on the type of promoter used in the reporter construct, because using a minimal promoter (GRE-TATA) (glucocorticoid

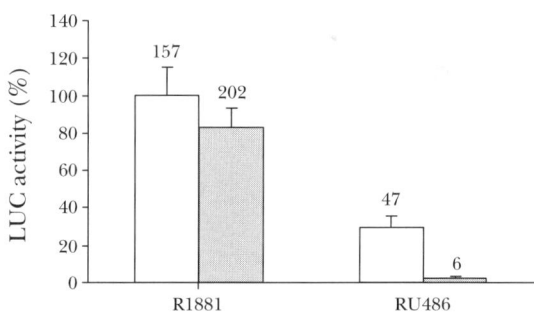

Figure 3 Repression by the nuclear receptor corepressor (N-CoR) of transcriptional activity of the androgen receptor (AR) complexed with the partial agonist RU486. Chinese hamster ovary (CHO) cells were transfected with AR-VP16 cDNA and the reporter plasmid MMTV-LUC together with either N-CoR cDNA plasmid (shaded bars) or empty vector plasmid as a control (open bars). Transcriptional activation of the androgen-responsive promoter was expressed in relative light units (RLU). The fold induction, measured as the ratio of the activities in the presence and absence of ligand (1 nmol/l R1881 or 1 μmol/l RU486), is indicated above each bar

responsive element) resulted in comparable repression to that with the MMTV promoter.

These results indicate that the corepressor N-CoR represses RU486- and CPA-induced AR activity, most likely as a consequence of inducing a conformational change of the AR-LBD, allowing recruitment of N-CoR.

To investigate the consequences of the LNCaP mutation (T877A) in the AR-LBD on the recruitment of N-CoR by an antiandrogen-complexed AR, cotransfections were performed with wild-type and mutant AR–VP. Bicalutamide, which induced a different conformational change of the mutant receptor, has been shown recently to recruit N-CoR to the prostate-specific antigen (PSA) promoter in LNCaP cells expressing the T877A mutant AR[38].

Results from the present study indicated that, in the mutant receptor, N-CoR was no longer able to suppress activity-induced CPA and hydroxyflutamide, while RU486-complexed mutant receptor could still be repressed by N-CoR. This suggests that the conformational changes induced by CPA and hydroxyflutamide

of the LBD of the mutant AR no longer allow recruitment of the corepressor N-CoR. This is further supported by the previously shown conformational changes induced by the antiandrogens in the mutant receptor, which were indistinguishable from those by R1881.

Conclusions

Based on the conformational changes of the AR-LBD induced by androgens or anti-androgens, it can be concluded that the different transcriptional activities displayed by full agonists (testosterone, 5α-dihydrotestosterone, methyltrienolone), partial agonists (RU486 and CPA) or full antagonists (hydroxyflutamide, bicalutamide) are the result of recruitment of a different repertoire of coregulators (co-activators or corepressors) as a consequence of these conformational changes. The differential recruitment of coregulators can be considered a special form of ligand-selective modulation of the AR-LBD, and can be applied in a broader sense also to the tissue-selective modulation of

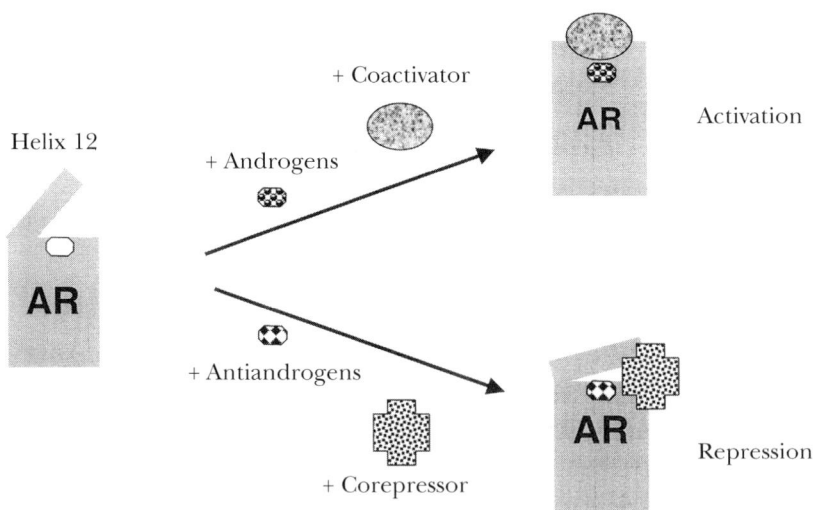

Figure 4 Ligand-selective modulation of the androgen receptor (AR) ligand-binding domain (LBD) by agonists and antagonists: role of coactivators and corepressors in the mechanism of action of androgens and antiandrogens, respectively. In the agonist-bound state, the AR-LBD is folded according to the mousetrap model in which helix 12 forms an essential part of a surface allowing binding of coactivators, resulting in activation of transcriptional activity. In the presence of an AR antagonist such as RU486, the AR-LBD is folded in such a way that the position of helix 12 no longer allows interaction of a coactivator with the LBD, but instead a corepressor can bind, resulting in repression of transcriptional activity

androgen action, where levels of coactivators and corepressors may ultimately determine the final activity. A simplified model representing the selective modulation of the AR-LBD in the mechanism of action of androgens and anti-androgens is shown in Figure 4.

Acknowledgements

The authors wish to acknowledge the valuable contributions of Dr Cor Kuil and Dr Jos Veldscholte. The authors would also like to thank Dr C. K. Glass and Dr M. G. Rosenfeld for the generous supply of N-CoR plasmid.

References

1. George FW, Wilson JD. Sex determination and differentiation. In Knobil E, Neill JD, eds. *The Physiology of Reproduction.* New York: Raven Press, 1994:Chapter 1
2. Chang C, Kokontis J, Liao S. Molecular cloning of human and rat complementary DNA encoding androgen receptors. *Science* 1988;240: 324–6
3. Lubahn DB, Joseph DR, Sullivan PM, *et al.* Cloning of human androgen receptor complementary DNA and localization to the X chromosome. *Science* 1988;240:327–30
4. Tilley WD, Marcelli M, Wilson JD, *et al.* Characterization and expression of a cDNA encoding the human androgen receptor. *Proc Natl Acad Sci USA* 1989;86:327–31
5. Trapman J, Klaassen P, Kuiper GGJM, *et al.* Cloning, structure and expression of a cDNA encoding the human androgen receptor. *Biochem Biophys Res Commun* 1988;153:241–8
6. Brinkmann AO, Trapman J. Genetic analysis of androgen receptors in development and disease. *Adv Pharmacol* 2000;47:317–41
7. Matias PM, Donner P, Coelho R, *et al.* Structural evidence for ligand specificity in the binding domain of the human androgen receptor: implications for pathogenic gene mutations. *J Biol Chem* 2000;275:26164–71
8. Sack JS, Kish KF, Wang C, *et al.* Crystallographic structures of the ligand binding domains of the androgen receptor and its T877A mutant complexed with the natural agonist dihydro-testosterone. *Proc Natl Acad Sci USA* 2001;98: 4904–9
9. Neumann F, Topert M. Pharmacology of anti-androgens. *J Steroid Biochem* 1986;25:885–95
10. Raynaud JP, Ojasoo T. The design and use of sex-steroid antagonists. *J Steroid Biochem* 1986; 25:811–33
11. Furr BJ, Valcaccia B, Curry B, *et al.* ICI 176 334: a novel non-steroidal, peripherally selective anti-androgen. *J Endocrinol* 1987;113:R7–9
12. Kuil CW, Mulder E. Mechanism of antiandrogen action: conformational changes of the receptor. *Mol Cell Endocrinol* 1994;102:R1–5
13. Kuil CW, Berrevoets CA, Mulder E. Ligand-induced conformational alterations of the androgen receptor analyzed by limited trypsinization – studies on the mechanism of antiandrogen action. *J Biol Chem* 1995;270: 27569–76
14. Visakorpi T, Hyytinen E, Koivisto P, *et al. In vivo* amplification of the androgen receptor gene and progression of human prostate cancer. *Nat Genet* 1995;9:401–6
15. Veldscholte J, Ris-Stalpers C, Kuiper GGJM, *et al.* A mutation in the ligand binding domain of the androgen receptor of human LNCaP cells affects steroid binding characteristics and response to antiandrogens. *Biochem Biophys Res Commun* 1990;173:534–40
16. Taplin ME, Bubley GJ, Shuster TD, *et al.* Mutation of the androgen receptor gene in metastatic androgen-independent prostate cancer. *N Engl J Med* 1995;332:1393–8
17. Schuurmans ALG, Bolt J, Veldscholte J, *et al.* Stimulatory effects of antiandrogens on LNCaP human prostate tumor cell growth, EGF-receptor level and acid phosphatase secretion. *J Steroid Biochem Mol Biol* 1990;37:849–53
18. Veldscholte J, Berrevoets CA, Brinkmann AO, *et al.* Antiandrogens and the mutated androgen receptor of LNCaP cells: differential effects on binding affinity, heat-shock protein interaction, and transcription activation. *Biochemistry* 1992; 31:2393–9
19. Steketee K, Timmerman L, Ziel-van der Made ACJ, *et al.* Broadened ligand responsiveness of androgen receptor mutants obtained by random amino acid substitution of H874 and mutation

hot spot T877 in prostate cancer. *Int J Cancer* 2002;100:309–17

20. Hörlein AJ, Näär AM, Heinzel T, *et al.* Ligand-independent repression by the thyroid hormone receptor mediated by a nuclear receptor co-repressor. *Nature (London)* 1995;377:397–403

21. Chen JD, Evans RM. A transcriptional co-repressor that interacts with nuclear hormone receptors. *Nature (London)* 1995;377:454–7

22. Jackson TA, Richer JK, Bain DL, *et al.* The partial agonist activity of antagonist-occupied steroid receptors is controlled by a novel hinge domain-binding coactivator L7/SPA and the corepressors N-CoR or SMRT. *Mol Endocrinol* 1997;11:693–705

23. Lavinsky RM, Jepsen K, Heinzel T, *et al.* Diverse signaling pathways modulate nuclear receptor recruitment of N-CoR and SMRT complexes. *Proc Natl Acad Sci USA* 1998;95:2920–5

24. Voegel JJ, Heine MJ, Zechel C, *et al.* TIF2, a 160 kDa transcriptional mediator for the ligand-dependent activation function AF-2 of nuclear receptors. *EMBO J* 1996;15:3667–75

25. Yeh S, Chang C. Cloning and characterization of a specific coactivator, ARA70, for the androgen receptor in human prostate cells. *Proc Natl Acad Sci USA* 1996;93:5517–21

26. Jenster G, Spencer TE, Burcin MM, *et al.* Steroid receptor induction of gene transcription: a two-step model. *Proc Natl Acad Sci USA* 1997; 94:7879–84

27. Petre CE, Wetherill YB, Danielsen M, *et al.* Cyclin D1: mechanism and consequence of androgen receptor co-repressor activity. *J Biol Chem* 2002; 277:2207–15

28. Sun Z, Pan J, Hope WX, *et al.* Tumor susceptibility gene 101 protein represses androgen receptor transactivation and interacts with p300. *Cancer* 1999;86:689–96

29. Lee SR, Ramos SM, Ko A, *et al.* AR and ER interaction with a p21-activated kinase (PAK6). *Mol Endocrinol* 2002;16:85–99

30. Yuan X, Lu ML, Li T, *et al.* SRY interacts with and negatively regulates androgen receptor transcriptional activity. *J Biol Chem* 2001;276:46647–54

31. Sharma M, Zarnegar M, Li Z, *et al.* Androgen receptor interacts with a novel MYST protein, HBO1. *J Biol Chem* 2000;275:35200–8

32. Yu X, Li P, Roeder RG, *et al.* Inhibition of androgen receptor-mediated transcription by amino-terminal enhancer of split. *Mol Cell Biol* 2001;21:4614–25

33. Lee Y-F, Shyr C-R, Thin TH, *et al.* Convergence of two repressors through heterodimer formation of androgen receptor and testicular orphan receptor-4: a unique signaling pathway in the steroid receptor superfamily. *Proc Natl Acad Sci USA* 1999;96:14724–9

34. Dotzlaw H, Moehren U, Mink S, *et al.* The amino terminus of the human AR is target for corepressor action and antihormone agonism. *Mol Endocrinol* 2002;16:661–73

35. Chang CY, McDonnell DP. Evaluation of ligand-dependent changes in AR structure using peptide probes. *Mol Endocrinol* 2002;16:647–60

36. Massiello D, Cheng S, Bubley GJ, *et al.* Bicalutamide functions as an androgen receptor antagonist by assembly of a transcriptionally inactive receptor. *J Biol Chem* 2002;277:26321–6

37. Cheng S, Brzostek S, Lee SR, *et al.* Inhibition of the dihydrotestosterone-activated androgen receptor by nuclear receptor corepressor. *Mol Endocrinol* 2002;16:1492–501

38. Shang Y, Myers M, Brown M. Formation of the androgen receptor transition complex. *Mol Cell* 2002;9:601–10

Profiling protein interactions in angiogenesis

21

R. Pasqualini and W. Arap

Introduction, overview and future directions

We are developing integrated, combinatorial library platform technologies that will enable the identification, validation and prioritization of molecular targets in human blood vessels. Expanding our understanding of this complex system will lead to insights into the biology of the tumor circulatory microenvironment, changes in blood vessels during tumor progression, and the localization of novel markers in cancer and in other diseases with an angiogenesis component. The vascular endothelium expresses differential receptors depending on the functional state and tissue localization of its lining cells. We have developed technologies to characterize functionally this receptor heterogeneity with phage display random peptide libraries[1,2]. We have isolated several peptide ligands that home to tissue-specific endothelial cell receptors following intravenous administration. Such peptide ligands can be used to target therapeutic compounds or imaging agents to endothelial cells *in vitro* and *in vivo*.

Recent advances in the field include identification of endothelial receptors expressed differentially in normal and pathological conditions, and the isolation of peptides or antibody ligands to such receptors in *in vitro* assays, in animal models and in patients. These milestones, which extend the 'functional map' of the vasculature, should lead to mechanistic insights into diseases that exhibit distinct vascular characteristics such as cancer and inflammation. Our research program is comprehensive because it is based on a series of platform technologies for discovery of ligand–receptor pairs that can be used for the development of targeted therapies. Target identification is intrinsically based on a functional selection; mechanistic studies surrounding these molecules result in strategies for intervention in disease. A ligand–receptor system has been identified directly in a patient screening, and has already been validated in human samples (Zurita and colleagues, unpublished observations). In summary, as future directions, we plan first, to create a molecular map of the human vasculature and second, to accelerate the translation of such diversity into clinical applications.

Phage display libraries and vascular targeting technology

Our work shows that peptide libraries can be used to probe organ- and tumor-specific markers. The library system we use is based on phage particles engineered so that random oligonucleotides are individually fused to cDNAs encoding a phage surface protein, and large collections of phage particles (10^9 individual clones) displaying unique peptides are generated[3,4]. Phage capable of homing to certain organs or tumors following an intravenous injection are selected from the libraries; the ability of individual peptides to target a tissue can also be evaluated by using different strategies[5–9]. Furthermore, this system provides a powerful way of identifying endothelial cell surface markers. Thus, in addition to the isolation of novel tools for selective vascular targeting of therapies, we have made progress towards furthering our understanding of tumor endothelium specificity and the definition of the role that endothelial cell markers play in angiogenesis. The targeting peptides that we have so far identified bind to different receptors selectively expressed on the endothelium of target tissues. Some of these vascular markers are proteases that not only serve as receptors for circulating ligands but also modulate angiogenesis. Moreover, certain vascular receptors are also involved in tumor cell homing during the metastatic process (unpublished observations).

Preclinical applications in animal models

The potential of *in vivo* phage display to identify vascular targeting peptides has not yet been fully explored. It is currently of particular interest to target sites involved in cancer. These probes will be useful in peptide-guided therapy against tumors; we also hope to shed light on the vascular biology and heterogeneity of blood vessels in cancer metastasis. Peptides that home to tumor vasculature have been used as carriers to deliver cytotoxic drugs[6], pro-apoptotic peptides[10], cytokines[11], protease inhibitors[12] and gene therapy vectors[3,13] (Marini and colleagues, unpublished observations). The coupling of homing peptides can yield targeted agents that, when compared with the parental compounds, show improved therapeutic index. *In vivo* phage screenings in humans will be developed that use probes for targeting therapies and to identify diagnostic and prognostic factors. Moreover, the diversity of the vasculature may affect responses to therapies, in particular antiangiogenic drugs. In order to map vascular receptors, we had relied for some time on isolating ligands and receptors in mice to find the putative human homologs. However, when such homologs are found, the question remains whether targeting will be observed in the context of human vasculature. In humans, cell surface receptors may have a very different distribution and function than in mice. The existence of differences among species means that any data derived from mouse studies must be carefully validated before being translated to human studies.

Fingerprinting antibodies from cancer patients

We have developed a phage display-based screening to select peptide sequences recognized by the repertoire of circulating tumor-associated antibodies. We isolated peptides recognized by antibodies purified from the serum of cancer patients. Consensus peptide motifs showed marked selective binding to circulating antibodies from cancer patients over control antibodies from blood donors. We next validated such motifs by showing that serum reactivity to the peptide can be specifically linked to disease progression and to patient survival. Finally, we isolated a corresponding tumor antigen eliciting the immune response. These results show that it is possible to identify tumor antigens by fingerprinting the pool of antibodies from the serum of cancer patients. Exploiting the differential humoral response to cancer through such an approach may identify molecular targets for therapy (Mintz and colleagues, unpublished observations).

Mapping human vasculature directly in patients

Recently, we have reported the first *in vivo* screening of a peptide library in a patient. We surveyed close to 50 000 motifs that localized to different organs. This large-scale screening shows that the tissue distribution of circulating peptides is non-random[13]. High-throughput analysis of the motifs revealed similarities to ligands for differentially expressed cell surface proteins. We isolated a potential mimic peptide of interleukin-11 (IL-11) from the human prostate. The immunostaining pattern obtained with an antibody against human IL-11 receptor on normal prostate tissue was indistinguishable from that of the Il-11 phage mimic overlay; a control antibody showed no staining in prostate tissue. Finally, using a ligand–receptor binding assay *in vitro*, we demonstrated the interaction of the CGRRAGGSC-displaying phage with immobilized IL-11Rα at the protein–protein level. The receptor–ligand system IL-11 : Il-11R may be useful for clinical translation. We are now expanding our studies and hope to validate multiple receptor–ligand pairs based on this strategy, as the potential of phage display to identify targeting sequences and receptors has hardly been fully explored. In soon to be published work, we have proposed ethical guidelines to allow patient-oriented research in end-of-life subjects[15].

Targeting urothelium *ex vivo*

We designed and optimized a receptor/ligand-binding assay on whole urothelium *ex vivo*. This strategy may form the molecular basis for clinical development of peptide- or peptidomimetic-guided intravesical compounds. We standardized an *ex vivo* binding assay, validated binding of selected phage to whole urothelium and evaluated whether receptor-mediated internalization into urothelium-derived cells occurred. Finally, we tested the influence of glycosaminoglycan layer on the urothelium-binding process. Phage selected and recovered in the screening were isolated and sequenced. Displayed peptide sequences were searched against online protein databases. Several classes of motifs were identified that bind to normal urothelial but not to control cells. Thus, we have introduced a strategy for screening combinatorial peptide libraries on bladder mucosa, a standard model for *ex vivo* whole urothelium binding assays and a panel of urothelium-binding peptides that may be suitable for translation into targeted intravesical therapy applications[9].

Angiogenesis in non-malignant diseases

Apart from cancer, abnormal angiogenesis accompanies many pathological conditions including inflammation and eye diseases. We have recently shown that neonatal mice with classic inherited retinal degeneration fail to mount reactive retinal neovascularization in a mouse model of oxygen-induced proliferative retinopathy. We have also found a comparable human paradigm: spontaneous regression of retinal neovascularization associated with long-standing diabetes mellitus occurs when retinitis pigmentosa becomes clinically evident. Our data show that reactive retinal neovascularization either fails to develop or regresses when the number of photoreceptor cells is markedly reduced. These findings support that a functional mechanism underlying this anti-angiogenic state is failure of the predicted up-regulation of vascular endothelial growth factor, although other growth factors may also be involved. Therapeutic strategies against retinopathies may emerge from this work[16].

Transplacental targeting

We have also performed sophisticated *in vivo* screenings to characterize the vasculature of highly specialized tissues such as the placenta[8]. In mammals, the interconnection between maternal and fetal molecules takes place through multiple distinct cell layers within the placenta[17]. Teratogens that affect the placenta seem to function by inhibiting selective transporters that are necessary for the transfer of nutrients to the embryo[18]. The functional role of the molecules that mediate maternal–fetal exchange in development is yet to be established. We have adapted, in phage display, a method for studying interactions between receptors expressed preferentially in an organ of interest and their ligands for the study of targets relevant in placental transport. We have selected teratogenic ligands that bind non-endothelial receptors expressed on the placental epithelium, the site where the molecular exchange occurs between the mother and the fetus. This study represents the first *in vivo* screening of a phage display library on non-endothelial tissues. Future implications of these findings include the basis for high-throughput identification of placental receptors prone to be affected by teratogenic compounds and also the design of safer drugs that could be used during pregnancy.

Conclusions

Recognition of molecular diversity in human disease is required for the development of targeted therapies. Validated ligands may be used as carriers for imaging or therapeutic agents. Moreover, the ligands themselves may be used either as drug discovery leads or for therapeutic modulation of their corresponding receptor(s). Finally, another application of the selected targeted ligands is identification of their vascular receptors. Discovery of functional targets in specific tissues and organs is likely to establish a platform for the development of a new pharmacology and the design of targeted therapies that will be more effective and less toxic in the context of cancer and other diseases.

Acknowledgements

This work was supported by the National Institutes of Health (CA90270 and CA82976 to R.P.; CA90270 and CA90810 to W.A.) and by a Gillson–Longenbaugh Foundation Award (to R.P. and W.A.).

References

1. Kolonin MG, Pasqualini R, Arap W. Molecular addresses in blood vessels as targets for therapy. *Curr Opin Chem Biol* 2001;5:308–13
2. Trepel M, Grifman M, Weitzman MD, *et al.* Molecular adaptors for vascular targeted adenoviral gene delivery. *Hum Gene Ther* 2000; 11:1971–81
3. Smith GP, Scott JK. Searching for peptide ligands with an epitope library. *Science* 1985; 228:1315–17
4. Smith GP, Scott JK. Libraries of peptides and proteins displayed in filamentous phage. *Meth Enzymol* 1993;21:228–57
5. Arap W, Pasqualini R, Ruoslahti E. Chemotherapy targeted to tumor vasculature. *Curr Opin Oncol* 1998;10:560–5
6. Arap W, Pasqualini R, Ruoslahti E. Cancer treatment by targeted drug delivery to tumor vasculature. *Science* 1998;279:377–80
7. Rajotte D, Ruoslahti E. Membrane dipeptidase is the receptor for a lung-targeting peptide identified by *in vivo* phage display. *J Biol Chem* 1999;274:11593–8
8. Kolonin M, Pasqualini R, Arap W. Teratogenicity induced by targeting a placental immunoglobulin transporter. *Proc Natl Acad Sci USA* 2002;99:13055–60
9. Ardelt PU, Wood, CG, Chen L, *et al.* Targeting urothelium: *ex-vivo* assay standardization and selection of internalizing ligands. *J Urol* 2002; in press
10. Ellerby M, Arap W, Andrusiak R, *et al.* Targeted proapoptotic peptides for cancer therapy. *Nat Med* 1999;9:1032–8
11. Curnis F, Sacchi A, Borgna L, *et al.* Enhancement of tumor necrosis factor α antitumor immunotherapeutic properties by targeted delivery to aminopeptidase. *Nat Biotechnol* 2000;18:1185–90
12. Koivunen E, Arap W, Valtanen H, *et al.* Tumor targeting with a selective gelatinase inhibitor. *Nat Biotechnol* 1999;8:768–74
13. Wickham TJ, Haskard D, Segal D, *et al.* Targeting endothelium for gene therapy via receptors up-regulated during angiogenesis and inflammation. *Cancer Immunol Immunother* 1997;45:149–51
14. Arap W, Kolonin MG, Trepel M, *et al.* Steps toward mapping human vasculature by *in vivo* phage display. *Nat Med* 2002;8:121–7
15. Pentz RD, Flamm AL, Pasqualini R, *et al.* Revisiting ethics guidelines for research in terminal wean and brain dead participants. *Hasting Center Rep* 2002;in press
16. Giordano R, Cardó-Vila M, Lahdenranta J, *et al.* Biopanning and rapid analysis of selective interactive ligands. *Nat Med* 2001;11:1249–53
17. Rugh R. *The Mouse: Its Reproduction and Development.* Oxford, England: Oxford Science Publications, 1990
18. Maranghi F, Macri C, Ricciardi C, *et al.* Evaluation of the placenta: suggestions for a greater role in developmental toxicology. *Adv Exp Med Biol* 1998;444:129–36

The immunotherapy of prostate cancer

22

A. G. Dalgleish

Introduction

The dawn of modern immunology probably started with William Coley, a New York surgeon at the turn of the 19th–20th century, who noticed that patients with residual postoperative disease who developed severe septicemia sometimes became disease-free and long-term survivors. He tried to mimic the immune response to the bacteria by making cell wall preparations, which became known as Coley's toxins. He reported a large number of long-term responses to this therapy, although the tumor types were limited to melanoma and a few others. Attempts by others to reproduce his work were often unsuccessful, and details of the approach were clearly critical. Further evidence that the immune response can contain cancer comes from the infrequent but persistent reports of spontaneous remissions, which are usually limited to melanoma and renal cell cancer. Complete remissions of superficial melanomas are common following intra-tumoral administration of bacille Calmette–Guerin (BCG), which has little effect on non-injected lesions, although BCG combined with cell lines would appear to be able to induce systemic responses as well as increasing long-term survival in stage IV melanoma[1].

A dramatic increase in virally driven cancers, such as lymphoma, Karposi's sarcoma and cervical cancer, in immune-deficient states is further evidence of the ability of the immune response (IR) to contain these cancers. This is entirely consistent with MacFarlane Burnett's immune surveillance theory.

Of great current interest is that the above remarks do not support a role for the IR in prostate cancer (nor other common solid tumors)! However, other evidence suggests a role for the IR.

It has been recognized for over two decades that patients with advanced prostate cancer have a reduced delayed T-cell hypersensitivity response[2]. More recently, a reduced cell-mediated response, as judged by reduced Th-1 (T helper-cell) cytokine production following whole-cell stimulation *in vivo*, has been noted by several groups. Our group became interested in the importance of this observation following the demonstration that non-specific stimulation with BCG or its close relative, *Mycobacterium vaccae*, could protect in animal models as well as induce a Th-1 response in patient volunteers[3].

Non-specific immune response and cytokine milieu

The reduced cell-mediated immune (CMI) response or Th-1 response seen in advanced prostate cancer is a feature of most chronic infections, such as human immunodeficiency virus (HIV) and tuberculosis (TB), as well as most human cancers. The reduced CMI or Th-1 response is probably due to the cancer secreting immunosuppressive cytokines, such as interleukin-10 (IL-10) and transforming growth factor-β (TGF-β), as it often reverses following total surgical resection. The most dramatic effect of this is in colorectal cancer, where small Duke's A cancers also lead to marked CMI and Th-1 suppression, a feature that is totally reversed following tumor removal[4].

The immune response appears to revolve around the delicate balance of the CMI/Th-1 system and the humoral or Th-2 system. Th-1 cytokines include IL-2, IL-12 and γ-interferon (γ-IFN), whereas Th-2 cytokines include IL-4, IL-6 and IL-10 (Figure 1). Chronic diseases appear to suppress the Th-1 response, which is probably vital for infectious agents to survive. Hence, enhancing the Th-1 response may be a crucial first step in inducing an effective IR. A small study in 1982 reported better survival in patients with prostate cancer who had BCG as well as standard therapy, compared with those who did not[5].

Prostate antigens

A major problem in developing cancer vaccines is that there is no specific tumor antigen to target. Prostate cancer has several specific antigens that may be targeted, as even if non-tumor cells are also killed the result would be no worse than with radiotherapy or surgery, and as such would be a medical prostatectomy. Such antigens include prostate-specific antigen (PSA), prostate-specific membrane antigen (PSMA) and prostatic acid phosphatase (PAP). In addition, prostate cancer expresses a number of tumor-associated antigens such as gangliosides and mucins.

Given the beneficial effect of inducing a Th-1 response in a few patients with *M. vaccae*, there is every reason to hope that the effect of adding a few relevant tumor antigens could be at least additive if not synergistic. There are a large number of approaches aimed at inducing an immune response, and they fall loosely into the following categories:

(1) Non-specific immune stimulants, e.g. BCG, *M. vaccae*; also includes granulocyte-macrophage colony-stimulating factor (GM-CSF) administration alone or with thalidomide;

(2) Autologous and allogeneic cells used as vaccines alone or transfected with GM-CSF and other cytokines;

(3) Cells may also provide lysates, which can be used to pulse dendritic cells (DCs), which can also be pulsed with peptides from PSMA, PAP, etc.;

(4) Direct viral delivery, using either suicide gene therapy, such as herpes simplex virus thymidine kinase (HSV-TK), or directly with oncolytic viruses. A large number of variations on this theme have been proposed, which have already entered the clinic.

Immunotherapy and prostate cancer: evidence so far

There is a trend for patients who improve their Th-1/Th-2 ratio with *M. vaccae*, BCG and allogeneic cells to survive longer than those who do not[6]. Lymph node cancer of the prostate (LNCaP) cells transfected with GM-CSF (cell genesis) also appear to have a beneficial effect on PSA as a surrogate marker, and in 56 patients followed to date, the survival time appears to be approximately twice that for similar non-treated patients[7]. This survival improvement has also been reported in an 80-patient trial using DCs pulsed with PAP (Dendreon™), which also reports a dose-dependent effect on PSA and survival response[7].

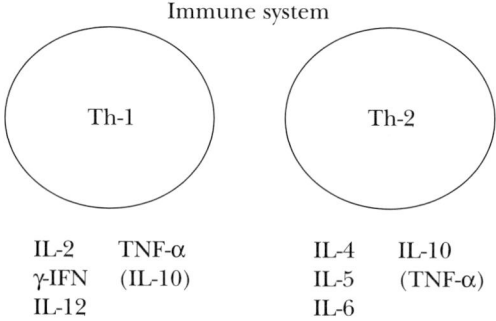

Immune system

Th-1

Th-2

IL-2	TNF-α	IL-4	IL-10
γ-IFN	(IL-10)	IL-5	(TNF-α)
IL-12		IL-6	

Figure 1 The immune system consists of cell-mediated (Th-1) and humoral-mediated (Th-2) systems, which are in balance in most healthy states. Chronic infections and cancer selectively suppress Th-1 and enhance Th-2 cytokines and functions. IL, interleukin; γ-IFN, γ-interferon; TNF-α, tumor necrosis factor-α

The Onyvax approach

Following the realization that prostate cancer may respond to immunotherapy, we have explored the possibility that prostate allogeneic cells offer an extra 'danger' signal to the immune system, which is associated with improved tumor-free and survival responses as compared with autologous vaccines. Using the Copenhagen and Lobund Wister rat models, we were impressed with a marked protective effect of allogeneic vaccination in these models[8].

Having had considerable experience using the Donald Morton triple whole-cell melanoma vaccine, which induces responses to a wide number of melanoma antigens, we raised a number of prostate cancer cell lines[1]. The Morton melanoma vaccine is associated with a significant improvement in 2–5-year survival for both stage III and stage IV disease in large phase II studies, and it was hoped that a similar approach would be effective in prostate cancer. Onyvax was formed to develop a prostate cancer vaccine based on non-specific immune stimulation in conjunction with allogeneic cell lines, and to gain expertise in cell line development and tumor immunology. A four-arm phase I study using different cell line combinations was completed in patients with advanced prostate cancer[9]. An optimum vaccine was selected for a CTX trial in hormonally resistant but low-volume metastatic disease, which has just recruited.

A considerable amount of basic research has been conducted to optimize this approach. The most important conclusion is that allogeneic cell lines are not significantly enhanced with regard to antigenicity or immunogenicity with gene transfer of a wide variety of cytokines including GM-CSF, unlike autologous cells[10]. Antigenicity and immunogenicity can be readily enhanced with specific and appropriate cell culture techniques and special adjuvant regimens.

New approaches: dendritic cells and gene therapy

The use of dendritic cells remains a popular technique to enhance antigen presenting. However, as it appears that successful cancer vaccination in advanced disease regimens, use of repeated vaccination and, hence, preparation of DCs pulsed with antigen are labor intensive, to make this approach practical it is necessary to freeze DC/vaccine preparations for future use/administration. We have recently developed a technique to freeze–thaw DC vaccines that have enhanced tumor antigen presentation. We have used this approach in patients with advanced prostate cancer with encouraging PSA responses. Several further trials are planned.

With regard to gene therapy approaches, we have explored HSV-TK transfer mechanisms and reported their beneficial effect on the immune system, having induced immune responses against non-transfected tumors in the rat prostate model[11]. We have now shown that similar approaches can be used *ex vivo* to enhance antigenicity and immunogenicity of whole-cell vaccines. (Greenhalgh and colleagues, unpublished data).

Future approaches

The success of monoclonal antibodies (MAbs) against breast cancer and lymphoma (herceptin and rituximab) strongly suggests that this approach could be applied to prostate cancer, which shares the herceptin target in some cases in addition to expressing some broad tumor-specific antigens, such as the ganglioside GM2, mucin-1 (MUC-1) and epidermal cellular adhesion molecule (EpCAM). MAbs could readily be combined with vaccine approaches, providing a mechanism to kill tumor bulk as well as induce immune surveillance. Vaccines may also synergize with other treatments, such as thalidomide, which in addition to being anti-angiogenic is also immunostimulatory. Some of the new analogs made by Celgene–Revemid and Actimed induce considerable synergy with vaccines in animal models, and will soon be tried in the clinic[12].

In a number of human cancers there is a trend that patients who respond to vaccination have a better quality of life and survival and toleration of chemotherapy and radiotherapy than non-vaccinated people. It will be important to translate lessons learned from successful prostate cancer vaccines into an overall management strategy. Prostate cancer leads itself to the consideration of sequential managed therapy (SMT), with different approaches being tried in a logical order following disease progression. Currently, most vaccine trials are in hormone-resistant patients. Logically, it would make most sense to use vaccines after radical treatments as adjuvant therapy, and to add other treatments only after evidence of progression.

Conclusion

There is now considerable evidence that prostate cancer will join the other urological malignancies to be deemed immunologically responsive (such as bladder cancer (local BCG) and renal cell carcinoma which responds to α-INF and IL-2). The potential for a sophisticated and effective approach is very real, given the breadth of technologies available to achieve this.

References

1. Morton DL, Foshag LJ, Hoon DS, *et al.* Prolongation of survival in metastatic melanoma after active specific immunotherapy with a new polyvalent melanoma vaccine. *Ann Surg* 1992;216:463–82

2. Schellhammer PF, Bracken RB, Bean MA, Pinsky CM, Whitmore WF Jr. Immune evaluation with skin testing. A study of testicular, prostatic, and bladder neoplasms. *Cancer* 1976;38:149–56

3. Hrouda D, Baban B, Dunsmuir WD, Kirby RS, Dalgleish AG. Immunotherapy of advanced prostate cancer: a phase I/II trial using *Mycobacterium vaccae* (SRL172). *Br J Urol* 1998;82:568–73

4. Heriot AG, Marriott JB, Cookson S, Kumar D, Dalgleish AG. Reduction in cytokine production in colorectal cancer patients: association with stage and reversal by resection. *Br J Cancer* 2000; 82:1009–12

5. Guinan PD, John T, Baumgartner G, *et al.* Adjuvant immunotherapy (BCG) in stage D prostate cancer. *Am J Clin Oncol* 1982;5:65–8

6. Maraveyas A, Baban B, Kennard D, *et al.* Possible improved survival of patients with stage IV AJCC melanoma receiving SRL172 immunotherapy: correlation with induction of increased levels of intracellular interleukin-2 in peripheral blood lymphocytes. *Ann Oncol* 1999;10:817–24

7. Press Release. Cell Gene system. Dendreon Corporation, Corporation Delaware, Mountain View, CA

8. Hrouda D, Todryk SM, Perry MJ, *et al.* Allogeneic whole-tumour cell vaccination in the rat model of prostate cancer. *BJU Int* 2000;86:742–8

9. Eaton JD, Perry MJ, Nicholson S, *et al.* Allogeneic whole-cell vaccine: a phase I/II study in men with hormone-refractory prostate cancer. *BJU Int* 2002;89:19–26

10. Todryk SM, Birchall LJ, Erlich R, Halanek N, Orleans-Lindsay JK, Dalgleish AG. Efficacy of cytokine gene transfection may differ for autologous and allogeneic tumour cell vaccines. *Immunology* 2001;102:190–8

11. Eaton JD, Perry MJ, Todryk SM, *et al.* Genetic prodrug activation therapy (GPAT) in two rat prostate models generates an immune bystander effect and can be monitored by magnetic resonance techniques. *Gene Ther* 2001;8:557–67

12. Dredge K, Marriott JB, Todryk SM, *et al.* Protective antitumor immunity induced by a costimulatory thalidomide analog in conjunction with whole tumor cell vaccination is mediated by increased Th1-type immunity. *J Immunol* 2002;168:4914–19

Prognostic tissue factors for prostate cancer: recent developments and pitfalls

23

M. A. Noordzij

Introduction

Prostate cancer has become the most prevalent malignant non-skin tumor in Western men during recent decades. Its mortality rate is only surpassed by that due to lung cancer[1]. This dramatic increase in incidence and prevalence is largely attributable to the introduction of prostate-specific antigen (PSA) testing, trans-rectal ultrasound (TRUS)-guided biopsy techniques and increased awareness of prostate cancer in the general population, notably in the USA, but also, albeit to a lesser extent, in other Western countries[2]. Data from the American National Cancer Database show that these developments have resulted in a decline in age at diagnosis of 2 years, combined with more favorable clinical parameters[3]. As a result, the number of newly diagnosed prostate cancer patients eligible for definite treatment has increased[3]. The incidence showed a peak in 1992, and has been declining since. Despite these developments, prostate cancer mortality rates have shown only small differences; in some countries a small decline has been seen, whereas in others it has increased[4,5].

Natural course of prostate cancer

It has been known for many years from autopsy studies, and studies of radical cystoprosta-tectomy specimens removed in bladder cancer, that the prevalence of latent prostate cancer increases dramatically with age to more than 50% in men over 80 years old. Sakr and colleagues[6] found foci of adenocarcinoma in 28% and 34% of men who died in their 30s and 40s, respectively. However, it has been estimated that no more than about one of four prostate cancers will become clinically apparent, and that about one of three men with clinical prostate cancer will eventually die from it[7]. On the one hand, it may therefore be argued that detection of clinically unapparent, slowly growing prostate cancers may lead to over-diagnosis and overtreatment, and may pose an avoidable psychological burden to the 'patient'[8]. On the other hand, prostate cancer kills patients, and is, in that respect, only second to lung cancer. Therefore, we have to answer a number of questions. Which tumor is *significant* and how can we identify such a tumor? Which patient should be treated and how should he be treated? The question of whether prostate cancer screening is benificial is clearly very important, but goes beyond the scope of this chapter.

The natural course of prostate cancer is highly variable and difficult to predict. Knowledge of the natural course, however, is essential if the above questions are to be answered. In a number of studies, Swedish inves-tigators have shown that long-term disease-specific survival can be expected in most conservatively managed patients (80% at a follow-up of 10–15 years)[9,10]. These studies have been criticized for a number of favorable selec-tion criteria applied to the study population. Chodak and colleagues[11] performed a meta-analysis of results from a total of 828 expectantly managed patients in six studies (including the Swedish ones). Tumor-specific survival for grade 1 and grade 2 tumors was identical to the life expectancy of the general population, but decreased significantly for grade 3 tumors. Metastasis-free survival at 10 years was about 70%, 55% and 20% for grade 1, 2 and 3 tumors, respectively. This meta-analysis was based on studies that all suffered from methodological problems, and it remains questionable whether definite conclusions can be drawn. However, these studies can provide some conclusions. First, the majority of prostate cancers have the potential to progress if left untreated, and may eventually lead to the death of the patient. Second, it usually takes years before prostate cancer leads to the death of the patient. It is clear that in elderly patients with small, well-differentiated tumors the likelihood of tumor progression is determined mainly by factors not related to the tumor itself (such as the presence of cardiovascular disease, diabetes mellitus or another malignancy). This discussion focuses only on tumor characteristics, however.

Prognostic factors

As described above, it is very important that relatively indolent tumors can be distinguished from potentially lethal tumors; therefore, prognostic factors are necessary. The term *prognosis* for patients with established prostate cancer can be defined as the prediction of future behavior of the tumor, either in the absence or after application of therapy. With the assessment of prognostic factors, attempts are being made to predict the clinical course of the disease in a specific patient. A *prognostic factor* can be defined as a qualitative or quantitative alteration or deviation from normal of a molecule, substance or process that can be detected by some kind of assay and that is correlated with prognosis[12]. The term response factor is used for a prognostic factor that predicts the response to a certain therapy. Ideally, knowledge of a prognostic factor should lead to clinical decisions that, in turn, should result in improved clinical outcome as defined by overall survival, quality of life or costs of care.

Prognostic factors in prostate cancer

In 1994, the College of American Pathologists organized a conference on the application of prognostic factors to common malignancies (breast, colon and prostate cancer). During this conference a hierarchic classification of prognostic factors was designed that made it easy to compare these factors[13]. Table 1 indicates this classification for prostate cancer factors as proposed by the prostate cancer working group during this conference. The conference was repeated in 1999 (although with some different members of the prostate cancer working group); Table 1 also gives the revised classification[14]. The American Joint Committee on Cancer also organized a consensus conference about prognostic factors in common malignancies (breast, colorectum, ovary and prostate)[15]. This conference was organized to discuss whether the TNM (tumor, nodes, metastasis) system for these tumors should be expanded to include non-anatomical factors (such as serum factors or molecular factors). The final conclusion was that, for all tumors, at present the TNM system should not be extended to include serum factors or other non-anatomical factors, although this may change in the near future for prostate cancer with serum PSA. Because serum PSA is not a tissue factor, it is not discussed here.

Table 1 indicates a number of striking observations:

(1) Two of the three factors from group I (i.e. the routinely used factors), pathological TNM (pTNM) stage and involvement of the surgical margins, can be established only following a radical prostatectomy. If the definitions are followed strictly, these factors are response factors for radical prostatectomy and not prognostic factors. Multiple studies have shown that pTNM stage and prostatectomy Gleason sum score have the strongest correlation with disease

Table 1   College of American Pathologists classification of prognostic prostate cancer factors

1994	1999
I Well supported by the literature; generally used in patient management	
(Pathological) TNM stage	pathological TNM stage
Histological grade	Gleason grade
Serum PSA	serum PSA
	surgical margins
II Extensively studied biologically and/or clinically	
DNA ploidy	DNA ploidy
Proliferation	histological tumor type
Nuclear morphometry	tumor volume (biopsy or radical prostatectomy)
Tumor angiogenesis	
Tissue PSA	
Apoptosis	
Tumor suppressor genes	
III Currently do not meet criteria for category I or category II	
HER-2/neu oncogene	perineural invasion
Proteases	lymph node micrometastasis
Cytogenetic analysis	neuroendocrine cells
Neuroendocrine cells	microvessel density
Growth factors	nuclear morphometry
Circulating tumor cells	other karyometric factors
	proliferation markers

TNM, tumor, nodes, metastasis; PSA, prostate-specific antigen

outcome. Also, many studies have shown that there is only a weak correlation between clinical TNM and pTNM stage, and only a modest correlation between biopsy Gleason sum score and prostatectomy Gleason sum score (although the correlation increases with increasing stage and/or grade). As a consequence, the relationship between clinical stage and grade and prognosis is also limited. This is even more so because a large percentage of currently detected prostate cancers are clinically at stage T1c.

What we need as clinicians are factors that can be established reliably prior to any therapy. For this reason, category I should contain *clinical* stage instead of *pathological* stage, and should not contain surgical margin status. Possibly, the classification reflects the fact that these conferences were organized by pathologists. Because the variables that are currently being used prior to therapy are only loosely correlated to prognosis (notably stage T1c), there is a great need for additional factors.

(2) Except for DNA ploidy, all tissue factors belonging to groups I and II are more or less standard pathological variables. The term 'standard pathological variable' in this respect does not mean that these variables are beyond discussion, as described above. It only implies that assessment of these variables is generally straightforward and can be performed without expensive or difficult techniques. For many tumor types, volume measurement is part of the TNM system. Owing to several factors this is more complicated for prostate cancer: prostate cancer is often difficult to recognize macroscopically using imaging techniques, it usually invades and grows in between benign glands and it is multifocal in about half of the cases. Nevertheless, prostate tumor volume can be predicted using some kind of measurement of involvement of the biopsy specimens, such as the number of biopsies with tumor or the total length of tumor in the biopsies, or some other method. Which method best predicts tumor volume is not discussed here. Some

studies have shown good correlation between biopsy-predicted tumor volume and prostatectomy tumor volume[16,17], whereas others have not[18]. Even in most of the studies that showed good correlation it was not possible to predict total tumor volume reliably for an individual patient.

The prognostic value of tumor type will probably be very limited, as by far the most common malignant tumor is adenocarcinoma, although it is of course very important that the presence of an uncommon tumor type is reported by the pathologist.

(3) All molecular and genetic factors that currently receive considerable attention in the literature are in group III.

(4) It appears that during the 5-year interval between the first and the second conference hardly any progress was made. During the above-mentioned 1999 College of American Pathologists conference it was found that the prognostic factor classification of breast and colon cancer had not changed significantly, either. Therefore, this conference focused more on the reasons why so little progress had been made and possibilities to overcome this. One of the main conclusions of the plenary session was: '. . . stagnation in the field of prognostic factors had occurred because the amount and quality of data concerning prognostic factors was so poor that no consensus of value could be achieved'[19]. To avoid the risk that the same cynical conclusion would be drawn during the 2004 conference, a number of recommendations were made, the most important of which are:

(a) New promising factors should be rapidly identified and tested;

(b) Much effort should be put into the standardization of patient populations, factor assays and data collection;

(c) Methods should be developed to aggregate data in large databases, once again emphasizing the need for standardization;

(d) New statistical techniques should be developed to allow especially for multifactor testing; probably, neural network techniques should be developed further;

(e) Co-ordinated collaboration will be necessary to plan activities based on prioritization of the most important issues.

It may appear that thinking about prognostic factors at a higher level is new, but this is certainly not the case. This topic has been receiving attention for more than a decade, notably in breast cancer research. In 1993 and 1995, Burke and co-workers[20,21] described criteria that outcome studies on prognostic factors should fulfil. In these articles, most of the criticism discussed during the 1999 College of American Pathologists conference was already mentioned. According to these criteria, which are still valid, articles should contain:

(1) A description of the sampling method;

(2) Inclusion and exclusion criteria;

(3) Characteristics of the subjects;

(4) Numbers of subjects and events;

(5) Duration of the follow-up period;

(6) A description of the assay;

(7) A description of the different types of variability of the assay, if applicable;

(8) Cut-off point criteria and whether the cut-off point was assessed before or during data analysis;

(9) Justification of the multivariate model that was used.

If these criteria are met, journal editors and reviewers should be able to judge the scientific quality of a submitted paper in this field.

The current prognostic system (TNM plus grade) is, on the one hand, easy to apply, widely used and well studied. On the other hand, because it is mutually exclusive and categorical, the system itself makes it very difficult to include new prognostic factors, for a number of reasons. The total number of possible categories increases exponentially with an increasing number of parameters: $T(0–4)N(0–2)M(0–1)$ gives $5 \times 3 \times 2 = 30$ categories (without subcategories) and even $10 \times 4 \times 3 = 120$ (with subcategories). If Gleason grading is incorporated, the number of categories becomes $30 \times 9 = 270$ or $120 \times 9 = 1080$, respectively (although many categories are very unlikely to appear). If stage grouping is used (I–IV), the number of categories is $4 \times 9 = 36$. The accuracy of the system is directly proportional to the number of patients per category; thus, with an increasing number of parameters, the accuracy may fall dramatically. In addition, the categories are ordered by worsening prognosis. The only way to include a new prognostic factor would be to study a large patient sample and to create a new classification based on all the factors tested. Finally, and probably most importantly, but somewhat difficult to understand, the system is static; when there is a change in the data underlying the system, the system itself has to be adapted[22]. For example, with the introduction of the reverse transcriptase-polymerase chain reaction (RT-PCR) technique to detect circulating PSA-expressing cells, it was thought that metastatic prostate cancer could be identified reliably[23]. If this had been true, patients that otherwise would have been classified as M0 would now have been at stage M1. This, in turn, would have changed the prognosis of *all* categories and would make a new classification necessary. This emphasizes the need for innovative statistical techniques and prognostic systems that, on the one hand, are easy to apply and appreciate, but, on the other hand, do not show the disadvantages of the current system.

Prognostic factor research in prostate cancer

A substantial part of prostate cancer research is dedicated to the identification of clinically applicable prognostic factors. If only prognostic tissue factors are considered, about 800 articles have been published since 1990. With increasing knowledge of the molecular biology of malignant tumors, more and more factors are being identified that may be related to the prognosis of a tumor. A malignant tumor is (almost by definition) genetically unstable, and, with the advance of the disease, increasing alterations and disturbances are to be expected in all kinds of cellular processes. It is therefore not surprising that many of those new 'factors' are related to stage and/or grade of the tumor, which does not imply that an independent prognostic value can be expected. Moreover, independent prognostic value does not necessarily imply clinical relevance.

As mentioned above, serum PSA is not discussed here, but it should be realized that it is a strong prognostic factor for prostate cancer outcome, which has implications for prognostic tissue factor research as well. First, studies of prognostic tissue factors should also include serum PSA (besides clinical stage and grade) as an outcome parameter. Second, because serum PSA is strongly related to prognosis, it will be 'difficult' for a new potential factor to have independent prognostic value.

Table 2 very briefly gives, in alphabetical order, almost all experimental prognostic factors that have been studied in prostate cancer. It shows whether a factor is related to grade and/or stage of the tumor and whether it has a prognostic value at the univariate or multivariate level. Only outcome studies are incorporated in the table. As can clearly be seen, many factors have a prognostic value if studied at the univariate level, which is subsequently lost if, in a multivariate model, grade and stage are considered as well. It goes far beyond the scope of this chapter to present all factors in full detail; the table is intended to give a quick overview of what has been studied in this field during the past 12 years. Several comprehensive reviews have been published[24–26]. In an increasing number of studies two or more factors are investigated simultaneously; in the table these data are split. Sometimes in these studies a combination of new factors gave better results, but these data are not given. It is also not indicated which factors were included in

Table 2 Overview of experimental prognostic tissue factors in prostate cancer (positive studies/total number of studies)

Factor	Type of study	Grade	Stage	u-var	m-var	Remarks
Argyrophilic nucleolar organizer regions (AgNOR)	prognostic			2/2	1/1	
	response HT			1/1		
α-Catenin	prognostic	3/4	2/2	3/5	1/3	
Androgen receptor	prognostic	0/2	0/2	0/1	0/2	
	response HT			5/8	4/6	
Apoptosis	prognostic	1/1		4/5	2/5	one study only Gleason sum 6 tumors, no multivariate analysis performed
β-Microseminoprotein	response HT			1/1	1/1	
Bcl-2	prognostic	1/2	1/3	6/10	4/12	in two studies, RP specimens had bcl-2 prognostic value, but biopsy specimens did not
	response HT			0/3	0/3	
	response RT			4/5	3/4	one study: better prognosis with higher bcl-2 expression (?)
Bone-sialoprotein	prognostic	1/1	1/1	2/2	0/1	
c-erbB-2	prognostic	4/5	3/4	5/5	3/5	
	response RT			1/1	1/1	
CD44	prognostic	6/6	5/6	6/6	3/5	
CD68 (tumor-associated macrophages)	prognostic	1/1	1/1	1/1	1/1	
Chondroitin sulfate	prognostic	1/1	1/1	2/2	2/2	
Chromosomal abnormalities						
7 (loss of 7q31)	prognostic			2/3	1/2	one case–control study
7 and/or 17 and/or X	prognostic			1/1	1/1	
8c, 8p (loss of 8p22)	prognostic			4/6	2/4	one study: only prognostic value if combined with c-myc
8, Y	prognostic				1/1	
13q	prognostic			0/1		
16q	prognostic			1/2	0/1	
c-myc	prognostic			1/1	1/1	see above, only if combined with 8p22 loss
Cyclin A	prognostic	1/1	1/1	1/2	0/2	
Cyclin D	prognostic	2/2	2/2	2/2	1/2	
E-cadherin	prognostic	8/8	8/8	3/6	2/3	
Epidermal growth factor receptor	prognostic	3/4	3/4	1/3	0/3	
Estrogen receptor (ER)	prognostic	2/2	1/2	2/3	2/2	expression of wild-type ERβ and ERβCX
	response HT			1/1		
Galectin-I	prognostic	1/1	1/1	1/1	1/1	expression in surrounding stroma, not in tumor cells

continued

Table 2 *Continued*

Factor	Type	Results (significant/total)	Comments
High-grade inflammation	prognostic	1/1 1/1 1/1	
HMSH2	prognostic	1/1 1/1 0/1 0/1	
Heat-shock protein 27	prognostic	0/1 0/1 0/1	
Inducible NO-synthetase	prognostic	1/1 1/2 1/2 0/1	
67-kDa Laminin receptor	prognostic	0/1 1/1 0/1 0/1	prognostic value only if assessed in RP specimens, not biopsy specimens
Minichromosome maintenance protein 2	prognostic	0/1 0/1 1/1 1/1	
Microvessel density	prognostic	10/13 10/13 9/13 11/16	good correlation between RP and biopsy values
	response RT	2/2 2/2	
Morphogenetic protein 6	prognostic	1/1 1/1 1/1	
Neuroendocrine differentiation	prognostic	4/8 3/5 4/13 2/12	
	response HT	1/2 1/1	
Nuclear morphometry (many different parameters)	prognostic	2/5 2/4	
	response HT	3/3 3/3 1/3	
	response RT	1/1 1/1 1/1	
p16	prognostic	2/2 2/2 3/3 2/2	
p21 (waf/cip-1)	prognostic	5/6 5/6 6/7 3/3	
	response HT	1/1 1/1 1/1	
	response RT	0/1 0/1 0/1	
p27kip1	prognostic	7/7 6/7 6/7 5/7	good correlation between RP and biopsy expression
p34cdc2	prognostic	1/1 1/1 2/2 2/2	
p53 (different techniques)	prognostic	8/15 6/14 14/21 9/24	in two studies: RP p53 prognostic value, biopsy p53 not, weak correlation between RP and biopsy expression
Perineural invasion	response HT	1/1 1/1 3/5 3/5	
	response RT	2/2 2/2 6/8 3/6	
Ploidy	prognostic	25/30 16/22 21/23 7/12	good correlation between RP and biopsy value
	response HT	7/7 7/7 5/9	
	response RT	1/2 1/3	
Proliferation (many different techniques)	prognostic	15/20 12/17 19/27 13/25	
	response RT	5/5 5/5 2/5	
Tissue PSA	prognostic	2/4 2/4 2/4	
	response HT	2/2 2/2 2/2	
PSA RT-PCR	prognostic	5/6 5/6 3/5	in one study: prognostic value of PSA RT-PCR in lymph nodes
Rb1	prognostic	0/1 0/1 0/3 2/4	
TGF-β1	prognostic	2/2 2/2 2/2 2/2	
TGF-β1 receptor I	prognostic	1/1 1/1 2/2	
Vascular endothelial growth factor	prognostic	2/2 2/2 2/2 1/1	

u-var, univariate analysis; m-var, multivariate analysis; HT, hormonal therapy; RP, radical prostatectomy; RT, radiotherapy; PSA, prostate-specific antigen; RT-PCR, reverse transcriptase-polymerase chain reaction; TGF, transforming growth factor multivariate analyses. In most studies only grade and stage were considered, but sometimes serum PSA or other experimental markers were included as well.

Thus, on the one hand, over 800 articles have been published about more than 40 different prognostic tissue factors. On the other hand, as discussed above, the clinically applied tissue factors have not changed significantly during recent decades. Therefore, the question arises whether there are any real recent developments at all to discuss, as the title of this chapter suggests. In the opinion of the author, however, certain improvements have been made:

(1) Basic prostate cancer research and basic oncological research identify many potential prognostic factors. These factors are rapidly being studied for their prognostic significance.

(2) In the majority of studies, the experimental prognostic factor is now compared with the standard factors as described above, and in most cases an appropriate multivariate analysis is performed. However, articles are still being published with inappropriate statistics. If the criteria of Burke and co-workers as described above are checked during the review process, this should not happen.

(3) More and more prognostic factors are now being studied using biopsy specimens after a prognostic value has been found in radical prostatectomy specimens. As Table 2 indicates, a number of prognostic factors 'lose' their prognostic value if biopsy specimens are used. For other factors, good correlation between biopsy and radical prostatectomy assessments has been described, however. The drawbacks described above for determination of total tumor volume using biopsy specimens most probably also hold true for other prognostic tissue factors. This implies that much effort has to be put into the improvement of biopsy techniques. In the future, this may very well prove to be the largest

obstacle in the routine application of new tissue factors to prostate cancer. But, if biopsy techniques can indeed be improved, this also will enhance the prognostic value of the 'standard factors'.

(4) An increasing number of studies are being performed to identify tissue response factors that may predict the response to radiation therapy or hormonal therapy (see also Table 2).

(5) An increasing number of studies investigate several tissue factors together. These studies are hampered, however, by the fact that, as yet, statistical techniques have to be developed to appreciate these data fully. Cox's proportional hazards model is currently most widely used to analyze these data[27]. Although this is a strong statistical technique, for a number of reasons which are not discussed here, it cannot be used to answer all relevant questions. Possibly, neural network-based techniques will be able to overcome the problems associated with classical statistical techniques. Several studies have shown that this method indeed may be superior to Cox's model. It is a complex technique, however, and the underlying (hidden) model is difficult to interpret.

Future directions of prognostic factor research in prostate cancer

It is not the intention of the author to indicate which potential prognostic factors are promising and which are not; any factor that might have additional value should be studied in a co-ordinated fashion. The general recommendations that were made during the 1999 College of American Pathologists conference are not repeated here. A number of other issues should receive attention as well:

(1) As indicated above, biopsy techniques must improve, to account for the inherent heterogeneity and multifocality of prostate cancer.

(2) Consensus should be reached about how prostate tumor volume should be assessed in biopsy specimens.

(3) It is essential that basic scientists, pathologists and urologists work closely together in this field. Statisticians should be involved as well, although this is not specifically in relation to prostate cancer. Besides this, it is important that meetings on prognostic factors in cancer in general are organized not only to solve the problems and avoid the pitfalls that are specific for a certain malignancy, but also to enhance the cross-talk between scientists working on different malignancies.

(4) The possibilities for using new and innovative techniques such as cDNA chips, protein chips and tissue arrays should be explored. These techniques may be used to test a large number of potential factors from a large number of patient samples in a high-throughput fashion, but may also be used to identify new prognostic factors. Some recent studies have indeed shown that these techniques may be of value in prostate cancer[28–30].

It is recommended that studies of prognostic tissue factors be performed according to the following scheme (some steps may be performed together):

(1) Identification of a potential factor;

(2) Development, testing and standardization of the assay;

(3) Application of the factor to easily accessible and well-defined samples (e.g. radical prostatectomy specimens) to study the distribution in benign, premalignant and malignant tissues, to study tissue heterogeneity and to study the relationship with tumor stage and grade;

(4) Assessment of the prognostic value in radical prostatectomy specimens, assessment of the cut-off point;

(5) If a prognostic value is found, assessment of the prognostic value with biopsy samples using clinical stage, grade and preoperative PSA; investigation of whether the factor can be used as a response marker for radiation or hormonal therapy, or to select patients who can be offered watchful waiting;

(6) If the prognostic value is confirmed by several well-performed studies, performance of prospective multicenter studies using a consensus technique and cut-off value;

(7) Performance of clinical trials in which the patients are grouped according to the new marker.

In conclusion, although a substantial part of prostate cancer research is dedicated to the identification of valuable prognostic factors, this has not led to an improved prognostic system as yet. This is partially due to several methodological problems, but the heterogeneous nature of prostate cancer and the fact that the biological behavior of a malignant tumor is very difficult to predict/assess also play a very important role. It cannot be predicted whether a better prognostic system will be available in the very near future if the recommendations are followed, but the best opportunities will be provided to reach this goal in an efficient manner.

References

1. Greenlee RT, Hill-Harmon MB, Murray T, *et al.* Cancer statistics, 2001. *CA Cancer J Clin* 2001; 51:15–36
2. Potosky AL, Miller BA, Albertsen PC, *et al.* The role of increasing detection in the rising incidence of prostate cancer. *J Am Med Assoc* 1995;273:548–52
3. Mettlinn CJ, Murphy GP, Rosenthal DS, *et al.* The National Cancer Database report on prostate carcinoma after the peak in incidence rates in the US. The American College of Surgeons Commission on Cancer and the American Cancer Society. *Cancer* 1998;83:1679–84
4. Merill RM, Stephenson RA. Trends in mortality rates in patients with prostate cancer during the era of prostate specific antigen screening. *J Urol* 2000;163:503–10
5. Oliver SE, May MT, Gunnel D. International trends in prostate-cancer mortality in the 'PSA era'. *Int J Cancer* 2001;92:893–8
6. Sakr WA, Haas GP, Cassin BF, *et al.* The frequency of carcinoma and intraepithelial neoplasia of the prostate in young male patients. *J Urol* 1993; 150:379–85
7. Coffey DS. Prostate cancer – an overview of an increasing dilemma. *Cancer* 1993;71(Suppl): 880–6
8. Adami HO, Baron JA, Rothman KJ. Ethics of a prostate cancer screening trial [Review]. *Lancet* 1994;343:958–60
9. Johansson JE, Adami HO, Andersson SO, *et al.* Natural history of localised prostatic cancer: a population-based study in 223 untreated patients. *Lancet* 1989;1:799–803
10. Johansson JE, Holmberg L, Johansson S, *et al.* Fifteen years survival in prostate cancer. A prospective, population-based study in Sweden. *J Am Med Assoc* 1997;277:467–71
11. Chodak GW, Thisted RA, Gerber GS, *et al.* Results of conservative management of clinically localized prostate cancer. *N Engl J Med* 1994;330: 242–8
12. Hayes DF, Bast RC, Desch CE *et al.* Tumor marker grading system: a framework to evaluate clinical utility of tumor markers. *J Natl Cancer Inst* 1996;88:1456–68
13. Grignon DJ, Hammond H. College of American Pathologists conference XXVI on clinical relevance of prognostic markers in solid tumors. Report of the prostate cancer working group. *Arch Pathol Lab Med* 1995;119:1122–6
14. Bostwick DG, Grignon DJ, Hammond EH, *et al.* Prognostic factors in prostate cancer: College of American Pathologists consensus statement 1999. *Arch Pathol Lab Med* 2000;124:995–1000
15. Yarbro JW, Page DL, Fielding LP, *et al.* American Joint Committee on Cancer prognostic factors consensus conference. *Cancer* 1999;86:2436–45
16. Peller PA, Young DC, Marmaduke DP, *et al.* Sextant prostate biopsies. A histopathologic correlation with radical prostatectomy specimens. *Cancer* 1995;75:530–8
17. Haggman M, De la Torre M, Brandstedt S, *et al.* Pre- and postoperative DNA ploidy patterns correlated to pT-stage, histological grade and tumor volume in total prostatectomy specimens. *Scand J Urol Nephrol* 1994;28:59–66
18. Cupp MR, Bostwick DG, Myers RP, *et al.* The volume of prostate cancer in the biopsy specimen cannot reliably predict the quantity of cancer in the radical prostatectomy specimen on an individual basis. *J Urol* 1995;153:1543–8
19. Hammond EH, Fitzgibbons PL, Compton CC, *et al.* College of American Pathologists conference XXXV: solid tumor prognostic factors – which, how and so what? *Arch Pathol Lab Med* 2000;124:958–65
20. Burke HB, Henson DE. Criteria for prognostic factors and for an enhanced prognostic system. *Cancer* 1993;72:3131–5
21. Burke HB, Hutter RVP, Henson DE. Breast carcinoma. In Hermanek P, Gospodarowicz MK, Henson DE, *et al.*, eds. *Prognostic Factors in Cancer.* Berlin: Springer, 1995:165–76
22. Black WC, Welch HG. Advances in diagnostic imaging and overestimations of disease prevalence and the benefits of therapy. *N Engl J Med* 1993;328:1237–43
23. Katz AE, Olsson CA, Raffo AJ, *et al.* Molecular staging of prostate cancer with the use of an enhanced reverse transcriptase-PCR assay. *Urology* 1994;43:765–75
24. Putzi MJ, De Marzo AM. Prostate pathology: histologic and molecular perspectives. *Hematol Oncol Clin North Am* 2001;15:407–21
25. Veltri RW, O'Dowd GJ, Orozco R, *et al.* The role of biopsy pathology, quantitative nuclear morphometry, and biomarkers in the preoperative prediction of prostate cancer staging and prognosis. *Semin Urol Oncol* 1998;16:106–17
26. Verhagen PCMS, Tilanus MGJ, de Weger RA, *et al.* Prognostic factors in localised prostate cancer with emphasis on the application of molecular techniques. *Eur Urol* 2002;41:363–71
27. Cox DR. Regression models and life-tables. *J R Stat Soc* 1972;34:187–220

28. Skacel M, Ormsby AH, Pettay JD, *et al.* Aneusomy of chromosomes 7, 8, and 17 and amplification of HER-2/neu and epidermal growth factor receptor in Gleason score 7 prostate carcinoma: a differential fluorescent *in situ* hybridization study of Gleason pattern 3 and 4 using tissue microarray. *Hum Pathol* 2001;32:1392–7

29. Dhanasekaran SM, Barrette TR, Ghosh D, *et al.* Delineation of prognostic biomarkers in prostate cancer. *Nature (London)* 2001;412:822–6

30. Bubendorf L, Kolmer M, Kononen J, *et al.* Hormone therapy failure in human prostate cancer: analysis by complementary DNA and tissue microarrays. *J Natl Cancer Inst* 1999;91: 1758–64

Diagnostic markers for prostate cancer detected in serum, plasma or blood: prostate-specific antigen forms and human kallikrein 2 for early detection and staging

A. Haese, H. Huland and H. Lilja

Prostate-specific antigen and adenocarcinoma of the prostate

Increased use of prostate-specific antigen (PSA) for early detection of prostate cancer has resulted in a continuous increase in the incidence of localized disease over more than a decade, while that of locally extensive or metastatic disease has steadily declined[1]. PSA has had such an impact on prostate cancer detection that the concern has arisen that its use may detect and cause treatment of clinically insignificant tumors. More recently, a decrease in prostate cancer incidence has been observed, and today the incidence is only minimally higher than in the era before PSA testing was available[2]. An effective screening method will increase the detection of a certain disease; however, the incidence should decrease over time, if significant disease is detected through that screening method. If, however, the incidence does not decline, the concern is that insignificant disease may be being detected.

Owing to extensive PSA testing, today the majority of newly diagnosed prostate cancers are detected only because of an elevated PSA level (T1c cancers)[3,4]. These cancers have a far better prognosis after treatment as compared with those detected on digital rectal examination. Thus, PSA has already improved early detection of prostate cancer considerably. Still, since only about 60% of all T1c prostate cancers are pathologically organ-confined[5,6], there is a need for improvement in the early detection of clinically significant prostate cancer.

PSA occurs in a variety of forms in human plasma. In this chapter, we describe the clinically relevant forms of PSA for early detection, staging and surgical management of prostate cancer.

Total PSA in the early detection of prostate cancer

Background

Diagnosis of prostate cancer requires microscopic evaluation of a specimen of the prostate, obtained by biopsy, preferably under ultrasound guidance. The likelihood of prostate cancer increases with increasing serum PSA concentrations, but is also related to the presence or absence of a palpable lesion. From retrospective studies, it has been estimated that an elevated PSA concentration due to prostate cancer occurs a mean 6.2 years before a palpable lesion can be identified[7].

A common concern of PSA use in the early detection of prostate cancer is the assumption that cancers which could be clinically insignificant may be diagnosed and subsequently treated. First descriptions[8] of clinically insignificant cancers assessed the volume of tumors found in prostates of patients who underwent cystoprostatectomy for bladder cancer and assigned them a volume of < 0.5 cm³. Other, more recent definitions take into account not only the volume but also the differentiation of the cancer[9]. Insignificant cancers detected on autopsy are in more than 90% of cases of low volume (e.g. less than 0.5 cm³) and of low grade (Gleason sum score less than 4)[10]. Comparing these results with the pathological features of prostate cancers detected through screening and removed surgically, less than 10% of these cancers show the criteria of insignificance[11,12]. Therefore, at present, there is only limited evidence that PSA leads to treatment of insignificant prostate cancer.

Despite its above-mentioned advantages for early detection of prostate cancer, PSA is still not a perfect tumor marker. The three most common disorders of the prostate – prostate cancer, benign prostatic hyperplasia and prostatitis – can increase serum PSA concentrations. Other factors (physical activity, ejaculation[13], cystoscopy, prostate biopsy[14]) can increase serum PSA too. The 5α-reductase inhibitor finasteride, used for treatment of symptomatic bladder outlet obstruction due to benign prostatic hyperplasia, on the other hand decreases serum PSA by approximately 50%, while maintaining the ratio of free/total PSA unchanged[15].

PSA in the early detection of prostate cancer using PSA ranges

Total PSA below 4 ng/ml Analysis of prostate cancer incidence in the range below 4 ng/ml and non-suspicious finding on digital rectal examination (DRE) has shown that up to 22% of men with total PSA in the range 2.6–4 ng/ml harbor significant disease. Moreover, the cancers removed – while still being clinically significant – were pathologically organ-confined in 81%[16]. Results from the European Randomized Study of Screening for Prostate Cancer (ERSPC) for patients with the same characteristics demonstrated a detection rate of 19% of prostate cancers when total PSA was 2.0–3.9 ng/ml[17]. Here 84% of all cancers were confined to the prostate, as opposed to 62% when total PSA was 4–10 ng/ml. Lodding and

colleagues found an increased detection of prostate cancer by 30%, with the majority of the cancers detected being clinically significant after radical prostatectomy[18].

Total PSA in the range 4–10 ng/ml The PSA range between 4 and 10 ng/ml is commonly referred to as the diagnostic gray zone, where PSA determination does not give valuable information as to the presence or absence of cancer. Analysis of screening studies of men 50 years or older shows that up to 10% of these men have a PSA of 4 ng/ml or higher. Biopsy results showed a positive predictive value between 12 and 32%[19–22] in the case of a non-suspicious DRE. A biopsy, associated with costs and some degree of morbidity, would reveal no evidence of malignancy in about three out of four men biopsied because of a PSA level from 4 to 10 ng/ml.

Total PSA above 10 ng/ml Patients with a total PSA above 10 ng/ml and a non-suspicious DRE have a likelihood of more than 40% of harboring prostate cancer[12]. It is therefore accepted that a biopsy should be undertaken owing to the high likelihood of detection of cancer. It is noteworthy, however, that the likelihood of pathologically organ-confined cancer may be as low as 25%.

Free PSA in the early detection of prostate cancer

A very large proportion of PSA in the extracellular fluids (e.g. blood) is found in stable complex with antiproteases, most notably α₁-antichymotrypsin (ACT). However, there are also significant concentrations of free, noncomplexed forms of PSA in the blood circulation, which are essentially unreactive with the very large excess of extracellular antiproteases[23]. The most valuable application of free PSA measurement is identification of the unique free PSA-specific antigenic epitope structures, unavailable when PSA forms stable covalent complexes with antiproteases such as ACT[23–25], which are the molecular basis for generation of the ratio free/total PSA (%fPSA)[26]. For reasons yet poorly understood, a higher %fPSA occurs in patients without, than in those with, prostate cancer[26]. This is consistent with the finding that the proportion of complexed PSA is higher in patients with prostate cancer than in those without[26,27]. By measuring both free and total PSA, the calculated %fPSA improves the armamentarium of prostate cancer detection[26]. Numerous studies have been published evaluating sensitivity and specificity of %fPSA for prostate cancer detection. These studies demonstrated that, using %fPSA cut-offs between 14 and 28%, between 19 and 64% of unnecessary biopsies could have been avoided while maintaining a sensitivity of prostate cancer detection of 71–100%[28–30]. A large, prospective, multicenter trial was able to confirm retrospective studies. In these studies, a cut-off value for %fPSA below 25% detected 95% of cancers and reduced the biopsy rate by 20% in the total PSA range of 4–10 ng/ml[31]. The range of total PSA at which %fPSA should be determined, approved for clinical use, is 4–10 ng/ml. However, an estimated 20% of men with total PSA in the 2.6–4-ng/ml range also harbor significant prostate cancer. Evaluation of %fPSA in this group demonstrated that a cut-off for %fPSA of 27% was able to detect 90% of cancers. Some 18% of unnecessary biopsies could have been avoided in these patients, thus encouraging the use of %fPSA in this total PSA range as well[16].

Moreover, percentage free PSA has been shown to be useful in identifying those patients who will develop highly aggressive cancer in the future. Measurement of free and total PSA was performed up to 10 years before diagnosis of prostate cancer with extraprostatic extension, lymph node or bone metastases, and compared with those in a group of patients who had prostate cancer with a more favorable pathology. These researchers demonstrated a statistically significant difference in %fPSA between disease entities ($p = 0.008$) 10 years prior to diagnosis. Total PSA failed to demonstrate this difference[32].

Several aspects must be kept in mind when using %fPSA in a clinical situation[33]. First, as with total PSA, results of free PSA detection vary owing to a lack of uniform standardization of the assay. Results for free PSA and subsequently calculated %fPSA may be different. In addition, assays for the detection of total and free PSA can be divided into two groups based on their relative ability to detect both PSA forms. Equimolar PSA assays detect free PSA and ACT–PSA equally, and the results are largely independent of the relative amounts of free PSA and ACT–PSA in serum. Skewed response assays measure preferably the free PSA. Thus, when the proportion of free PSA increases, a higher amount of total PSA is the result. The higher amount of total PSA is the denominator in the calculation of %fPSA; therefore, the free PSA appears to be lower, which in turn changes the %fPSA ratio to a lower level, falsely suggesting prostate cancer. Hence, the use of a standard assay calibrator, preferably an equimolar assay for total PSA and free PSA detection and %fPSA calculation is of utmost importance.

Prostatic manipulation increases total PSA concentrations owing to an increase in free PSA. Analysis of the subfractions of total PSA in a preoperative versus intraoperative comparison of radical prostatectomy patients demonstrated that virtually all increase in total PSA level during surgery is due to the release of free PSA. %fPSA increased from a mean 11.9% preoperatively to 52.5% as a consequence of prostatic manipulation[34]. The same has been observed for DRE, prostate biopsy and urethral instrumentation, which should consequently be avoided at least 48–72 h before free PSA and %fPSA calculation.

Moreover, prostatic volume also affects %fPSA in patients with prostate cancer[35]. In smaller prostates, there was a statistically significant difference in the %fPSA ratio when patients with benign disease and prostate cancer patients were compared. However, with increasing total prostate volume, differences in %fPSA between patients with cancer and those without cancer diminished, and at large volumes %fPSA concentrations may be indistinguishable. A similar result was found when prostates < 35 cm^3 and ≥ 35 cm^3 were compared: a cut-off of 14%

for small prostates and a cut-off of 25%fPSA for larger prostates detected prostate cancer with 95% sensitivity[36].

A reference value for %fPSA cannot be precisely recommended, since it is affected by multiple factors. Commonly, a range between 14 and 25% is applied[26,29–31]. However, narrowing this range to an optimal, widely accepted cut-off value has not been possible to date. It is therefore the decision of the individual physician and patient to be either more aggressive to detect the cancer and consequently perform more unnecessary biopsies (e.g. trend to higher sensitivity), or more restrictive and perform fewer biopsies revealing benign results while risking overlooking patients with prostate cancer.

It can be concluded that %fPSA improves specificity while maintaining a high sensitivity for prostate cancer in men with a total PSA of 2.6–10 ng/ml.

Complex PSA in the early detection of prostate cancer

As described above, PSA is able to form stable covalent complexes with several of the major extracellular antiproteases such as ACT[24], α_2-macroglobulin[24], protein C inhibitor[37] and, to a much lesser extent and very slowly, α_1-protease inhibitor (API–PSA) in blood[38]. The sum of ACT–PSA, API–PSA (which corresponds to only 0.5–2% of total PSA) and other currently unknown PSA complexes are termed complex PSA or cPSA. This is the major form of PSA, which is also most strongly influenced by prostate cancer, as first reported from two simultaneous and independently performed studies in Sweden and Finland[26,27]. Much later, commercially available immunoassays were developed that render it possible to measure cPSA without any significant non-specific interference from other protease–ACT complexes (e.g. granulocyte-derived cathepsin G), which limit the accuracy of the specific PSA–ACT assays[39,40].

As outlined, total PSA cannot reliably separate benign from malignant disease in the

PSA range below 10 ng/ml. Percentage free PSA may be more exposed to day-to-day variation considering its considerably shorter elimination rate from *in vivo*, i.e. reported half-life of 12–18 h[34], compared with the PSA–ACT complex[41], as well as significant *in vitro* instability[42,43]. By contrast, cPSA levels are less affected than the levels of free PSA by severe renal impairment, DRE, cystoscopy, prostate biopsy or manipulation of the prostate during surgery, compared with free PSA[41].

Several studies have been able to show that detection of cPSA in total PSA ranges of 2.5–4 ng/ml[44], 2.6–20 ng/ml[45], 0.37–117 ng/ml[46] and 4.1–10 ng/ml[47] demonstrated cPSA specificities better than those seen for total PSA. At sensitivity levels of 92–95% (accepting oversight of only 5–8% of cancers), the specificity for cPSA ranged between 23 and 42%, while at the same sensitivity, the specificty for total PSA was 14–18%. Another aspect is that cPSA values can be obtained by two methods. It can be measured by immunoassay: the results of the above studies were all obtained in this way. An alternative is the generation of calculated complex PSA levels. These can be obtained by subtracting free PSA from total PSA. Okihara and colleagues[44] evaluated these calculated cPSA results in the total PSA range 2.5–4 ng/ml, and concluded that results were comparable to measured cPSA values with respect to sensitivity/specificity. This study also confirmed the improved cancer detection rate in the narrowly low PSA range 2.5–4 ng/ml achieved by cPSA, in comparison with %fPSA.

It may be concluded that the reported data suggest that measurement of cPSA in serum is a reliable tool which contributes a statistically significant improved specificity at high sensitivity levels in men with suspected prostate cancer, compared with conventional testing for total PSA. In the total PSA range between 4 and 10 ng/ml, percentage free PSA contributes statistically significant enhancement to the diagnostic efficacy of cPSA. cPSA can be calculated from pre-existing free and total PSA assays, without any major drawback in comparison with other means of performing cPSA measurements.

Subfractions of free PSA in the early detection of prostate cancer

Subfractions of free PSA are modifications of the free, uncomplexed PSA molecule. Several types of modifications have been distinguished:

(1) Internally cleaved, nicked or multichain PSA forms have been described, most notably an isoform showing cleavages at Lys145–Lys146 and Lys182–Ser183 positions (BPSA).

(2) Pro-PSA is enzymatically inactive and consists of 237 amino acids plus a seven-amino acid polypeptide that is cleaved to activate pro-PSA into its active form. Variations in the numbers of amino acids that are clipped to activate pro-PSA occur, leading to variable sizes of the molecule (e.g. (−2) pPSA).

(3) Intact PSA is a non-reactive single-chain isoform of free PSA isolated from lymph node cancer of the prostate (LnCaP) cells.

The nature of these isoforms of free PSA, and whether they will improve prostate cancer detection, are reviewed below.

The typical feature of BPSA is a double peptide cleavage at Lys145–Lys146 and Lys182–Ser183; hence, it is a multichain peptide of free PSA. BPSA has been described in seminal plasma and nodular tissue samples of the transition zone of benign prostatic hyperplasia (BPH)[48]. A comparison of tissue from enlarged prostates due to BPH, normal prostates and prostate cancer showed that BPSA was exclusively expressed in the transition zone. The expression of BPSA in normal prostates and in prostate cancer tissue was much less intense. The development of an immunoassay for the detection of BPSA in serum revealed a significant concentration of BPSA in the serum of men with BPH, whereas it was undetectable in normal control males. An estimated 15–50% of all free PSA in serum was shown to be BPSA[49]. While it seems likely that BPSA reflects, at least to some extent, BPH, and has potential for monitoring BPH under surgical or medical treatment, its role in the early diagnosis of prostate cancer remains to be clarified. This is because prostate cancer and BPH are commonly found in the same organ.

(−2)pPSA was found as a variant of free PSA expressed in large amounts in prostate cancer tissue[50]. It is a single-chain polypeptide characterized by incomplete cleavage of the seven amino acids that are normally removed to activate pro-PSA. Two amino acid residues remain in place, giving it a total size of 239 amino acids, and hence its designation as (−2)pPSA. Again, it was first described in prostate cancer tissue. When serum of prostate cancer (total PSA 6–24 ng/ml) was analyzed for (−2)pPSA, it could be shown that 25–95% of free PSA consisted of (−2)pPSA. Serum levels of men with no evidence of disease read an average of five-fold lower (−2)pPSA concentrations. An important aspect of (−2)pPSA is that it is detectable at total PSA concentrations typically encountered when the differential diagnosis of BPH versus prostate cancer is made. It is premature to speculate on the impact of (−2)pPSA on early detection of prostate cancer.

A subgroup of free PSA, a cancer-specific form called intact PSA isolated from LnCaP cells, was evaluated for distinguishing benign from malignant prostatic tumors[51]. As opposed to multichain PSA, intact PSA is a single-chain polypeptide. A research assay for this PSA isoform was developed, and analysis of 383 men (141 with no evidence of disease and 242 patients scheduled for radical prostatectomy for prostate cancer) was performed. Determination of intact PSA and its application as the ratio of intact/free PSA improved the distinction of patients with a negative systematic prostate biopsy from those with biopsy-proven prostate cancer[52].

In summary, subfractions of free PSA to date present encouraging results; however, further evaluation is mandatory, not only with reference to refinements in detection techniques, but also, the exact number and nature of subfractions of free PSA must be determined.

PSA derivates in the detection of prostate cancer

PSA derivates are permutations of total serum PSA used in an attempt to improve sensitivity and specificity of prostate cancer detection. These permutations are PSA density, PSA velocity and age-specific PSA ranges. Their meaning in the early detection of prostate cancer is described in the following.

PSA density

The concept of PSA density was first described by Benson and colleagues[53]. The rationale of PSA density is the observation of a positive relationship between serum PSA and prostatic volume. The background is that the majority of prostatic enlargement is due to benign hyperplastic tissue of the transition zone. Normalization by prostate volume might enhance cancer specificity. PSA density determination divides the serum PSA level by prostatic volume. It was created to normalize a certain PSA for the volume of a particular prostate, assuming that a certain volume of prostate cancer would increase PSA to a greater extent than the same volume of BPH. However, two aspects limit the use of PSA density. First, it relies on the examiner to estimate the prostatic volume correctly. Second, the ratio of stroma to epithelium varies considerably between individuals. Since only the epithelium produces PSA and the stroma cannot be estimated from transrectal ultrasound, this influences PSA density to an unforeseeable extent[54,55]. Therefore, results of PSA density have been discordant. A cut-off of $0.15 \, \text{ng/ml/cm}^3$ for PSA density has been reported, and it was found that PSA density enhanced prostate cancer detection when PSA was below 10 ng/ml[56]. Other studies, however, found that about 50% of all prostate cancers would have been missed, when a cut-off of $0.15 \, \text{ng/ml/cm}^3$ was used[57]. Others could not find any statistically significant difference between 107 men with positive or negative biopsy result when PSA density was employed[58]. Therefore, at present, the role of PSA density in the early detection of prostate cancer has not

been proved to be useful when PSA is 4–10 ng/ml and DRE is unremarkable.

A modification of PSA density, transition zone density (PSA-TZD) is the normalization of PSA level to the transition zone volume[59]. It focuses on the assumption that, histologically, hyperplasia occurs almost exclusively in the transition zone. PSA from the peripheral zone and central zone is assigned to be a constant and less substantial source of PSA in the absence of cancer. In an initial study with a cut-off of $0.35 \, \text{ng/ml/cm}^3$, the highest positive predictive value for prostate cancer detection was found using PSA-TZD (74%)[60]. However, methodological problems of volume measurement and epithelial/stromal ratio affect PSA-TZD in the same way as for simple PSA density. Since other centers have failed to reproduce the advantage of PSA-TZD, to date it cannot be considered a routine tool for prostate cancer detection.

PSA velocity

PSA velocity describes changes in PSA concentration over time. It was introduced to enhance the ability of the isolated PSA measurement to improve prostate cancer detection[61]. PSA velocity uses the formula $1/2 \times (\text{PSA2} - \text{PSA1}/\text{time1}$ in years $+ \text{PSA3} - \text{PSA2}/\text{time2}$ in years). PSA1 is the first PSA measurement, PSA2 the second and PSA3 the third serum PSA measurement. These three measurements should be obtained in a 2-year period or at least 12–18 months apart. Clinically, a PSA velocity of $\geq 0.75 \, \mu\text{g/ml/year}$ has been described to suggest the presence of prostate cancer, with 72% sensitivity and 95% specificity. These significant differences in PSA velocity between BPH and prostate cancer were detectable up to 9 years before prostate cancer was diagnosed.

Disadvantages of PSA velocity are attributable to the fact that PSA is not cancer-specific, that an intraindividual day-to-day variation of PSA concentration can be observed. A study showed that when an increase in total PSA was less than 20–46%, it was more likely to be attributable to biological and assay variation than to prostate cancer development[62]. Moreover, short event-related episodes of PSA rise (e.g. associated with inflammatory processes) may interfere with the normal natural elevation of PSA over time[63,64]. Finally, it is known that PSA results are different when measured on different PSA assays and add some degree of imprecision to PSA velocity determinations[33]. Despite these limitations, a PSA velocity greater than 0.75 ng/ml/year may still be of guidance in assessing the need for a prostate biopsy in patients with a total PSA below 10 ng/ml and unremarkable DRE, when following the guidelines of PSA velocity determination.

Age-specific PSA ranges

As outlined above, the upper limit of normal PSA concentration commonly assigned is 4 ng/ml. This, however, does not compensate for increasing prostate volume with increasing age. Hence, the principle of age-specific PSA ranges has been introduced[65] to improve sensitivity of prostate cancer detection in patients of younger age (e.g. age 50) with a PSA that might be of no concern in a patient at the age of 70, and vice versa, hence improving specificity by avoiding detection of insignificant cancers in the elderly. Several studies have evaluated age-specific PSA ranges. In the evaluation of almost 4600 men, age-specific PSA ranges detected 74 additional cancers in men 60 years or younger. Pathological work-up was favorable (Gleason score below 7, organ-confined or capsular penetration, no lymph node metastases and seminal vesicle invasion) in 80% of cancers. In younger men the detection of prostate cancer increased by 18%, but decreased by 22% in older men[66]. The comparison of age-specific PSA ranges with the normal PSA cut-off of 4 ng/ml in a screening population showed that the number of cancers detected increased by 8% using age-specific ranges in men below 59 years when DRE was unremarkable. Moreover, in men older than 60 years, 21% of biopsies could have been spared while missing only 4% of organ-confined cancers. It was concluded that age-specific PSA ranges improved sensitivity in the younger population[67]. Other studies, however, concluded that the standard PSA cut-off of 4 ng/ml was optimal for all age

groups[19] and, in addition, was the most cost-effective tool[68].

Race-corrected age-specific PSA ranges take into account reports that describe higher PSA in black as compared with white or Asian men, even when controlled for age, Gleason grade or clinical stage, which has been associated with a larger tumor volume in black compared with white men (1.3–2.5 times larger). It was reported that 40% of cancers in a black population would have been missed if traditional age-specific ranges had been used[65,69,70].

Human glandular kallikrein in the early detection of prostate cancer

Human glandular kallikrein (hK2) and PSA (which is systematically termed human glandular kallikrein 3) share an extensive 80% identity in protein sequence[71]. Both hK2 and PSA are expressed under androgen control[72]. Despite similarities in organ specificity, some differences between these proteins can be observed. Some immunohistochemical studies have suggested different tissue expression of hK2 compared with that of PSA[73,74], whereas such data have not been confirmed by others[75]. In body fluids, hK2 levels correspond to only ≈ 1% of those of PSA[76], and therefore it is crucial that assays for immunodetection of hK2 contribute reproducible data at very low limits of detection (e.g. < 20% coefficient of variation at hK2 levels ≤ 8–10 pg/ml), and manifest insignificant cross-reactivity with different forms of PSA (e.g. < 0.05–0.1% cross-reaction with PSA)[77]. The covariance of hK2 and total PSA concentrations is frequently less than 60%, which suggests that hK2 might provide additional, independent information compared with PSA[76–79]. This difference implicates hK2 as a potential tumor marker for prostate cancer.

Serum concentrations of hK2, free hK2 and ACT–hK2 have shown to be elevated in patients with prostate cancer[79–83]. However, after measurement of total and free PSA, the gain in clinical information is moderate for hk2, since PSA provides similar information[84]. Nevertheless, two scenarios for early diagnosis of prostate cancer exist.

First is an increase of specificity in the total PSA range between 4 and 10 ng/ml where only 25% of men harbor prostate cancer and biopsy should be recommended. The specificity for cancer of the ratio free/total PSA is about 31%. Hence, unnecessary biopsies are performed in about 70% of patients, a procedure that is costly and is associated with some morbidity[28].

Second is an increase in sensitivity. Of interest is the patient group with PSA levels below 4 ng/ml. In this PSA range, up to 25% of men harbor clinically significant prostate cancer[16] which PSA fails to detect.

Saedi and colleagues[82] described an increased concentration of pro-hK2 in sera of patients with prostate cancer, compared with BPH patients, female sera and healthy controls. Several other studies reported total hK2 concentrations using different research assays. In 937 archived serum samples of men with histologically confirmed prostate cancer or negative biopsy and a total PSA of 2–10 ng/ml, hK2, total PSA and free PSA were measured[80]. The ratio of total hK2/fPSA gave additional specificity in prostate cancer detection: in the PSA range of 4–10 ng/ml the risk of cancer was 23%, and in the PSA range of 2–4 ng/ml it was 13%. A classification into three risk groups was made using %fPSA (cut-off 25%), resulting in a likelihood of cancer of between 10 and 43%. A further subclassification was made using hK2/fPSA. By this means, the crude risk groups defined by %fPSA could be refined, yielding positive predictive values for cancer of between 9 and 62%. Cumulatively, if %fPSA and hK2/fPSA were used, 40% of cancers could have been detected, requiring a biopsy in only 16.5% of men in the PSA range 2–4 ng/ml. Magklara and colleagues[85] analyzed hk2 and total and free PSA, and merged hk2 and free PSA into the same algorithm, hK2/fPSA. On receiver operating characteristic (ROC) analysis, hK2/fPSA (area under the curve (AUC) 0.69) was a stronger predictor of cancer than %fPSA (AUC 0.64). Moreover, at 95% specificity, hK2/fPSA identified 30% and 25% of cancers when PSA was 2.5–10 ng/ml and 2.5–4 ng/ml, respectively. The above authors found the use of hK2 valuable for identifying a subset of patients with low PSA but still high likelihood of cancer.

Kwiatkowski and associates[86] calculated a median hK2/fPSA of 0.139 in prostate cancer patients versus 0.075 in BPH patients. At a sensitivity of almost 95%, the specificity of hK2/fPSA was 60.4% compared with 27.6% for %fPSA.

Becker and co-workers[87] evaluated hK2 concentrations in a population-based study of 604 men with total PSA > 3 ng/ml to evaluate discriminative power of additional hK2 measurement in prostate cancer detection. They merged hK2 and total and free PSA into an algorithm (hK2 × tPSA/fPSA). ROC analysis revealed that the AUC for hK2 × tPSA/fPSA was greater than that for total PSA and %fPSA. Moreover, at a specificity of 90%, sensitivity was 55%, compared with 41% for %fPSA

A cross-sectional study of 324 men performed by Nam and colleagues[83] referred for prostate biopsy revealed significantly higher hK2 and hK2/fPSA levels in men with cancer, compared with patients with a negative biopsy. The authors found a 5–8-fold increased risk of prostate cancer with elevated hK2 levels and elevated ratio of hK2/fPSA, hence improving selection criteria for patients referred for prostate biopsy.

Studies performed so far show a moderate clinical potential for hK2, but should not for the time being replace total and free PSA detection for early diagnosis of prostate cancer.

The most efficient way to use hK2 (alone or in combination with total and/or free PSA) still remains to be clarified. All restrictions of immunodetection in the case of free PSA (different types of immunoassays, no standardization) also need to be considered when hK2 is studied.

Staging of prostate cancer

Correct staging in men with prostate cancer is crucial, not only to select the appropriate therapy in clinically localized prostate cancer but also for comparison of outcome of different treatment approaches. While surgical procedures offer the possibility of evaluating a histological specimen and, as such, give exact information on the stage of tumor, other therapies, e.g. radiation, do not offer such a possibility, and hence rely to a much larger extent on accurate clinical staging of the disease. This is necessary not only to compare results of radiation therapy from different centers, but also to compare radiation therapy with radical prostatectomy. The TNM (tumor, nodes, metastasis) classification describes local, lymphatic and distal extension of prostate cancer. However, serious limitations of transrectal ultrasound and DRE significantly compromise the precision to which patients harboring prostate cancer can be staged. Cancers confined to the prostate have far better prognosis than those showing extraprostatic extension[88,89]. However, since extraprostatic extension may be detectable only on microscopic evaluation, it is logical that clinical assessment fails to detect this crucial step in cancer spread.

Total PSA in the staging of prostate cancer

PSA and local staging

With the introduction of PSA into clinical use, PSA has outperformed DRE-based stage prediction, which showed unsuspected extraprostatic spread in up to 63%[90]. The application of PSA in the staging of prostate cancer has demonstrated that serum PSA levels in a group of patients correlate with tumor volume and advancing clinical and pathological stage[54,91]. When PSA ranges and staging results are analyzed, it can be shown that PSA in ranges below 4 ng/ml and above 10 ng/ml correlates reasonably well with organ-confined or extraprostatic cancer. Namely, when PSA was below 4 ng/ml, the likelihood of an organ-confined cancer was shown to be 81–84%[16,17], when DRE was negative. Organ-confined rates dropped to 53–67% in the total PSA range 4–10 ng/ml[92] and to 31–55.9% when PSA was between 10 and 20 ng/ml[18,93]. Hence, in the most frequently encountered PSA range of 4–10 ng/ml, PSA does not provide valuable staging information. Therefore, on an individual basis, single PSA levels are not specific enough to permit pre-

diction of pathological stage. This has led to the development of multiparameter staging tools (nomograms and predictive algorithms) to improve the accuracy of staging. These are described elsewhere in this book.

PSA and distant staging

PSA has been shown to be a good predictor of a positive bone scan in patients with prostate cancer. The correlation of PSA, prostatic acid phosphatase (PAP), tumor grade and clinical stage revealed that PSA was most accurate in predicting bone scan results. Namely, if PSA was below 20 ng/ml, the negative predictive value was 99.7%. This resulted in a decrease in the number of bone scans performed in patients with a PSA < 20 ng/ml[94]. However, some urologists still perform these as part of their preoperative work-up.

Ratio of free/total PSA for staging of prostate cancer

In contrast to its wide acceptance for the detection of prostate cancer, comparisons of studies that have analyzed the ratio of free/total PSA (%fPSA) in the staging of prostate cancer have produced conflicting results, with the main parameter of outcome being whether or not the tumor was organ-confined. While some studies reported %fPSA to provide useful staging information, others failed to demonstrate such findings. Lerner and colleagues found statistically significant differences only in substages of prostate cancer[95], which is supported by data from the University of Hamburg where no difference between organ- and non-organ-confined cancers was seen; however, a significantly lower %fPSA distinguished prostate cancers that already had seminal vesicle invasion from those that did not[96]. It is important to stress that patient selection, study design, and the various immunoassays and %fPSA cut-off values used influence the conclusions of each study. Owing to methodological differences among these studies, a definitive answer can only be provided by a multicenter trial. Therefore, to date, no established use of %fPSA for the staging of prostate cancer exists.

ACT–PSA complex for staging of prostate cancer

While ACT–PSA studies evaluating early detection of prostate cancer are numerous, only a limited number of studies have evaluated ACT–PSA as a staging parameter for prostate cancer. Recently, PSA, PSA density, ACT–PSA and ACT–PSA density were assessed in 62 patients with clinically localized prostate cancer before radical prostatectomy. It was found that values for all variables increased significantly from organ-confined cancers to extraprostatic cancers and in each pathological stage, and, hence, ACT–PSA and ACT–PSA density only complemented PSA and PSA density. Calculation of ROC curves showed that both ACT and ACT–PSA density had a larger, but not significantly larger, AUC, compared with PSA and PSA density. However, at a sensitivity of 100% to detect prostate cancer, specificity was 37% and 42% for ACT–PSA and ACT–PSA density, compared with 19% and 24% for PSA and PSA density[97]. This is in agreement with an earlier study looking at 652 patients, which concluded that ACT–PSA might replace PSA as a staging tool for prostate cancer[98]. However, owing to the limited amount of data available, no conclusions as to the utility of ACT–PSA for staging purposes of prostate cancer can be drawn.

PSA in the staging of prostate cancer: algorithms and nomograms

The above-outlined weaknesses of PSA use have led to the construction of nomograms, which combine a number of clinically available variables that provide independently prognostic significance (e.g. clinical stage, PSA, Gleason sum or grade of prostatic biopsies), to provide a more accurate preoperative estimation of pathological stage. PSA is an important contributing factor in predictive nomograms for lymphatic spread, pathological stage or outcome of clinically localized prostate cancer. A widely accepted tool for predicting pathological stage is the Partin nomogram, which takes into account PSA, clinical stage and the Gleason sum score of the biopsy obtained. The Partin nomogram has been recently updated and validated[6]. Another algorithm was developed and validated by Graefen and colleagues, based on a CART analysis (classification and regression tree). This model performed a side-specific prediction of pathologically organ-confined prostate cancer based on serum PSA and Gleason grade 4/5 in prostatic biopsies[99].

Human glandular kallikrein 2 in the staging of prostate cancer

Human glandular kallikrein 2 has been studied in the early detection of prostate cancer and proven to have potential to complement the information of PSA and %fPSA, but at present not to replace either of them in terms of diagnostic accuracy. More recently, studies evaluated the use of hK2 as a staging parameter for clinically localized prostate cancer. Detection of hK2 and total and free PSA in 68 sera from men scheduled for radical retropubic prostatectomy revealed that hK2 and a derived algorithm that combined hK2 with total PSA and free PSA (hK2 × tPSA/fPSA) significantly improved the prediction of organ-confined versus non-organ-confined prostate cancer, in a total PSA range up to 66 ng/ml[100].

With increased sample size, the same group analyzed the PSA range below 10 ng/ml in 161 patients, and found results consistent with earlier observations, in that hK2 or the derived algorithm was significantly better in the prediction of pathological stage 2a/b prostate cancer than PSA[101].

Another study confirmed the improvement in staging accuracy described above. The authors found hK2 to be the only single serum analyte that highly significantly discriminated pT2a/b from ≥ pT3a prostate cancers (extraprostatic extension). Moreover, hK2 distinguished aggressive grade 3 prostate cancers from less aggressive grades 1 and 2 prostate cancers[102].

These results encourage further studies to improve prostate cancer staging. As with the use of %fPSA for detection of prostate cancer (lack of standardization, research assays, different assay principles), potential uncertainties must be kept in mind when hK2 is analyzed. Therefore, results from different centers, and the performance of different assays, ideally as a multicenter trial, must be awaited before the role of hK2 as a potential staging tool for prostate cancer can be clarified.

PSA and radical prostatectomy

PSA has been proven to be the most powerful tool to identify those men in whom aggressive local therapy offers the best disease control[12]. It has been reported that PSA levels can stratify men in whom radical prostatectomy may result in high cure rates[6,12,99].

Following radical prostatectomy, PSA displays a truly unique feature: once the prostate is removed, the contributing factors mentioned above are excluded, and hence PSA, if detectable, is derived from remaining prostate cancer cells.

Failure to reach undetectable PSA levels is evidence for persisting prostate cancer. An undetectable PSA after radical prostatectomy is synonymous with being disease-free. In the case of recurrent disease, PSA can be detected more than 5 years earlier than any clinical symptom, and, as such, is by far the most sensitive marker for prostate cancer relapse. Recurrence of prostate cancer typically occurs first as a PSA recurrence, which means that PSA levels are rising from an undetectable level to levels accessible to conventional or ultrasensitive PSA assays[103–105]. In the absence of clinical signs of recurrence (palpable lesion on DRE, histological evidence of prostate cancer cells when a biopsy is taken from the former prostate location, positive bone scan, etc.), this is called biochemical recurrence. It has been shown that DRE or imaging studies in the case of a biochemical failure provide little additional information as to the type of recurrence (local recurrence or distal metastatic disease). Biochemical recurrences are due to PSA elevation from a negative postoperative baseline PSA. The 'ultrasensitive' PSA assays with detection limits < 0.01 ng/ml PSA provide an additional lead time of almost 2 years[104,105].

References

1. Mettlin CJ, Murphy GP, Ho R, *et al.* The National Cancer Data Base report on longitudinal observations on prostate cancer. *Cancer* 1996;77:2162–6
2. Wingo PA, Landis S, Ries LA. An adjustment to the 1997 estimate for new prostate cancer cases. *Cancer* 1997;80:1810–13
3. Ito K, Kubota Y, Suzuki K, *et al.* Correlation of prostate-specific antigen before prostate cancer detection and clinicopathologic features: evaluation of mass screening populations. *Urology* 2000;55:705–9
4. Plawker MW, Fleisher JM, Vapnek EM, *et al.* Current trends in prostate cancer diagnosis and staging among United States urologists. *J Urol* 1997;158:1853–8
5. Partin AW, Kattan MW, Subong EN, *et al.* Combination of prostate-specific antigen, clinical stage, and Gleason score to predict pathological stage of localized prostate cancer. A multi-institutional update. *J Am Med Assoc* 1997;277:1445–51
6. Partin AW, Mangold LA, Lamm D, *et al.* Contemporary update of prostate cancer staging nomograms (Partin Tables) for the new millenium. *Urology* 2001;58:843–8
7. Gann PH, Hennekens CH, Stampfer MJ. A prospective evaluation of plasma prostate-specific antigen for detection of prostatic cancer. *J Am Med Assoc* 1995;273:289–94
8. Stamey TA, Freiha FS, McNeal JE, *et al.* Localized prostate cancer. Relationship of

tumor volume to clinical significance for treatment of prostate cancer. *Cancer* 1993;71:933–8

9. Epstein JI, Chan DW, Sokoll LJ, *et al.* Nonpalpable stage T1c prostate cancer: prediction of insignificant disease using free/total prostate specific antigen levels and needle biopsy findings. *J Urol* 1998;160:2407–11

10. Belville WD. Are T1c tumors different from incidental tumors found at autopsy? The risk and reality of overdetection. *Semin Urol Oncol* 1995;13:181–6

11. Mettlin C, Murphy GP, Lee F, *et al.* Characteristics of prostate cancer detected in the American Cancer Society–National Prostate Cancer Detection Project. *J Urol* 1994;152:1737–40

12. Catalona WJ, Smith DS, Ratliff TL, *et al.* Detection of organ-confined prostate cancer is increased through prostate-specific antigen-based screening. *J Am Med Assoc* 1993;270:948–54

13. Herschman JD, Smith DS, Catalona WJ. Effect of ejaculation on serum total and free prostate-specific antigen concentrations. *Urology* 1997;50:239–43

14. Oesterling JE, Rice DC, Glenski WJ, *et al.* Effect of cystoscopy, prostate biopsy, and transurethral resection of prostate on serum prostate-specific antigen concentration. *Urology* 1993;42:276–82

15. Pannek J, Marks LS, Pearson JD, *et al.* Influence of finasteride on free and total serum prostate specific antigen levels in men with benign prostatic hyperplasia. *J Urol* 1998;159:449–53

16. Catalona WJ, Smith DS, Ornstein DK. Prostate cancer detection in men with serum PSA concentrations of 2.6 to 4.0 ng/ml and benign prostate examination. Enhancement of specificity with free PSA measurements. *J Am Med Assoc* 1997;277:1452–5

17. Schroder FH, van der Cruijsen-Koeter I, de Koning HJ, *et al.* Prostate cancer detection at low prostate specific antigen. *J Urol* 2000;163:806–12

18. Lodding P, Aus G, Bergdahl S, *et al.* Characteristics of screening detected prostate cancer in men 50 to 66 years old with 3 to 4 ng/ml prostate specific antigen. *J Urol* 1998;159:899–903

19. Catalona WJ, Richie JP, Ahmann FR, *et al.* Comparison of digital rectal examination and serum prostate specific antigen in the early detection of prostate cancer: results of a multicenter clinical trial of 6630 men. *J Urol* 1994;151:1283–90

20. Cooner WH, Mosley BR, Rutherford CL Jr, *et al.* Prostate cancer detection in a clinical urological practice by ultrasonography, digital rectal examination and prostate specific antigen. *J Urol* 1990;143:1146–52

21. Hammerer P, Huland H. Systematic sextant biopsies in 651 patients referred for prostate evaluation. *J Urol* 1994;151:99–102

22. Ellis WJ, Chetner MP, Preston SD, *et al.* Diagnosis of prostatic carcinoma: the yield of serum prostate specific antigen, digital rectal examination and transrectal ultrasonography. *J Urol* 1994;152:1520–5

23. Lilja H, Christensson A, Dahlen U, *et al.* Prostate-specific antigen in serum occurs predominantly in complex with α_1-antichymotrypsin. *Clin Chem* 1991;37:1618–22

24. Christensson A, Laurell CB, Lilja H. Enzymatic activity of prostate-specific antigen and its reactions with extracellular serine proteinase inhibitors. *Eur J Biochem* 1990;194:755–63

25. Piironen T, Villoutreix BO, Becker C, *et al.* Determination and analysis of antigenic epitopes of prostate specific antigen (PSA) and human glandular kallikrein 2 (hK2) using synthetic peptides and computer modeling. *Protein Sci* 1998;7:259–69

26. Christensson A, Bjork T, Nilsson O, *et al.* Serum prostate specific antigen complexed to α_1-antichymotrypsin as an indicator of prostate cancer. *J Urol* 1993;150:100–5

27. Stenman UH, Leinonen J, Alfthan H, *et al.* A complex between prostate-specific antigen and α_1-antichymotrypsin is the major form of prostate-specific antigen in serum of patients with prostatic cancer: assay of the complex improves clinical sensitivity for cancer. *Cancer Res* 1991;51:222–6

28. Luderer AA, Chen YT, Soriano TF, *et al.* Measurement of the proportion of free to total prostate-specific antigen improves diagnostic performance of prostate-specific antigen in the diagnostic gray zone of total prostate-specific antigen. *Urology* 1995;46:187–94

29. Prestigiacomo AF, Lilja H, Pettersson K, *et al.* A comparison of the free fraction of serum prostate specific antigen in men with benign and cancerous prostates: the best case scenario. *J Urol* 1996;156:350–4

30. Bjork T, Piironen T, Pettersson K, *et al.* Comparison of analysis of the different prostate-specific antigen forms in serum for detection of clinically localized prostate cancer. *Urology* 1996;48:882–8

31. Catalona WJ, Partin AW, Slawin KM, *et al.* Use of the percentage of free prostate-specific antigen to enhance differentiation of prostate cancer from benign prostatic disease: a prospective multicenter clinical trial. *J Am Med Assoc* 1998;279:1542–7

32. Carter HB, Partin AW, Luderer AA, *et al.* Percentage of free prostate-specific antigen in

sera predicts aggressiveness of prostate cancer a decade before diagnosis. *Urology* 1997;49: 379–84

33. Semjonow A, De Angelis G, Schmidt HP. Variability of immunoassays for PSA. In Brawer MK, ed. *Prostate-Specific Antigen*. New York: Dekker, 2001;1:217–21

34. Lilja H, Haese A, Bjork T, *et al.* Significance and metabolism of complexed and noncomplexed prostate specific antigen forms, and human glandular kallikrein 2 in clinically localized prostate cancer before and after radical prostatectomy. *J Urol* 1999;162:2029–34

35. Haese A, Graefen M, Noldus J, *et al.* Prostatic volume and ratio of free-to-total prostate specific antigen in patients with prostatic cancer or benign prostatic hyperplasia. *J Urol* 1997;158:2188–92

36. Partin AW, Catalona WJ, Southwick PC, *et al.* Analysis of percent free prostate-specific antigen (PSA) for prostate cancer detection: influence of total PSA, prostate volume, and age. *Urology* 1996;48:55–61

37. Christensson A, Lilja H. Complex formation between protein C inhibitor and prostate-specific antigen *in vitro* and in human semen. *Eur J Biochem* 1994;220:45–53

38. Leinonen J, Zhang WM, Paus E, *et al.* Reactivity of 77 antibodies to prostate-specific antigen with isoenzymes and complexes of prostate-specific antigen. *Tumour Biol* 1999;20(Suppl 1): 28–31

39. Pettersson K, Piironen T, Seppala M, *et al.* Free and complexed prostate-specific antigen (PSA): *in vitro* stability, epitope map, and development of immunofluorometric assays for specific and sensitive detection of free PSA and PSA–α_1-antichymotrypsin complex. *Clin Chem* 1995;41:1480–8

40. Allard WJ, Zhou Z, Yeung KK. Novel immunoassay for the measurement of complexed prostate-specific antigen in serum. *Clin Chem* 1998;44:1216–21

41. Bjork T, Ljungberg B, Piironen T, *et al.* Rapid exponential elimination of free prostate-specific antigen contrasts the slow, capacity-limited elimination of PSA complexed to α_1-antichymotrypsin from serum. *Urology* 1998; 51:57–61

42. Piironen T, Pettersson K, Suonpaa M, *et al. In vitro* stability of free prostate-specific antigen (PSA) and prostate-specific antigen (PSA) complexed to α_1-antichymotrypsin in blood samples. *Urology* 1996;48:81–7

43. Woodrum D, French C, Shamel LB. Stability of free prostate-specific antigen in serum samples under a variety of sample collection and sample storage conditions. *Urology* 1996;48:33–9

44. Okihara K, Fritsche H, Ayala A, *et al.* Can complexed prostate-specific antigen enhance prostate cancer detection in men with total prostate specific antigen between 2.4 and 4 ng/ml. *J Urol* 2001;165:1930–6

45. Mitchell IDC, Croal BL, Dickie A, *et al.* A prospective study to evaluate the role of complexed prostate-specific antigen and free/total prostate-specific antigen ratio for the diagnosis of prostate cancer. *J Urol* 2001;165: 1549–53

46. Brawer MK, Cheli CD, Neaman IE, *et al.* Complexed prostate specific antigen provides significant enhancement of specificity compared with total prostate specific antigen for detecting prostate cancer. *J Urol* 2000;163: 1476–80

47. Okegawa T, Noda H, Nutahara K, *et al.* Comparison of two investigative assays for the complexed prostate-specific antigen in total prostate-specific antigen between 4.1 and 10 ng/ml. *Urology* 2000;55:700–4

48. Mikolajczyk SD, Millar LS, Wang TJ, *et al.* 'BPSA', a specific molecular form of free prostate-specific antigen is found predominantly in the transition zone of patients with nodular benign prostatic hyperplasia. *Urology* 2000;55:41–5

49. Mikolajczyk SD, Rittenhouse HG. BPSA and pPSA are complementary forms of PSA that are found, respectively, in the serum of men with benign and malignant prostate disease. *J Clin Lig Assay* 2002;in press

50. Mikolajczyk SD, Millar LS, Wang TJ, *et al.* A precursor form of prostate-specific antigen is more highly elevated in prostate cancer compared with benign transition zone prostate tissue. *Cancer Res* 2000;60:756–9

51. Nurmikko P, Vaisanen V, Piironen T, *et al.* Production and characterisation of novel anti-prostate-specific antigen (PSA) monoclonal antibodies that do not detect internally cleaved Lys145–Lys146 inactive PSA. *Clin Chem* 2000; 46:1610–18

52. Steuber T, Haese A, Becker C, *et al.* Determination of a cancer-specific form of free PSA – intact PSA – discriminates by statistical significance patients with a negative systematic prostate biopsy from those with biopsy proven prostate cancer. *J Urol* 2001;165(Suppl):1162A

53. Benson MC, Whang IS, Olsson CA, *et al.* The use of prostate specific antigen density to enhance the predictive value of intermediate levels of serum prostate specific antigen. *J Urol* 1992;147: 817–21

54. Partin AW, Carter HB, Chan DW, *et al.* Prostate specific antigen in the staging of localized prostate cancer: influence of tumor differentiation,

tumor volume and benign hyperplasia. *J Urol* 1990;143:747–52

55. Stamey TA, Kabalin JN, McNeal JE, *et al.* Prostate specific antigen in the diagnosis and treatment of adenocarcinoma of the prostate. II. Radical prostatectomy treated patients. *J Urol* 1989;141:1076–83

56. Seaman E, Whang IS, Olsson CA, *et al.* PSA-density (PSAD). Role in patient evaluation and management. *Urol Clin North Am* 1993; 20:635–42

57. Catalona WJ, Richie JP, de Kernion JB, *et al.* Comparison of prostate-specific antigen concentration versus prostate-specific antigen density in the early detection of prostate cancer: receiver operator characteristic curves. *J Urol* 1994;152:2031–6

58. Brawer MK, Aramburu EAG, Chen GL, *et al.* The inability of prostate-specific antigen index to enhance the predictive value of prostate specific antigen in the diagnosis of prostatic carcinoma. *J Urol* 1993;150:369–73

59. Djavan B, Zlotta AR, Byttebier G, *et al.* Prostate specific antigen density of the transition zone for early detection of prostate cancer. *J Urol* 1998;160:411–18

60. Djavan B, Marberger M, Zlotta AR, *et al.* PSA, f/tPSA, PSAD, PSA-TZ and PAS-velocity for prostate cancer prediction: a multivariate analysis. *J Urol* 1998;159:898(A)

61. Carter HB, Pearson JD. PSA velocity for the diagnosis of early prostate cancer. A new concept. *Urol Clin North Am* 1993;20:665–70

62. Nixon RG, Wener MH, Smith KM. Biological variation of prostate specific antigen levels in serum: an evaluation of day-to-day physiological fluctuations in a well-defined cohort of 24 patients. *J Urol* 1997;157:2183–90

63. Nadler RB, Humphrey PA, Smith DS, *et al.* Effect of inflammation and benign prostatic hyperplasia on elevated serum prostate specific antigen levels. *J Urol* 1995;154:407–13

64. Hoekx L, Jeuris W, Van Marck E, *et al.* Elevated serum prostate specific antigen (PSA) related to asymptomatic prostatic inflammation. *Acta Urol Belg* 1998;66:1–2

65. Oesterling JE. Age-specific reference ranges for serum PSA. *N Engl J Med* 1996;335:345–51

66. Partin AW, Criley SR, Subong EN, *et al.* Standard versus age-specific prostate-specific antigen reference ranges among men with clinically localized prostate cancer: a pathological analysis. *J Urol* 1996;155:1336–41

67. Reissigl A, Pointner J, Horniger W, *et al.* Comparison of different prostate-specific antigen cutpoints for early detection of prostate cancer: results of a large screening study. *Urology* 1995;46:662–7

68. Littrup PJ, Kane RA, Mettlin C, *et al.* Cost-effective prostate cancer detection. Reduction of low-yield biopsies. *Cancer* 1994;74:3146–50

69. Morgan TO, Jacobsen SJ, McCarthy WF, *et al.* Age-specific reference ranges for prostate-specific antigen in black men. *N Engl J Med* 1996;335:304–9

70. Oesterling JE, Kumamoto Y, Tsukamoto T, *et al.* Serum prostate-specific antigen in a community based population of healthy Japanese men: lower values than for similarly aged white men. *Br J Urol* 1995;75:347–51

71. Schedlich LJ, Bennetts BH, Morris BJ. Primary structure of a human glandular kallikrein gene. *DNA* 1987;6:429–37

72. Young CY, Andrews PE, Montgomery BT, *et al.* Tissue-specific and hormonal regulation of human prostate-specific glandular kallikrein. *Biochemistry* 1992;31:818–24

73. Darson MF, Pacelli A, Roche P, *et al.* Human glandular kallikrein 2 (hK2) expression in prostatic intraepithelial neoplasia and adeno-carcinoma: a novel prostate cancer marker. *Urology* 1997;49:857–62

74. Darson MF, Pacelli A, Roche P, *et al.* Human glandular kallikrein 2 expression in prostate adenocarcinoma and lymph node metastases. *Urology* 1999;53:939–44

75. Siivola P, Pettersson K, Piironen T, *et al.* Time-resolved fluorescence imaging for specific and quantitative immunodetection of human kallikrein 2 and prostate-specific antigen in prostatic tissue sections. *Urology* 2000;56:682–8

76. Piironen T, Lovgren J, Karp M, *et al.* Immuno-fluorometric assay for sensitive and specific measurement of human prostatic glandular kallikrein (hK2) in serum. *Clin Chem* 1996;42:1034–41

77. Becker C, Piironen T, Kiviniemi J, *et al.* Sensitive and specific immunodetection of human glandular kallikrein 2 in serum. *Clin Chem* 2000;46:198–206

78. Klee GG, Goodmanson MK, Jacobsen SJ, *et al.* Highly sensitive automated chemilumino-metric assay for measuring free human glandular kallikrein-2. *Clin Chem* 1999;45:800–6

79. Becker C, Piironen T, Pettersson K, *et al.* Discrimination of men with prostate cancer from those with benign disease by measurements of human glandular kallikrein 2 (HK2) in serum. *J Urol* 2000;163:311–16

80. Partin AW, Catalona WJ, Finlay JA, *et al.* Use of human glandular kallikrein 2 for the detection of prostate cancer: preliminary analysis. *Urology* 1999;54:839–45

81. Grauer LS, Finlay JA, Mikolajczyk SD, *et al.* Detection of human glandular kallikrein, hK2, as its precursor form and in complex with

protease inhibitors in prostate carcinoma serum. *J Androl* 1998;19:407–11

82. Saedi MS, Hill TM, Kuus-Reichel K, *et al.* The precursor form of the human kallikrein 2, a kallikrein homologous to prostate-specific antigen, is present in human sera and is increased in prostate cancer and benign prostatic hyperplasia. *Clin Chem* 1998;44:2115–19

83. Nam RK, Diamandis EP, Toi A, *et al.* Serum human glandular kallikrein-2 protease levels predict the presence of prostate cancer among men with elevated prostate-specific antigen. *J Clin Oncol* 2000;18:1036–42

84. Klee GG, Young CY, Tindall DJ. Human glandular kallikrein protein. In Brawer MK, ed. *Prostate-Specific Antigen.* New York: Dekker, 2001;1:283–96

85. Magklara A, Scorilas A, Catalona WJ, *et al.* The combination of human glandular kallikrein and free prostate-specific antigen (PSA) enhances discrimination between prostate cancer and benign prostatic hyperplasia in patients with moderately increased total PSA. *Clin Chem* 1999;45:1960–6

86. Kwiatkowski MK, Recker F, Piironen T, *et al.* In prostatism patients the ratio of human glandular kallikrein to free PSA improves the discrimination between prostate cancer and benign hyperplasia within the diagnostic 'gray zone' of total PSA 4 to 10 ng/ml. *Urology* 1998; 52:360–5

87. Becker C, Piironen T, Pettersson K, *et al.* Clinical value of human glandular kallikrein 2 and free and total prostate-specific antigen in serum from a population of men with prostate-specific antigen levels 3.0 ng/ml or greater. *Urology* 2000;55:694–9

88. Epstein JI, Pizov G, Walsh PC. Correlation of pathologic findings with progression after radical retropubic prostatectomy. *Cancer* 1993; 71:3582–93

89. Pound CR, Partin AW, Epstein JI, *et al.* Prostate-specific antigen after anatomic radical retropubic prostatectomy. Patterns of recurrence and cancer control. *Urol Clin North Am* 1997;24:395–406

90. McNeal JE, Villers AA, Redwine EA, *et al.* Capsular penetration in prostate cancer. Significance for natural history and treatment. *Am J Surg Pathol* 1990;14:240–7

91. Oesterling JE, Chan DW, Epstein JI, *et al.* Prostate specific antigen in the preoperative and postoperative evaluation of localized prostatic cancer treated with radical prostatectomy. *J Urol* 1988;139:766–72

92. Narayan P, Gajendran V, Taylor SP, *et al.* The role of transrectal ultrasound-guided biopsy-based staging, preoperative serum prostate-specific antigen, and biopsy Gleason score in prediction of final pathologic diagnosis in prostate cancer. *Urology* 1995;46:205–12

93. Partin AW, Yoo J, Carter HB, *et al.* The use of prostate specific antigen, clinical stage and Gleason score to predict pathological stage in men with localized prostate cancer. *J Urol* 1993;150:110–14

94. Chybowski FM, Keller JJ, Bergstralh EJ, *et al.* Predicting radionuclide bone scan findings in patients with newly diagnosed, untreated prostate cancer: prostate specific antigen is superior to all other clinical parameters. *J Urol* 1991;145:313–18

95. Lerner SE, Jacobsen SJ, Lilja H, *et al.* Free, complexed, and total serum prostate-specific antigen concentrations and their proportions in predicting stage, grade, and deoxyribonucleic acid ploidy in patients with adenocarcinoma of the prostate. *Urology* 1996;48: 240–8

96. Noldus J, Graefen M, Huland E, *et al.* The value of the ratio of free-to-total prostate specific antigen for staging purposes in previously untreated prostate cancer. *J Urol* 1998;159:2004–7

97. Hara I, Miyake H, Hara S, *et al.* Value of the serum prostate-specific antigen–α_1-antichymotrypsin complex and its density as a predictor for the extent of prostate cancer. *BJU Int* 2001; 88:53–7

98. Kuriyama M, Ueno K, Uno H, *et al.* Clinical evaluation of serum prostate-specific antigen–α_1-antichymotrypsin complex values in diagnosis of prostate cancer: a cooperative study. *Int J Urol* 1998;5:48–54

99. Graefen M, Haese A, Pichlmeier U, *et al.* A validated strategy for side specific prediction of organ confined prostate cancer: a tool to select for nerve sparing radical prostatectomy. *J Urol* 2001;165:857–63

100. Haese A, Becker C, Noldus J, *et al.* Human glandular kallikrein 2: a potential serum marker for predicting the organ confined versus non-organ confined growth of prostate cancer. *J Urol* 2000;163:1491–7

101. Haese A, Graefen M, Steuber T, *et al.* Human glandular kallikrein 2 levels in serum for discrimination of pathologically organ-confined from locally-advanced prostate cancer in total PSA-levels below 10 ng/ml. *Prostate* 2001;49:101–9

102. Recker F, Kwiatkowski MK, Piironen T, *et al.* Human glandular kallikrein as a tool to improve discrimination of poorly differentiated and non-organ-confined prostate cancer compared with prostate-specific antigen. *Urology* 2000;55:481–5

103. Lange PH, Ercole CJ, Lightner DJ, *et al.* The value of serum prostate specific antigen determinations before and after radical prostatectomy. *J Urol* 1989;141:873–9

104. Haese A, Huland E, Graefen M, *et al.* Ultra-sensitive detection of prostate specific antigen in the followup of 422 patients after radical prostatectomy. *J Urol* 1999;161:1206–11

105. Stamey TA, Graves HC, Wehner N, *et al.* Early detection of residual prostate cancer after radical prostatectomy by an ultrasensitive assay for prostate specific antigen. *J Urol* 1993;149: 787–92

Expected impact of new technologies on prostate cancer research

25

G. W. Jenster

Introduction

Prostate cancer is the most common cancer and the second leading cause of cancer death in men. Although considerable progress in the clinical setting has been made in recent decades, early detection, reliable prognosis, and more and improved treatment options are needed to decrease mortality and morbidity from this disease significantly. The basis of the development and progression of cancer is an accumulation of genetic changes within the genomic DNA of the cancer cells. These chromosomal deletions, amplifications, mutations and rearrangements lead to differences in expression of genes (to be measured on the RNA level) and, subsequently, expression and modification of their protein products. Identification of these changes at the DNA, RNA and protein level is the first step towards the discovery of markers for the presence and progression of cancer. The combination of our expanded knowledge of the human genome, and the introduction of technologies to perform high-throughput DNA, RNA and protein analyses, has led to a refined understanding of cancer progression and the discovery of novel markers and therapeutic targets. Moreover, expression profiles of tumor RNA and serum proteins might become the latest tools to diagnose patients reliably, predict disease outcome and advise patient-tailored treatment regimens.

Genomics

The field of 'gene-research' advanced exponentially with the availability of the sequence of the human genome. The number of genes currently predicted to be encoded by the human genome is somewhere between 30 000 and 45 000. This knowledge of the entire human sequence would be much less significant were it not for the introduction of novel techniques to screen for the presence and expression of thousands of genes within a single experiment. cDNA microarray technology has made it possible to analyze the mRNA expression of most or all human genes simultaneously[1,2]. In this technology, thousands of spots are deposited on a glass slide. Each spot harbors a unique fragment of a gene: each spot represents a different gene. RNAs from the cancer sample and a normal reference are isolated and labelled with two different fluorescent dyes (for example, green for the tumor sample and red for the normal reference). These samples are mixed and hybridized on the cDNA microarray (Figure 1). The microarray is washed and the signal intensity of the individual fluorescent dyes in each spot is measured. If the expression of a gene is higher in the cancer sample, the spot will contain more green label, while genes down-regulated during cancer development will have relatively more red signal. The resulting comprehensive gene expression analyses have led to the identification of genes and pathways involved in prostate cancer progression and development and, therefore, new markers and therapeutic targets[3–10]. In principle, a set of genes can be selected that discriminate between normal and cancer, or even between clinically relevant and latent non-aggressive cancers. These types of

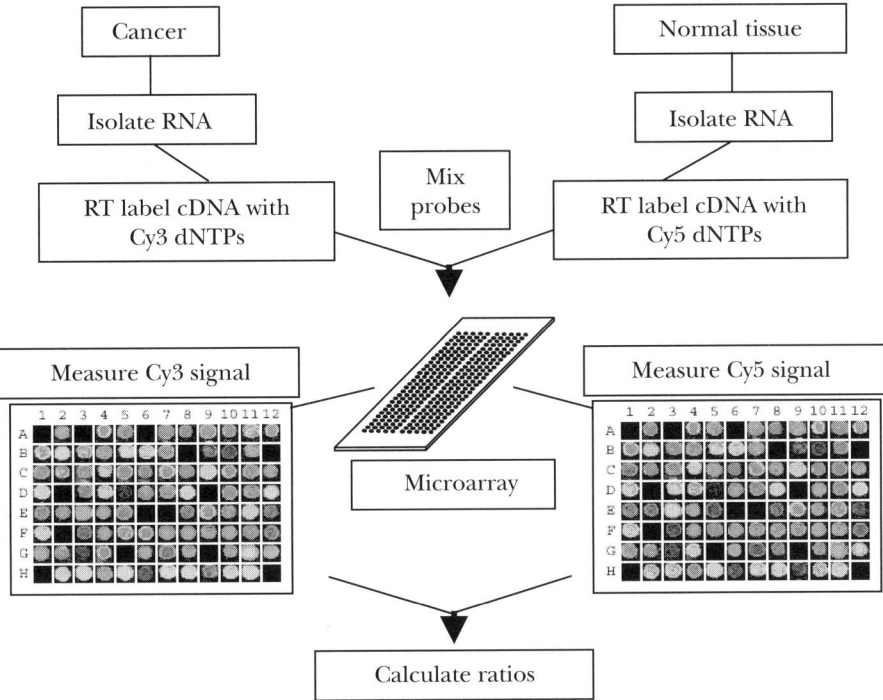

Figure 1 DNA microarray technology. RNA isolated from cancer and normal tissue is labelled with Cy3 or Cy5 fluorescent dye, respectively. The labelled samples are mixed and hybridized to a DNA microarray, harboring thousands of spots of DNA representing different genes. The microarray is washed and the Cy3 (representing cancer expression) and Cy5 (representing normal tissue expression) signals for each individual spot are separately measured using a microarray laser scanner. The ratio of Cy3/Cy5 signals for each individual spot delineates relative expression of the particular spot/gene in cancer as compared with normal tissue. RT, reverse transcriptase; dNTP, 2′-deoxyribonucleoside triphosphate

expression profiles can be useful tools to perform prognostic evaluations and decide on patient-tailored treatment.

As well as the expression of genes (measured on the RNA level), chromosomal imbalances on the genomic DNA level can be identified using cancer versus reference DNA as starting material. These comparative genomic hybridization (CGH) microarrays are useful tools to identify deletions or amplifications of genes and hint of potential tumor suppressor genes and oncogenes[11].

Proteomics

In the past, protein assays were mainly focused on expression analysis of a single protein of interest. The technology to identify marker proteins and study protein modifications has been refined, and has become more accessible to cancer researchers. The main progress has been made in the application of mass spectrometry (MS) for high-resolution protein mass separation, low-quantity detection and sequencing. Using MALDI-TOF and SELDI-TOF MS (matrix-assisted and surface-enhanced laser desorption ioninization – time of flight), hundreds to thousands of proteins can be detected in a microliter of serum or tissue extract. This has enabled researchers to perform two types of analyses: identify proteins of interest, and generate protein profiles in a high-throughput manner.

When the purpose is to identify a few novel markers or therapeutic targets, it is possible first to separate, visualize and compare proteins from extracts using two-dimensional polyacrylamide gel electrophoresis (2-D PAGE) and then identify differentially expressed proteins using MS applications[12,13]. 2-D PAGE technology is very laborious and not appropriate for high-throughput research, but can prove valuable for identification of markers in a small set of samples. These potential markers can then be tested (for example by immunohistochemistry) in larger sets of patient material to validate their usefulness.

The strength of the second type of analysis, MS protein profiling, is not direct protein identification, but the potential to link the presence or height of multiple individual protein peaks to clinical parameters (Figure 2).

In these types of assays, proteins from normal and cancer samples are separated by MS, and complete protein profiles are compared to identify differences in protein peaks. SELDI-TOF MS has been successfully applied to ovarian, prostate and breast cancer detection, in which cancer could be diagnosed with a sensitivity/specificity of 100/95%, 83/97% and 93/91%, respectively[14–16]. The sensitivities and specificities of these analyses are high, mainly because they are based on the combination of multiple protein peaks within the profile. Each individual peak only marginally differentiates between normal and cancer. Although the specificity is

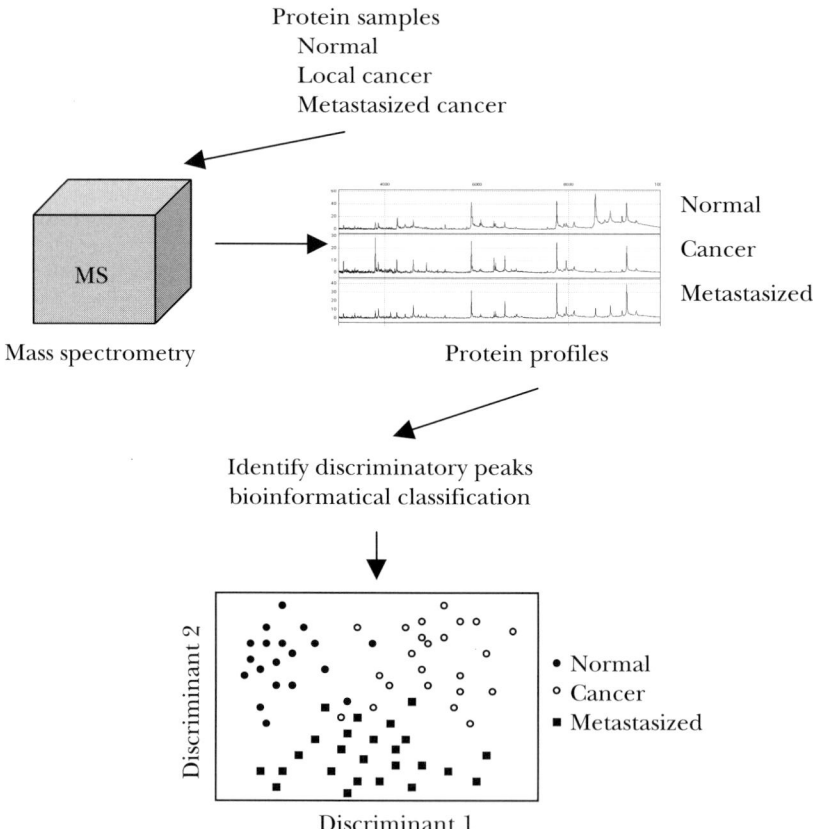

Figure 2 Protein profiling using mass spectrometry (MS). Proteins are isolated from serum or prostate tissue from men without cancer or with local or metastasized disease. Proteins are separated and detected using MS, such as SELDI-TOF or MALDI-TOF (surface-enhanced or matrix-assisted laser desorption ionization – time of flight) MS. The protein peaks from the three different groups are compared and discriminatory peaks determined for optimal classification. The classification from such a training set is then verified using a separate blinded test set to determine sensitivity and specificity of the classification system

high, it is still too low to use SELDI-TOF MS as a single diagnostic assay for low-incidence diseases such as cancer[17]. A very important feature of these SELDI-TOF MS analyses is that they were performed on serum, an easily accessible body fluid.

Microarray technology has also been applied to protein expression analyses. Antibodies directed against specific proteins were spotted on the glass slide, and fluorescently labelled protein extracts hybridized to the micro-array[18,19]. In another application, individual cellular proteins were synthesized *in vitro*, spotted and hybridized to fluorescently dyed proteins[20]. This assay can be utilized to visualize protein–protein interactions and is, like the antibody arrays, in an experimental phase (reviewed in reference 21).

Tissue

Although many tools have been developed and implemented to discover novel markers and therapeutic targets, their properties and significance still need to be validated in larger patient studies. An important tool has been established to perform high-throughput immunohisto-chemical protein staining: the tissue microarray (TMA). In order to link marker expression in prostate cancer sections to patient characteristics, many different slides have to be stained with the antibody directed against the marker. Each slide contains a tumor section from a single patient. In the tissue array, hundreds of small tissue cylinders acquired from different tumor blocks are inserted as an array into holes of an empty paraffin block using a thin-walled needle[22]. This paraffin tissue-array block can be cut into hundreds of sections with a microtome. Each section will harbor a microarray of the hundreds of small circular fragments of tumor or control samples. With a single immunohisto-chemical staining of a tissue microarray, protein expression in many different samples can be assessed.

Another technical development related to tissue is the microdissection of specific cells from tissue sections. Using this laser capture microdissection (LCM) technology, it is possible for example, to collect only the cancer cells from a heterogeneous tissue section for DNA, RNA or protein extraction, thereby eliminating contamination from normal epithelial or surrounding stromal cells[23,24]. This laborious technology is particularly useful for more targeted marker discovery in one of the cell types present in tumors. The DNA, RNA or protein extracted from the microdissected cells can be used for microarray or mass spectro-metry analysis[25].

Bioinformatics

The high-throughput analyses of DNA, RNA and protein have generated an enormous wealth of data that need to be: processed, managed, integrated and stored; analyzed and mined; and visualized. The interpretation of this flood of information has been the origin of a new field, bioinformatics, which combines elements of biology, mathematics and computer science[26].

One of the most challenging parts, and the power of bioinformatics, lies within the potential to link and mine data of different formats. Novel facts might be discovered by, for example, combining the mRNA expression data of a series of cancer-related genes (from cDNA microarrays) with: everything known about these genes within the complete literature (semantic searches of PubMed); homology information within their promoter sequences (from the human genome project); protein–protein interaction data (from protein micro-arrays); and so on. Tools are currently being developed to perform these types of tasks in an automated, batch-wise fashion. Limitations of this approach are the incompleteness and incorrectness of databanks. Since each data resource will harbor some mistakes, combined data from multiple resources will eventually be full of errors. Another important challenge faced by bioinformaticians is visualization of the large quantity of data, particularly after analysis and data mining. The ultimate goal is to summarize all informative data in a single figure that can, at a glance, be comprehended by the biologist and clinician.

Table 1 Summary of the potential impact of new technologies on prostate cancer research and their potential for clinical implementation

Technique	Input	Patient sample	Potential impact for research	Potential impact for clinic
Genomics				
CGH microarray	DNA	cancer	high, discovery of suppressor genes/oncogenes	medium, less informative, laborious
cDNA microarray	RNA	cancer	very high, discovery of markers/targets, pathway mapping	low, impractical
Proteomics				
Protein microarray	protein	cancer	medium, discovery of markers/targets, pathway mapping	low, impractical
Mass spectrometry				
2-D PAGE	protein	cancer	medium, discovery of markers/targets	low, impractical
protein profiles	protein	cancer	high, discovery of markers/targets	low, impractical
protein profiles	protein	serum	medium, discovery of markers/targets	high
Tissue				
Tissue microarray	tissue	cancer	high, high-throughput marker screening	not applicable
Laser capture microdissection	tissue	cancer	medium, targeted marker discovery	low, impractical

CGH, comparative genomic hybridization; 2-D PAGE, two-dimensional polyacrylamide gel electrophoresis

Significance for cancer research and clinical implications

In the past few years, we have seen a number of new developments for analyses of DNA, RNA, protein and tissues (Table 1 and Figure 3). Almost all of these new technologies will prove to be very useful in basic cancer research, and will yield new markers and therapeutic targets for drug development and clinical applications. The value of genomics and proteomics in a clinical setting, however, is questionable owing to the more stringent requirements. Diagnostic and prognostic assays must be cost-effective, reproducible and uncomplicated. Microarray technology applied to DNA, RNA or protein is complex and expensive, and unlikely to become a standard assay in diagnostic laboratories.

The use of patient-derived material for performing assays will also enforce restrictions. The tissue must preferentially be easily accessible and invariable. Extracting the easily degraded RNA or protein from prostate biopsies for further analysis is quite complicated for standard practice. Moreover, prostate biopsies will generally harbor a lot of normal tissue that can obscure the abnormalities in the cancerous part. Although LCM could circumvent this problem, this procedure is too laborious ever to outgrow its experimental phase. If, however, more easily accessible body fluids such as blood, urine, saliva, sweat or tear fluid can be utilized instead of prostate tissue, it would greatly facilitate population screening studies. From all technologies discussed above, mass

Figure 3 (*on facing page*) Overview of new technologies implemented in prostate cancer research. Different samples can be extracted from a prostate cancer patient including prostate cancer tissue and serum. DNA, RNA or protein can be extracted directly from the tissue or from purified cancer cells using laser capture microdissection technology. The DNA, RNA and protein can be used for microarray analyses to identify potential markers or generate expression profiles to classify patients. Formalin-fixed, paraffin-embedded tissue samples can be used to generate tissue microarrays (TMA) to analyze gene/protein expression in a high-throughput manner. Protein fractions from tissue or serum can be analyzed and separated using 2D-PAGE (two-dimensional polyacrylamide gel electrophoresis) and SELDI/MALDI-TOF (surface-enhanced or matrix-assisted laser desorption ionization – time of flight) mass spectrometry (MS) protein profiling. Protein spots and peaks can be identified using MS applications and further validated as potential markers or therapeutic targets

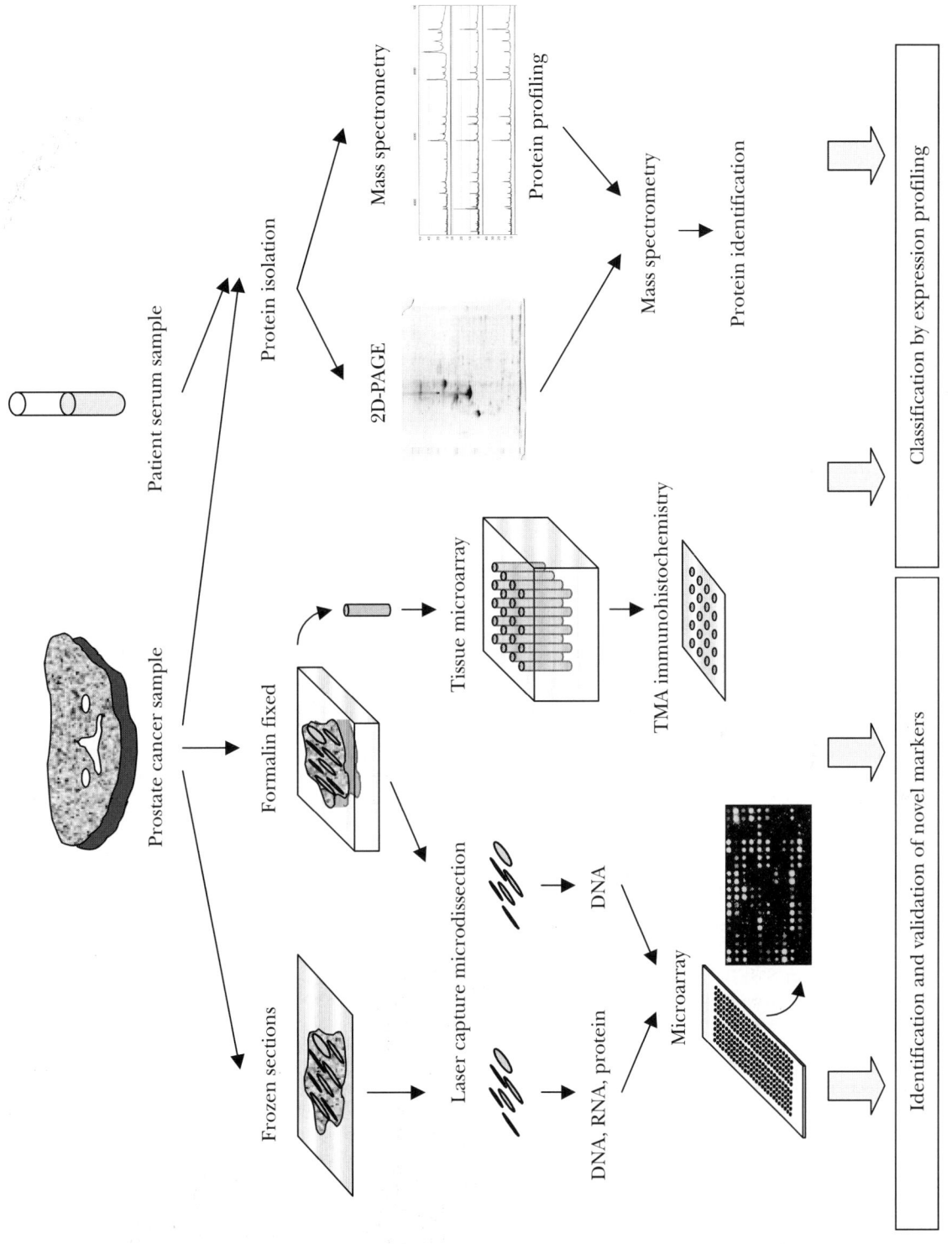

spectrometry of serum to generate complex protein profiles for diagnostic and prognostic evaluation seems the most promising development for widespread clinical implementation. A 1-h, simple and cost-effective assay on the easily accessible serum could become a valuable tool to diagnose patients, predict disease outcome and advise on patient-tailored treatment regimens. An essential drawback with respect to the use of body fluids that are not directly associated with the cancer (such as saliva or sweat) is the absence of diagnostic/prognostic cancer markers. Serum or prostate fluid seem the best candidates in which prostate cancer markers can be detected. Interestingly, it still needs to be proven whether the protein peaks that differentiate between normal and cancer from SELDI-TOF MS analysis are tumor-derived products or epiphenomena of metabolic changes due to the presence of the tumor[27].

As has become clear, the starting material from which the DNA, RNA or protein is to be extracted must be of high quality. DNA is the most stable of the three, and can even be reliably extracted from formalin-fixed, paraffin-embedded tissues. To isolate intact RNA or protein, however, the tissue must be fresh or directly deep-frozen upon removal from the patient. This is quite complicated for prostate biopsies or prostate fragments after radical prostatectomies, since it requires special procedures and can be in conflict with the pathologist's needs for formalin-fixed material for diagnosis. Utilizing RNA or protein from prostate samples is therefore less suitable for screening large numbers of patients for diagnosis, prognosis or therapy recommendations. For research purposes, however, a well-equipped laboratory, with support from pathologists and urologists, can easily implement high-throughput RNA and protein technologies.

References

1. Duggan DJ, Bittner M, Chen Y, *et al.* Expression profiling using cDNA microarrays. *Nat Genet* 1999;21:10–14
2. Brown PO, Botstein D. Exploring the new world of the genome with DNA microarrays. *Nat Genet* 1999;21:33–7
3. Xu J, Stolk JA, Zhang X, *et al.* Identification of differentially expressed genes in human prostate cancer using subtraction and microarray. *Cancer Res* 2000;60:1677–82
4. Dhanasekaran SM, Barrette TR, Ghosh D, *et al.* Delineation of prognostic biomarkers in prostate cancer. *Nature* (*London*) 2001;412:822–6
5. Luo J, Duggan DJ, Chen Y, *et al.* Human prostate cancer and benign prostatic hyperplasia: molecular dissection by gene expression profiling. *Cancer Res* 2001;61:4683–8
6. Magee JA, Araki T, Patil S, *et al.* Expression profiling reveals hepsin overexpression in prostate cancer. *Cancer Res* 2001;61:5692–6
7. Welsh JB, Sapinoso LM, Su AI, *et al.* Analysis of gene expression identifies candidate markers and pharmacological targets in prostate cancer. *Cancer Res* 2001;61:5974–8
8. Ernst T, Hergenhahn M, Kenzelmann M, *et al.* Decrease and gain of gene expression are equally discriminatory markers for prostate carcinoma: a gene expression analysis on total and micro-dissected prostate tissue. *Am J Pathol* 2002;160: 2169–80
9. LaTulippe E, Satagopan J, Smith A, *et al.* Comprehensive gene expression analysis of prostate cancer reveals distinct transcriptional programs associated with metastatic disease. *Cancer Res* 2002;62:4499–506
10. Singh D, Febbo PG, Ross K, *et al.* Gene expression correlates of clinical prostate cancer behavior. *Cancer Cell* 2002;1:203–9
11. Cai WW, Mao JH, Chow CW, *et al.* Genome-wide detection of chromosomal imbalances in tumors using BAC microarrays. *Nat Biotechnol* 2002; 20:393–6
12. Alaiya AA, Oppermann M, Langridge J, *et al.* Identification of proteins in human prostate tumor material by two-dimensional gel electrophoresis and mass spectrometry. *Cell Mol Life Sci* 2001;58:307–11

13. Meehan KL, Holland JW, Dawkins HJ. Proteomic analysis of normal and malignant prostate tissue to identify novel proteins lost in cancer. *Prostate* 2002;50:54–63

14. Adam BL, Qu Y, Davis JW, *et al.* Serum protein fingerprinting coupled with a pattern-matching algorithm distinguishes prostate cancer from benign prostate hyperplasia and healthy men. *Cancer Res* 2002;62:3609–14

15. Li J, Zhang Z, Rosenzweig J, *et al.* Proteomics and bioinformatics approaches for identification of serum biomarkers to detect breast cancer. *Clin Chem* 2002;48:1296–304

16. Petricoin EF, Ardekani AM, Hitt BA, *et al.* Use of proteomic patterns in serum to identify ovarian cancer. *Lancet* 2002;359:572–7

17. Elwood M. Proteomic patterns in serum and identification of ovarian cancer. *Lancet* 2002;360:170, discussion

18. Haab BB, Dunham MJ, Brown PO. Protein microarrays for highly parallel detection and quantitation of specific proteins and antibodies in complex solutions. *Genome Biol* 2001;2:0004

19. Sreekumar A, Nyati MK, Varambally S, *et al.* Profiling of cancer cells using protein microarrays: discovery of novel radiation-regulated proteins. *Cancer Res* 2001;61:7585–93

20. Zhu H, Bilgin M, Bangham R, *et al.* Global analysis of protein activities using proteome chips. *Science* 2001;293:2101–5

21. Schweitzer B, Kingsmore SF. Measuring proteins on microarrays. *Curr Opin Biotechnol* 2002;13:14–19

22. Kononen J, Bubendorf L, Kallioniemi A, *et al.* Tissue microarrays for high-throughput molecular profiling of tumor specimens. *Nat Med* 1998;4:844–7

23. Emmert-Buck MR, Bonner RF, Smith PD, *et al.* Laser capture microdissection. *Science* 1996;274:998–1001

24. Krizman DB, Chuaqui RF, Meltzer PS, *et al.* Construction of a representative cDNA library from prostatic intraepithelial neoplasia. *Cancer Res* 1996;56:5380–3

25. Rubin MA. Use of laser capture microdissection, cDNA microarrays, and tissue microarrays in advancing our understanding of prostate cancer. *J Pathol* 2001;195:80–6

26. Bayat A. Science, medicine, and the future: bioinformatics. *Br Med J* 2002;324:1018–22

27. Diamandis EP. Proteomic patterns in serum and identification of ovarian cancer. *Lancet* 2002;360:170, discussion

Predictive algorithms and their clinical relevance

26

M. Graefen and H. Huland

Introduction

In the past few years, many nomograms and algorithms have been published predicting stage and outcome of clinically localized prostate cancer treated with radical prostatectomy or radiation therapy[1-8]. External validation of published nomograms is essential, because otherwise it remains unclear whether the predictive accuracy reported in the original study can be expected elsewhere. Different prostate-specific antigen (PSA) assays and differences in Gleason grading, surgical experience, number of surgeons and pathologists involved are just a few potential confounders that might disturb the performance of a nomogram when applied to a different cohort of patients. Therefore, differences related to the geographic region, country or continent that may impact upon each of the steps related to diagnosing prostate cancer may affect the performance of a nomogram that incorporates such diagnostic variables. In theory, in a stable nomogram, such differences should result in minimal predictive accuracy variations, as a truly generalizable nomogram should adjust properly for any such differences.

We assessed the accuracy of several published *preoperative* predictive tools addressing lymph node stage, pathological stage and outcome following aggressive treatment for localized prostate cancer. As only algorithms with readily available predictor variables such as clinical stage, PSA or Gleason sum score in the biopsy allow a common use in each institution, we focused on tools that are based on these parameters.

Prediction of lymph node stages and pathological stage

In recent years, many predictive tools have been published to predict pathological stage and treatment outcome in patients with clinically localized prostate cancer. However, the only predictive tools published to date that were validated on external multi-institutional data sets are the prediction of pathological stage by Partin and colleagues[3] and the prediction of disease recurrence by Kattan and associates[1].

Partin and co-workers compiled tables predicting the probability of organ confinement, extracapsular extension, seminal vesicle invasion and lymph node involvement using a pooled database of 4133 men who underwent radical prostatectomy between 1982 and 1996. The validity of these tables in external patients was demonstrated recently using 2475 patients operated on at the Mayo Clinic in Rochester, Minnesota[9]. The area under the receiver operating characteristic curve (AUC) for the analysis, comparing the predicted probability and the actual incidence of organ-confined disease in those patients, was 0.84, which demonstrates a high predictive accuracy. However, this predictive tool has yet not been tested in a non-US population, and it therefore remains unclear whether accuracy of the Partin tables is acceptable in European patients. We therefore applied the Partin tables in a validation study to 1278 patients with localized prostate cancer treated only by radical prostatectomy in Hamburg, Germany.

We chose the Partin tables for our validation study as this predictive tool is based on a multi-institutional date set, and has already been externally validated in US patients[9]. Multi-institutionally derived predictive tools have the potential to overcome limitations inherent to single-center based nomograms. The external validation performed in the USA by Blute and colleagues from the Mayo Clinic, Rochester, Minnesota, confirmed reliability of this tool in an institution with similar detection and treatment strategies and similar pre-selection of the patients[9]. Despite the good performance of the tables in those patients, we were interested whether its predictive accuracy might deteriorate when it was applied to patients where detection strategies are different, compared with the USA.

For statistical assessment of the discriminative ability of the Partin tables, we performed receiver operating characteristic (ROC) curve analyses for the most important pathological features such as organ confinement and lymph node involvement.

Despite apparent differences in pretreatment variables of our patients compared with the derivation cohort, the Partin tables were able accurately to predict organ confinement and lymph node metastases in the European patient cohort from Hamburg. This was demonstrated by high AUCs, with values of 0.817 for organ confinement and 0.807 for metastatic disease. In fact, accuracy of the tables for prediction of organ-confined cancer was higher in our patients than in the study published by Blute and colleagues from the Mayo Clinic. The AUC for the Partin tables in their study was 0.727 when applied to the Mayo patients. There was a higher similarity of pretreatment variables, compared with our patients, except that low Gleason scores (less than 5) were found more frequently in the Mayo patients compared with the Partin cohort (17% vs. 5%). The rate of pathologically organ-confined disease in the Mayo cohort (67%) was substantially higher than in our cohort (56%) and in the Partin data set (48%). However, this difference in prevalence of organ-confined cancers does not affect ROC analyses, and should not account for a lesser (even though still accurate) predictive ability of the Partin

tables in the Mayo series, compared with our patients. Predictive accuracy was similar when lymph node metastases were addressed: the AUC for the Partin tables in the Mayo series was 0.818, compared with 0.807 in Hamburg patients. This demonstrates that the Partin tables have similar accuracies in patients from different geographic regions when similarities in diagnostic and treatment strategies are apparent.

The incidence of lymph node metastases has substantially decreased in modern patient series, and routine lymphadenectomy prior to radical prostatectomy has recently been questioned by several investigators[10,11]. As the incidence of positive nodes is low in all reported contemporary series, it seems to be important to identify those men with an extremely low likelihood of metastases, as these patients are candidates in whom diagnostic lymphadenectomy could potentially be spared. Accepting a likelihood for lymph node metastases of ≤ 3% for patients in whom a lymphadenectomy could be omitted, the Partin tables could identify 682 patients (53.4%) in our series. The incidence of positive nodes was 1.6% in these men, which again confirms the reliability of this predictive tool. Nevertheless, in a prospectively validated predictive model from our own institution addressing the same topic, we could stratify 82% of investigated patients in a low-risk group using the same predicted likelihood of ≤3% for metastatic spread of the cancer (Figure 1)[11]. The incidence of positive nodes was similarly low in these patients at 2.8%; however, almost 30% more of the initial patients could be correctly assigned to the favorable group when this predictive tool was applied.

In that series, systematic biopsy results were included in the nomogram derivation, and it is conceivable that patient stratification can be improved by this information at a similar level of accuracy. This was furthermore confirmed by Haese and colleagues when our algorithm for prediction of lymph node metastases was applied to prostate cancer patients from the Johns–Hopkins University in Baltimore, with a striking concordance between predicted and actual incidence of metastases[12]. We would

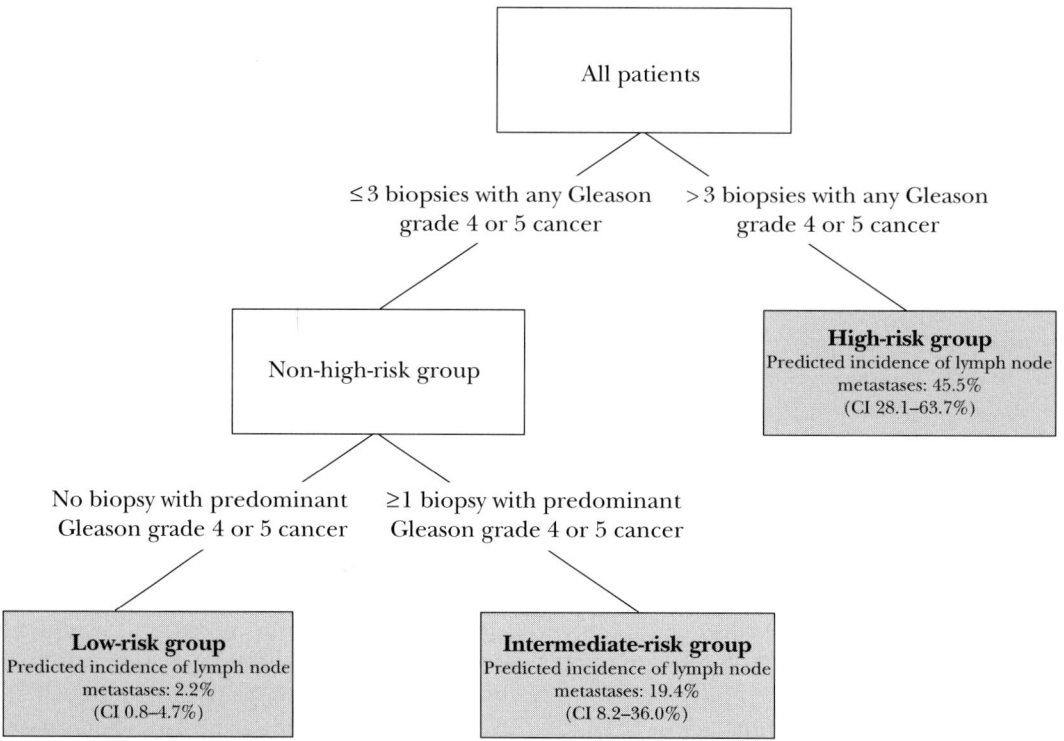

Figure 1 Retrospectively developed and prospectively validated decision tree for predicting lymph node status. From reference 11. CI, confidence interval

therefore recommend use of our decision tree if systematic biopsy data are available to maximize the number of patients in whom a lymph node dissection can safely be omitted. However, considering recent reports of a higher incidence of lymph node metastases after an extended lymph node dissection, algorithms that focus on the prediction of metastases only in the obturator fossa might need an update once clinical consequences are apparent[13,14].

Partin and colleagues used the readily available clinical features of pretreatment PSA, clinical stage and biopsy Gleason sum for prediction. The advantage of this approach is that this predictive tool can potentially be applied at all centers, as these three features constitute the current mainstay in the diagnosis of prostate cancer patients. Including systematic biopsy features[11,15], new molecular or serum markers[5] or information on angiogenesis[3] has the potential to enhance predictive accuracy of tools based on the three traditional parameters. Yet, including additional features will limit

applicability to those few centers where these factors are obtained. Furthermore, in accordance with the findings of Blute and associates, we could demonstrate that high predictive accuracy was achieved by combination of these three basic variables as used in the Partin tables. Our study suggests that the Partin tables provide accurate predictions when applied to heterogeneous data sets in geographic regions where diagnostic and treatment strategies might differ from those in the USA.

Even though highly reliable, the Partin tables might not be the ideal prognostic instrument for treatment planning and patient counselling. It is important to realize that these tables do not provide information beyond pathological stage, and therefore do not predict therapeutic outcome. The tables do not indicate the probability of recurrence or need for further treatment for cancer, since organ confinement (or lack thereof) is not synonymous with surgical cure (or failure)[1]. For this reason, nomograms were developed which address likelihood of disease recurrence, and we therefore focus on such nomograms in the second part of this chapter.

Predicting organ confinement can be useful to indicate a nerve-sparing radical prostatectomy, as preservation of the neurovascular bundles appears to be safe in patients without extraprostatic disease[15]. Yet the Partin tables do not provide side-specific information, which is desirable as a neurovascular bundle can be spared on each side of the prostate. Predictive tools that provide this specific information are therefore superior to the Partin tables when used to indicate a nerve-sparing technique[15]. Furthermore, the Partin tables do not include features from systematic biopsies but use the simple Gleason sum for prediction. In a recent multi-institutional study based on 1200 patients, Ohori and colleagues could demonstrate that systematic biopsy features were highly significant independent predictors of organ confinement when considered together with the three traditional Partin variables in multivariate Cox models[14]. They could furthermore show that, in the same data set, the predictive accuracy of a Cox model-derived nomogram including systematic biopsy features was higher than in a nomogram which ignored these features as predictor variables.

If an algorithm should be used to predict the side-specific likelihood of organ confinement for indicating a nerve-sparing radical prostatectomy, we recommend applying the decision tree published by our own institution in 2001[15]. This algorithm uses the preoperative information in a side-specific manner, and therefore allows indication of uni- or bilateral preservation of the neurovascular bundle (Figure 2).

To develop this algorithm we performed a retrospective regression analysis to maximize the positive predictive value associated with predicting side-specific organ confinement in a maximized patient group. From nine included preoperative parameters, the number of biopsies with high-grade cancer, serum PSA concentration and number of cores positive for cancer were considered in the multivariate tree-structured regression analysis. The other included parameters did not add independent information and were rejected. Note that the

results of a systematic sextant biopsy achieve highest predictive value. However, this decision tree can only be applied in a population where this information is available. The analysis resulted in four risk groups with different likelihoods of organ-confined disease (Figure 2).

The regression tree (Figure 2) starts with all prostate lobes, and alongside the arrows are those parameters that have the highest impact on distinguishing whether the tumor growth is organ-confined or not. The resulting subgroups are shown in the boxes. This allows stratifying each prostate lobe individually to the likelihood for organ-confined disease. Only displayed parameters reached significance levels in the analyses. In the most favorable group, the predicted likelihood of organ-confined disease was 86% (95% confidence interval (CI) 81.5–89.9%) when characterized by ≤ 1 biopsy with Gleason grade 4 or 5 cancer and serum PSA < 10 ng/ml. If serum PSA was > 10 ng/ml, it was important whether more than one biopsy core was positive for cancer. In lobes in which, at most, one positive core was found, organ-confined disease was still found in 72.1% (95% CI 62.8–80.2%). If more than one positive core was detected, the likelihood of organ-confined disease dropped to 44.8% (95% CI 32.6–57.4%). Patients with more than one biopsy with high-grade cancer had a likelihood of 22.3% (95% CI 14.4–32.1%) of organ-confined tumor growth regardless of serum PSA. Pooling the two most favorable groups (see Figure 1) leads to $n = 391$ (70.8% of investigated) prostate lobes with a positive predictive value of 82.1% (95% CI 77.9–85.8%). This collapsed decision rule is suggested for routine application in the sequel.

This retrospectively developed decision tree was prospectively validated in patients who were operated on between 1997 and 2000 in Hamburg. Organ-confined disease was found in 65.7% of the patients ($n = 232/353$) in the validation data set. In the side-specific analysis, organ-confined tumor growth was found in 552 of 706 investigated prostate lobes (78%). Stratification of the lobes was performed according to the retrospective decision rule. The increased incidence of organ-confined

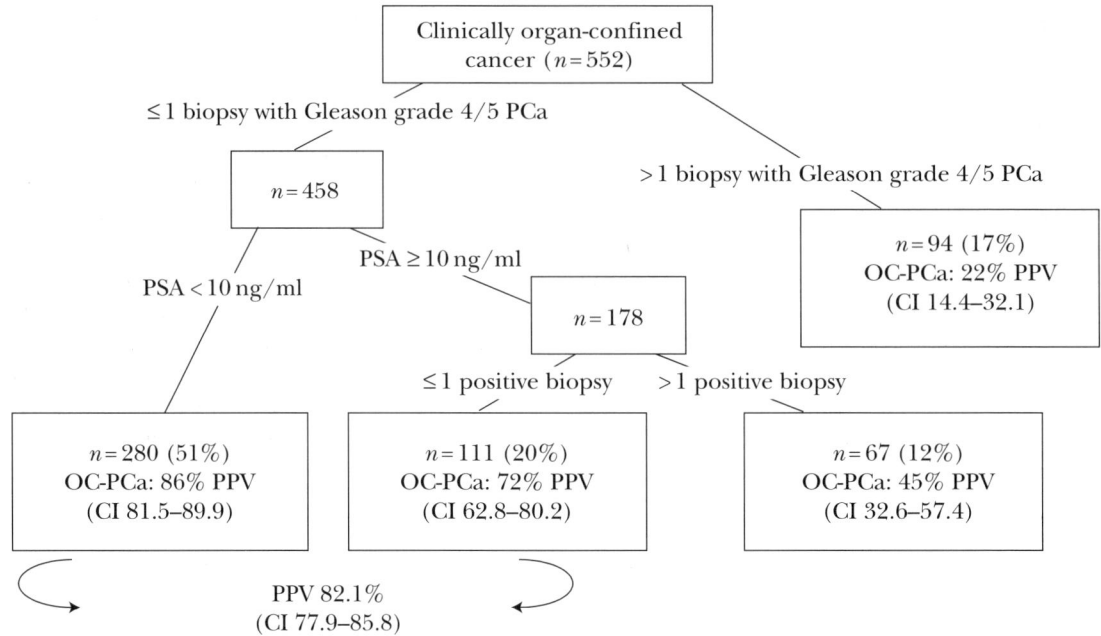

Figure 2 Classification of likelihood of organ-confined prostate cancer (OC-PCa) in the training data set. Data are expressed for each lobe of the prostate. Positive predictive value (PPV) and 95% confidence interval (95% CI) are displayed for each risk group. PSA, prostate-specific antigen

disease in all risk groups may be explained by stage migration towards more favorable findings preoperatively, which was confirmed by higher incidence of organ-confined cancer in the prospective data set compared with the retrospective data set. In addition, more patients were stratified to the favorable group in the prospective validation data set than in the retrospective study. Retrospectively, 50.7% ($n = 280/552$) of the prostate lobes fulfilled the criteria for an 86% likelihood of organ-confined cancer, and in the validation data set 60.4% ($n = 427/706$) of prostate lobes were stratified to that risk group. The actual incidence of organ-confined disease characterized by PSA of < 10 ng/ml and not more than one biopsy with Gleason grade 4 or 5 cancer was 88.3% (95% CI 85.1–91.4%). The retrospectively estimated positive predictive value of 72% carried over into an actual incidence of 81.5% (95% CI 73.9–87.6%), the likelihood of 45% into an actual incidence of 59.4% (95% CI 47.9–70.4%) and the likelihood of 22% into an actual incidence of 26.9% (95% CI 16.6–39.7%).

Pooling the two most favorable risk groups (as suggested in the retrospective data set), organ-confined disease occurred in 86.8% (95% CI 83.8–89.5%) of prostate lobes; 69% ($n = 488/706$) of investigated prostate lobes were assigned to this group.

In summary, the Partin tables provide high accuracy for the prediction of organ confinement and lymph node stage across different patient cohorts. However, more patients can safely be stratified to a low-risk group for lymph node metastases if an algorithm based on systematic biopsy results is utilized[11]. The Partin tables do not provide side-specific information on organ-confined tumor growth. We recommend using the side-specific prediction published by Graefen and colleagues if an algorithm should be used to indicate a nerve-sparing radical prostatectomy[13].

Algorithms to predict outcome

The above-mentioned predictive tools focus on pathological features, which can be used as surrogate markers for the estimation of outcome after a definitive treatment for localized prostate cancer. While the accuracy of these tables has been demonstrated, it is important to realize that no information beyond predicted pathological stage is provided, and therapeutic outcome is not predicted. Therefore, information about the likelihood of PSA recurrence may be of greater benefit to urologists and patients than pathological stage. Treatment outcome can nowadays be directly predicted using PSA recurrence or other evidence of disease progression as an end-point.

We tested the performance characteristics of two such tools, the Kattan nomogram[1] (Figure 3) prediction likelihood of being free from recurrence 5 years after radical prostatectomy, and the D'Amico nomogram (Table 1), which uses the same end-point 2 years following radical surgery[4]. Again, predicted likelihoods by

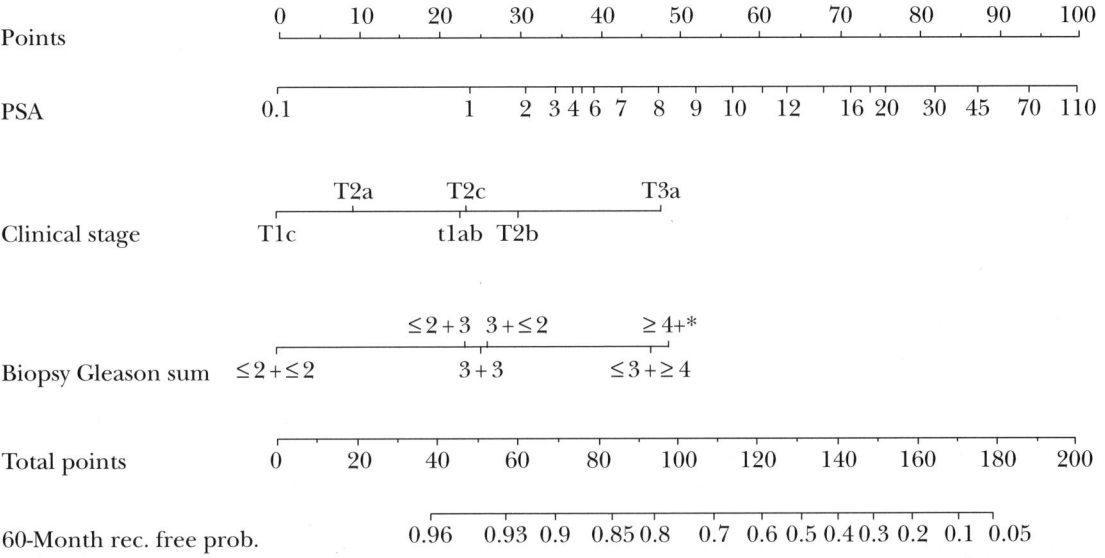

Instructions for physician: Locate the patient's PSA on the **PSA** axis. Draw a line straight upwards to the **Points** axis to determine how many points towards recurrence the patient receives for his PSA. Repeat this process for the **Clinical stage** and **Biopsy Gleason sum** axes, each time drawing straight upward to the **Points** axis. Sum the points achieved for each predictor and locate this sum on the **Total points** axis. Draw a line straight down to find the patient's probability of remaining recurrence free (rec. free prob.) for 60 months assuming he does not die of another cause first.

Note: This nomogram is not applicable to a man who is not otherwise a candidate for radical prostatectomy. You can use this only on a man who has already selected radical prostatectomy as treatment for his prostate cancer.

Instruction to patient: 'Mr. X, if we had 100 men exactly like you we would expect between <predicted percentage from nomogram - 10%> and <predicted percentage + 10%> to remain free of their disease at 5 years following radical prostatectomy, and recurrence after 5 years is very rare.'

© 1997 Michael W. Kattan and Peter T. Scardino

Figure 3 Preoperative nomogram based on 983 patients treated at Baylor College of Medicine, Houston, Texas, for predicting prostate-specific antigen (PSA) recurrence after radical prostatectomy. Adapted from reference 1

Table 1 Percentage prostate-specific antigen (PSA) failure at 2 years (and 95% confidence intervals), stratified by pretreatment PSA, American Joint Committee on Cancer clinical stage and biopsy Gleason score of surgically managed patients at Harvard Medical School ($n = 892$). Adapted from reference 4

Pretreatment PSA (ng/ml)	Biopsy Gleason score	T1c	T2a	T2b	T2c
0–4.0	2–4	4(2–7)	5(3–7)	8(4–13)	10(16–17)
	5	8(5–11)	9(6–11)	15(8–21)	18(12–25)
	6	10(6–15)	11(8–14)	19(11–27)	24(17–31)
	7	14(8–20)	15(11–19)	25(15–35)	31(22–40)
	8–10	24(13–37)	26(16–36)	42(24–59)	50(34–65)
4.1–10	2–4	5(3–8)	6(4–9)	10(5–16)	13(8–20)
	5	10(6–14)	11(8–13)	18(11–25)	22(16–30)
	6	13(8–18)	14(11–17)	24(15–32)	29(22–37)
	7	17(11–24)	19(14–23)	31(20–42)	37(28–46)
	8–10	29(17–44)	32(20–44)	50(31–67)	58(43–72)
10.1–20.0	2–4	7(4–12)	8(5–13)	15(8–23)	18(11–29)
	5	14(9–20)	15(11–19)	25(17–34)	31(23–40)
	6	18(11–26)	20(15–25)	33(22–43)	39(31–48)
	7	24(15–34)	26(20–30)	42(29–54)	49(40–59)
	8–10	39(24–58)	43(29–58)	63(44–80)	72(56–84)
20.1–50.0	2–4	18(10–34)	20(12–36)	33(19–54)	40(25–64)
	5	31(18–52)	34(23–53)	52(36–73)	61(46–81)
	6	40(24–63)	43(30–63)	63(47–83)	72(60–88)
	7	50(32–74)	53(39–75)	75(58–91)	82(71–95)
	8–10	72(48–94)	76(57–94)	92(77–99)	96(88–100)

the tested nomograms were compared with follow up information from patients operated on in Hamburg for localized prostate cancer. The derivation criteria of the two nomograms were identical to the selection criteria used for the validation cohort.

Accuracy of the nomograms was assessed by camparing the probabilities of recurrence predicted by the nomograms with actual disease progression. Specifically, we performed an ROC curve analysis comparing the D'Amico nomogram-derived 2-year probability of freedom from PSA recurrence with the actual follow-up, and a similar analysis comparing the Kattan nomogram-derived 5-year probability of freedom from PSA recurrence with actual follow-up. With censored data, the ROC calculation needs to be modified from its conventional form. Therefore, Harrell's transformation was calculated[15]. Its interpretation is similar to the conventional ROC analysis. The AUC for censored data is the probability that, for any random patients, the patient whose

disease recurs first had the greater predicted probability of recurrence.

The AUC in the ROC curve analysis was 0.80 when the D'Amico nomogram was applied to the patients from Hamburg ($n = 932$) who met the same criteria as the patients in the derivation data set from that study. The AUC for comparison of the probability of 5-year recurrence-free survival predicted by the Kattan nomogram with the actual follow-up reached 0.83 when applied to the 1003 men fitting the inclusion criteria used at the Baylor College of Medicine, Houston, Texas. The AUC of the Kattan nomogram for those 932 men used for the D'Amico nomogram validation was 0.81, slightly better than 0.80 for the D'Amico nomogram ($p = 0.0274$). The ability of the Kattan nomogram to predict outcome in our patients was slightly better than that of the D'Amico nomogram ($p = 0.0274$). This small difference may derive from differences in statistical methodology used to derive these predictive tools. The Kattan nomogram uses preoperative

PSA as a continuous variable, while in the D'Amico nomogram PSA is categorized. This is because the D'Amico nomogram creates tables based on risk groups to which a patient is assigned, and then gives the likelihood of recurrence for each group (see Table 1). In contrast, the Kattan nomogram predicts outcome for each patient individually (see Figure 3). While being slightly less precise, the D'Amico tables offer a more user-friendly approach as the probabilities may easily be obtained from these 'look-up' tables. Although a paper-based version is available, the Kattan nomogram, owing to its complexity, is best used with a palm digital assistant (see www.nomograms.org). Since many physicians already use this equipment, the accuracy gain achieved from computational complexity appears warranted and of minor disadvantage. Another potential factor for the improved ability of the Kattan nomogram to predict outcome in our patients could be the way the Gleason grades in the biopsy were considered. The D'Amico nomogram uses Gleason sum while the Kattan nomogram takes the primary and secondary Gleason grades into account. Several investigators have demonstrated additional prognostic information when using primary and secondary Gleason grades rather than the overall Gleason sum. This is especially the case in patients with Gleason sum $7^{11,15}$. In these patients the Kattan nomogram differentiates between men with biopsy Gleason grades of $3 + 4$ and $4 + 3$, while the D'Amico nomogram considers them the same. Additionally, PSA failure in the Harvard nomogram is defined as three consecutive rises. This definition is unusual for surgically managed patients, and may create difficulty in determining the exact date of failure. Despite these subtle differences, it must be emphasized that both nomograms could accurately predict outcome in our patients as demonstrated by the AUCs of 0.80 and 0.83 for the D'Amico and the Kattan nomograms, respectively. Furthermore, the Kattan nomogram has recently demonstrated a high predictive accuracy in a multi-institutional validation study, underlining its generalizability.

Evidence indicates that nomograms that quantitatively assess cancer in systematic biopsies, for example the percentage of positive cores or cores positive for high-grade cancer, can improve predictive accuracy[11,15,16]. However, for this chapter we have focused on two nomograms employing the most widely used predictors, pretreatment PSA, clinical stage and biopsy Gleason grade. The advantage of this approach resides in universally wide availability of these variables. Furthermore, the AUCs derived from the nomograms demonstrate that a combination of these basic tumor characteristics predicts outcome after radical prostatectomy with a high degree of accuracy.

This validation study has demonstrated that predictive tools which rely on the combined information from three commonly used clinical variables can predict outcome in a highly accurate fashion. The D'Amico nomogram predicts 2-year freedom of recurrence, and might be an important tool to stratify patients for neoadjuvant or adjuvant therapeutic trials. The Kattan nomogram predicts longer-term outcome, and could be better used for conselling patients on treatment options. It appears that both nomograms accurately predict recurrence, but the nomograms may potentially be improved with the addition of novel predictor variables such as tumor quantification in the biopsy specimens.

References

1. Kattan MW, Eastham JA, Stapleton AMF, *et al.* A preoperative nomogram for disease recurrence following radical prostatectomy for prostate cancer. *J Natl Cancer Inst* 1998;90:766–71

2. Kattan MW, Stapleton AMF, Wheeler TM, *et al.* Evaluation of a nomogram for predicting pathological stage of men with clinically localized prostate cancer. *Cancer* 1997;79:528–37

3. Partin AW, Kattan MW, Subong ENP, *et al.* Combination of prostate-specific antigen, clinical stage, and Gleason score to predict pathological stage in men with localized prostate cancer: a multi-institutional update. *J Am Med Assoc* 1997;277:1445–51

4. D'Amico AV, Whittington R, Malkowicz SB, *et al.* Pretreatment nomogram for prostate-specific antigen recurrence after radical prostatectomy or external beam radiation therapy for clinically localized prostate cancer. *J Clin Oncol* 1999;17:168–72

5. Snow PB, Smith DS, Catalona WJ. Artificial neural networks in the diagnosis and prognosis of prostate cancer: a pilot study. *J Urol* 1994;1525:1923–8

6. Graefen M, Noldus J, Pichlmeier U, *et al.* Early prostate-specific antigen relapse after radical retropubic prostatectomy: prediction on the basis of preoperative and post-operative tumor characteristics. *Eur Urol* 1999;361:21–30

7. D'Amico AV, Whittington R, Malkowicz SB, *et al.* Clinical utility of the percentage of positive prostate biopsies in defining biochemical outcome after radical prostatectomy for patients with clinically localized prostate cancer [see Comments]. *Mol Urol* 2000;4:171–5

8. Kattan MW, Zelefsky MJ, Kupelian P, *et al.* Pretreatment nomogram for predicting the outcome of three-dimensional conformal radiotherapy in prostate cancer. *J Clin Oncol* 2000;19:3352–9

9. Blute ML, Bergstrahl EJ, Partin AW, *et al.* Validation of Partin tables for predicting pathologic stage of clinically localized prostate cancer. *J Urol* 2000;164:1591–5

10. Soh S, Kattan MW, Berkman S, *et al.* Has there been a recent shift in the pathological features and prognosis of patients treated with radical prostatectomy? *J Urol* 1997;157:2212–18

11. Conrad S, Graefen M, Pichlmeier U, *et al.* Systematic sextant biopsies improve preoperative prediction of pelvic lymph node metastases in patients with clinically localized prostatic carcinoma. *J Urol* 1998;159:2023–8

12. Haese A, Epstein JI, Huland H, Partin AW. Validation of a biopsy-based pathologic algorithm for predicting lymph node metastases in patients with clinically localized prostate carcinoma. *Cancer* 2002;95:1016–21

13. Graefen M, Haese A, Pichlmeier U, *et al.* A validated strategy for side specific prediction of organ confined prostate cancer: a tool to select for nerve sparing radical prostatectomy. *J Urol* 2001;165:857–63

14. Ohori M, Graefen M, Karakiewicz PI, *et al.* Improved predictive accuracy in algorithms including systematic biopsy features. *J Urol* 2001;165:abstr 721

15. Harrell FE Jr, Califf RM, *et al.* Evaluating the yield of medical tests. *J Am Med Assoc* 1982;247:2543

16. Stamey TA, McNeal JE, Yemoto CM, *et al.* Biological determinants of cancer progression in men with prostate cancer. *J Am Med Assoc* 1999;15:1395–400

17. Graefen M, Karakiewicz PI, Cagiannos I, *et al.* International validation of a preoperative nomogram for prostate cancer recurrence after radical prostatectomy. *J Clin Oncol* 2002;20:3206–12

Defining the proper 'window of opportunity' in the early detection of prostate cancer

27

A. N. Vis and the European Randomized Study of Screening for Prostate Cancer, Study Group Rotterdam

Introduction

Major efforts are currently being made to improve the outcome of patients with prostate cancer by investigating the value of early detection of the disease. As is known from screening efforts directed at two other high-incidence cancers, i.e. those of the breast and lung, screening for malignancy can have serious negative side-effects. For instance, cancers thought to have a silent or latent natural course of disease may be detected, which are believed never to progress clinically. Obviously, the detection of these cancers will not lead to a reduction of disease-related mortality. On the other hand, cancers that would have soon progressed clinically may be detected by early screening, and such detection programs will only give the host the earlier knowledge of having an incurable, lethal disease. In previous reports we have already attempted to define the 'window of opportunity' in population-based screening for prostate cancer, i.e. for those men in whom the application of screening tests, subsequent diagnostics and early treatment is believed to be truly beneficial[1]. In this particular study, the tumor characteristics of those who underwent radical prostatectomy were compared with the recurrence of prostate-specific antigen (PSA) after surgery. Unfortunately, the median follow-up was short (33.0 months) and

the number of events was small. Furthermore, as PSA relapse is known to be an intermediate end-point after surgery, and in itself does not predict the occurrence of clinically progressing disease, firm conclusions on the prognostic value of radical prostatectomy tumor features could not be drawn. As time passes, and the European screening study continues its course towards completion, the exact (tumor) characteristics of those who may be cured definitively by radical prostatectomy, and alternatively of those who may not be helped by this operative procedure, may be defined and outlined more precisely. Still, we must understand that the precise window of opportunity in screening for prostate cancer can only be determined when large-scale randomized clinical trials have been completed and properly analyzed. Using the prostate cancer death rate as a definitive outcome measure of screening, the exact 'window of curability' may be defined in retrospection.

With extended follow-up and with a larger study cohort, this chapter again investigates the prognostic value of conventional pathological tumor features as assessed in the radical prostatectomy specimen. Some preoperative tumor features (e.g. PSA level, palpability and biopsy Gleason score) were also studied in terms of their association with intermediate prognostic

The European Randomized Study of Screening for Prostate Cancer (ERSPC), Study Group Rotterdam is a cooperative venture between the Department of Urology (C. H. Bangma, I. W. van der Cruijsen-Koeter, W. J. Kirkels, M. J. Roobol-Bouts, F. H. Schröder, M. F. Wildhagen), Department of Pathology (Th. H. van der Kwast, R. F. Hoedemaeker), Department of Clinical Chemistry (B. G. Blijenberg), the Comprehensive Cancer Center (R. A. M. Damhuis) and the Department of Public Health (G. Draisma, H. J. de Koning, P. J. van der Maas, S. Otto).

outcome measures as well as the recurrence of PSA (PSA relapse) after radical prostatectomy. More definitive outcome measures such as local recurrence of disease and the presence of metastatic disease have also been investigated. Thus, the aim of this chapter was to define further the boundaries of curable and incurable disease, and to gain more insight into the characteristics of cancers within the window of opportunity in the early detection of prostate cancer.

Materials and methods

Patient selection

We investigated 281 men who underwent radical prostatectomy at the Erasmus Medical Center Rotterdam (formerly, University Hospital Rotterdam) between June 1994 and December 1999. All men were participants in the screening arm of our randomized screening trial, i.e. the European Randomized study of Screening for Prostate Cancer (ERSPC), section Rotterdam. The first 218 surgically treated men had been subjects of an earlier investigation by our department[1], and their clinical, biochemical and biopsy tumor characteristics are outlined in detail elsewhere[1]. In brief, cancer diagnosis was made after the evaluation of an elevated PSA level (i.e. PSA $\geq$ 3.0 ng/ml), or a digital rectal examination (DRE) or transrectal ultrasound (TRUS) scan indicating 'suspicious for cancer' at low PSA values (0.0–2.9 ng/ml). In the case of an elevated PSA level and/or a suspicious rectal examination, a diagnostic biopsy was performed to obtain prostatic tissue. The biopsy procedure consisted of a systematic sextant biopsy as described in detail by Rietbergen and colleagues[2]. Additional biopsies were taken from hypoechoic or palpable lesions when present. The decision to undergo radical prostatectomy was made by the patient and his treating urologist, considering the patient's age, his comorbidities, biopsy tumor features and personal preferences. All patients underwent bilateral pelvic lymph node dissection prior to radical prostatectomy, and none received (hormonal) treatment prior to operation.

Patient follow-up and definition of intermediate end-points

All patients were followed at intervals of 3 months for the first year after radical prostatectomy, semi-annually for the second year, and yearly thereafter for evidence of PSA relapse and clinical progression. Two definitions of PSA relapse were used. The first definition was strict at two sequential detectable PSA levels of 0.1 ng/ml and higher, whereas the second definition demanded that serum PSA had to reach a level of 0.4 ng/ml at least. This latter definition was chosen to identify cases believed to be at high risk (or that already showed evidence) of clinical disease progression. Time to biochemical progression was defined as the time from radical prostatectomy to the time of (first) recurrence of serum PSA, or until last follow-up, if the patient did not experience PSA relapse. Clinical progression was defined as local recurrence of disease as proven by a positive prostate cancer histology finding near the vesicourethral anastomosis site, and/or the presence of metastatic disease as indicated by hot spots on bone scintigraphy and/or suspicious-for-prostate-cancer lesions on abdominal computerized tomography (CT), magnetic resonance imaging (MRI), thoracic X-ray imaging or ultrasound imaging of the liver. Time to clinical recurrence was defined as the time from radical prostatectomy to the time of first recording of clinical recurrence, or to the date of last follow-up if the subject did not have evidence of clinical progression. No patient received adjuvant hormonal or radiation therapy, until eventual PSA relapse or clinical progression occurred. Two patients died within 1 year after radical prostatectomy without evidence of recurrent prostate cancer.

Conventional pathology

All radical prostatectomy specimens were fixed, totally embedded and processed according to well-established protocols[3,4]. For each case, a biopsy and radical prostatectomy Gleason score was determined, the number of positive-for-malignancy cores was determined and the tumor was staged according to the TNM 1997 classification (tumor, nodes, metastasis) by a single genitourinary pathologist. Considering the proportion of high-grade cancer (Gleason growth pattern 4/5), three main prognostic categories were distinguished: I, no high-grade cancer; II, 0–50% high-grade cancer; III, ≥ 50% high-grade cancer. The presence of tumor cells at the inked margin of resection was considered a positive surgical margin. All tumor areas were traced and outlined on the slides, and subsequent morphometric analysis was performed to determine the tumor volume as described in detail by Hoedemaeker and colleagues[5].

Evaluation and validation of tumor classification model

Cancers were classified based on combined conventional tumor characteristics into minimal, moderate and advanced disease according to the definition reported elsewhere[1] (Figure 1). This categorization model combines independent prognostic tumor features such as pathological tumor stage, tumor volume and proportion of high-grade cancer. *Minimal* cancers are those tumors that, although cured by radical prostatectomy, justify that treatment is delayed without endangering the host. These cancers are thought to be organ-confined (pT$_2$), have a tumor volume of less than 0.5 ml and lack high-grade tumor components. *Advanced* cancers are those tumors that recur quickly after radical prostatectomy, have mostly adverse prognostic tumor characteristics and are not expected to be cured by radical prostatectomy alone. These are thought to be cancers that grow into adjacent organs such as the bladder (pT$_4$) or seminal vesicles (pT$_{3b}$), or which contain more than 0.5 ml of high-grade cancer. *Moderate* cancers are those tumors that are cured by operative intervention, have some adverse prognostic tumor features as well and are believed to be treated in time. In the absence of early detection programs, these cancers would show signs and lead to complaints, and to mortality later on. The features of moderate cancers fall in between those of minimal and advanced cancers.

Cancers were also classified according to their specimen-confinability. In this procedure, the surgical margin status of the cancers was considered, and this independent prognostic parameter was combined with the tumor classification model.

Statistical analysis

Statistical analysis was performed using the Statistical Package for the Social Sciences (SPSS 9.0; SPSS Inc., Chicago, IL). Cox proportional regression analysis was used to assess the relationship between postoperative variables and PSA relapse and clinical progression (i.e. local recurrence, metastatic disease) after radical prostatectomy. Gleason score, pathological tumor stage, proportion of high-grade cancer, tumor volume and surgical margins were categorized according to Table 1. Kaplan–Meier curves were constructed to show the probability of remaining free of PSA relapse and clinical progression of disease, as a function of time after radical prostatectomy.

Results

Patient characteristics

For the cohort of 281 included patients, the mean age was 64 years (standard deviation, SD ± 4.6), and the median PSA level at the time of biopsy was 5.2 ng/ml (range 0.8–29.5). The median follow-up was 50 months (range 5–89). No patient had positive lymph nodes on fresh–frozen tissue examination intraoperatively, while just one patient experienced metastatic lymph node disease after the evaluation of paraffin slides (i.e. pT$_{3b}$pN$_1$). The median tumor volume was 0.65 ml (range 0.001–13.48). PSA relapse, i.e. ≥ 0.1 ng/ml and ≥ 0.4 ng/ml, occurred in 34 (12.1%) and 25 (8.9%) patients, respectively, after a median follow-up of 15.5 months (range 1–68) and 12.0 months (range 1–41) after radical prostatectomy. Evidence of clinical progression of disease occured in eight patients (2.8%) after a median follow-up of 28.0 months (range 17–38) after treatment. Four of these had local

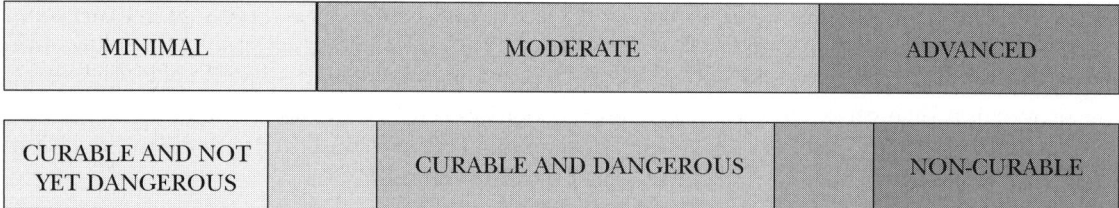

Figure 1 According to the tumor classification model, tumors with features corresponding to minimal disease are assessed as curable and not yet dangerous, while tumors with features of advanced disease are already beyond the reach of cure. All cancers with features in between those of minimal and advanced (i.e. moderate) disease are assumed to cause severe prostate cancer complaints and mortality in the absence of screening and treatment. Still, these cancers may be cured with the current treatment options

recurrent disease and five experienced dissemination of disease at distal sites, whereas one man had both locally and distally progressing disease. All clinically progressing patients had PSA levels of more than 0.4 ng/ml (and rising) after treatment. None of the patients who progressed clinically progressed without a prior or concomitant PSA relapse.

Prognostic impact of conventional postoperative tumor features

Table 1 gives the distribution of postoperative tumor features and their correlation to PSA relapse (≥ 0.1 ng/ml and ≥ 0.4 ng/ml), and clinical progression of disease. For PSA relapse, only a proportion of men within the various prognostic groups had evidence of biochemical recurrent disease, e.g. 7.1–52.4% for pT_2 to pT_{3b-4} disease, and 32.8% for men with positive surgical margins, for PSA ≥ 0.1 ng/ml. An adverse prognostic postoperative parameter constituted a higher risk of progression, although did not imply that progression of disease was to be expected.

Of the eight men who progressed clinically, six were found to have tumors that invaded adjacent organs such as the bladder or the seminal vesicles. Four of these had evidence of metastatic disease later on, while two had disease that recurred locally only. One patient who progressed had a tumor with extraprostatic extension and a large volume of high-grade cancer (i.e. > 3.0 ml), and showed intraosseal metastases after 19 months after radical prostatectomy. The last progressing man had organ-

confined cancer with clear positive surgical margins at the lateral confines of the prostate, with intrapelvic recurrence after 23 months.

Tumor classification model

Table 2 indicates the risk of progression (PSA, clinically) when tumors were categorized according to the tumor classification model (minimal, moderate, advanced disease), and when the surgical margin status of the tumors was also assessed (see also Figure 2).

Preoperative tumor features and progression of disease

Of the men who had PSA relapse, defined as ≥ 0.1 ng/ml and ≥ 0.4 ng/ml, one (4.8%) and one (4.8%) had a PSA level of 1.0–1.9 ng/ml preoperatively, one (7.7%) and none (0.0%) had a PSA 2.0–2.9 ng/ml, one (2.4%) and one (2.4%) had a PSA 3.0–3.9 ng/ml, 23 (13.9%) and 16 (9.7%) had a PSA 4.0–9.9 ng/ml and eight (23.5%) and seven (20.6%) had a PSA level above 10.0 ng/ml, respectively. These figures were 14 (6.9%) and 10 (4.9%) for Gleason scores 2–6, 16 (24.2%) and 12 (18.2%) for Gleason score 7 and four (33.3%) and three (25.0%) for Gleason scores 8–10, respectively. Twenty-four (19.7%) and 19 (15.6%) of the progressing tumors were palpable when ≥ 0.1 ng/ml and ≥ 0.4 ng/ml were considered as PSA relapse, respectively.

All clinically progressing men had a preoperative PSA level above 4.0 ng/ml, which prompted biopsy, three of whom had a PSA level

Table 1 Distribution of postoperative tumor features of screened participants of the European Randomized study of Screening for Prostate Cancer (ERSPC), section Rotterdam ($n = 281$), and the number of men who had prostate-specific antigen (PSA) progression and clinically recurrent disease after radical prostatectomy

Variable	Progression after radical prostatectomy			
	PSA (≥ 0.1 ng/ml) (n (% of total))	PSA (≥ 0.4 ng/ml) (n (% of total))	Clinically (n (% of total))	Total (n)
Pathological stage				
pT_2	15 (7.1)	9 (4.3)	1 (0.5)	211
pT_{3a}	8 (16.3)	6 (12.2)	1 (2.0)	49
pT_{3b-4}	11 (52.4)	10 (47.6)	6 (28.6)	21
Gleason score				
2–6	8 (4.8)	7 (4.2)	1 (0.6)	165
7	21 (19.3)	14 (12.8)	4 (3.7)	109
8–10	5 (71.4)	4 (57.1)	3 (42.9)	7
Percentage high-grade				
0–50	20 (7.8)	14 (5.5)	3 (1.2)	256
≥ 50	14 (56.0)	11 (44.0)	5 (20.0)	25
Tumor volume (ml)				
< 0.5	3 (2.8)	2 (1.8)	0 (0.0)	109
0.5–1.0	6 (8.5)	4 (5.6)	1 (1.4)	71
≥ 1.0	25 (24.8)	19 (18.8)	7 (6.9)	101
Surgical margin				
Positive	22 (32.8)	14 (20.9)	3 (4.5)	67
Negative	12 (5.6)	11 (5.1)	5 (2.3)	214
Total	34 (12.1)	25 (8.9)	8 (2.8)	281

Table 2 Distribution of screened participants of the European Randomized study of Screening for Prostate Cancer (ERSPC), section Rotterdam ($n = 281$), when these were categorized according to the tumor classification model, and its association with prostate-specific antigen (PSA) progression and clinically recurrent disease after radical prostatectomy. For definition of minimal, moderate and advanced disease, see text

Variable	Progression after radical prostatectomy			
	PSA (≥ 0.1 ng/ml) (n (% of total))	PSA (≥ 0.4 ng/ml) (n (% of total))	Clinically (n (% of total))	Total (n)
Tumor classification (1)				
Minimal	1 (1.4)	1 (1.4)	0 (0.0)	73
Moderate	11 (7.6)	6 (4.1)	1 (0.7)	145
Advanced	22 (34.9)	18 (28.6)	7 (11.1)	63
Tumor classification (2)				
Min/Mod + SC	1 (0.6)	1 (0.6)	0 (0.0)	176
Min/Mod + Non-SC	11 (26.2)	6 (14.3)	1 (2.4)	42
Advanced + SC	11 (28.2)	10 (25.6)	5 (12.8)	39
Advanced + Non-SC	11 (45.8)	8 (33.3)	2 (8.3)	24
Total	34 (12.1)	25 (8.9)	8 (2.8)	281

Min, minimal; Mod, moderate; SC, specimen-confined, i.e. with negative surgical margins; Non-SC, non-specimen-confined, i.e. with positive surgical margins

above 10.0 ng/ml. All men had palpable lesions, three had a biopsy Gleason score of 6, three had a biopsy Gleason score of 7 (all, 3 + 4), and one had high-grade components on biopsy only (i.e. Gleason score 8).

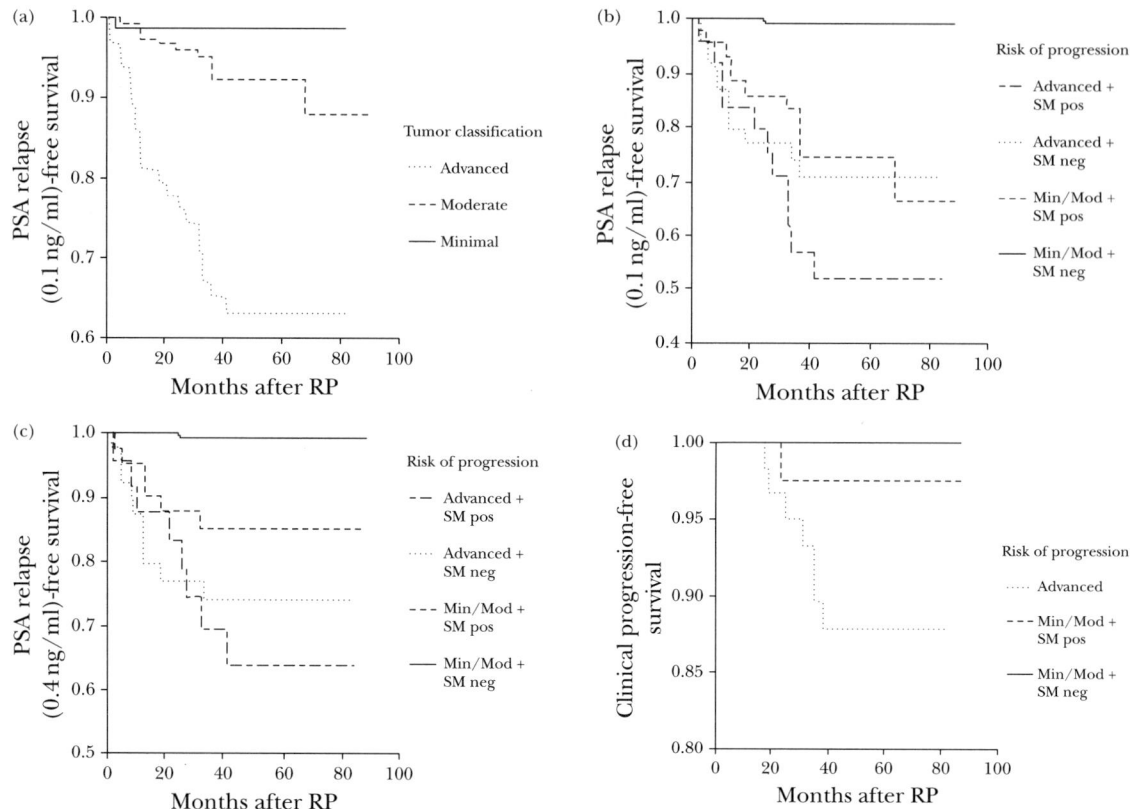

Figure 2 Kaplan–Meier curves of the probability of disease recurrence after radical prostatectomy (RP) as a function of the tumor classification model, divided into: minimal disease (Min), moderate disease (Mod) and advanced disease, and specimen-confinability, divided into: surgical margin (SM) positive (pos) and surgical margin negative (neg). (a) Prostate-specific antigen (PSA) relapse (≥ 0.1 ng/ml) as a function of the tumor classification model. (b) PSA relapse (≥ 0.1 ng/ml) as a function of the tumor classification model and specimen-confinability. (c) PSA relapse (≥ 0.4 ng/ml) as a function of the tumor classification model and specimen-confinability. (d) Clinical progression of disease as a function of the tumor classification model and specimen-confinability

Discussion

Screening for prostate cancer remains a widely disputed area of scientific research. At present, large-scale screening trials for prostate cancer with approximately 300 000 men randomized are being performed in Western Europe and the USA to investigate the sense (or non-sense) of such early detection programs. Recent reports on breast cancer have questioned the earlier reported benefits of screening for breast cancer with mammography, with respect to the decline in breast cancer mortality[6]. As a consequence of these intense disputes about breast cancer screening, the outcomes of yet unfinished early

detection studies of prostate cancer will be viewed closely and suspiciously. Thus, efforts should be made to scrutinize and analyze these early detection programs properly and unambiguously. The potential negative side-effects of screening are not easily tolerated, and are justified only when an unequivocal decrease in the number of cases with metastatic (incurable) disease is proven as a result of the application of screening tests and subsequent early treatment. However, as the results of large-scale randomized controlled trials with prostate cancer death rate as an end-point are awaited, it is anticipated that a proportion of these screen-detected prostate cancers may still be detected and treated unnecessarily as they have seemingly innocuous tumor characteristics. In the absence of treatment, these prostate cancers might not have caused clinical signs and symptoms in their host. Again, the disputes about breast cancer screening made clear that detection (and treatment) of these 'clinically insignificant' or 'overdiagnosed' cases should be avoided at all costs. Conversely, it is likely that some men diagnosed with prostate cancer in early detection programs are treated with erroneous curative intent, since the treated tumors have features associated with poor prognosis, and these cancers recur quickly after radical prostatectomy or radiation therapy. These cancers could have been better treated with antihormonal therapy initially. If prostate cancer screening were to be introduced as a general health-care measure, in which many asymptomatic men would be subjected to screening tests, cancers detected should be those that are potentially aggressive (in the absence of screening), although which may still be cured with radical treatment (in the presence of screening). These cancers, treatment of which will eventually reduce the prostate cancer mortality rate, are said to be in the 'window of opportunity' in studies of screening for prostate cancer, or otherwise, in the 'window of curability' when treatment of prostate cancer (both screen-detected or non-screen-detected) is meant.

In an attempt to define the boundaries of curable and incurable prostate cancer in yet unfinished screening trials, the (PSA) recurrence rate after treatment with curative intent is indicative of the aggressiveness of disease and its final outcome. In our study, the rate of a detectable serum PSA level after radical prostatectomy was low, especially when compared with figures reported in literature[7–9]. When a serum level of 0.1 ng/ml was used to define PSA relapse, only 12.1% of men showed evidence of biochemical disease recurrence at a median of 50.0 months (i.e. 4.2 years) of follow-up, and this figure was 8.9% when a PSA of 0.4 ng/ml and higher was used as the definition of failure. The chance of remaining free of disease at 3 years and 5 years of follow-up was 177 of 208 (85.1%) and 77 of 92 (83.7%), respectively. Thus, most relapses

occurred within 3 years after radical prostatectomy. In line with Pound and colleagues[9], we propose that radical prostatectomy provides for excellent (long-term) cancer control in most cases with clinically confined prostate cancer. Furthermore, the vast majority of men who experienced clinical progression of disease had first evidence of biochemical recurrence within 2 years after radical prostatectomy, i.e. 87.5% of men. The chance of staying free of disease in cases with an undetectable PSA level after radical prostatectomy was 178 of 184 (96.7%) and 77 of 78 (98.7%) at 3 and 5 years of follow-up, respectively. This implies that these men may be considered more and more likely to be curatively treated as these time points after surgery are reached. The present study also showed that the number of men who progressed clinically (i.e. locally and/or distally) after radical prostatectomy was small, i.e. eight of 281 men (2.8%). Moreover, clinical progression of disease never occurred without a prior PSA relapse, and in our study did not occur when a postoperative PSA level of at least 0.4 ng/ml was measured. Our low reported figure of clinically progressing cases after curative treatment may be explained by the knowledge that the lead time for prostate cancer, which is expected to be at least 4–8 years, was only just passed. The number of cases progressing clinically might thus further increase in forthcoming years. In fact, there are 17 men in follow-up in whom the PSA level has already risen above the 0.4 ng/ml threshold, although in whom we were not able to prove progression of disease clinically. These cases are scrutinized in follow-up. Another explanation for our low reported figure of clinically progressing cases is the finding that some of the men who failed biochemically had already started antiandrogen treatment (i.e. orchidectomy, treatment with luteinizing hormone-releasing hormone agonists) after the first indication of a detectable (and rising) PSA level. It is evident that the application of early hormonal treatment in these cases caused PSA to fall below the 0.4-ng/ml level, and even to undetectable levels in some men. Early application of endocrine treatment after the first evidence of PSA failure has been a matter of debate in the peer-reviewed literature. Suppression of the male endocrine system is known to have a drastic negative influence on a man's quality of life with, for example, loss of libido, sexual dysfunction and loss of energy and drive, and does not by any means give certainty that years are added to life. Until clear evidence is presented, early hormonal treatment in men with a rising PSA after radical prostatectomy is a matter of personal preference for doctor and patient. To date, endocrine treatment has been applied only infrequently at our institution in cases with PSA relapse only.

Our results again indicate that a clear association exists between conventional prognostic tumor features as assessed in the radical prostatectomy specimen and disease outcome after radical prostatectomy. Pathological tumor stage, volume of cancer with Gleason grades 4 and 5 and surgical margin status all had independent prognostic value when either of the intermediate outcome measures was concerned (data not given). Of the cases that progressed after treatment, the vast majority had one or more of the adverse prognostic tumor features, such as invasion into periprostatic organs (i.e. bladder, seminal vesicles), a volume of more than 0.5 ml high-grade cancer and/or a positive surgical margin (Tables 1 and 2). We have also shown that the preoperative prediction of relapse using preoperative variables is of only little additional value. For instance, the positive predictive value of an adverse preoperative prognostic factor for PSA relapse ≥ 0.1 ng/ml was relatively low, for example 23.5% for PSA ≥ 10.0 ng/ml, 33.3% for biopsy Gleason scores of 8–10 and 18.8% for 3–6 positive-for-prostate-cancer biopsies. Moreover, surgical margin status (an important independent prognostic factor) has no preoperative equivalent, and can only be considered after surgery. As a consequence, we are not in any way able to predict the natural course of disease in those diagnosed with the disease. As conventional radical prostatectomy tumor features are far more superior in predicting patient outcome than preoperative clinical, biochemical and biopsy tumor parameters, single or combined, future efforts should be directed towards

predicting tumor features in the radical prostatectomy specimen using these pretreatment variables. The use of nomograms that combine different prognostic factors for the determination of a specific outcome parameter might assist in adequate individual assessment of the extent of disease, or the risk of progression and metastases[8,10]. Also, artificial neural network (ANN) analysis and computer and regression tree (CART) analysis are being investigated, regarding their use in the prediction of prostate cancer outcome measures.

We provide a tumor classification model using prognostically independent pathological features in the radical prostatectomy specimen. In this, we show that a subdividing of cancers into prognostic subgroups:

(1) Not yet dangerous;

(2) Dangerous but still curable;

(3) Dangerous, but not curable;

is feasible, and that patients can be advised of appropriate treatment, such as:

(1) Close surveillance;

(2) Curative treatment;

(3) Palliative treatment and support;

in line with their particular needs and the tumor classification model (Figure 1). We realize that the tumor classification model is not in any way 'waterproof', and remains to be investigated further. Cases with presumably innocuous tumor features should be followed with care, as it is known that prostate cancer is an unpredictable disease, and some of the 'harmless' cancers may still progress clinically. Also, it might well be that cases with advanced disease at the time of screen detection will benefit from early detection, for instance, by means of radical prostatectomy with or without the application of adjuvant radiotherapy or antihormonal treatment. In our study, only 35% of men with features of advanced disease progressed, implying that other yet unknown host and tumor-related factors also play a role in the final outcome of disease. With reference to the good work of Albertsen and colleagues, it must again be emphasized that the age of a screened man, and the severity of his comorbidities, are as much predictors of outcome as are the characteristics of the tumor[11].

In conclusion, the question whether screening for prostate cancer is truly beneficial at a population level, and could be accepted as a general health-care measure, can only be finally answered after randomized clinical trials have been completed and analyzed. Data will not be available until half-way through the present decade. Eventually, features of screen-detected prostate cancers leading to metastatic disease and prostate cancer mortality, and, conversely, features of those that may be cured definitively with the currently available treatment options, will only be defined in retrospection.

Acknowledgements

We wish to thank Mrs Monique Roobol for collecting ERSPC data with respect to the clinical follow-up of men who underwent radical prostatectomy at the Erasmus Medical Center Rotterdam (EMCR). We also wish to thank Professor Theo van de Kwast, pathologist, for his continuous support and enthusiasm, his careful review of the present chapter and his prior efforts in grading and staging the radical prostatectomy specimens. Last, we wish to thank Professor Fritz Schröder, urologist, for his support, his scientific comments and of course his invitation to participate in and speak at the PACIOU VII and DUA VII congress.

References

1. Vis AN, Hoedemaeker RF, Van der Kwast ThH, *et al*. Defining a window of opportunity in screening for prostate cancer; validation of a predictive tumor classification model. *Prostate* 2001;46: 154–62

2. Rietbergen JBW, Boeken Kruger AE, Kranse R, *et al*. Complications of transrectal ultrasound (TRUS) guided systematic sextant biopsies of the prostate: evaluation of complication rates and risk factors within a population based screening program. *Urology* 1997;49:875–80

3. Stamey TA, McNeal JE, Freiha FS, *et al*. Morphometric and clinical studies on 68 consecutive radical prostatectomies. *J Urol* 1988;139:1235–41

4. Hoedemaeker RF, Ruijter ETG, Ruizeveld-de Winter JA, *et al*. The Biomed II MPC Study group. Processing radical prostatectomy specimens. *J Urol Pathol* 1998;9:211–22

5. Hoedemaeker RF, Rietbergen JBW, Kranse R, *et al*. Comparison of pathological characteristics of T1c and non-T1c cancers detected in a population-based screening study, the European Randomized study of Screening for Prostate Cancer. *World J Urol* 1997;15:339–45

6. Gotzsche PC, Olsen O. Is screening for breast cancer with mammography justifiable? *Lancet* 2000;355:124–34

7. Zincke H, Oesterling JE, Blute ML, *et al*. Long-term (15 years) results after radical prostatectomy for clinically localized (stage T2c or lower) prostate cancer. *J Urol* 1994;152:1850–7

8. Kattan MW, Wheeler TM, Scardino PT. Postoperative nomogram for disease recurrence after radical prostatectomy for prostate cancer. *J Clin Oncol* 1999;17:1499–507

9. Pound CR, Partin AW, Eisenberger MA, *et al*. Natural history of progression after PSA elevation following radical prostatectomy. *J Am Med Assoc* 1999;281:1591–7

10. Partin AW, Kattan MW, Subong EN, *et al*. Combination of prostate-specific antigen, clinical stage, and Gleason score to predict pathological stage of localized prostate cancer. A multi-institutional update. *J Am Med Assoc* 1997; 277:1445–51

11. Albertsen PC, Hanley JM, Gleason DF, *et al*. A competing risk analysis of men aged 55 to 74 years at diagnosis managed conservatively for clinically localized prostate cancer. *J Am Med Assoc* 1998;280:975–80

Screening for prostate cancer: views from the UK and the rest of the world

28

F. C. Hamdy

'Primum non nocere'...

Hippocrates

Introduction

Prostate cancer is a significant cause of morbidity and mortality in the USA and Europe. In the USA alone, an estimated 189 000 new prostate cancer cases will be diagnosed in 2002, with 30 200 deaths attributable to the disease[1]. The natural aging of the population, combined with the continued and widespread use of improved diagnostic tests such as that for serum prostate-specific antigen (PSA), is resulting in an increase in the numbers of men diagnosed with localized prostate cancer. Screening to identify organ-confined prostate cancer has provoked much public and scientific attention, and there is intense debate about its role in improving men's health. While there are strong advocates of screening, the findings from most reviews of the scientific evidence conclude that it is insufficient, at present, to recommend routine population screening because of the lack of evidence that this would improve survival and the quality of men's lives. Particular concerns in these reviews relate to the lack of knowledge about the natural history of screen-detected disease, and the lack of evidence about the effectiveness of treatments. In particular, to date, no survival advantage has been shown in screen-detected cases for any of the major treatments (radical prostatectomy, radical radiotherapy including brachytherapy and 'watchful waiting'), and each can result in damaging iatrogenic complications and outcomes, including various levels of incontinence and impotence for radical interventions and

anxiety relating to the presence of cancer in 'watchful waiting'.

The purpose of screening is to identify a group of asymptomatic men with early-stage, organ-confined prostate cancer who would benefit from early radical intervention. 'Benefit' from radical intervention can be expressed only in terms of prolonged survival and/or improved quality of life. To date, there is no evidence from any data available in the literature that these benefits can be obtained by the establishment of mass screening programs.

General criteria for establishing a screening program

In 1968, Wilson and Jungner[2] established key principles that a disease should satisfy before introducing screening as a public-health policy. The most important of these criteria are discussed in the light of available evidence in prostate cancer.

The disease should be an important health problem

With the incidence and mortality figures quoted above, there is little doubt that prostate cancer represents a significant public-health burden in Western countries. In the USA, men have a lifetime risk of 1 : 6 for developing prostate cancer[1]. However, the disease will not necessarily cause their death, which in many cases will occur from other causes, such as cardiovascular disease. The burden to the community is significant, and although a clear stage migration is observed as a consequence of screening[3], men who are diagnosed with advanced prostate cancer develop metastatic disease at the rate of 8% per year, reaching 40% at 5 years. These metastases affect the skeleton predominantly, causing high levels of morbidity, hospitalization and expensive palliation. In addition, treatment of advanced disease, largely hormonal in nature, causes known iatrogenic morbidity by reducing bone density and inducing osteoporosis, again leading to skeletal-related events requiring either prophylaxis using agents such as bisphosphonates, or treatment to correct the complications. Although the ultimate aim of a screening program is to reduce mortality by treating the disease early, consideration must be given to consequences of initiating immediate treatment in early advanced disease, as a result of stage migration. It would be improper to initiate a screening program if immediate treatment of these men is likely to reduce their quality of life, increase the burden on health resources and exceed the benefits obtained from screening for truly localized disease, if any.

There should be a preclinical state more amenable to successful treatment than clinical disease

This remains unclear in prostate cancer, largely because of the rather loose definition attributed to 'clinically significant' disease. Beyond stage migration, methods of detection are being refined continually in prostate cancer[4–8]. The majority of cases detected are T1c cancers with low serum PSA values. Different molecular forms of PSA are being evaluated to enhance detection, and the exact ability of these tests to detect inconsequential cancers found at autopsy remains unknown. Furthermore, the well-known histopathological entity of high-grade prostatic intraepithelial neoplasia (HGPIN), associated in approximately 50% of cases with invasive carcinoma, is thought to be a precursor of prostate cancer[9]. However, insufficient proof prevents HGPIN from representing the 'preclinical' state as required by screening principles.

There should be an acceptable screening instrument for the disease

The advent of PSA measurement in the late 1980s as a simple blood test to suspect prostate cancer has revolutionized its diagnosis. While the combination of PSA, digital rectal examination (DRE), transrectal ultrasound (TRUS) and biopsies remains conventional for confirming the diagnosis and staging the disease[10], it is now accepted that neither DRE nor TRUS should be included in screening for prostate cancer[11]. Many pilot and larger-scale studies have demonstrated the wide acceptability of screening by PSA. However, an infrequently asked question remains unanswered: what is the psychological effect of PSA screening in men whose PSA is raised, but cancer cannot be found? There is a paucity of quality-of-life studies addressing these important issues.

There should be an accepted and effective treatment

Until very recently, there was a significant lack of first-degree evidence that aggressive treatment of localized prostate cancer improves survival and/or quality of life. This missing evidence can only emerge from well-conducted large randomized controlled trials, comparing treatment options. Such a trial has indeed been performed in Scandinavia, and first results were published recently[12,13]. The trial randomized 695 men with clinically localized prostate cancer to either watchful waiting or radical prostatectomy (RP). Median follow-up was 6.2 years. The most important findings were a 50% reduction in disease-specific mortality from prostate cancer, in favor of RP, and a 14% increased risk of progression to metastatic disease in patients receiving watchful waiting, as well as a 40% increase in local progression. There was no difference, however, in overall mortality between the two groups, and morbidity from the surgery was significant, with 49% incontinence and 100% erectile dysfunction rates – results which are incompatible with current standard surgical practice in institutions dealing with large numbers of patients[14]. The study has a number of limitations:

(1) It precedes the PSA testing era;

(2) More than 50% of men were symptomatic, an unusual finding in contemporary practice, where most men have T1c disease with low PSA levels;

(3) The criteria for local progression in the watchful waiting arm were unreliable, defined by subjective DRE and bladder outflow obstruction symptoms;

(4) Seventeen patients needed to be treated to prolong one man's disease-specific survival;

(5) There was no difference in overall survival between the two groups.

In addition, the authors did not present detailed pathological staging of patients receiving RP, i.e. rates of positive margins and up-staging, and it is not known whether patients found to have positive nodes at surgery were given hormone manipulation. One may therefore conclude that the effectiveness of treatment in screen-detected prostate cancer remains unproven. In the USA, the Prostate Cancer Versus Observation Trial (PIVOT) has been recruiting and randomizing men under the age of 75 to a trial of treatment, comparing radical prosta-tectomy with expectant management, with all-cause mortality as a primary end-point. The trial has closed recently, having recruited 731 men, and results are awaited[15]. Researchers in the UK have recently launched a large random-ized trial of treatment, following the success of a feasibility study performed over the past 2 years. The ProtecT (Prostate testing for cancer and Treatment) study will recruit 130 000 men aged 50–69 years over a period of 5 years from nine regions of the UK, and randomize approxi-mately 2000 patients with clinically localized prostate cancer to a trial of treatment com-paring active monitoring, radical prostatectomy and three-dimensional conformal external beam radiotherapy. The main aim is to investigate the effectiveness of treatment in terms of survival at 10 years and quality of life. It is likely that screening issues will also be

informed by the trial[16]. Preliminary results will become available by 2008, at the same time as the much-awaited results from screening studies in Europe: the European Randomized Screening for Prostate Cancer (ERSPC) trial, and in the USA: the Prostate, Lung, Colon and Ovary cancer trial (PLCO).

The natural history of the disease should be known

The natural history of prostate cancer is known only, to some extent, in relation to the pre-PSA era, which makes any data difficult to translate in contemporary terms. In clinical practice, it has become customary to state that unless a man has a minimum 10-year life expectancy, he is unlikely to benefit from treatment. This first observation – which still holds true – appears to have originated in the late 1960s[17], when it was recognized that competing medical co-morbidity is more likely to cause patient death than prostate cancer. Other studies from Sweden analyzed the natural history of the disease, following up patients for an average of 14 years[18,19]. The studies demonstrated that the higher were the stage and grade of the disease, the more likely were the patients to die of prostate cancer, with many men with well- and moderately differentiated, low-volume disease showing a favorable outcome. A further multi-center and international analysis of outcomes in patients receiving no active treatment showed similar findings, with poorly differentiated cancers being particularly fatal[20]. Two further interesting studies, one analyzing the SEER (Surveillance, Epidemiology and End Results) database, and the other the Connecticut Tumor Registry, confirmed that men with well-differentiated cancers did best, while patients with moderately to poorly differentiated disease had their survival curtailed by 4–8 years if treated conservatively[21,22]. The PSA era is likely to revolutionize these previous observations. Most men detected through PSA testing have T1c disease, and contemporary lead times are long (6–8 years). Lead time biases may there-fore influence the perception of prolonged survival of contemporary men with screen-detected prostate cancer.

Does screening for prostate cancer reduce mortality from the disease?

Following the development of the PSA test, screening for early prostate cancer has become prevalent in the USA, with a sharp rise in incidence of the disease in the early 1990s (Figure 1). This was paralleled by a static incidence rate in countries where screening was not practiced, such as the UK. By 1996, the USA started to experience a slow but constant decrease in mortality rate associated with prostate cancer, which was advocated by some as resulting from the intensive screening program, associated with early aggressive intervention. This conclusion is flawed with a number of problems. First, in view of the protracted natural history of the disease, it is unlikely that the effect of treatment caused this reduction in mortality. Second, a similar reduction in mortality rates was observed in countries where screening had not been adopted, such as England and Wales, suggesting that other factors must have been involved in this continuing reduction in mortality from the disease, including diet and environmental factors, yet to be determined[23] (Figure 2). Similarly, in the Tyrol region of

Austria, intensive screening and treatment of early disease has been associated with a 42% reduction in mortality. Again this 'cause and effect' association has yet to be confirmed, and it is clear that the current reduction in mortality in Tyrol cannot be attributed to screening alone[3].

More recently, Lu-Yao and colleagues[24] analyzed rates of screening and treatment as well as outcome in two different areas of the USA: 94 000 men in Seattle and 120 621 men in Connecticut, using the SEER database. Over an 11-year period of follow-up, in Seattle, intensive PSA screening (5.39-fold compared with Connecticut) and treatment (5.9-fold for radical prostatectomy and 2.3-fold for radiotherapy) did not lead to an improved disease-specific survival rate for prostate cancer, compared with the Connecticut practice.

How can we study screening?

Screening for prostate cancer can be studied by randomized controlled trials, which are under way in Europe and the USA. This involves randomizing a population of men at risk of harboring the disease, with a good life expectancy, to either an intensive screening program or no screening. The outcome is measured by analyzing differences in mortality between the

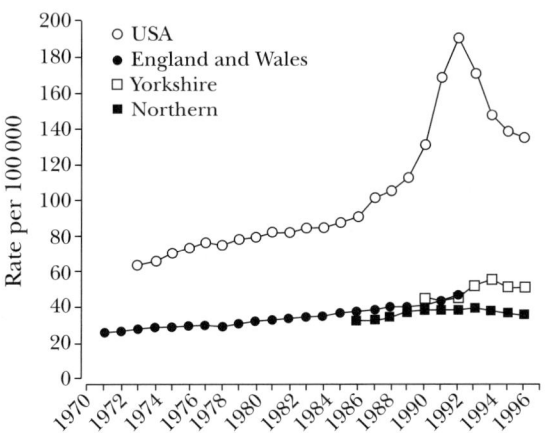

Figure 1 Age-standardized incidence of prostate cancer. Reprinted with permission from Elsevier (*Lancet* 2000;355:1788–9)

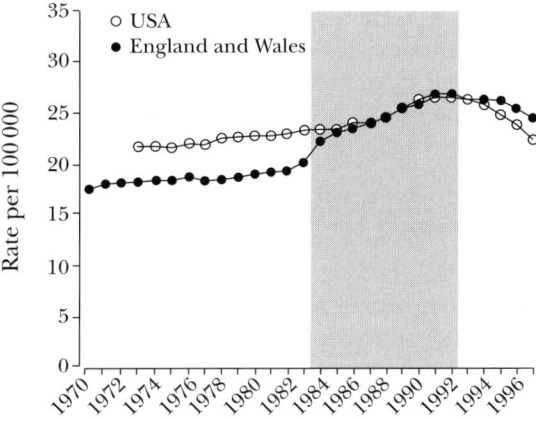

Figure 2 Age-standardized mortality from prostate cancer. Reprinted with permission from Elsevier (*Lancet* 2000;355:1788–9)

two groups, on the assumption that the screened group would have received early aggressive intervention, compared with the non-screened group. The ERSPC trial and the PLCO cancer trial in the USA represent such examples[25]. Data from the two studies are being merged, and results are expected by approximately 2008. The ERSPC trial was planned with a total sample of 190 000 men aged 55–74 years, involving The Netherlands, Belgium, Finland, Italy, Sweden, Spain and Switzerland. However, over time targets have changed, and it is now estimated that 120 000 men will be required in the intervention arm, and 140 000 in the control arm. Age range was also altered to 55–69 years. These changes were implemented to take into account the variability of countries involved, and the increasing rate of contamination (i.e. men in the control arm seeking PSA screening for prostate cancer and potentially receiving treatment), which has been ranging from 10 to 30%. The aim of the study is to detect a 20% difference in prostate cancer mortality between the two groups, with a statistical power of 90%. However, treatments are not defined in these studies, and a significant proportion of men may elect for watchful waiting. This is compounded by the uncertainty of treatment effectiveness, and ever-increasingly sensitive methods of detection, which may not allow the screening studies to show differences sufficient to have an impact on public-health policies. Despite these reservations, results are awaited eagerly, and will represent a phenomenal milestone in determining the value of screening in reducing mortality from prostate cancer.

What do men with prostate cancer think of screening for the disease?

Men's perception of screening for prostate cancer varies. A recent interesting study by Chapple and colleagues[26] highlights these feelings, following accurate and elegant qualitative research. Fifty-two men with prostate cancer were interviewed in various geographic areas of the UK. Some true conceptions, but also many misconceptions, were revealed, such as:

'Early diagnosis brings better chances of cure', '5-year survival figures in America are higher than in Britain because of PSA screening programs', 'PSA testing is not taking place because of lack of resources in the National Health Service', 'Men should be tested for prostate cancer as women are for breast cancer', 'Men with urinary tract symptoms should all be tested for prostate cancer', 'The government is not spending enough money on prostate cancer treatment'. These examples of arguments from men with the disease can be mostly refuted, and reflect a profound lack of knowledge about prostate cancer in the general population, compounded by misleading information from the media. The study also showed clearly how ill prepared men are to suffer the consequences of screening and the surrounding controversies over treatment issues. The public does not appear to perceive an important aspect and consequence of screening, as highlighted by Thornton and Dixon-Woods in a recent editorial: that screening is about changing identities and becoming a patient, which is no trivial matter[27]. It is therefore our duty not only to inform and educate men about these difficult issues, but also to engage them firmly in decision- and policy-making in the management of prostate cancer.

Screening policies world-wide

Because of the uncertainties described above, it is not surprising to find that screening policies for prostate cancer differ considerably in most countries of the world, where prevalence is high. A recent survey of a large number of countries requested three specific pieces of information:

(1) Does the country have a mass screening program?

(2) Does the country encourage and allow early detection?

(3) Is the PSA test reimbursable[28]?

Interestingly, no single country in the world has a mass-screening program for prostate cancer. A large proportion of other countries allow early detection, and a few reimburse the cost of PSA testing. Even within certain countries, opinions and practices are divided. For instance, in the USA, the American Cancer Society and American Urological Association have recommended screening, since 1990, by DRE and PSA testing from the age of 50 years, while the US Preventive Services Task Force, American Academy of Family Physicians and American College of Physicians recommend not screening for prostate cancer[28-31] (and Perrin, personal communication). In the UK, opinions are divided. Some clinicians and a large part of the public, driven by patient-support groups and the media, advocate screening for prostate cancer as a public-health policy[26]. Others promote joining ongoing trials of screening in Europe, or advocate testing treatment effectiveness before screening[16]. In the early 1990s, a pilot study of screening was undertaken in the south-west, suggesting that British men would be amenable to a mass-screening program[32]. In 1996, the British Government commissioned two key systematic reviews of the literature[33,34]. These reviews led to the recommendation by health ministers that there was currently insufficient evidence to establish screening as a public-health policy in the UK, and that PSA measurement in asymptomatic men should be discouraged. In the year 2000, however, further recommendations were made, allowing men who request a PSA test to receive it, providing that adequate counselling is delivered regarding the uncertainties about the detection and treatment of prostate cancer[35]. Furthermore, in an attempt to improve delivery of cancer services generally in the UK, the Department of Health requested that all men whose PSA is elevated over 4 ng/ml should be seen by a urological surgeon within 2 weeks, for further management. The intellectual incompatibility between these rules and existing evidence about screening and the treatment of prostate cancer is flagrant, adding confusion to the existing uncertainties for physicians and patients alike.

Conclusions

The dilemmas surrounding the value of screening and treatment in clinically localized prostate cancer remain unresolved. Recently published work from Scandinavia has shed some light onto potential benefits of radical prostatectomy in preventing patients from dying of prostate cancer, although aggressive treatment did not improve overall survival compared with watchful waiting. Results from the now merged ERSPC in Europe and PLCO in the USA, as well as from the ProtecT study in the UK and PIVOT study in the USA, are awaited eagerly. It is reassuring for the medical community and prostate cancer patients world-wide that these longstanding dilemmas in the management of prostate cancer are being resolved through large, and robust, randomized controlled trials supported by governments and funding institutions in Europe and the USA. Having introduced this chapter with a famous quote by the venerable Greek philosopher Hippocrates, it is appropriate to end the discussion with the wise words of a contemporary North American colleague[36]:

'*Individual doctors must fulfill their responsibilities to patients. Men aged over 50 have a right to know about screening, regardless of whether health service providers fund it, and to decide for themselves which option to pursue. Whether patients will, or can, act on the information bears little on this duty.*'

Steven Woolf

References

1. Ahmedin J, Thomas A, Murray T, Thun M. Cancer statistics, 2002. *CA Cancer J Clin* 2002; 52:23–47

2. Wilson JMG, Jungner G. *Principles and practice of screening for disease.* Public health papers no. 34. Geneva: World Health Organization, 1968

3. Bartsch G, Horninger W, Klocker H, *et al.* Tyrol Prostate Cancer Screening Group. Prostate cancer mortality after introduction of prostate-specific antigen mass screening in the Federal State of Tyrol, Austria. *Urology* 2001;58:417–24

4. Catalona WJ, Smith DS, Ratliff TL, *et al.* Measurement of prostate specific antigen in serum as a screening test for prostate cancer. *N Engl J Med* 1991;324:1156–61

5. Brawer MK, Cheli CD, Neaman IE, *et al.* Complexed prostate specific antigen provides significant enhancement of specificity compared with total prostate specific antigen for detecting prostate cancer. *J Urol* 2000;163:1476–80

6. Recker F, Kwiatkowski MK, Piironen T, *et al.* Human glandular kallikrein as a tool to improve discrimination of poorly differentiated and non-organ confined cancer compared with prostate specific antigen. *Urology* 2000;55:481–5

7. Barry MJ. Clinical practice. Prostate-specific-antigen testing for early diagnosis of prostate cancer. *N Engl J Med* 2001;344:1373–7

8. Lilja H. Role of hK2, free PSA, and complexed PSA measurements in the very early detection of prostate cancer. *Eur Urol* 2001;39(Suppl 4):47–8

9. Häggman MJ, Macoska JA, Wojno KJ, Oesterling JE. The relationship between prostatic intra-epithelial neoplasia and prostate cancer: critical issues. *J Urol* 1997;158:12–22

10. Wilkinson BA, Hamdy FC. State-of-the-art staging in prostate cancer. *BJU Int* 2001;87:423–30

11. Holmberg L, Bill-Axelson A, Helgesen F, *et al.* A randomized trial comparing radical prostatectomy with watchful waiting in early prostate cancer; Scandinavian Prostatic Cancer Group Study Number 4. *N Engl J Med* 2002;347:781–9

12. Steineck G, Helgesen F, Adolfsson J, *et al.* Quality of life after radical prostatectomy or watchful waiting; Scandinavian Prostatic Cancer Group Study Number 4. *N Engl J Med* 2002;347:790–6

13. Schröder FH, van der Maas P, Beemsterboer P, *et al.* Evaluation of the digital rectal examination as a screening test for prostate cancer. Rotterdam section of the European Randomized Study of Screening for Prostate Cancer. *J Natl Cancer Inst* 1998;90:1817–23

14. Begg CB, Riedel ER, Bach PB, *et al.* Variations in morbidity after radical prostatectomy. *N Engl J Med* 2002;346:1138–44

15. Wilt TJ, Brawer MK. The Prostate Cancer Intervention Versus Observation Trial (PIVOT). *Oncology (Huntingt)* 1997;11:1133–9

16. Donovan J, Mills N, Smith M, *et al.* Improving design and conduct of randomised trials by embedding them in qualitative research: ProtecT (Prostate testing for cancer and Treatment) study. *Br Med J* 2002;325:766–70

17. Barnes RW. Survival with conservative therapy. *J Am Med Assoc* 1969;210:331

18. Johansson JE, Adami HO, Andersson SO, Bergstrom R, Krusemo UB, Kraaz W. Natural history of prostate cancer: a population based study of 223 untreated patients. *Lancet* 1989; 1:799–803

19. Johansson JE, Holmberg L, Johansson S, Bergstrom R, Adami HO. Fifteen-year survival in prostate cancer. A prospective, population-based study in Sweden. *J Am Med Assoc* 1997;277:467–71

20. Chodak GW, Thisted RA, Gerber GS, *et al.* Results of conservative management of clinically localized prostate cancer. *N Engl J Med* 1994;330: 242–8

21. Albertsen PC, Frybeck DG, Storer BE, Kolon TF, Fine J. Long-term survival among men with conservatively treated localized prostate cancer. *J Am Med Assoc* 1995;274:626–31

22. Albertsen PC, Hanley JA, Gleason DF, Barry MJ. A competing risk analysis of men age 55–74 years at diagnosis managed conservatively for clinically localized prostate cancer. *J Am Med Assoc* 1998; 280:975–80

23. Oliver SE, Gunnell D, Donovan JL. Comparison of trends in prostate-cancer mortality in England and Wales and the USA. *Lancet* 2000; 355:1788–9

24. Lu-Yao G, Albertsen PC, Stanford JL, Stukel TA, Walker-Corkery ES, Barry MJ. Natural experiment examining impact of aggressive screening and treatment on prostate cancer mortality in two fixed cohorts from Seattle area and Connecticut. *Br Med J* 2002;325:740–3

25. de Koning HJ, Auvinen A, Berenguer Sanchez A, *et al.*, European Randomized Screening for Prostate Cancer (ERSPC) trial, International Prostate Cancer Screening Trials Evaluation Group. Large-scale randomized prostate cancer screening trials: program performances in the European Randomized Screening for Prostate Cancer trial and the Prostate, Lung, Colorectal and Ovary cancer trial. *Int J Cancer* 2002; 97:237–44

26. Chapple A, Ziebland S, Shepperd S, Miller R, Herxheimer A, McPherson A. Why men with prostate cancer want wider access to prostate

specific antigen testing: qualitative study. *Br Med J* 2002;325:737–9

27. Thornton H, Dixon-Woods M. Prostate specific antigen testing for prostate cancer. *Br Med J* 2002;325:725–6

28. Mettlin C, Jones G, Avetett H, *et al.* Defining and updating the American Cancer Society guidelines for the cancer-related check-up: prostate and endometrial cancers. *Cancer J Clin* 1993; 43:42–6

29. American Urological Association. Early detection of prostate and cancer use of transrectal ultrasound. In AUA, ed. *American Urological Association 1992 Policy Statement Book.* Baltimore, MD: American Urological Association, 1992; 4–20

30. US Preventive Service Task Force. Screening for prostate cancer. In USPSTF, ed. *Guide to Clinical Preventive Services*, 2nd edn. Baltimore, MD: Williams and Wilkins, 1996;119

31. American College of Physicians. Screening for prostate cancer. *Ann Intern Med* 1997;126:480–4

32. Chadwick DJ, Kemple T, Astley JP, *et al.* Pilot study of screening for prostate cancer in general practice. *Lancet* 1991;338:613–16

33. Selley S, Donovan J, Faulkner A, Coast J, Gillatt D. Diagnosis, management and screening of early localised prostate cancer. *Health Technol Assess* 1997;1(2):i, 1–96

34. Chamberlain J, Melia J, Moss S, Brown J. The diagnosis, management, treatment and costs of prostate cancer in England and Wales. *Health Technol Assess* 1997;1(3):i–vi, 1–53

35. Milburn A. http://www.doh.gov.uk/cancer, 2000

36. Woolf SH. Should we screen for prostate cancer? *Br Med J* 1997;314:989–90

Outcome after radical prostatectomy: how predictive are biopsies versus radical prostatectomy specimens?

29

L. Boccon Gibod, L. Nicolas, O. Dumonceau, V. Ravery, M. Toublanc and Li Boccon Gibod

Introduction

The ultimate outcome of radical treatment of localized prostate cancer is directly related to the organ confinement of the disease, which in turn is closely dependent on tumor volume. Unfortunately, there is currently no imaging technique (ultrasonography, magnetic resonance imaging (MRI), spectroscoscopic MRI, etc.) able to demonstrate the entire tumor and its actual relationship with the prostatic capsule and surrounding structures/adjacent organs. Therefore, the evaluation of these characteristics, i.e. the staging of the tumor, relies on indirect assessment of the tumor volume based mostly on digital rectal examination (DRE), serum prostate-specific antigen (PSA) testing and careful analysis of prostate biopsy features.

The ability of prostate biopsies to predict accurately the final pathological stage of the tumor and, consequently, the risks of further biochemical/clinical relapse is therefore of critical importance.

Indeed, accurate local staging of the disease should help the clinician to decide whether the tumor:

(1) Is still organ-confined and therefore amenable to radical local therapy with curative intent, and, if surgery is considered, whether nerve-sparing is feasible;

(2) Has extended beyond the prostate capsule to surrounding structures/adjacent organs and will probably no longer be amenable to local monotherapy but will require some form of combination treatment;

(3) Is of such a low volume that it can be submitted safely to watchful waiting, in other words whether the cancer be considered 'insignificant'.

How important is the understaging of clinically localized prostate cancer?

Although extensive PSA testing followed by agressive biopsy protocols has led to a dramatic stage migration, characterized by an increasing imbalance between T1c and T2 tumors in favor of the former, the incidence of unexpected discovery of extraprostatic extension upon pathological examination of the radical prostatectomy specimen remains around 15–25%, even in the most prestigious institutions where highly experienced surgeons operate on a highly selected patient population[1-4]. Concurrently, the incidence of lymph node-positive disease has decreased to 0–2% and seminal vesicle invasion to 5–10%.

The current staging systems are based on a combination of analysis of tissue morphology, expressed using the Gleason scoring system, and what is currently known as 'quantitative histology', in conjunction with PSA and clinical findings. This chapter aims to review their efficacy and practical utility for the clinician.

How reliable is the biopsy Gleason score compared with the specimen Gleason score?

The reliability of the biopsy Gleason score is critical for two reasons: first, the biopsy Gleason score is the only available measure for patients submitted to non-extirpative radical treatment of their tumor; and second, the biopsy Gleason score is the basis, along with PSA and clinical staging, of Partin's table[5], which is one of the most extensively popularized nomograms used to predict pathological stage.

Unfortunately, there are significant variations between the biopsy and specimen Gleason scores, explained partially by the heterogeneity and multifocality of the tumor, the limited amount of tissue sampled even using extensive prostate sampling techniques and the heterogeneity of various pathologists. Over the years, the discrepancies observed have tended to decrease from 40 to 25%[6,7], probably in relation to the wider use of extensive aggressive biopsy techniques, and the increased familiarity of uropathologists with the Gleason scoring system (the possibility for pathologists to assess their understanding on the Hopkins pathology website is extremely useful).

The discrepancy between a 'Hopkins' and a 'non-Hopkins' pathologist 5 years ago was around 25%[8]. A recent study from the Cancer of the Prostate Strategic Urologic Research Endeavor (CAPSURE)[7], shows that undergrading without a central referee pathologist is still about 25%, with an error of 13% on the primary and 29% on the secondary Gleason grade. The discrepancy between specimen and biopsy Gleason scores explains why Partin's nomogram is not as efficient as initially thought, at least in the community setting, as shown by recent data from the CAPSURE study[9]. However, it is important to emphasize that, in spite of these imperfections, the Gleason score retains a very significant prognostic ability[7].

Two important points were recently stressed by the Hopkins group. First, the Gleason score of 4 (2 + 2) often mentioned in biopsy reports is never seen in the final specimen[8], and therefore reports mentioning such a score should be

considered with extreme caution. A new evaluation of the slides is strongly recommended in these cases, particularly if, on the basis of such a Gleason score, the option of watchful waiting is considered. Second, determination of the primary grade in Gleason score 7 (3 + 4 versus 4 + 3) is of the utmost prognostic importance; the risk of ignoring a predominant grade 4 is highly significant[10].

What is the practical input of quantitative histology?

The suboptimal efficacy of staging systems based on the sole utilization of DRE, PSA and Gleason score is indicated by the increased incidence of T1c disease, the questionable sensitivity and specificity of DRE findings, and the relative unreliability of the biopsy Gleason score. Therefore, attention has moved towards what can be termed 'quantitative histology', i.e. the consideration of easily accessible measurable parameters extracted from the examination of prostate biopsy cores. In the past, several systems based on complicated equations using parameters of questionable validity were published; none of them was submitted to external validation, and their high sophistication probably explains their low dissemination in the urological community[11,12].

Considering the number of positive cores, as well as the percentage of cancer in each core or in the total length of biopsy cores, quantitative histology can be used:

(1) To predict the pathological stage;

(2) To select the patient for nerve-sparing surgery;

(3) To consider the patient for watchful waiting (?).

Ravery and colleagues[13] were the first to show that when two-thirds or more of the biopsy cores of a set of sextant transrectal ultrasound (TRUS)-guided biopsies were positive for cancer, the incidence of extraprostatic extension was well over 70%. This indeed makes for sound clinical judgement, as one can assume that the larger the tumor for a given prostate volume, the higher the number of potential positive biopsies. Since that initial report, several groups have discussed the importance of integrating the number of positive biopsies in the staging process[14–17]; taking into consideration the proportion of cores invaded by cancer can help further stratify patients into accepted risk groups based on PSA and biopsy Gleason score, the critical values being less than 30, 30–50 and more than 50% of the cores invaded by cancer.

The finding of a single positive biopsy totally invaded by cancer is highly predictive of extracapsular extension, reflecting again the presence of a large tumor volume. We have shown[18], along with several other groups[19–21], that the percentage of core length involved in prostate cancer, as it reflects roughly the tumor volume, is also an important feature to consider, the critical cut-off value being between 15 and 20%. Therefore, the integration of this parameter in staging systems should be considered. However, using multivariate analysis, other groups have shown that this variable adds little information[22]; therefore, the issue is not at present entirely settled. The staging system can further be refined, integrating the percentage of grade 4–5 in the biopsy; however, the reliability of the biopsy Gleason grade again comes into question.

Because of the dramatic stage migration observed in recent years, it is obvious that a non-negligible number of patients with extraprostatic extension will not experience an early biochemical relapse, and therefore the focus has moved away from the pathological prediction of actual extraprostatic extension towards the prediction of the occurrence of biochemical relapse. Several nomograms have been devised for various treatment options, the most accomplished being that developed by the group of Kattan, based on clinical findings, PSA and Gleason score, which has been successfully internally, externally and internationally validated[23].

Quantitative histology can also help to fine-tune surgical technique, particularly in the area of nerve-sparing surgery: the average, overall and per-side percentages of biopsy cores are highly predictive of extracapsular extension; the sextant-specific percentage of positive biopsies is predictive of sextant side extraprostatic extension with a very high negative predictive value, and can thus help to select adequately the surgical technique[24,25] for the individual patient.

The prediction of unifocal, 'insignificant' prostate cancer is probably one of the best ways to study the actual predictability of biopsy features versus radical prostatectomy specimens. Several authors have emphasized the difficulty of predicting the presence of microfocal insignificant prostate cancer (a single positive focus less than 3 mm in size, no Gleason grade 4) on the sole basis of biopsy features and PSA[26,27]. Therefore, although it has been shown that over a short period of 2 years the clinical and pathological features of such tumors do not tend to deteriorate, treatment decisions are not always easy to make. In our personal experience of 420 patients submitted to radical prostatectomy for clinically (T1–T2) localized prostate cancer between 1988 and 2002, 38 met the criteria for 'insignificant' prostate cancer: they had a single focus of Gleason grade ≤ 6, ≤ 3 mm in size. Of these, four had extraprostatic extension, 26 had Gleason grade 7 cancer in their specimen and 33 had multifocal tumors with 30 harboring contralateral tumors, six of whom had grade 4 in the contralateral lobe. The median tumor volume was 0.8 ml. Of these 38 patients, 27 had a PSA < 10 ng/ml, two of whom had extraprostatic extension (pT3a), 16 had Gleason score 7 and 23 had multifocal tumors, 21 with involvement in the contralateral lobe with two of grade 4 (Table 1). Therefore, it is extremely difficult to use strict criteria, considering that a microfocal prostate tumor on biopsy is indeed a non-significant prostate cancer.

Further pathological features

In the past, several other predictive factors have been considered: perineural invasion, microvessel density, various immuno-DNA ploidies and various immunohistochemical markers.

Table 1 Pathological features of 'insignificant' prostate cancers predicted according to different criteria

	Gleason ≤ 6, Ca ≤ 3 mm (n = 38)	Gleason ≤ 6, Ca ≤ 3 mm, PSA < 10 ng/ml (n = 27)
pT3	4	2
Gleason 7	25	16
Gleason > 7	1	
Multifocal cancer	33	23
Contralateral cancer	30	21
Grade 4 contralateral	6	2
PSM	9	4

Ca, cancer focus size; PSA, prostate-specific antigen; PSM,

Perineural invasion has been considered in the past to be an independent prognostic factor of extraprostatic extension and ultimate biochemical relapse. However, it seems that with the contemporary stage migration, perineural invasion is losing its previous importance[28].

DNA ploidy has been extensively studied. However, it seems that with accurate needle Gleason grading, it does not add useful information to standard histopathology[29].

Immunostaging with p53 and Bcl-2 is probably a useful adjunct in the evaluation of radical prostatectomy specimens[30,31], although the additional information does not consistently appear in multivariate analyses. There is currently no practical indication to use these markers in prostate biopsies, the major reason being the heterogeneity of prostate cancer, and the semiquantitative character of the analysis.

Prostate biopsy has also been used to evaluate surrounding structures and adjacent organs, for example extraprostatic spaces and seminal vesicles. The presence of cancer in the extra-prostatic spaces has a very high sensitivity but a low specificity[11]. Biopsy of the seminal vesicles was extremely popular a decade ago. It is now very seldom used for at least three reasons. First, biopsy of the seminal vesicles is extremely painful. Also, at surgery, dissection of the seminal vesicles is undoubtedly made more difficult by hematoma surrounding the prostate gland. Finally, stage migration has very much reduced the incidence of seminal vesicle invasion.

Conclusions

Adequately performed and interpreted prostate biopsies, along with PSA assessment and digital rectal examination, remain the cornerstone of the modern staging of clinically localized prostate cancer. The pathology report from the biopsy should mention:

(1) The Gleason score with characterization of the predominant Gleason grade;

(2) The number of cores positive for cancer;

(3) The length of cancer per core or in the total cores.

It should be kept in mind that bad news (high Gleason score, associated with high PSA, more than 60% of biopsies positive for cancer, more than 30% of the length of cores invaded per cancer) is always bad news, implying the presence of extraprostatic extension and ultimate biochemical failure; however, good news is not always good news: microfocal cancer is extremely rarely microfocal and insignificant, the actual Gleason score is often under-estimated and there still remains a risk of 15–20% of extraprostatic extension at the final pathological examination, even in the best of hands.

References

1. Veltri RW, Miller Mangold LA, O'Dowd, Epstein JI, Partin AW. Prediction of pathological stage in patients with clinical stage T1c prostate cancer: the new challenge. *J Urol* 2002;168:100–4
2. Elliott SP, Shinohara K, Logan S, Carroll PR. Sextant prostate biopsies predict side and sextant site of extracapsular extension of prostate cancer. *J Urol* 2002;168:105–9
3. Freedland SJ, Wieder JA, Jack GS, Dorey F, deKernion JB, Aronson WJ. Improved risk stratification for biochemical recurrence after radical prostatectomy Gleason score. *J Urol* 2002;168:110–15
4. Sofer M, Hamilton Nelson KL, Civantos F, Soloway MS. Positive surgical margins after radical retropubic prostatectomy: the influence of site and number on progression. *J Urol* 2002; 168:2453–6
5. Partin AW, Kattan MW, Subong ENP, *et al.* Combination of prostate specific antigen, clinical stage and Gleason score to predict pathological stage of localized prostate cancer. *J Am Med Assoc* 1997;277:1445–51
6. Cookson MS, Fleshner NE, Soloway SM, Fair WR. Correlation between Gleason score of needle biopsy and radical prostatectomy specimen: accuracy and clinical implications. *J Urol* 1997; 157:559–62
7. Grossfled GD, Chang JJ, Broering JM, *et al.* Under staging and under grading in a contemporary series of patients undergoing radical prostatectomy: results from the cancer of the prostate strategic urologic research endeavor database. *J Urol* 2001;165:851–6
8. Steinberg DM, Sauvageaut J, Piantodosi S, Epstein JI. Correlation of prostate needle biopsy and radical prostatectomy Gleason grade in academic and community settings. *Am J Surg Pathol* 1997;21:566–76
9. Penson DF, Grossfeld GD, Li YP, Henning JM, Lubeck DP, Carroll PR. How well does the Partin nomogram predict pathological stage after radical prostatectomy in a community based population? Results of the Cancer of the Prostate Strategic Urological Research Endeavor. *J Urol* 2002;167:1653–8
10. Makarov DV, Sanderson H, Partin AW, Epstein JI. Gleason score 7 prostate cancer on needle biopsy: is the prognostic difference in Gleason cores 4 + 3 and 3 + 4 independent of the number of involved cores? *J Urol* 2002;167:2440–2
11. Pisansky TM, Kahn MJ, Bostweck DG. An enhanced prognostic system for clinically localized carcinoma of the prostate. *Cancer* 1997; 79:2154–61
12. D'Amico AV, Whittington R, Schultz D, Malkowicz B, Tomazeewski JE, Wein A. Outcome based staging for clinically localized adenocarcinoma of the prostate. *J Urol* 1997;158: 1422–6
13. Ravery V, Boccon-Gibod LA, Dauge-Geffroy MC, *et al.* Systematic biopsies accurately predict extracapsular extension of prostate cancer and persistent/recurrent detectable PSA after radical prostatectomy. *Urology* 1994;44:371
14. Sebon TJ, Bock BJ, Cheville JC, Lhose C, Wollan P, Zincke H. The percent of cores positive for cancer in prostate needle biopsy specimens is strongly predictive of tumor stage and volume at radical prostatectomy. *J Urol* 2000;163:174–8
15. D'Amico A, Whittington R, Malkowicz SB, *et al.* Combination of the preoperative PSA level, biopsy Gleason score, percentage of positive biopsies and MRI T-stage to predict early PSA failure in men with clinically localized prostate cancer. *Urology* 2000;55:572–7
16. Grossfeld GD, Latini DM, Lubeck DP, *et al.* Predicting disease recurrence in intermediate and high risk patients undergoing radical prostatectomy using percent positive biopsies: results from CAPSURE. *Urology* 2002;59:560–5
17. D'Amico AV, Whittington R, Malkowicz SB, *et al.* Clinical utility of the percentage of positive prostate. Biopsies in defining biochemical outcome after radical prostatectomy for patients with clinically localized prostate cancer. *J Clin Oncol* 2000;18:1164–72
18. Ravery V, Chastang C, Toublanc M, Boccon-Gibod L, Delmas V, Boccon-Gibod L. Percentage of cancer on biopsy cores accurately predicts extracapsular extension and biochemical relapse after radical prostatectomy for T1–T2 prostate cancer. *Eur Urol* 2000;37:449–55
19. Grosklaus DJ, Coffey CS, Shappell SB, Jack GS, Chang SS, Cookson MS. Percent of cancer in the biopsy set predicts pathological findings after prostatectomy. *J Urol* 2002;167:2032–6
20. Freedland SJ, Csathy GS, Dorey F, Aronson WJ. Percent prostate needle biopsy tissue with cancer is more predictive of biochemical failure or adverse pathology after radical prostatectomy than prostate specific antigen or Gleason score. *J Urol* 2002;167:516–20
21. Freedland SJ, Csathy GS, Dorey F, Aronson WJ. Clinical utility of percent prostate needle biopsy tissue with cancer cutpoints to risk stratify patients before radical prostatectomy. *Urology* 2002;60:84–8
22. Lonson PW, Lee AK, Doytchinova T, *et al.* Percentage of core lengths involved with prostate

cancer; does it add to the percentage of positive prostate biopsies in predicting postoperative prostate specific antigen outcome for men with intermediate risk prostate cancer? *Urology* 2002; 59:704–8

23. Graefen M, Karakiewicz PI, Bogiannos I, *et al.* International validation of a preoperative nomogram for prostate cancer recurrence after radical prostatectomy. *J Clin Oncol* 2002;20: 3206–12

24. Graefen M, Haese A, Pichlmeier U, *et al.* A validated strategy for side specific prediction or organ confined prostate cancer: a tool to select for nerve sparing radical prostatectomy. *J Urol* 2001;165:857–63

25. Elliot SP, Shinohar K, Logan SL, Carroll PR. Sextant prostate biopsies predict side and sextant site of extracapsular extension of prostate cancer. *J Urol* 2002;168:105–9

26. Gardner TA, Lemer ML, Schlegel PN, Waldbaum RS, Baugha ED, Stecker J. Microfocal prostate cancer: biopsy cancer volume does not predict actual tumour volume. *Br J Urol* 1998; 81:839–43

27. D'Amico AV, Wu Y, Chen MH, Nash M, Renshaw AA, Richie JP. Pathologic findings and prostate specific antigen outcome after radical prostatectomy for patients diagnosed on the basis of a single microscopic focus of prostate carcinoma with a Gleason score ≥ 7. *Am Cancer Soc* 2000; 1810–17

28. Potter SR, Epstein JI, Wartin AW. What are the implications of perineural invasion on prostate biopsy? *Contemp Urol* 2001;21–6

29. Brinke DA, Ross JS, Tran TA, Jones DM, Epstein JI. Can ploidy of prostate carcinoma diagnosed on needle biopsy predict radical prostatectomy stage and grade? *J Urol* 1999;162:2036–9

30. Leibovich BC, Chen L, Weaver AL, Myers RP, Bostwick DG. Outcome prediction with p53 immunostaging after radical prostatectomy in patients with locally advanced prostate cancer. *J Urol* 2000;163:1756–60

31. Stackhouse GB, Sesterhenn IA, Bauer JJ, *et al.* p53 and Bcl-2 immunohistochemistry in pretreatment prostate needle biopsies to predict recurrence of prostate cancer after radical prostatectomy. *J Urol* 1998;162:2040–5

A randomized trial comparing radical prostatectomy with watchful waiting in early prostate cancer

30

M. Häggman for the Scandinavian Prostatic Cancer Group 4 (SPCG4) study group

Introduction

The management of early prostate cancer is controversial. Radical prostatectomy is widely used, but its effect on the course of the disease has not been proven in a randomized trial. Earlier observational studies have indicated a lower rate of progression in patients treated by surgery than in cases treated by external radiation, but no gain in overall survival at long-term follow-up compared with watchful waiting. Systematic review of available studies reveals a lack of reliable data to support any specific treatment recommendations[1–7].

Side-effects of radical prostatectomy may affect the quality of life in men undergoing the procedure, and the choice of whether to have radical treatment or not will also be dependent on such issues.

We conducted a randomized trial in 695 men with early prostate cancer, assigning them to either radical prostatectomy or watchful waiting. Median follow-up was 6.2 years. The main aim of the study was to determine whether prostate cancer-specific mortality was lower among men treated with radical prostatectomy than among patients treated with watchful waiting. Secondary aims were to assess metastasis-free survival and the risk of local tumor progression. Later on, an analysis of total mortality was added.

Methods

In total, 695 men under 75 years of age with newly diagnosed, previously untreated adeno-carcinoma of the prostate, World Health Organization (WHO) grade 1 or 2, stage T1b–T2c (T1c added after 1994), were randomized during a 10-year period. Some 376 men from the participating centers in Sweden were offered enrolment in a concomitant study on quality of life after radical prostatectomy or during watchful waiting.

Men assigned to watchful waiting received no immediate treatment except the transurethral resection of the prostate (TURP) that some had already undergone. In the radical prostatectomy group, the operative procedure was begun with an obturator lymph node dissection, and only if frozen section did not reveal metastasis was a retropubic radical prostatectomy performed[8,9]. No adjuvant treatments were administered. If dissemination of disease occurred, orchiectomy or gonadotropin-releasing hormone (GnRH) agonist treatment was recommended.

All diagnostic biopsy specimens, core or fine-needle, were blindly reviewed by four pathologists, re-evaluated and scored according to the Gleason system[10].

All patients were routinely followed up twice a year for the first 2 years, and then annually, with clinical examination and assessment of hemoglobin, alkaline phosphatase, creatinine and prostate-specific antigen (PSA). Bone scans were done annually. From 1998 to 2001 all patient records from the Departments of Urology and Oncology were reviewed, and an extended search for all medical records of deceased subjects was carried out.

Outcomes and definitions of clinical events

In relation to cause of death, two of the investigators extracted standardized relevant clinical data for all deceased participants. Group assignment and primary treatment mode was blinded. An independent end-point committee or two urologists and one pathologist classified all deaths individually.

Metastases were diagnosed when a bone scan or skeletal radiogram was positive, when computed tomography (CT) or a chest X-ray showed metastases and when lymph nodes beyond the regional nodes showed cytological or histological evidence of prostate cancer.

Local progression in the watchful waiting group was defined as palpable transcapsular growth or infravesical obstruction necessitating intervention, or both. In the radical prostatectomy group, the criterion for progression and local recurrence was a histologically confirmed local tumor.

End-points

Three end-points were used. Disease-specific mortality was defined by the time to death from prostate cancer. Rate of distant metastasis was defined as the time to diagnosis of such. Overall mortality was defined as the time to death, regardless of cause.

Sample size

To demonstrate a 10% difference in disease-specific survival at 5 years, the initial target sample size was 520 patients. Two interim analyses, after enrolment of 300 and 520 patients, respectively, showed a lower overall mortality rate than expected. The sample size was thus increased to 700 patients. This would enable the detection of an absolute survival rate difference of 6% between the two groups.

Statistical analysis

All analyses were performed according to the intention-to-treat principle and were based on the complete follow-up of all enrolled eligible men. At the end of follow-up on 31 December 2000, 520 men had been followed for at least 5 years, when the first according-to-protocol open analysis was to be undertaken. Cumulative cause-specific hazard rates were calculated with negative log transformation of the Kaplan–Meier estimator for each end-point.

Ninety-five per cent confidence intervals for point estimate differences at 5 and 8 years for the cumulative hazard rates are reported. The log-rank test was used for comparisons between groups, p values of less than 0.05 indicating statistical significance. Cox proportional hazards models were used to estimate relative hazards with 95% confidence intervals. A multivariate Cox model was used to check influences from any imbalances in age, tumor distribution or Gleason score.

Quality of life assessment

After an introductory letter and contact by telephone, patients agreeing to participate were mailed a questionnaire, comprising 77 questions and two psychometric tests. The questionnaire was based on instruments previously used and tested for face validity on a subgroup of 30 men.

Results

Survival analysis

From a total of 698 enrolled subjects, 695 fulfilled all criteria for participation; 348 were assigned to watchful waiting and 347 to radical prostatectomy. During follow-up, 30 men in the watchful waiting group were treated with curative intent and 25 men in the radical prostatectomy group were followed without radical treatment. No one was lost to follow-up, with a median duration of 6.2 years. Characteristics at baseline were similar in the study groups, albeit with a somewhat higher proportion of T1b tumors in the watchful waiting group. Most men had T2 tumors.

During follow-up 115 men died, 62 in the watchful waiting group and 53 in the radical prostatectomy group. The end-point committee reached a consensus in all cases regarding the causes of death. Of the 115 deceased men, 47 died of prostate cancer; all had received hormonal treatment. In the watchful waiting arm, 31 men died of prostate cancer, compared with 16 in the radical prostatectomy group. There were 31 deaths from other causes in the watchful waiting arm, and 37 in the radical prostatectomy arm.

The cumulative hazard for death from prostate cancer showed a difference increasing over time to an absolute difference of 6.6% at 8 years. The relative hazard for men assigned to radical prostatectomy was 0.50 ($p = 0.02$).

The cumulative hazard for distant metastases also increased over time, with an absolute difference of 14% at 8 years in favor of radical prostatectomy ($p = 0.03$).

The rate of local progression was also significantly different between the groups, with a 20% biopsy-proven rate in the radical prostatectomy group at 8 years compared with approximately 60% in the watchful waiting group ($p < 0.001$).

The relative hazard of death from any cause was 0.83 in the radical prostatectomy group (not significant).

Overall, 116 men in the watchful waiting group and 80 men in the radical prostatectomy group received hormonal treatment. Palliative irradiation was given to 22 men in the watchful waiting arm and 13 men in the radical prostatectomy arm, and laminectomy was performed in eight men and one man, respectively.

Quality of life analysis

The frequency of sexual thoughts was similar in the two groups (40% in the radical prostatectomy group versus 34% in the watchful waiting group). The prevalence of satisfactory erectile function was higher in the watchful waiting group. A total of 45% of men in the watchful waiting group reported erectile dysfunction, compared with 80% in the radical prostatectomy group. Forty per cent of men in the watchful waiting group were distressed by a compromised sexuality, versus 56% of those operated on.

A weak urinary stream was less prevalent in the radical prostatectomy group (28%) than in the watchful waiting group (44%). However, all variables concerning urinary leakage were more prevalent in the operated group versus the watchful waiting group. Almost half the men in the radical prostatectomy group had urinary leakage at least once weekly; 18% had a moderate or severe leakage against 2% in the watchful waiting group. Also, 27% of men operated on were distressed by urinary problems, compared with 18% in the watchful waiting group.

All psychological variables evaluated had a lower prevalence in the radical prostatectomy group, but no statistically significant differences were noted.

Discussion

This trial was designed to determine whether radical prostatectomy reduces the risk of death from prostate cancer. We found a statistically significant difference in the risk of death due to prostate cancer after radical prostatectomy, compared with watchful waiting, yet there was no statistically significant difference in overall survival. At 8 years the absolute difference in both overall and disease-specific death rate was approximately 6%. For distal metastasis this difference was 14%. This implies that 17 patients would need a radical prostatectomy to prevent one prostate cancer death over an 8-year period.

Within the first 5 years after inclusion into the study there was only a small difference between the groups. This may be explained by a similar proportion of cases in both groups with undetectable disseminated disease. These patients may account for the majority of deaths from prostate cancer during early follow-up. Removal of the primary tumor would only provide cure in men with truly localized disease at diagnosis; the results indicate that this effect would be apparent beyond 5 years after surgery.

The study was initiated before the era of PSA screening. The assigned men thus had clinically detected well- to moderately well-differentiated prostate cancer, in contrast with tumors that may be detected in a screening population. A substantial lead-time may be expected in such a population over clinically detected cases, and the reduction in disease-specific mortality may take several more years to emerge[11].

Men assigned to radical prostatectomy had a higher prevalence of erectile dysfunction and urinary leakage, but a lower prevalence of obstructive urinary symptoms. On average, well-being and subjective quality of life were similar in the two groups.

Erectile dysfunction is a well-documented complication of radical prostatectomy. However, 45% of patients in the watchful waiting arm were also affected by this, a higher figure than the 32% observed among population controls of the same age-group in a previous Swedish study[12-14].

It cannot be said that radical prostatectomy is better than watchful waiting for all men with localized prostate cancer. These alternatives are associated with complex and incommensurable outcomes, and each man must judge for himself which treatment he prefers.

Acknowledgements

The members of the Scandinavian Prostatic Cancer Group 4 were:

Steering committee H.-O. Adami, A. Bill-Axelson, F. Helgesen, L. Holmberg, J.-E. Johansson, B. J. Norlen (principal investigator).

Statisticians L. Holmberg, J. Nilsson, J. Palmgren.

Monitoring committee A. Bill-Axelson, B. Goben, F. Helgesen.

Study group J. Adolfsson, S. O. Andersson, A. Bill-Axelson, S. Bratell, G. Einarsson, P. Ekman, P. Elfving, P. Folmerz, G. Hagberg, P. O. Hedlund, M. Häggman, J. E. Johansson, L. Karlberg, T. Lindeborg, O. Lukkarinen, M. Norberg, B. J. Norlen, M. Ruutu, J. Salo, A. Spångberg, H. Wijkström, B. Zackrisson.

Reference pathologists C. Busch (chairman), M. de la Torre, A. Lindgren, S. Nordling.

End-point committee J. E. Damber, A. Lindgren, E. Varenhorst (chairman).

External review committee P. F. Schellhammer, U. E. Studer, R. Sylvester.

Quality of life study group G. Steineck, F. Helgesen, J. Adolfsson, P. W. Dickman, J.-E. Johansson, B. J. Norlen, L. Holmberg.

References

1. Paulson DF, Lin GH, Hinshaw W, Stephani S. Radical surgery versus radiotherapy for adenocarcinoma of the prostate. *J Urol* 1982;128:502–4
2. Graversen PH, Nielsen KT, Gasser TC, Corle DK, Madsen PO. Radical prostatectomy versus expectant primary treatment in stages I and II prostatic cancer: a fifteen-year follow up. *Urology* 1990;36:493–8
3. Iversen P, Madsen PO, Corle DK. Radical prostatectomy versus expectant treatment for early carcinoma of the prostate: twenty-three-year follow up of a prospective randomized study. *Scand J Urol Nephrol* 1995;172(Suppl):65–72
4. Chodak GW, Thisted RA, Gerber GS, *et al.* Results of conservative management of clinically localized prostate cancer. *N Engl J Med* 1994; 330:242–8
5. Gerber GS, Thisted RA, Scardino PT, *et al.* Results of radical prostatectomy in men with clinically localized prostate cancer. *J Am Med Assoc* 1996;276:615–19
6. Middleton RG, Thompson IM, Austenfeld MS, *et al.* Prostate cancer clinical guidelines panel summary report on the management of clinically localized prostate cancer. *J Urol* 1995;154:2144–8
7. Fleming C, Wasson JH, Albertsen PC, Barry MJ, Wennberg JE. A description analysis of alternative treatment strategies for clinically localized prostate cancer. *J Am Med Assoc* 1993; 269:2650–8

8. Brendler CB, Cleeve LK, Anderson EE, Paulson DF. Staging pelvic lymphadenectomy for carcinoma of the prostate: risk versus benefit. *J Urol* 1980;124:849–50

9. Walsh PC, Lepor H. The role of radical prostatectomy in the management of prostatic cancer. *Cancer* 1987;60:526–37

10. Gleason DF. Histologic grading and clinical staging of prostatic carcinoma. In Tannenbaum M, ed. *Urologic Pathology: the Prostate.* Philadelphia: Lea & Febiger, 1977:171–98

11. Pearson JD, Luderer AA, Metter EJ, *et al.* Longitudinal analysis of serial measurements of free and total PSA among men with and without prostatic cancer. *Urology* 1996;48(Suppl):4–9

12. Stanford JL, Feng Z, Hamilton AS, *et al.* Urinary and sexual function after radical prostatectomy for clinically localized prostate cancer: the prostate cancer outcomes study. *J Am Med Assoc* 2000;283:354–60

13. Litwin MS, Flanders SC, Pasta DJ, Stoddard ML, Lubeck DP, Hanning JM. Sexual function and bother after radical prostatectomy or radiation for prostate cancer: multivariate quality of life analysis from CaPSURE: Cancer of the Prostate Strategic Urologic Research Endeavor. *Urology* 1999;54:503–8

14. Helgason AR, Adolfsson J, Dickman P, *et al.* Sexual desire, erection, orgasm and ejaculatory functions and their importance to elderly Swedish men: a population-based study. *Age Ageing* 1996;25:285–91

Prostate cancer mortality and screening

S. E. Oliver

31

Background

Prostate cancer is the second most common life-threatening cancer in men in the majority of Western countries[1], and accounted for over 31 000 deaths in the USA in 2000. Despite its major impact on public health, the etiology of prostate cancer is poorly understood, with the only recognized risk factors being age, family history and ethnicity[2]. The paucity of identified risk factors limits the opportunity for primary prevention, and attempts to reduce the burden of prostate cancer morbidity and mortality have increasingly focused on secondary prevention through early detection and treatment. Early detection is now largely achieved through use of the prostate-specific antigen (PSA) test, augmented with digital rectal examination and transrectal ultrasound. The aim of this form of cancer screening is avoidance of prostate cancer as a cause of death, and this chapter therefore focuses on this end-point.

While the PSA test makes population screening possible, the question of whether early detection will lead to a sufficient reduction in deaths from prostate cancer, to outweigh adverse consequences of over-detection, remains open. The only meaningful method to answer this question is through well-conducted randomized controlled trials (RCTs), and two such studies are under way in North America[3] and Europe[4].

Why do trends in mortality matter?

Given that the results of RCTs are going to be the only reliable source of evidence on the effectiveness of screening, what can we learn from examining trends in mortality? The variation in PSA testing intensity both over time and between populations provides a number of 'natural experiments', and an opportunity for observational epidemiological study. While these studies may give an insight into what might occur at a population level in the event of screening, they are open to bias, and it is always important to recall that non-randomized populations may differ in other ways than in uptake of screening. However, in the final event, the true impact of screening can only be measured through changes in mortality at a population level. An understanding of how mortality patterns are changing over time is therefore vital in putting the results of experimental studies in context. Mortality trends also have an impact on the design of RCTs of screening; death rates in the control population are an important determinant of the power of any screening study.

Recent trends in prostate cancer mortality

Until the late 1980s, prostate cancer incidence and mortality were both rising in most countries[5]. However, from the late 1990s onwards it became clear that death rates were falling in some parts of the world[6,7]. The greatest interest has focused on mortality trends in the USA, where a dramatic peak in prostate cancer incidence followed the introduction of the PSA test in 1985[7–9]. Since 1991, a fall in mortality has been seen in the USA, and there has been debate over the extent to which this may be a consequence of PSA screening[9]. In England and Wales, where national health policy has discouraged PSA screening[6], similar declines in mortality have also been observed[10]. Reports of

267

falling prostate cancer death rates have also come from Scotland[11] and Canada[12].

A systematic review of mortality trends in industrialized countries

In 2000 we conducted a systematic review of trends in mortality from prostate cancer within industrialized countries[13]. Mortality and population data were extracted from the World Health Organization (WHO) Mortality Database for the period 1979–97. Countries were included in analyses if:

(1) They had at least 200 deaths from prostate cancer per year;

(2) Mortality data were available for at least 9 years in the period 1979–97;

(3) They had systems of death certification in which cause of death was assigned by a medical practitioner in $\geq 95\%$ of cases, and coverage was considered good.

Deaths coded to prostate cancer using the 9th revision of the International Classification of Disease were used in analyses (ICD9 185). Age-standardized death rates were calculated for the age range 50–79 years in 5-year age bands, using the European standard population. Deaths in the population aged over 79 years were excluded, as death certification is known to be less accurate in older individuals[14]. Mortality and population data from the former German Democratic Republic and the Federal Republic of Germany for the years 1979–89 were combined to give a single rate for Germany.

Trends in age-specific and age-standardized mortality were calculated using join point regression[15]. This is a form of regression analysis in which trend data can be described by a number of contiguous linear segments and 'join points' at which trends change. The regression model also estimates the annual percentage change (APC) in rates, the number and location of join points and confidence intervals (CIs) for these parameters.

There was a more than five-fold difference between the lowest (Japan 1994, 15.1 per 100 000) and highest (Sweden 1996, 81.5 per 100 000) age-standardized rates at the end of the time series. The lowest death rates were seen in Japan and the Southern European countries (Greece, Spain, Portugal, Italy), and the highest in Scandinavia and North America. Most countries experienced a constant increase in prostate cancer mortality over the years studied. In seven countries, Canada, the USA, Austria, France, Germany, Italy and the UK, mortality trends showed a down-turn in recent years. In Belgium and Hungary trends were static.

Estimates of the year when changes in the trend in prostate cancer mortality occurred, and of the APC in prostate cancer mortality between these years, are given in Table 1. Mortality rates increased at between 1 and 2% per year in most countries during the study period. Japan, with the lowest initial mortality rate, had one of the highest rates of increase at 2.6% per year. In those countries where a down-turn in trend was identified, join points for this being clustered in the time period 1988–91, the earliest reversal in trend was seen in Italy (1988, 95% CI 1986–1991). Following the reversal in trend, the APC ranged from falls of 2.1% per year in the UK (95% CI 1.3–2.9%) and Italy (95% CI 1.0–3.3%) to 6% (95% CI 0.1–11.5%) in Germany.

In Canada, the USA, France, Italy and the UK a reversal in mortality trends was seen in each 5-year age group from 60 to 79 years. The timing of these changes in age-specific trends ranged from 1986 to 1992, consistent with a calendar period effect. Trends in age-specific rates were less consistent in Germany and Austria, where changes were observed mainly in the 74–79-year age band.

Mortality trends within countries

Two recent articles have used the opportunities provided by 'natural experiments' in which the intensity of PSA testing has varied within countries to examine the possible impact of screening on mortality. In Austria, PSA testing was made freely available to men aged 45–75 in the Tyrol region in 1993[16]. In the following 5 years approximately two-thirds of the population of the region (c. 65 000 men in the age

Table 1 Summary of the annual percentage change (APC) and join points for trends in age-standardized prostate cancer mortality (50–79 years) in 24 countries. (When more than one join point was identified in the trend for a country, the APC between join points is given)

Country (range of years)	APC (95% CI)	Join point (95% CI)	APC (95% CI)	Join point (95% CI)	APC (95% CI)
Two join points					
USA (1979–87)	0.5 (0.1 to 1.0)	1988 (1981–1990)	3.6 (−1.0 to 8.4)	1991 (1989–1993)	−3.6 (−4.3 to −2.8)
UK (1979–97)	0.1 (−5.5 to 6.0)	1981 (1981–1992)	3.2 (2.7 to 3.7)	1991 (1989–1995)	−2.1 (−2.9 to −1.3)
One join point					
Canada (1979–97)	1.7 (1.2 to 2.3)	1991 (1988–1992)	−3.0 (−4.3 to −1.6)		
Austria (1980–97)	1.0 (0.2 to 1.9)	1991 (1989–1994)	−2.5 (−4.5 to −0.3)		
France (1979–95)	1.1 (0.6 to 1.6)	1989 (1987–1990)	−2.9 (−3.7 to −2.0)		
Germany (1980–97)	0.5 (0.3 to 0.8)	1995 (1993–1995)	−6.0 (−11.5 to −0.1)		
Italy (1979–95)	1.0 (0.1 to 1.7)	1988 (1986–1991)	−2.1 (−3.3 to −1.0)		
No join point					
Belgium (1979–97)	−0.1 (−0.5 to 0.4)				
Finland (1987–95)	1.1 (−0.4 to 2.6)				
Greece (1979–97)	1.0 (0.5 to 1.4)				
Ireland (1979–96)	1.8 (1.0 to 2.7)				
Netherlands (1979–95)	0.9 (0.5 to 1.2)				
Norway (1986–95)	0.4 (−0.3 to 1.1)				
Portugal (1980–97)	1.4 (1.0 to 1.8)				
Spain (1980–95)	0.3 (0.01 to 0.5)				
Sweden (1987–96)	1.3 (0.5 to 2.2)				
Bulgaria (1979–95)	0.9 (0.5 to 1.2)				
Hungary (1979–95)	−0.02 (−0.4 to 0.4)				
Poland (1980–96)	1.8 (1.4 to 2.1)				
Romania (1979–97)	1.0 (0.5 to 1.4)				
Israel (1979–96)	1.8 (0.8 to 2.8)				
Japan (1979–94)	2.6 (2.3 to 3.0)				
Australia (1979–95)	1.7 (1.3 to 2.1)				
New Zealand (1979–96)	1.1 (0.4 to 1.8)				

CI, confidence interval

range 45–75 years) had at least one PSA test. Mortality rates within the region were seen to fall significantly faster than in the rest of Austria. The authors of the study concluded that PSA testing and subsequent management of screen-detected cancer was probably the cause for the decline in mortality. However, they also concluded that the very short lead time between introduction of PSA testing and changes in mortality suggested that improved death rates might result from down-staging and successful treatment, rather than through detection and treatment of early cancers.

In contrast, a recent paper from North America observed no difference in mortality trends between regions with very different intensities of PSA testing and aggressive treatment. On the basis of data on men over the age of 65 years, Lu-Yao and colleagues compared mortality rates among men living in Seattle and Connecticut[17]. In Seattle, rates of PSA testing in the period 1988–90 were over five times higher than in the region of Connecticut, and in addition, rates of biopsy and potentially curative treatment were also higher. However, a review of mortality rates over the period 1987–97 showed no evidence of a difference in death rates between these regions.

Mortality trends and screening

Recent trends in prostate cancer mortality reveal marked differences among industrialized nations. In most countries, the long-term trend of rising death rates has persisted over the past 20 years, and in others there is evidence of a decline over the past decade. These observed declines in mortality could result from any combination of artifact, reduction in prostate cancer incidence, rise in competing causes of death or changes in the risk of death from prostate cancer.

Artifact

Because of its relatively slow progression, and peak incidence in an elderly population, attribution of cause of death in men with prostate cancer poses particular difficulties.

Changes in the interpretation of WHO rules on assigning underlying cause of death have resulted in spurious changes in prostate cancer mortality trends in England and Wales[6]. Two recent studies from the USA suggest that 10–20% of prostate cancer deaths may be mis-attributed[18,19]. In a study comparing patterns of non-prostate cancer deaths in cohorts of men with and without prostate cancer, Newschaffer and colleagues reported that attribution of cause of death in men with prostate cancer could have been influenced by knowledge of previous treatment. Prior beliefs about the effectiveness of radical treatment may have led to a reluctance to attribute death to prostate cancer in men who had undergone 'aggressive' interventions[19].

Changes in incidence

Trends in mortality could fall if the underlying incidence of aggressive prostate tumors was decreasing, possibly in response to changes in environmental risk factors such as diet. Such changes are hard to detect, as overall estimates of incidence are heavily influenced by methods of case detection, particularly with the advent of PSA testing. However, age-specific death rates in most countries experiencing apparent falls in mortality appear to be consistent with a period effect, with rates declining at similar times in different age bands. Changes in chronic disease incidence are more commonly reflected in mortality trends as cohort effects, unless the latent time between exposure and outcome is short and all age groups experience a simultaneous change in exposure. Apart from the short-term changes in incidence driven by PSA testing, there is as yet little evidence that prostate cancer incidence is in decline in those countries where mortality trends have reversed[5].

Competing causes

It is also unlikely that reductions in prostate cancer mortality are due to a real increase in the incidence of competing causes of death. Life expectancy in the age range 50–79 is increasing in those countries experiencing a reversal in trend[20], and this hypothesis is not consistent with knowledge about trends in the other major life-threatening conditions.

Increased survival: impact of health care

Earlier detection of prostate cancer following the introduction of PSA testing distorts analyses of survival (lead-time bias), and makes comparisons of recent data on survival between countries and over time very difficult. However, as this study is based only on the timing of death, the observed changes could imply true reductions in disease-specific mortality. Given the apparent period effects in age-specific prostate cancer death rates, the most likely cause of the observed down-turns in mortality is the impact of some form of therapeutic intervention. Two recent changes in the management of prostate cancer could account for this. First, in countries such as the USA, the rapid rise in incidence was accompanied by an increase in the utilization of radical surgery and radiotherapy. However, it appears unlikely that the results of radical treatments alone could have caused the observed changes in death rates. Using a simulation model of prostate cancer mortality, including varying estimates of treatment efficacy and screening lead time, Etzioni and colleagues estimated the possible impact of radical treatments on death rates in the USA[21]. Only when the effectiveness of radical treatments was set at its highest level (relative risk reduction of 0.5) and lead time at its lowest (3 years) could use of such treatments account for the observed mortality change in the USA. In the UK the extent of radical treatment has been far lower, but a similar down-turn in mortality has been observed[6].

Second, developments in the management of advanced prostate cancer also occurred in the 1980s with the introduction of medical anti-androgen therapies. While the effectiveness of drug-induced androgen deprivation is similar to the traditional approach of surgical castration[22], increased uptake of more acceptable medical therapies could extend population survival by deferring death from prostate cancer sufficiently for competing causes to intervene. Initiation of hormone treatment earlier in the course of advanced disease might also have an influence on death rates[23]. However, it is also worth observing that any unrecognized adverse effects of therapy, if they induced competing causes of death such as thromboembolic disease or other malignancies, would be translated into reductions in prostate cancer-specific death rates. International and secular variation in health-care interventions for prostate cancer are not well described, and it is unclear whether the patterns in observed mortality trends are matched by differences in treatment.

Impact of PSA screening

The relationship between the observed national mortality trends and the known uptake of PSA testing raises some paradoxes. Mortality rates are falling in the USA where PSA screening is common[9], but not in Australia where uptake has also been high[24,25]. In contrast, in the UK where screening uptake is low[6], mortality rates are declining. Published reports of prostate cancer screening in other countries are limited. PSA testing was thought to have had an impact on prostate cancer incidence by 1988 in at least one area in France[26], while in the Italian region of Tuscany PSA was first being used in the early 1990s[27]. Feasibility studies for prostate cancer screening are also ongoing in Austria[28] and Italy[29], and centers in Belgium, Finland, Italy, The Netherlands and Sweden are participating in the European Randomized Study of Screening for Prostate Cancer[30]. The lack of a consistent association between PSA uptake and mortality trends highlights the limitations of observational data in assessing the effectiveness of cancer screening, which awaits the results of ongoing randomized trials.

Conclusion

Data on trends in death rates suggest that important changes have happened recently in several countries, which may be a result of health-care activity. However, evidence from mortality trends is not sufficient to answer the issue of the effectiveness of population screening, which can still only come from randomized controlled trials. The burden of prostate cancer morbidity and mortality continues to rise in most parts of the world, and research into isolating the contributing causes of observed declines in mortality should have high priority.

Acknowledgements

The analyses presented in this chapter were carried out with the help of David Gunnell, Margaret May and Jenny Donovan. Data on mortality were obtained from the WHO Mortality Database. All analyses, interpretations and conclusions based on these data are the responsibility of the author, not the WHO, which is responsible only for provision of the original information.

References

1. Jensen OM, Esteve J, Moller H, *et al. Cancer in Five Continents.* Lyon: IARC Press, 1997;VII
2. Selley S, Donovan J, Faulkner A, Coast J, Gillat D. *Diagnosis, Management and Screening of Early Localised Prostate Cancer.* Southampton: Health Technology Assessment, 1997
3. Gohagan JK, Prorok PC, Kramer BS, Cornett JE. Prostate cancer screening in the prostate, lung, colorectal and ovarian cancer screening trial of the National Cancer Institute. *J Urol* 1994;152: 1905–9
4. Auvinen A, Rietbergen JB, Denis LJ, Schroder FH, Prorok PC. Prospective evaluation plan for randomised trials of prostate cancer screening. The International Prostate Cancer Screening Trial Evaluation Group. *J Med Screen* 1996; 3:97–104
5. Hsing AW, Tsao L, Devesa SS. International trends and patterns of prostate cancer incidence and mortality. *Int J Cancer* 2000;85:60–7
6. Oliver SE, Gunnell D, Donovan JL. Comparison of trends in prostate-cancer mortality in England and Wales and the USA. *Lancet* 2000;355:1788–9
7. Mettlin CJ, Murphy GP. Why is the prostate cancer death rate declining in the United States? *Cancer* 1998;82:249–51
8. Farkas A, Schneider D, Perrotti M, Cummings KB, Ward WS. National trends in the epidemiology of prostate cancer, 1973 to 1994: evidence for the effectiveness of prostate-specific antigen screening. *Urology* 1998;52:444–8
9. Hankey BF, Feuer EJ, Clegg LX, *et al.* Cancer surveillance series: interpreting trends in prostate cancer – part I: Evidence of the effects of screening in recent prostate cancer incidence,

mortality, and survival rates. *J Natl Cancer Inst* 1999;91:1017–24
10. Majeed A, Babb P, Jones J, Quinn M. Trends in prostate cancer incidence, mortality and survival in England and Wales 1971–1998. *BJU Int* 2000; 85:1058–62
11. Brewster DH, Fraser LA, Harris V, Black RJ. Rising incidence of prostate cancer in Scotland: increased risk or increased detection? *BJU Int* 2000;85:463–72
12. Meyer F, Moore L, Bairati I, Fradet Y. Downward trend in prostate cancer mortality in Quebec and Canada. *J Urol* 1999;161:1189–91
13. Oliver SE, May MT, Gunnell D. International trends in prostate-cancer mortality in the 'PSA era'. *Int J Cancer* 2001;92:893–8
14. Grulich AE, Swerdlow AJ, dos Santos Silva I, Beral V. Is the apparent rise in cancer mortality in the elderly real? Analysis of changes in certification and coding of cause of death in England and Wales, 1970–1990. *Int J Cancer* 1995;63:164–8
15. Kim HJ, Fay MP, Feuer EJ, Midthune DN. Permutation tests for joinpoint regression with applications to cancer rates. *Stat Med* 2000;19: 335–51
16. Bartsch G, Horninger W, Klocker H, *et al.* Prostate cancer mortality after introduction of prostate-specific antigen mass screening in the Federal State of Tyrol, Austria. *Urology* 2001; 58:417–24
17. Lu-Yao GL, Albertsen PC, Stanford JL, Stukel TA, Walker-Corkery ES, Barry MJ. Natural experiment examining impact of aggressive screening and treatment on prostate cancer

mortality in two fixed cohorts from Seattle area and Connecticut. *Br Med J* 2002;325:740–3

18. Albertsen PC, Walters S, Hanley JA. A comparison of cause of death determination in men previously diagnosed with prostate cancer who died in 1985 or 1995. *J Urol* 2000;163:519–23

19. Newschaffer CJ, Otani K, McDonald MK, Penberthy LT. Causes of death in elderly prostate cancer patients and in a comparison nonprostate cancer cohort. *J Natl Cancer Inst* 2000;92:613–21

20. World Health Organization. *World Health Statistics Annual 1996.* Geneva: World Health Statistics, 1998

21. Etzioni R, Legler JM, Feuer EJ, Merrill RM, Cronin KA, Hankey BF. Cancer surveillance series: interpreting trends in prostate cancer – part III: Quantifying the link between population prostate-specific antigen testing and recent declines in prostate cancer mortality. *J Natl Cancer Inst* 1999;91:1033–9

22. Chamberlain J, Melia J, Moss S, Brown J. Report prepared for the Health Technology Assessment panel of the NHS Executive on the diagnosis, management, treatment and costs of prostate cancer in England and Wales. *Br J Urol* 1997; 79(Suppl 3):1–32

23. Anonymous. Immediate versus deferred treatment for advanced prostatic cancer: initial results of the Medical Research Council Trial. The Medical Research Council Prostate Cancer Working Party Investigators Group. *Br J Urol* 1997;79:235–46

24. Slevin TJ, Donnelly N, Clarkson JP, English DR, Ward JE. Prostate cancer testing: behaviour, motivation and attitudes among Western Australian men. *Med J Aust* 1999;171:185–8

25. Smith DP, Armstrong BK. Prostate-specific antigen testing in Australia and association with prostate cancer incidence in New South Wales. *Med J Aust* 1998;169:17–20

26. Menegoz F, Colonna M, Exbrayat C, Mousseau M, Orfeuvre H, Schaerer R. A recent increase in the incidence of prostatic carcinoma in a French population: role of ultrasonography and prostatic specific antigen. *Eur J Cancer* 1995;31A: 55–8

27. Barchielli A, Crocetti E, Zappa M. Has the PSA wave already crashed upon us? Changes in the epidemiology of prostate cancer from 1985 to 1994 in central Italy. *Ann Oncol* 1999;10:361–2

28. Reissigl A, Horninger W, Fink K, Klocker H, Bartsch G. Prostate carcinoma screening in the county of Tyrol, Austria: experience and results. *Cancer* 1997;80:1818–29

29. Ciatto S, Bonardi R, Mazzotta A, Zappa M. Evidence and feasibility of prostate cancer screening. *Cancer J* 1995;8:33–5

30. Schroder FH, Denis LJ, Kirkels W, de Koning HJ, Standaert B. European randomized study of screening for prostate cancer. Progress report of Antwerp and Rotterdam pilot studies. *Cancer* 1995;76:129–34

Expectant management with selective delayed intervention for favorable-risk prostate cancer

32

L. Klotz

Introduction

The optimal management of clinically localized prostate cancer remains unresolved. Management options are diverse, varying from a conservative approach (expectant management) to definitive treatment (radical prostatectomy or radiotherapy). Several studies have suggested that expectant management provides similar 10-year survival rates and quality-adjusted life-years compared with radical prostatectomy or radiotherapy[1–8]. Expectant management alone, however, clearly deprives some patients with potentially curable life-threatening disease of the opportunity for curative therapy. Lu-Yao and Yao[9] reported in a population-based study that particularly patients with a high Gleason score who had undergone radical prostatectomy or radiotherapy had improved 5-year overall and disease-specific survival, compared with those managed by expectant management alone.

The dilemma of management stems from the heterogeneity of the natural history of prostate cancer. Estimates from autopsy studies indicate that 30% of men over the age of 50 have prostate cancer. However, only 10% of men over 50 years old will have clinical progression of prostate cancer resulting in a diagnosis. Among those with clinically diagnosed prostate cancer, the likelihood of death from prostate cancer is one in three. While these statistics suggest a high incidence of 'latent' prostate cancer and a slow natural history of prostate cancer in many patients, they also indicate that the risk of dying from clinically diagnosed prostate cancer is substantial. This conundrum is the rationale for both conservative management and radical treatment.

The surveillance studies in the published literature are summarized in Table 1[1–8,10–16]. A number of observations can be made from these studies. Mortality from other causes is common in all cohorts, probably reflecting the average age of patients at entry. Cause-specific survival varies substantially, from 30 to 80% at 15 years. This reflects patient selection at study entry. All reflect natural history from the pre-prostate-specific antigen (PSA) era. The stage migration phenomenon of the past decade had not occurred when these studies were carried out. Second, none offered salvage radical therapy for local progression. Watchful waiting in these series consisted of no active treatment until symptomatic metastases developed, at which point androgen ablation was offered. Additionally, these series are characterized by problems of selection bias to varying degrees. Confounding issues include the use of aspiration cytology for diagnosis, exclusion of higher-risk patients, elderly cohorts and inclusion of T1a patients.

None the less, one striking similarity stands out: every series contains a substantial subset of long-term survivors, particularly in the group with favorable clinical parameters. This is a critical observation. In the absence of treatment, a substantial subset of patients with prostate cancer are not destined to die of the disease. The challenge, of course, is to identify that subset accurately.

Table 1 Summary of prostate cancer surveillance studies

Reference	Stage	Year last accrued	Patient n	Survival (%) 5 years	10 years	15 years
Hanash *et al.*, 1972	A	1942	50	86	52	22
	B		129	19	4	1
Lerner *et al.*, 1991	T1b–T2	1982	279	88	61	
				95(CSS)	80(CSS)	
Adolfsson *et al.*, 1992	T1–2	1982	122	82	50	
				99(CSS)	84(CSS)	
Johansson *et al.*, 1997	T1–2	1984	223		41/86(CSS)	21
						81(CSS)
Albertsen *et al.*, 1998		1984				
Handley *et al.*, 1988		1985	278			
Waaler and Stenwig, 1993	T2	1985	28	94(CSS)		
Whitmore *et al.*, 1991	T2	1986	37	95	90	62
George, 1988	Tx	1986	120	86	66	66
Aus *et al.*, 1995	T1–4	1991	301	80(CSS)	50(CSS)	30(CSS)

CSS, cause-specific survival

Rationale for an expectant approach

Since the advent of PSA testing in 1989, substantial resources have been directed towards the early detection and treatment of prostate cancer. Mortality rates have fallen by about 20% during this period. Whether this improvement in mortality is due to these efforts, or to other causes, is the subject of intense controversy. Other factors, including dietary and life-style modification, and a trend towards earlier initiation of androgen ablation for recurrent disease, may explain some or all of the fall in mortality. Indeed, Albertsen[17] has demonstrated that the fall in mortality in Connecticut, where screening is uncommon, is equivalent to the reduction in Oregon, a highly screened population. Thus, it remains uncertain whether our efforts at early diagnosis and local treatment have resulted in a decline in prostate cancer mortality.

The prevalence of prostate cancer far exceeds the incidence. In the PSA era, increasing efforts at screening, and the consequent rise in incidence, has resulted in about one of seven men being diagnosed. As well, the mortality rate has fallen. Thus, the chance of dying of prostate cancer in patients who are diagnosed has decreased steadily, from about one in three to one in five. While this may reflect improved treatment, it may also reflect increased diagnosis of indolent disease.

Prostate cancer is typically slow-growing. Work by Sakr and colleagues[18] has indicated that the disease develops in the 30s in the typical patient, and takes 20 years to become clinically detectable. Studies by Pound and co-workers[19] demonstrate that, in patients who fail radical prostatectomy and go on to die of prostate cancer, a median of 16 years elapses from surgery until death. The watchful-waiting studies also demonstrate that disease-related mortality in populations of prostate cancer patients only becomes substantial after 10 years. In addition, it is particularly clear that low-grade prostate cancer is associated with low progression rates and high survival rates in the intermediate term.

One indirect piece of evidence supporting the long window of curability can be derived from nomograms predicting the likelihood of biochemical recurrence on the basis of PSA, grade and stage. Using the Kattan nomogram for a patient with T1c and Gleason 6 prostate cancer, with PSA of 5 ng/ml, the 5-year biochemical disease-free survival (DFS) is 95%[20]. If one were to delay intervention until the PSA level reaches 10 ng/ml, the 5-year DFS is still 90%; and with further delay until the PSA is 15 ng/ml it is 85%. Thus, following such a patient during a period of PSA doubling or tripling is associated with a 5–10% reduction in the risk of progression.

Widespread use of PSA testing has also resulted in profound stage migration. Most patients newly diagnosed with prostate cancer have clinically impalpable, stage T1c disease. Additionally, these patients typically have a PSA which is only mildly elevated (< 10 ng/ml). These patients usually have slowly growing cancer with a long window of curability. This is also supported by the Albertsen data (Table 2)[16].

A meta-analysis of six surveillance series comprising 828 patients reported by Chodak indicated that, at 10 years, disease-specific survival was 87% for well- and moderately differentiated cancers, and metastasis-free survival was 81% and 58%, respectively[21]. These studies also incorporated an 'either–or' approach, and reflected a pre-stage-migration population. Thus, many patients with favorably prognostic factors, diagnosed considerably earlier in their disease process than the average patient in this surveillance population, are likely to have an incredibly long natural history.

The Prostate Cancer Intervention Versus Observation Trial (PIVOT), comparing radical prostatectomy with watchful waiting, has been an ambitious effort to compare these two approaches in a randomized design[22]. This trial,

against all expectations, is close to reaching its accrual target. The outcome will be of profound importance. However, one limitation of the trial is that the observation arm does not have an option for intervention for the subset with evidence of rapid biochemical or local progression early on in the course of the disease.

The art of the management of localized prostate cancer is to differentiate patients with biologically aggressive disease for whom curative therapy is strongly warranted from those with indolent malignancy for whom conservative management is equally efficacious. A blanket policy of observation for all results in under-treatment for some; similarly, a policy of treatment for all results in over-treatment for a subset.

Traditionally, watchful waiting has meant no treatment until progression to metastatic or locally advanced disease, followed by androgen ablation therapy. Today, in the PSA era, patients who are managed conservatively are typically still followed with periodic PSA tests. This raises the question: can treatment of favorable prostate cancer be deferred indefinitely in many while effective, albeit delayed, therapy is offered to those who progress rapidly?

Results of watchful waiting with selective intervention approach

We have been conducting a clinical study to evaluate a novel approach in which the choice between definitive therapy and a conservative policy is determined by the rate of PSA increase or the development of early, rapid clinical and/or histological progression. This strategy, which has never been previously described or evaluated, offers the powerful attraction of individualizing therapy according to the biological behavior of the cancer. This would mean that patients with slowly growing malignancy would be spared the side-effects of radical treatment, while those with more rapidly progressive cancer would still benefit from curative therapy.

This prospective study consisted of 250 patients followed with watchful waiting with selective delayed intervention. Patients had PSA

Table 2 Prostate cancer mortality in a watchful waiting cohort according to grade. Patients with low-grade prostate cancer, by and large, do not die of their disease. As grade increases, the risk of death also increases, but for Gleason 6, this remains at only 18–30%. From reference 16

Gleason score	Prostate cancer mortality at 15 years (%)
2–4	4–7
5	6–11
6	18–30
7	42–70
8–10	60–87

< 15 ng/ml, Gleason ≤ 7 and T ≤ 2b. Patients were followed with watchful waiting until they met specific criteria defining rapid or clinically significant progression. These criteria were as follows:

(1) PSA progression, defined by all of the following three conditions:

    (a) PSA doubling time < 2 years, based on at least three separate measurements over a minimum of 6 months;

    (b) Final PSA > 8 ng/ml;

    (c) *p* value < 0.05 from a regression analysis of ln(PSA) versus time.

(2) Clinical progression when one of the following conditions was met:

    (a) More than twice increase in the product of the maximum perpendicular diameters of the primary lesion as measured digitally;

    (b) Local progression of prostate cancer requiring transurethral resection of the prostate (TURP);

    (c) Development of ureteric obstruction;

    (d) Radiological and/or clinical evidence of distant metastasis.

(3) Histological progression: Gleason score ≥ 8 in the rebiopsy of prostate at 12–18 months.

Most of the patients in this series fulfilled the criteria for favorable disease (PSA < 10 ng/ml, Gleason ≤ 6, T ≤ 2a). Eighty per cent of patients had Gleason 6 or less, and the same proportion had PSA < 10 ng/ml. With a median follow-up of 42 months, 60 patients (30%) came off watchful observation while 140 have remained on surveillance. Of the patients coming off surveillance, 8% came off because of rapid biochemical progression; 8% for clinical progression; and 8% owing to patient preference. The remaining 6% came off surveillance for a variety of other reasons.

The distribution of PSA doubling times is seen in Figure 1. The median PSA doubling time was 10.15 years. Only 20% of patients had a PSA doubling time of < 3 years.

Patients were re-biopsied 1.5–2 years after being placed on the surveillance protocol. Grade remained stable in 92%; only 8% demonstrated significant (> 2) Gleason score rise. This is also consistent with the recent publication by Epstein and Walsh, demonstrating a 4% rate of grade progression over 2–3 years[23].

Nine patients (of 200) had a radical prostatectomy after they manifested a PSA doubling time of less than 2 years. All had Gleason 5–6,

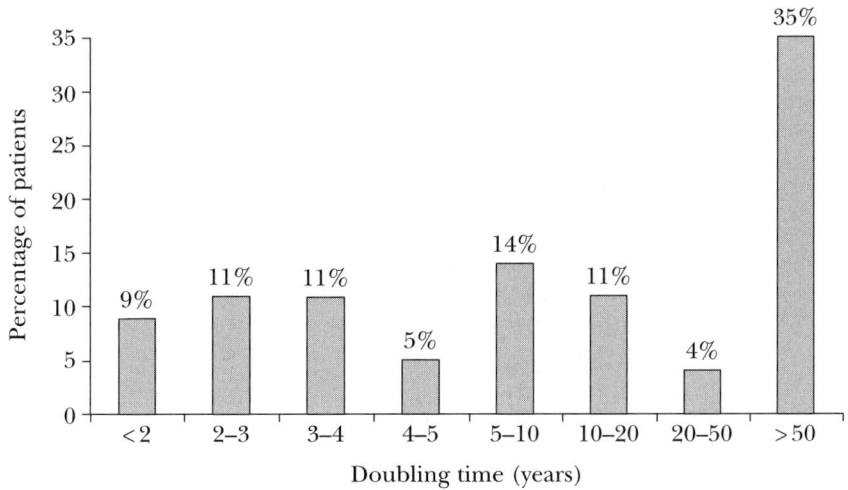

Figure 1 Doubling times of prostate-specific antigen (PSA) in patients on a watchful waiting protocol. Data are based on a median follow-up of 55 months. Median PSA doubling time was 10.15 years. Median number of measurements was 7 (range 3–19), 20% of patients had a PSA doubling time of < 3 years

PSA < 10 ng/ml, pT1–2 at study entry. Final pathology was as follows: three of nine were pT2, five were pT3a–c and one was N1. For a group of patients with favorable clinical characteristics, this is a high rate of locally advanced disease. This supports the view that a short PSA doubling time is associated with a more aggressive phenotype. A PSA doubling time of < 2 years, in patients with otherwise favorable clinical features, portents a high likelihood of advanced disease. Fortunately, this scenario is uncommon. This also suggests that, insofar as cure of the patients with early rapid biochemical progression is a goal, the optimal PSA doubling time threshold for intervention should be greater than 2 years. The optimal threshold is probably in the region of 3 years. In our series, that constituted 22% of patients.

Zeitman and colleagues recently published a retrospective review of 199 men with T1–2 prostate cancer and PSA < 20 ng/ml, managed with watchful waiting[24]. Median follow-up was 3.4 years. Overall survival at 5 and 7 years was 77% and 63%, and disease-specific survival was 99% and 99%, respectively. At 5 and 7 years, the proportion of patients who were alive and untreated was 43% and 26%. Sixty-three patients were treated radically. The median PSA rise from diagnosis to treatment was 2.9 ng/ml in the treated cohort, compared with 0.9 ng/ml in the untreated group.

This study raises the concern that watchful waiting may simply be a version of delayed therapy, unless patients die of comorbid illness in the interim. However, the indication for intervention in this series was a mild rise in PSA (< 3 ng) over a prolonged period. This emphasizes that conservative management in the modern PSA era requires 'buy-in' by the patient and the doctor. This involves an understanding that PSA will probably progress slowly over time, but that slow progression is not a reason for intervention.

One assumption on which the selective intervention approach is based is that the PSA rate of rise remains relatively stable over time. This is not the case in some patients; rapid rises in PSA after long periods of stability (PSA acceleration) have been clearly documented. The following critical unanswered questions with respect to PSA acceleration remain. When does it occur in the natural history of prostate cancer, in particular, relative to the point at which the disease becomes metastatic or locally incurable? How common is a sudden rapid increase? Are patients who manifest PSA acceleration still curable?

Conclusions

The approach of watchful waiting with selective intervention for patients with rapid biochemical or clinical progression is feasible. Most patients, who understand the basis for the approach, will remain on observation for the long term. Doubling time varies widely, and is not predicted by grade, stage or baseline PSA. Fifty per cent have a PSA doubling time of > 10 years. Doubling time appears to be a useful tool to guide treatment intervention for patients managed initially with expectant management. A doubling time of less than 2 years appears to identify patients at high risk for local progression in spite of otherwise favorable prognostic factors. The appropriate threshold for initiation of definitive therapy is a doubling time of around 3 years; approximately 20% of patients will fall into this category. The remainder have a high chance of remaining free of recurrence and progression for years.

Watchful waiting is clearly appropriate for patients who are elderly, have significant comorbidity and have favorable clinical parameters. The use of comorbidity indices such as the Index of Co-existent Disease facilitates the identification of patients whose life expectancy is diminished, relative to the natural history of their prostate cancer. The likelihood of prostate cancer death in these patients is low. Many patients, however, fall into a gray zone where the benefits of treatment are unclear. In these patients, a policy of close monitoring with selective intervention for the 15% who progress rapidly is appealing. This approach is currently the focus of several clinical trials.

References

1. Johansson JE, Adami HO, Andersson SO, *et al.* High 10 year survival rate in patients with early, untreated prostatic cancer. *J Am Med Assoc* 1992; 267:2191–6

2. Johansson JE, Holmberg L, Johansson S, *et al.* Fifteen-year survival in prostate cancer. A prospective, population-based study in Sweden. *J Am Med Assoc* 1997;277:467–71

3. Hanash KA, Utz DC, Cook EN, *et al.* Carcinoma of the prostate: a 15 year followup. *J Urol* 1972; 107:450–3

4. Cook GB, Watson FR. Twenty nodules of prostate cancer not treated by total prostatectomy. *J Urol* 1968;100:672–4

5. Barnes R, Hirst A, Rosenquist R. Early carcinoma of the prostate: comparison of stages A and B. *J Urol* 1976;115:404–5

6. Lerner SP, Seale-Hawkins C, Carlton CE, *et al.* The risk of dying of prostate cancer in patients with clinically localized disease. *J Urol* 1991;146: 1040–5

7. Handley R, Carr TW, Travis D, *et al.* Deferred treatment for prostate cancer. *Br J Urol* 1988; 62:249–53

8. Adolfsson J, Carstensen J, Lowhagen T. Deferred treatment in clinically localized prostate carcinoma. *Br J Urol* 1992;69:183–7

9. Lu-Yao GL, Yao SL. Population-based study of long-term survival in patients with clinically localised prostate cancer. *Lancet* 1997;349:906–10

10. Waaler G, Stenwig AE. Prognosis of localised prostatic cancer managed by 'watch and wait' policy. *Br J Urol* 1993;72:214–19

11. Whitmore WF, Warner IA, Thompson IM. Expectant management of localized prostatic cancer. *Cancer* 1991;67:1091–6

12. George NJR. Natural history of localised prostatic cancer managed by conservative therapy alone. *Lancet* 1988;1:494–6

13. Aus G, Hugosson I, Norlen L. Long-term survival and mortality in prostate cancer treated with noncurative intent. *J Urol* 1995;154:460–5

14. Sandblom G, Dufmats M, Varenhorst E. Long-term survival in a Swedish population-based cohort of men with prostate cancer. *Urology* 2000;56:442–7

15. Madsen PO, Graversen PH, Gasser TC, Corle DK. Treatment of localized prostatic cancer. Radical prostatectomy versus placebo. A 15-year follow-up. *Scand J Urol Nephrol* 1988;110(Suppl):95–100

16. Albertsen PC, Hanley IA, Gleason DF, Barry MJ. Competing risk analysis of men aged 55 to 74 years at diagnosis managed conservatively for clinically localized prostate cancer. *J Am Med Assoc* 1998;280:975–80

17. Albertsen PC. Prostate cancer mortality trends in Oregon and Connecticut. Presented at the *Whistler International Conference on Prostate Cancer*, March 2001, Whistler, Canada

18. Sakr WA, Haas GP, Cassin BF, Pontes JE, Crissman JD. The frequency of carcinoma and intraepithelial neoplasia of the prostate in young male patients. *J Urol* 1993;150:379–85

19. Pound CR, Partin AW, Eisenberger MA, Chan DW, Pearson JD, Walsh PC. Natural history of progression after PSA elevation following radical prostatectomy. *J Am Med Assoc* 1999;281: 1591–7

20. Kattan MW, Zelefsky MJ, Kupelian PA, Scardino PT, Fuks Z, Leibel SA. Pretreatment nomogram for predicting the outcome of three-dimensional conformal radiotherapy in prostate cancer. *J Clin Oncol* 2000;18:3352–9

21. Chodak GW. The management of localized prostate cancer. *J Urol* 1994;152:1766

22. Wilt TJ, Brawer MK. The Prostate Cancer Intervention Versus Observation Trial (PIVOT). *Oncology* 1997;11:1133–43

23. Epstein J, Walsh P, Carter H. Dedifferentiation of prostate cancer grade with time in men followed expectantly for stage T1c disease. *J Urol* 2001; 166:1688–91

24. Zeitman AL, Thakral H, Wilson L, Schellhammer P. Conservative management of prostate cancer in the prostate specific antigen era: the incidence and time course of subsequent therapy. *J Urol* 2001;166:1702–6

Is cure of prostate cancer possible in those in whom it is necessary?

33

P. C. Walsh

Background

For men in the USA, prostate cancer is the most common major cancer and the second most common cause of cancer death. In 2002, it is estimated that there will be 189 000 new cases and 30 200 deaths, a marked decline from 1993 when 43 000 died from the disease[1,2]. The cause for this dramatic decrease in mortality is not known for certain, but it is widely believed that it is secondary to diagnosis at an earlier stage with effective treatment. One would assume that with time these statistics would improve. Unfortunately, this is not the case. The 'baby boomers', children born immediately following the end of World War II, represent almost one-quarter of the population in the USA: 80 million men and women. In 4 years the first wave of individuals in this large group will turn 60 years of age, the year when the age-specific diagnoses of breast and prostate cancer are equal. Thereafter, with aging, the incidence of prostate cancer begins to exceed the incidence of breast cancer, and it is believed that within 20–40 years, unless there is a continued dramatic improvement in the management of prostate cancer, there will be an estimated 100 000 men who will die from prostate cancer, and prostate cancer will overtake breast cancer as a cause of death (Chan, unpublished observations). This observation emphasizes the urgency in addressing the question raised by the title of this chapter.

For many years Willet F. Whitmore, Jr, the father of urological oncology in the USA, was a thoughtful nihilist regarding the management of localized prostate cancer. He cleverly phrased his objections in a two-part question[3]: 'Is cure necessary in those in whom it may be possible and is cure possible in those in whom it is neces-

sary?' His criticism was based on three premises, which for many years were more or less true:

(1) Cure was most often not necessary because most men with the disease were old, and death from other causes, such as cardio-vascular disease, was most likely.

(2) Cure was most often not possible because there were no established screening procedures. Thus, most men were diagnosed with advanced disease because they presented with symptomatic, large, palpable lesions. Conversely, the only patients who presented with curable disease were most often diagnosed by transurethral resection of the prostate and had small well-differentiated transition zone tumors, which often required no treatment.

(3) Treatment in this era was also often associated with significant morbidity: incontinence, impotence and blood loss.

Given the risk/benefit ratio, Whitmore argued logically and strongly against the aggressive treatment of localized disease.

Over the past 20 years, there has been a revolution in the diagnosis and management of localized prostate cancer. It is reasonable now to ask whether the criticisms raised two decades ago are still valid today and, if Whitmore were alive today, what he would say.

Is cure necessary?

Over the past 25 years there has been a revolution in the medical and surgical management of cardiovascular disease, and a marked decrease in the number of men who smoke cigarettes. This has had a profound impact on the cause of death in men in the USA. In 1988, the most common cause of death in US men was heart disease: 385 402 deaths[4]. By 1999, this number had fallen by 10% to 351 617[1]. In 1988, heart disease was the number-one cause of death for all men older than 34 years of age. By the year 2000, however, cancer became the major cause of death in men between the ages of 60 and 79 years. Thus, there are many men who present today with prostate cancer in whom the disease may be the major cause of death if left untreated.

In the past, the majority of patients with localized curable prostate cancer had stage T1a disease. We now understand that these well-differentiated, transition zone tumors rarely required aggressive therapy. With modern screening techniques (see below) these small tumors are rarely diagnosed. Instead, most patients are identified with significant tumors that require treatment. However, with any new form of screening there is always a subset of patients who will be diagnosed 'too early'. This must be taken into consideration when any patient with localized prostate cancer is being evaluated. Patients with low-volume tumors characteristically have non-palpable T1c disease involving fewer than three cores of tissue, less than half of any core, a prostate-specific antigen (PSA) density of < 0.1 ng/ml and a free PSA level of > 15%[6]. Many of these patients are candidates for a watchful-waiting protocol, in which patients are carefully observed with PSA determinations and digital rectal examinations every 6 months and periodic needle biopsies. It is too early to know whether this logical approach to the disease will be effective in diagnosing patients who progress at a time when they are still curable, but early results appear promising[5].

Is cure possible?

With the advent of screening strategies based upon PSA determinations and digital rectal examinations there has been a dramatic shift in the stage at presentation towards men who have more curable disease. In 1979–84, 64% of men presented with clinically localized prostate cancer, 16% local extension and 20% distant metastasis[4]. However, of the patients with apparent clinically localized prostate cancer, less than 30% had organ-confined disease at the time of radical prostatectomy[6]. In contrast, between 1989 and 1995, 80% of men presented with localized/regional disease and only 8% with metastatic disease[1,4]. During this era, 50–60% of men undergoing radical prostatectomy had pT2 disease, and by 1998 this had risen to 80%[6]. This shift in the earlier diagnosis of the disease can also be seen in the Partin tables. The original tables were published in 1994, based upon 1000 men who underwent a radical prostatectomy at the Johns Hopkins Hospital between 1985 and 1992[7]. The most recent Partin tables are based on 5000 men who underwent a radical prostatectomy at the Johns Hopkins Hospital between 1994 and 2000[8]. If one looks at the patients who had the most aggressive disease (Gleason score ≥ 7, PSA > 10 ng/ml, palpable disease), in the original tables the chance of seminal vesicle invasion was 20–70% and the probability of lymph node involvement was 10–70%. In the 2002 Partin tables, the probability of seminal vesicle invasion fell to 10–19% and of positive lymph nodes to 14–38%. This has also translated into a dramatic improvement in biochemical recurrence-free survival. In men who underwent a radical prostatectomy between 1982 and 1988, their biochemical recurrence-free survival at 10 years was 68%, compared with 80% for patients who underwent a radical prostatectomy after 1992[6].

Who needs to be cured?

The ideal candidate for radical prostatectomy is a patient who is curable, who is going to live long enough to need to be cured and who has a tumor that has lethal potential during his lifetime. Thus, to answer this question, one needs to look at the cure rates in patients who are young and in patients who are at high risk for progression of disease.

Data from several studies indicate that younger men are more likely to have curable disease than older men. In a study of 444 patients with stage T2a and T2b disease, the probability of advanced pathological stage (extracapsular extension and involvement of the seminal vesicle) was statistically higher in men over age 60 than in younger men[9]. More recently, in 492 men with stage T1c disease, younger age was a strong predictor of the probability of curable cancer[10]. Finally, in men who underwent a radical prostatectomy, patients younger than 50 years had a significant improvement in biochemical recurrence-free survival at 10 years compared with older men[11]. Thus, not only are younger men more likely to live long enough to need to be cured, they are more curable.

Although it is well known that patients with high Gleason score (≥ 7), high PSA (≥ 20 ng/ml) and high clinical stage (T2c) are more likely to have progression of disease, what is the evidence that definitive treatment can have an impact on progression? The probability of PSA progression following external beam radiotherapy, interstitial radiotherapy and radical prostatectomy was evaluated in 590 men using the criteria of the American Society of Therapeutic Radiology and Oncology (ASTRO)[12]. At 5 years, men who underwent external beam radiotherapy or radical prostatectomy had a significant improvement in

biochemical recurrence-free survival over patients undergoing interstitial radiotherapy. Although this was not a randomized controlled trial, it demonstrates that effective control of the local lesion can prevent progression of disease.

It is widely recognized that patients with high-grade disease (Gleason 8–10) provide the greatest challenge for cure following definitive therapy. We have studied 94 men with Gleason 8–10 disease on needle biopsy who underwent a radical prostatectomy at the Johns Hopkins Hospital between 1982 and 2001 (50 patients from 1982 to 1991 and 44 patients from 1992 to 2001)[13]. The probability of biochemical recurrence-free survival for patients with tumor that was confined to the surgical specimen (organ-confined and extraprostatic extension with a negative surgical margin) was significantly better than for patients with positive surgical margins, positive seminal vesicles and positive lymph nodes (Figure 1). Furthermore, patients with specimen-confined disease treated in the most recent era (1992–2001) had a 60% probability of an undetectable PSA at 10 years, compared with 34% patients treated in the earlier era. This demonstrates that high-grade tumors, if detected early, can be treated effectively with surgery, providing significant long-term tumor-free survival.

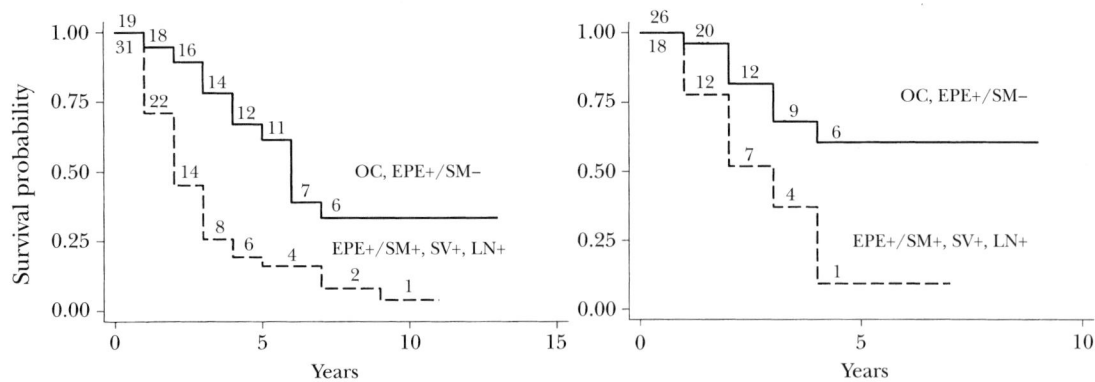

Figure 1 Biochemical recurrence-free survival following radical prostatectomy for Gleason 8–10 disease based on pathological stage: OC, organ-confined; EPE+/SM–, extraprostatic extension with negative surgical margins; SM +, positive surgical margins; SV +, seminal vesicle invasion; LN +, positive lymph nodes. Data divided into two eras: (a) 1982–91; (b) 1992–2001

Randomized controlled trial

The most convincing way to prove whether patients who are curable need to be cured is the gold standard of outcomes research: the randomized controlled trial. Until recently this information has not been available, and no argument, however compelling, influenced critics. However, the landmark study by Holmberg and colleagues has once and for all shown that definitive treatment of prostate cancer reduces deaths from the disease[14]. In a randomized clinical controlled trial, the Scandinavian Prostate Cancer Group randomized 695 men with newly diagnosed prostate cancer (clinical stage T1b, T1c or T2) to watchful waiting or radical prostatectomy. Eight years following randomization, progression to metastatic disease (27% in the watchful-waiting group and 13% in the surgical group) and deaths from prostate cancer (13.6% versus 7.1%) were reduced by 50% in the radical prostatectomy group. Although at this time point there was no difference in overall mortality, recognizing that men with metastatic disease have a median survival of only 2–3 years, it is clear that within a relatively short period of time the influence on prostate cancer-specific mortality will increase markedly and should have an impact on overall mortality.

Quality of life

Anyone who knew Dr Whitmore realized that his major objection to radical prostatectomy was its profound adverse impact on quality of life, especially sexual function. During his lifetime he introduced handheld interstitial radiotherapy placed at an open surgical procedure as a means to treat prostate cancer, in an effort to avoid this side-effect. However, he subsequently reported that local relapse and the development of distant metastasis 15 years following treatment were greater than expected[15]. During this same time it became clear that the major side-effects of radical prostatectomy (bleeding, incontinence and impotence) could be avoided, based upon new anatomical observations of the periprostatic anatomy[16]. Bleeding occurred because the anatomical location of the periprostatic venous plexus was unknown. Once this anatomy was clarified it was possible to perform the operation in a more controlled safe setting, where anatomical structures were more clearly delineated. This resulted in a better cancer operation which was safer, and over the next 20 years the mortality of radical prostatectomy fell from 2 to 0.4%. Impotence occurred because the location of the autonomic nerves to the corpora cavernosa was unknown. Once these nerves were identified and the concept of the neurovascular bundle was developed it became possible intraoperatively to preserve these nerves where possible, or excise them widely where necessary. Indeed, in reviewing radical prostatectomies in the pre-nerve-sparing era, it is clear that the neurovascular bundles were never completely excised with the specimen. Rather, because they are adherent to the rectum, they were cut and left in place. Today it is possible to preserve sexual function in most men under the age of 65. In a multicenter study involving five experienced surgeons, patient-reported potency using a confidential validated instrument at 12 months was 75%[17]. Finally, incontinence was common because the understanding of the sphincteric complex was incorrect. Once the concept of the striated sphincter was demonstrated it became possible during ligation of the dorsal vein complex to preserve it more completely. Today, in the hands of experienced surgeons, the long-term probability of significant urinary incontinence is less than 5%.

Epilogue

In 1980 only 7% of men with localized prostate cancer underwent surgical treatment. However, over the next 20 years the number of radical prostatectomies rose dramatically, peaking at 104 000 in 1992–93. A decade later the number of deaths from prostate cancer declined from 43 000 in 1993 to 30 200 in 2002. If one applies the 7% reduction in death rate from the Scandinavian randomized trial to the 1992–93 data in the USA (an era in which most patients were diagnosed with palpable disease like in the

Scandinavian trial), it is possible to assume that much of the reduction in deaths from prostate cancer in the USA arose from the increased application of surgery[18].

In 1983, Dr Whitmore wrote to me: 'Hopefully, one day in the not too distant future I will be able to break away from this cancer center long enough to come down to Hopkins and, with your permission, look over your shoulder while you do one of your classic dissections for the preservation of sexual potency during a radical retropubic prostatectomy! From those who watched you do it, from the reports of those who are doing it, and from your elegant publications on the subject, you appear to have made one of the first real breakthroughs that I can remember. Quite apart from the fact that [125]Iodine implantation may not stand the test of time, the possibility of preserving sexual function in the face of a radical cystectomy deserves our serious appraisal. I understand from unofficial reports that you have already had some success in this area.' In 1986, he was invited to provide a discussion for a fascicle that I had written on the operation. In it he stated: 'I enjoyed the privilege of assisting Dr Walsh in the performance of a nerve-sparing radical prostatectomy in Stockholm in 1984 and was impressed by the controlled anatomical exposure and technical precision possible with the procedure. I also realized that in doing literally hundreds of radical cystectomies over the years I had seen the neurovascular bundles countless times but had not recognized them.' Later that year he again wrote: 'After a lapse of 17+ years I finally accomplished a radical prostatectomy August 7, 1986! I did a Walsh nerve-sparing radical retropubic operation with bilateral pelvic lymph node dissection. The excisional part of the operation was uneventful but the urethrovesical anastomosis gave me a hard time. Under the influence of sedatives, the patient removed his catheter on the evening of the first postoperative day, but he had the good sense to deflate the balloon before doing so and a catheter was reinserted without difficulty and left in place for a total of 3 weeks. On removal of the catheter his urinary control was apparently normal. On follow-up examination on October 29 his urinary control was perfect, his urinary stream like a fire hose, and his sexual function was normal! I may close my "series" while my results are better than yours! Finally, I should add that the operation spared the patient's nerves but not mine!'

Conclusion

Today, most men who are candidates for the definitive treatment of localized prostate cancer are curable, are healthy enough to need to be cured and can be cured with fewer side-effects than in the past. Were Dr Whitmore alive today I believe that he would conclude that in this modern era, yes, cure is possible in those in whom it is necessary.

References

1. Greenlee RT, Murray T, Bolden S, et al. Cancer statistics, 2000. CA Cancer J Clin 2000;50:7–33
2. Boring CB, Squires TS, Tong T. Cancer statistics, 1993. CA Cancer J Clin 1993;43:7–26
3. Whitmore WF Jr. Natural history of low-stage prostatic cancer and the impact of early detection. Urol Clin North Am 1990;17:689–97
4. Silverberg E, Lubera BBA. Cancer statistics, 1988. CA Cancer J Clin 1988;38:5–22
5. Carter HB, Walsh PC, Landis P, et al. Expectant management of non-palpable prostate cancer with curative intent: preliminary results. J Urol 2002;167:1231–4
6. Han M, Partin AW, Piantadosi S, et al. Era specific biochemical recurrence-free survival following radical prostatectomy for clinically localized prostate cancer. J Urol 2001;166:416–19

7. Partin AW, Walsh PC. The use of prostate specific antigen, clinical stage, and Gleason score to predict pathologic stage in men with localized prostate cancer. *J Urol* 1994;152:172–3

8. Partin AW, Mangold LA, Lamm DM, *et al.* Contemporary update of prostate cancer staging nomograms (Partin tables) for the new millennium. *Urology* 2001;58:843–8

9. Alexander RB, Maguire MG, Epstein JI, *et al.* Pathological stage is higher in older men with clinical stage B1 adenocarcinoma of the prostate. *J Urol* 1990;143:586–7

10. Carter HB, Epstein JI, Partin AW. Influence of age and prostate-specific antigen on the chance of curable prostate cancer among men with nonpalpable disease. *Urology* 1999;53:126–30

11. Riopel MA, Polascik TJ, Partin AW, *et al.* Radical prostatectomy in men less than 50 years old. *Urol Oncol* 1995;1:80–3

12. D'Amico AV, Whittington R, Malkowicz B, *et al.* Biochemical outcome after radical prostatectomy, external beam radiation therapy, or interstitial radiation therapy for clinically localized prostate cancer. *J Am Med Assoc* 1998; 280:969–74

13. Han M, Partin AW, Zahurak M, *et al.* Biochemical (PSA) recurrence probability following radical prostatectomy for high-grade clinically localized prostate cancer. *J Urol* 2003;169:517–23

14. Holmberg L, Bill-Axelson A, Helgesen F, *et al.* A randomized trial comparing radical prostatectomy with watchful waiting in early prostate cancer. *N Engl J Med* 2992;347:781–9

15. Zelefsky M, Whitmore WF Jr. Long-term results of retropubic permanent ^{125}Iodine implantation of the prostate for clinically localized prostatic cancer. *J Urol* 1997;158:23–30

16. Walsh PC. Anatomic radical prostatectomy: evolution of the surgical technique. *J Urol* 1998; 160:2418–24

17. Walsh PC, Marschke P, Catalona WJ, *et al.* Efficacy of first-generation Cavermap to verify location and function of cavernous nerves during radical prostatectomy: a multi-institutional evaluation by experienced surgeons. *Urology* 2001;57:491–4

18. Walsh PC. Surgery and the reduction of mortality from prostate cancer [Editorial]. *N Engl J Med* 2002;347:839–40

Modern molecular classification of renal cell carcinoma: relevance for urologists

34

F. Algaba

Renal cell carcinoma histogenesis

Once we overcame the hypothesis that renal cell carcinoma (RCC) was the malignant transformation of intrarenal adrenal remnants, it was considered that all renal parenchymal neoplasias originated in the proximal tubules[1]. For this reason, only grading, staging and some morphological characteristics such as spindle cell phenotype are generally used to describe biological differences between patients. However, in the literature, various morphological forms are described, involving growth (papillary renal cell carcinoma) or cytological features (chromophobe cell carcinoma, chromophil cell carcinoma, granular cell carcinoma)[2]. Also described is the concept of oncocytoma as a benign biological neoplasia[3].

Initially, urologists did not take all these variables into account because they were considered to be part of a morphological process without clinical translation. Pathologists reinforced this attitude when they did not succeed in defining the immunophenotype for the above morphological variables because the different antibodies co-appear in several forms[4].

The situation would have remained the same were it not for the introduction of chromosomal studies. Research into chromosomal alterations soon found that a large proportion of RCC featured 3p deletion, while other cases featured trisomies 7, 12 and 17[5]. These findings helped to correlate morphology with chromosomal alterations. It was also recognized that within the different morphological forms of RCC there were several morphological variations that pathologists were wrongly classifying. Finally, for each RCC cellular subtype, a biological spectrum could be defined.

Relevance for urologists of modern molecular classification of renal cell carcinoma

More accurate pathological classification

Histological subtyping has had an impact on patient prognosis[6]. Nowadays, the pathologist is able to recognize RCC molecular subtypes (chromosomal) by means of morphology. The various forms of RCC are described in the following.

Conventional RCC   This belongs to the group of classic clear cell carcinomas (75% of RCC), so called because of the large amount of cytoplasmic mitochondria which contains eosinophils. Its chromosomal feature is loss of heterozygosity (LOH) 3p, which explains its relationship to von Hippel–Lindau (VHL) syndrome. However, it can also include deletions in chromosomes 8, 9, 13 and 14. Conventional RCC usually demonstrates a solid pattern, but in some cases a papillary arrangement is possible, and for this reason it would not be classified as papillary renal carcinoma[7].

Chromophil (papillary) RCC   The literature used to call this variant papillary, because this is the most frequent growth pattern. However, it can also be possible to observe a solid pattern[8]. The cells have scanty cytoplasm (chromophil cells), but in some circumstances a clear-like cytoplasm can be present in some areas. It is the second most frequent type of RCC, constituting 10–15%. The chromosomal features are trisomies 7, 17, 12, 16 and 20 but without LOH 3p, so this type is not correlated with VHL syndrome. There can be hereditary forms of this variant by mutation of the *MET* gene[9], which strengthens the oncogenic effect by selective duplication of chromosome 7.

Chromophobe RCC This form represents 5–10% of RCC, and was distinguished from conventional carcinoma by Thoenes and colleagues[10] who investigated the existence of neoplasias with clear cytoplasm. The cells of this variant of RCC have large dimensions, perfect delineation of the cytoplasmic membranes and fine granular appearance of the cytoplasm, secondary to the presence of microvesicles that are stained by colloidal iron (Hale tincture). Several cases have been identified, however, in which the abundance of mitochondria gave the cells an eosinophilic appearance[11]. Chromosomal features are multiple allele losses (monosomies 10, 13, 17 and 21, and also sometimes 1, 2, 6 and Y)[12].

Collecting duct (Bellini) RCC This variant has been widely discussed because, from a clinical point of view, high-grade carcinomas, usually of papillary pattern and associated with the medulla or hilus, have been attributed to a collecting duct origin. Chromosomal characterization is limited and conflicting, although apparently LOH involving 8p and 13q are the most frequent features[13]. Monosomies 1, 2, 6 and 19 have also been described, as well as gains in 1q21–23, especially in the metastatic tumor. This rare form represents only 1%, approximately, of RCC. Its growing pattern is variable and oscillates from tubular to papillary, with characteristic areas of prominent collagen reaction of the stroma.

Sarcomatoid differentiation in RCC Recent chromosomal studies have shown that carcinomas with a spindle-cell pattern are a further evolution of the morphological variants mentioned above, and the presence of this pattern is associated with a poor prognosis[14].

Unclassifiable RCC Some cases cannot be classified, and at the present time they are included under this heading[15].

Conclusions Based on recent chromosomal studies, the following conclusions can be drawn:

(1) Conventional (clear cell) carcinoma can be distinguished from chromophobe RCC;

(2) Chromophil RCC sometimes has a solid pattern and/or some cell areas with an unusual clear-like cytoplasm appearance;

(3) An eosinophilic aspect is considered an expression of a high concentration of cytoplasmic mitochondria, with no classification use;

(4) Chromophil RCC can be distinguished from conventional (clear) RCC and from collecting duct (Bellini) carcinomas;

(5) Spindle cell carcinomas are not considered a different entity from the others, because it is possible to find this morphology in various subtypes;

(6) Unclassifiable morphologies are awaiting the description of new entities, so that recognized variants can be classified into more homogeneous subtypes.

Problems with the adenoma–carcinoma relationship

Problems have arisen because, knowing the various chromosomal alterations in RCC, it has been possible to correlate them with lesions that are considered to be renal adenoma. The existence of clear cell adenoma is currently still not accepted, and, concerning other varieties of benign epithelial neoplasm, the following discussion focuses on metanephric adenoma and oncocytoma.

Metanephric adenoma A major finding in chromosomal studies, in papillary (chromophil) epithelial tumors, is the existence of trisomies in chromosomes 7 and 17 and loss of Y. Such tumors are considered benign, and therefore called papillary adenoma[16]. Recently, the concept of metanephric adenoma has been used in terms of a cell neoformation of chromophil phenotype, but with the formation of microtubules and myxoid stroma. Some cytogenetics studies of this tumor also show chromosomes 7 and 17 gain and Y loss, as with the papillary (chromophil) adenoma[17,18], which questions whether this is actually a different type of papillary adenoma. However, more recently, it has been suggested that the influence of a possible tumor suppressor gene on the short arm of chromosome 2 is necessary for metanephric adenoma[19].

Oncocytoma The oncocytoma is considered a benign neoplasia, despite its size, and even in some cases with nuclear atypia. It could originate from intercalated cells. Chromosomal studies of this tumor have shown the existence of two types: balanced translocation involving 11q13[20] and LOH 1p, 14q and Y[21], the latter suggesting possible precursor lesions for chromophobe RCC[21]. There are also some cases without chromosomal alterations.

Conclusion New methods have thrown into doubt the interpretation of some lesions that are considered benign, suggesting that not all oncocytomas are the same, and that some of them could be precursors of chromophobe RCC. However, at present, these hypotheses should not induce any change in therapeutic attitude.

Identification of a biological spectrum in some histological subtypes and definition of new entities

This has been observed especially in the case of the collecting duct carcinomas. These are conventionally considered as a homogeneous group of neoplasias, but various types can be recognized: low-grade collecting duct carcinomas[22] and very aggressive varieties such as medullary renal cell carcinomas[23], related to sickle cell disease. However, there are not sufficient molecular studies of such unusual renal neoplasias to be sure that they are a spectrum of the same entity.

In relation to this situation, a new morphological entity has been described, named low-grade myxoid RCC, with a possible origin in Henle's loop. It has low aggressiveness, even in cases with a spindle cell component[24]; but molecular studies are still lacking.

Conclusion Although we have acquired a large amount of knowledge from molecular studies, some morphological types still remain to be classified in the same way as the others mentioned above. However, this should not be an obstacle to applying the phenotypical, immunological and clinical knowledge that is emerging related to these new entities. We now await their molecular categorization.

Evolutionary model for prognosis and treatment

The purpose of the classification of RCC is to determine the different biologies, and hence prognostic factors for the identification of suitable treatments.

In any attempt to design an evolutionary model, a series of possible errors must be considered, taking into account the intrinsic tumor heterogeneity[25], as well as technical characteristics of the study method, for example, false positives in comparative genomic hybridization (CGH) analysis of guanine–cytosine-rich regions[26]; likewise, it is necessary to take into account the random genetic changes of natural cancer instability and use analysis methods considering clonal copy number aberration.

Bearing the above in mind, to date, two subtypes have been distinguished in conventional RCC, in accordance with chromosomal alterations: the group of tumors with −6q, +17q, +17p and cases with −9p, −13q, −18q. These two types are correlated neither with degree of differentiation nor with local extension, and the second group (LOH at chromosomes 9, 13, 18) is associated with poorer prognosis than that of the first group[27].

According to these studies, it is considered that in conventional RCC:

(1) There is a high frequency of different random genetic events;

(2) The path-like model (similar to colorectal cancer) is insufficient for a complete definition of RCC, and a tree-like model is proposed;

(3) The 3p loss is an early event in carcinogenesis transformation;

(4) Two different pathogenic processes can be distinguished, with different biologies;

(5) The 4q loss can represent a suppressor gene;

(6) The 8p loss is frequently seen in metastases using the fluorescence *in situ* hybridization (FISH) method, but not in the primary tumor.

In papillary (chromophil) RCC the 9p loss is associated with poor prognosis[28].

Conclusions

The role of tumor suppressor genes and oncogenes remains to be determined, since only partial details are known, for example:

(1) Alteration of gene *p53* (chromosome 17p) is frequent in papillary tumors, but occurs in only 15% of conventional RCC;

(2) The gene *c-erbB-1* (chromosome 7p12–13) is correlated with differentiation grade;

(3) In the case of gene *c-erbB-2* (chromosome 17q11.2–12), no relationship to RCC has been demonstrated;

(4) Alterations of c-*met*, K-*ras* and c-*myc* have scarcer incidence, but are very specific for the hereditary forms.

References

1. Delahunt B, Thornton A. Renal cell carcinoma. A historical perspective. *J Urol Pathol* 1996;4: 31–49

2. Thoenes W, Storkel S, Rumpelt HJ. Human chromophobe cell renal carcinoma. *Virchow's Arch (Cell Pathol)* 1985;155:277–87

3. Klein MJ, Valensi QJ. Proximal tubular adenomas of kidney with so-called oncocytic features: a clinicopathologic study of 13 cases of a rarely reported neoplasm. *Cancer* 1976;38: 906–14

4. Bander NH. Monoclonal antibodies to renal carcinoma antigens. *Eur Urol* 1990;18(Suppl 2): 10–12

5. Kovacs G. Molecular differential pathology of renal cell tumors. *Histopathology* 1993;22:1–8

6. Amin MB, Amin MB, Tamboli P, *et al.* Prognostic impact of histologic subtyping of adult renal epithelial neoplasms. An experience of 405 cases. *Am J Surg Pathol* 2002;26:281–91

7. Füzesy I, Gunawan B, Bergmann F, *et al.* Papillary renal cell carcinoma with clear cell cytomorphology and chromosomal loss of 3p. *Histopathology* 1999;35:157–61

8. Renshaw AA, Zhang H, Corless CL, *et al.* Solid variants of papillary (chromophil) renal cell carcinoma: clinicopathologic and genetic features. *Am J Surg Pathol* 1997;21:1203–9

9. Zbar B, Flenn G, Lubensky I. Hereditary papillary renal cell carcinoma: clinical study of 10 families. *J Urol* 1995;153:907–12

10. Thoenes W, Storkel ST, Rumpelt HJ, *et al.* Chromophobe cell renal carcinoma and its variants: a report on 32 cases. *J Pathol* 1988; 155:277–87

11. Latham B, Dickersin GR, Oliva E. Subtypes of chromophobe cell renal carcinoma. An ultra-structural and histochemical study of 13 cases. *Am J Surg Pathol* 1999;23:530–5

12. Mohamed AN, El-Naggar M, Koppitch FC, *et al.* Chromosome analysis of six chromophobe renal cell carcinomas. *J Urol Pathol* 1998;9:223–31

13. Polascik TJ, Cairns P, Eptstein JI, *et al.* Distal nephron renal tumors: microsatellite allelotype. *Cancer Res* 1996;56:1892–5

14. Peralta-Venturina M, Moch H, Amin M, *et al.* Sarcomatoid differentiation in renal cell carcinoma. A study of 101 cases. *Am J Surg Pathol* 2001;25:275–84

15. Fleming S, O'Donnell M. Surgical pathology of renal epithelial neoplasms: recent advances and current status. *Histopathology* 2000;36:195–202

16. Kovacs G, Fuzesi L, Emanual A, *et al.* Cytogenetics of papillary renal cell tumors. *Genes Chromosomes Cancer* 1991;3:249–55

17. Brown JA, Sebo TJ, Segura JW. Metaphase analysis of metanephric adenoma reveals chromosome Y loss with chromosome 7 and 17 gain. *Urology* 1996;48:473–475

18. Renshaw AA, Maurici D, Fletcher JA. Cytologic and fluorescence *in situ* hibridization (FISH) examination of metanephric adenoma. *Diagn Cytopathol* 1997;16:107–11

19. Stumm M, Koch A, Wieacker PF, *et al.* Partial monosomy 2p as the single chromosomal anomaly in a case of renal metanephric adenoma. *Cancer Genet Cytogenet* 1999;115:82–5

20. Neuhaus C, Dijkhuizen T, van den Berg E, *et al.* Involvement of the chromosomal region 11q13 in renal oncocytoma: case report and literature review. *Cancer Genet Cytogenet* 1997;94:95–8

21. van Poppel H, Nilsson S, Algaba F, *et al.* Pre-cancerous lesions in the kidney. *Scand J Urol Nephrol* 2000;34(Suppl 205):136–65

22. MacLennan G, Farrow GM, Bostwick DG. Low-grade collecting duct carcinoma of the kidney. Report of 13 cases of low-grade mucinous tubulocystic renal carcinoma of possible collecting duct origin. *Urology* 1997;50:679–84

23. Davis CJ, Mostofi FK, Sesterhenn IA. Renal medullary carcinoma: the seventh sickle cell nephropathy. *Am J Surg Pathol* 1995;19:1–11

24. Parwani AV, Husain AN, Epstein JI, *et al.* Low-grade myxoid renal epithelial neoplasms with distal nephron differentiation. *Hum Pathol* 2001; 32:506–12

25. Moch H, Schraml P, Bubendorf L, *et al.* Intratumoral heterogeneity of 3p deletions in renal cell carcinoma detected by fluorescence *in situ* hybridization. *Cancer Res* 1998;58:2304–9

26. Kallioniemi O, Kallioniemi A, Piper J, *et al.* Optimizing comparative genomic hybridization for analysis of DNA sequence copy number changes in solid tumors. *Genes Chromosomes Cancer* 1994;10:231–43

27. Jiang F, Desper R, Papadimitrou CH, *et al.* Construction of evolutionary tree models for renal cell carcinoma from comparative genomic hybridization data. *Cancer Res* 2000;60:6503–9

28. Schraml P, Muller D, Bednar R, *et al.* Allelic loss at the D9S171 locus on chromosome 9p13 is associated with progression of papillary renal cell carcinoma. *J Pathol* 2000;190:457–61

Prognostic factors for renal cell carcinoma

35

Z. Kirkali, E. Tuzel and M. U. Mungan

Introduction

Renal cell carcinoma (RCC) accounts for 3% of adult solid tumors, and each year 30 000 new cases in the USA and 20 000 in the European Union are detected[1]. Men are twice as often afflicted as women, usually between the ages of 50 and 70. Despite modern imaging techniques and early diagnosis, one-third of patients present with metastatic disease and up to 50% with localized disease progress after radical nephrectomy. An increase of more than 30% in incidence has been observed in the past decade, owing to better imaging, early diagnosis and environmental factors. The outcome of patients treated for RCC 10–20 years ago showed a substantially lower 5-year cancer-specific survival rate, but today patients with localized and advanced disease have an improved prognosis[2].

An ideal prognostic marker should have high specificity, sensitivity and reproducibility. It should be cancer-specific and have the power to predict the prognosis, and its assessment should be practical, easy and cost-effective. Although numerous factors have been examined for RCC prognosis, none of those has proved to have the aforementioned properties. Nevertheless, a comprehensive understanding and appreciation of the factors that have an impact upon the biological behavior of RCC are essential for understanding the natural history of the disease in patients with RCC. In 1997, the Union Internationale Contre le Cancer and American Joint Committee on Cancer evaluated the potential prognostic factors for RCC, including tumor-, patient- and treatment-related factors[3] (Table 1). In this chapter, the discussion of currently available prognostic markers is based on this classification.

Tumor-related prognostic factors

Pathological findings

Stage Currently, the anatomical extent of the tumor is the most important prognostic feature[4,5]. The two major staging schemes are the Robson classification and the tumor, nodes, metastasis (TNM) system. The TNM classification, widely used for its detailed stratification of findings, is predictive of patient survival and cancer-free interval[6]. Patients with organ-confined disease have the best prognosis, and patients with regional spread involving perinephric fat, venous structures and lymph nodes have worse outcomes. The 5-year survival rates by TNM stage for most recently reported cohorts range between 91 and 100% for stage I, 74 and 96% for stage II, 59 and 70% for stage III and 16 and 32% for stage IV disease[7-11]. TNM classification is a dynamic system undergoing regular revision. In 1997, the TNM staging system underwent some modification according to improved results in the management of RCC. The T1 stage was expanded from 2.5 to 7 cm, and tumor thrombus located above the diaphragm, which was previously staged T4, was changed to T3c. However, there is still controversy regarding the optimal cut-off point in size criteria for staging localized RCC[2,12,13]. A cut-off point of 4–5 cm has been proposed for differentiating T1a and T1b tumors for future classification[2].

Grade A large number of grading schemes have been proposed for RCC, and most of those emphasize nuclear features. Several studies have reported the independent prognostic value of grade in predicting long-term survival[14-17]. Nevertheless, grade is usually

Table 1 Patient-related and tumor-related prognostic factors according to the College of American Pathologists Working Classification[3]

Classification	Attribute	Findings
I: Generally used in patient management and well supported by the literature	patient-related	presentation (symptomatic) weight loss (> 10% of body weight) erythrocyte sedimentation rate (> 30 mm/h) anemia hypercalcemia increased alkaline phosphatase

	tumor-related	surgical margins
		metastases
		    number (multiple)
		    solitary (unresectable)
		    location (liver, lung, etc.)
		pTNM
		grade
		histological type
		    conventional (clear cell)
		    architecture (sarcomatoid)

II: Extensively studied in clinical trials or biological and correlative studies	patient-related	C-reactive protein

	tumor-related	histological type
		    collecting duct
		    nuclear morphometry

	biomolecular markers	DNA aneuploidy
		proliferative markers
		    Ki-67 (MIB-1)
		    AgNORs

III: Currently do not meet the criteria for categories I and II	biomolecular markers	proliferative markers
		    S-phase fraction
		    PCNA
		apoptotic markers
		    p53
		    Bcl-2
		    p21
		growth factors
		cell adhesion molecules
		angiogenesis
		tumor suppressor genes/oncogenes
		cytogenetic abnormalities

	demographic	age race socioeconomics

pTNM, pathological tumor, nodes, metastasis; AgNOR, silver-staining nucleolar organizing region; PCNA, proliferating cell nuclear antigen

secondary to stage in significance, because of subjectivity and the lack of uniformity in grading systems. No ideal grading method exists, although the four-tier Fuhrman nuclear grading system is used most commonly[18,19]. The 5-year survival rates of patients according to Fuhrman grade range between 65 and 76%, 30 and 72%, 21 and 51% and 10 and 35% for grade I, II, III and IV tumors, respectively[6]. Although this grading system is based on nuclear size, shape and content, there is still considerable interobserver variability. To resolve this problem, the development of a new three-tier grading system was proposed at an international consensus meeting[18].

Tumor histology Advances in the understanding of the genetics underlying the pathogenesis of RCC have led to a new histopathological classification[20] (Table 2). The most common subtype is conventional (clear cell) RCC, which has an overall 5-year survival rate of 55–60%[21]. Collecting duct carcinoma (also known as Bellini duct carcinoma) and medullary carcinoma are two uncommon but most aggressive forms of RCC[6,22]. Patients usually present with local extension or widespread metastasis, and almost all cases are high-grade[6]. Chromophobe and papillary RCCs are more indolent than conventional RCC. In general, these tumors remain well-differentiated and confined to the kidney, and the prognosis is favorable[23,24]. In a recent large series, survival rates of pT1 papillary and chromophobe RCCs were compared with that of pT1 conventional RCC[25]. Cancer-specific survival rates of conventional, papillary and chromophobe RCCs were 89.1%, 95.5% and 100%, respectively, and patients with conventional RCC had a significantly worse prognosis. Sarcomatoid RCC represents a relatively rare, high-grade form of RCC characterized by a spindle cell growth pattern, and can be encountered in most types of RCC. Recent genetic studies of the histogenesis of RCC revealed that sarcomatoid histology is not a distinct disease entity but a de-differentiated histological component which can arise from any subtype. Clinically, patients with sarcomatoid histology have a poor prognosis, with most patients dying within 1 year[26].

Microvascular invasion Microvascular invasion (MVI) within cancer is of prognostic significance in RCC. It has been demonstrated that, in patients undergoing radical nephrectomy for clinically non-metastatic RCC with MVI, the chance of progression is significantly increased[27,28]. MVI is more frequent in larger (> 10 cm), high-grade and high-stage tumors[27,28]. In one study, survival of patients with localized RCC following surgery was found to decrease from 89 to 59% in patients with MVI, and the presence of MVI was found to be an independent prognosticator after curative radical nephrectomy for RCC[27]. Detection of MVI in localized RCC is highly suggestive of disease progression after curative surgery; therefore, this group of patients may require further adjuvant treatment.

Table 2 Classification of renal tumors[20]

Tumor type	Incidence (%)	Cell of origin	Genetic abnormalities
Malignant tumors			
Conventional (clear cell) RCC	60–62	proximal convoluted tubule	3p deletions, VHL gene mutation
Papillary RCC	7–14	distal convoluted tubule	trisomies 7 and 17, Y deletions
Chromophobe RCC	6–11	intercalated cells	hypodiploidy (monosomies)
Collecting duct carcinoma	< 1	collecting ducts of renal medulla	1, 6, 14, 15, 22, 8p, 13q deletions
Medullary carcinoma	—	distal collecting ducts of renal medulla	unknown
RCC, unclassified	6–7		
Tumors of unknown malignant potential			
Multilocular cystic RRC	—	—	
Benign tumors			
Papillary tubular adenoma	—	—	
Oncocytoma	7–10	intercalated cells	Y, 14 deletions, t(14)
Metanephric adenoma	—	—	normal karyotype, 7+, 17+, Y–, X–

RCC, renal cell carcinoma; VHL, van Hippel–Lindau

Biomolecular markers

There are a number of promising techniques that allow the assessment of tumor cell proliferation: DNA flow-cytometry proliferation analysis (S phase), counting of nucleolar organizer regions (AgNORs), and measurement of proliferating cell nuclear antigen and immunohistochemically detectable cell-cycle proteins. Appreciation of the associations among nuclear grade, nucleolar morphometry and prognosis has generated interest in these techniques, to identify nuclear aberrations associated with prognosis.

Nuclear DNA content (ploidy) DNA ploidy is measured by single-cell DNA cytometry and describes the chromosome number of tumor cells, differentiating diploid tumor cells characterized by a normal set of chromosomes from aneuploid tumor cells showing irregular DNA content. Several groups have reported that tumor DNA content as measured by flow cytometry may have prognostic value in patients with RCC, with aneuploid tumors being associated with poor outcome. Aneuploid DNA content pertains to a cell population in which the DNA index differs from diploid (DNA index 1) by at least 10–15%[29]. Determinations may be made by flow cytometry or image analysis. Some studies contradict its usefulness in RCC[30,31], whereas other studies support the role of DNA content analysis in predicting outcome[32–34]. Owing to tumor heterogeneity, ploidy patterns can vary within the same tumor. Investigation of aneuploid RCC revealed that approximately 43% presented a mixture of both aneuploid and diploid cell lines[32]. In a previous study in which eight samples were taken from each tumor to identify all aneuploid RCC correctly, DNA ploidy was a significant and independent predictor for survival of RCC patients[34]. In two recent studies that included only organ-confined RCC patients, a statistically significant association was found between tumor size and DNA content[32,33], and a 22-fold increased relative risk of disease progression was noted for aneuploid tumors compared with diploid ones[33].

Proliferation markers Cellular proliferation may be a measure for predicting the biological aggressiveness and the prognosis of RCC.

(1) AgNOR Nucleolar organizing regions are chromosomal DNA loops encoding ribosomal RNA detectable by silver staining (AgNOR). Silver-staining AgNOR counts are increased in malignant cells and are an indirect measure of interphase duration[29]. Like many histological methods, the assessment of AgNOR counts suffers from subjectivity. In one study, a mean AgNOR count greater than 4.4 per nucleus was shown to be a significant independent prognostic indicator of overall survival, even when corrected for stage and grade[35]. In another study, although there was good correlation between AgNOR count and tumor grade, it was not an independent prognostic factor[36].

(2) Proliferating cell nuclear antigen (PCNA) PCNA, which is synthesized in the late G_1 phase and S phase of the cell cycle, is a marker of active cell proliferation. High levels of PCNA are associated with poor prognosis, independent of stage and grade[37]. In some studies, PCNA expression was significantly associated with tumor grade, and a significant survival advantage is observed in tumors with lower PCNA indices[36–38]. However, significant intratumor variability and altered expression related to factors other than cell proliferation are usually considered possible limiting factors of this method[39]. Recently, another cell proliferation marker, the proliferation-associated nuclear antigen p105, which is present in interchromatin granules, was found to be an independent prognostic factor in RCC patients[40].

(3) Mitotic index A mitotic index is the number of mitoses per field counted under the microscope. The mitotic rate is low in many RCCs, but gives prognostic information[37,41]. Mitotic figures were not seen in lower-grade tumors and mitotic activity was found to be limited to higher grades[41,42]. Mitotic activity is common in aggressive RCC subtypes, such as with sarcomatoid changes, but rare in lower-grade

papillary RCC[6]. Although in one study mitotic frequency per mm^2 was found to be an independent prognostic factor in RCC[42], it seems that assessment of mitotic rate provides inferior prognostic information to that obtained from evaluation of cell proliferative markers.

(4) Ki-67 (MIB-1) Ki-67 is a proliferation-associated nuclear antigen present in the G_1, S, G_2 and M phases of all cycling human cells[43]. The percentage of Ki-67-positive cells within a tumor is thought to be a reflection of the proliferative rate of the tumor. Many investigators have demonstrated that the Ki-67 index retains a significant association with survival, independent of both histological grade and tumor stage[38,41,43–46]. In some studies the Ki-67 index was an independent predictor of survival[38,43,44,46], but contradictory results were noted by other investigators[31]. The fraction of Ki-67 positivity varies within a wide scale between different tumors, but also within the same tumor, indicating the tumor proliferative heterogeneity. Ki-67 expression correlates with survival, and may provide additional information beyond stage. Also, it may identify patients who are prone to recurrence despite having initially localized cancer, and patients with disseminated cancer who may have a long survival. Nevertheless, further multicenter studies in larger numbers of patients with longer follow-up are needed to conclude that the Ki-67 labelling index can augment or replace conventional prognostic indicators such as grade and stage.

Angiogenesis Tumor growth and metastasis depend on both angiogenesis and certain signals from the tumor cells inducing rapid growth of the endothelial cells[47]. Determination of microvessel density (MVD) using routine methods of immunochemistry with antibodies directed against the endothelial cells allow light microscopic evaluation and precise morphometric assessment of MVD as a marker of angiogenesis. Previously, the significance of tumor angiogenesis has been studied by various investigators, but the results are conflicting[31,46,48,49]. It has been suggested that the increased neovascularity in renal cancer compared with other neoplasms (more than three-fold) accounts for the lack of clinical utility of angiogenesis as a prognostic marker[49]. On the other hand, in one study, tumor microvessel count independently predicted survival in 36 patients with RCC[48]. More recently, angiogenesis was assessed using stereology, but no correlation was observed between the vascular surface density and microvessel number per mm^3 stroma and survival[46]. Therefore, further studies to measure absolute vascular surface area within a defined volume of tumor are necessary to clarify the role of angiogenesis in RCC.

Nuclear morphometry The subjectivity of nuclear grading, particularly in the intermediate grades, has fostered quantitative morphometric approaches to evaluate nuclear features[50]. The quantitative assessment of nuclear morphometry is possible with computer imaging systems, providing a useful and reproducible method of prognosis for RCC[32,45,50–53]. The results of previous studies indicate that nuclear morphometry provides important prognostic information for patients with localized RCC treated by radical nephrectomy. The predictive power of nuclear morphometry is based on the assumption that a large nucleus is a morphological manifestation of anomalous DNA content, since a group of patients with tumors containing foci of cells with larger nuclei had a consistently shorter length of survival[51]. Nuclear descriptors such as nuclear perimeter, nuclear area, convexity and ellipticity have significant correlation with stage and grade[51]. This correlation is reasonable because larger tumors contain more areas with highest-grade cells, and those with larger nuclei[42]. Because the nuclei are three-dimensional structures, estimation of nuclear enlargement in terms of volume-weighted mean nuclear volume (MNV) using stereological analysis has been investigated[54,55]. Although the MNV was positively correlated with tumor grade, its clinical usefulness is controversial in RCC because of contradictory results of previous studies. In one study, MNV was shown to be an independent prognostic factor for survival; however, in another, no difference was observed between patients with good and poor prognosis[54,55]. Among many morphometric parameters examined, mean nuclear area has been considered to be one of the most valuable prognostic factors[32,45,50–53]. However, the proposed threshold values of mean nuclear area for the discrimination of patients with good and poor prognosis are not consistent among investigators (ranging from 32 to 39 μm^2). These observations are not suprising, because nuclear morphometric features such as nuclear size and nucleolar prominence are the key qualitative features of most grading systems.

Tumor suppressor genes/oncogenes

(1) *p53* The tumor suppressor gene *p53*, located on chromosome 17p13.1, encodes a nuclear phosphoprotein involved in the cell cycle that allows cellular DNA repair and/or apoptosis to occur by controlling cellular progression from the G_1 to the S phase[56]. Point mutations of the *p53* gene result in p53 protein overexpression, and are found in many human cancers including RCC[57]. Mutant p53 proteins have a longer half-life, accumulate and can easily be detected by immunohistochemistry. The resulting decreased affinity for DNA leads to cell proliferation. RCC has been shown by several investigators to have infrequent *p53* mutations[58–60], but, in some studies, reported expression rate of p53 varied between 32 and 41%[57,61–63]. Only a few studies have shown that overexpression of p53 is associated with poor prognosis[57,59], whereas others have shown no correlation between p53 expression and survival[58,61–63]. According to the current literature, mutations of *p53* are believed to lead to tumor progression in some cancers but do not seem to be important in most RCCs.

(2) *Bcl-2* Bcl-2 is an intracellular membrane protein capable of blocking programmed cell death induced by several stimuli, and over-expression is associated with prolongation of cell survival[64]. In some series, increased Bcl-2 expression as high as 80% has been demonstrated and correlated with tumor grade[58,59]. However, no association has been observed between Bcl-2 overexpression and an adverse outcome[58,59].

(3) *Murine double minute-2 (mdm-2)* The oncoprotein murine double minute-2 gene encodes a nuclear protein capable of forming complexes with wild-type and mutant p53 protein, and can inhibit *p53*-mediated tumor suppressor function[64]. Co-expression of p53/mdm-2 has been suggested as a useful prognostic marker in RCC, in a recent study[59]. The authors proposed that the functional role of mdm-2 contributes to a loss of p53 function such that tumor development and/or progression occurs.

(4) *p21* The p21 protein is a main mediator of *p53* tumor suppressor gene effects, and elevated levels of p21 protein in response to both *p53*-dependent and -independent signals mediate cell cycle arrest predominantly at the G_1 phase[65]. It is normally present in high levels in renal tubules. In previous studies, p21 positivity was not associated with the expression of PCNA or other indicators of accelerated cell proliferation[65,66]. These studies indicated that p21 and combined p21/p53 positivity does not have a prognostic value in RCC.

(5) *Other oncogenes* Myc refers to a family of proteins normally found in the nucleus but also in the cytoplasm. An association between high tumor grade and overexpression of protein product of the c-*myc* oncogene has been demonstrated, but such data provide no additional clinical useful information[67]. Unlike c-*myc*, c-*fos* oncogene expression was found to be decreased in RCC[68]. The *ras* family of oncogenes were frequently identified in solid tumors including RCC, but it does not appear that the *ras* oncogene plays an important role in RCC[69].

Growth factors Epidermal growth factor receptor (EGFR) binds epidermal growth factor and transforming growth factor-α (TGF-α), and is associated with tyrosine kinase activity and mitosis. A significant difference in EGFR contents was observed among nuclear grades of RCC[70], and expression of EGFR and TGF-α alone was associated with a poor clinical outcome[70].

Adhesion molecules and proteases

(1) *CD44* Adhesion molecules in cell–matrix interactions play a key role in the process of carcinogenesis. Among them, CD44, the main receptor of hyaluronan, plays a crucial role in tumor progression[71]. In one study, increased immunostaining of clear cell carcinomas was observed in 45% of tumors compared with no staining in lower-grade tumors[72]. In another study, 48% of tumors showed CD44 staining, and survival of CD44-positive patients was significantly lower than that of CD44-negative ones[71]. Although CD44 expression offered prognostic information independent of stage and grade in one series, Gilcrease and colleagues reported that CD44 expression was probably not an independent prognosticator in clear RCCs because it correlated closely with nuclear grade[71,72]. Larger trials with more patients are required to validate these early series.

(2) *E-cadherin,* α*-catenin* E-cadherin, a calcium-dependent epithelial cadherin, is considered a critical molecule for epithelium integrity. Cadherin function is modulated through cytoplasmic proteins called catenins. Although no multivariate analysis has shown independent characteristics of these parameters, immunohistochemical staining on renal cancer cells using specific antibodies revealed that the ratios of abnormal staining for E-cadherin and α-catenin were 77% and 37%, respectively[73,74].

(3) *Urokinase plasminogen activator (u-PA)* u-PA plays a key role in the metastatic process by promoting plasmin-mediated tissue degradation. Metastatic cell invasion requires localized proteolysis, which may be directed by the u-PA receptor[75]. Enzymatic activity can be blocked by natural specific inhibitor plasminogen activator inhibitor-1 (PAI-1)[75]. PAI-1 represents an efficient means of regulating the activity of the cell-surface plasminogen activating system. In a recent study, u-PA and PAI-1 were measured in renal cell tumor tissue and benign tissue in 152 patients using enzyme-linked immunosorbent assay (ELISA). It was demonstrated that high tissue levels of u-PA were associated with infiltration into the perirenal fat and development of distal metastases in the follow-up. Moreover, a poor prognosis with early relapse by metastatic disease after nephrectomy could be predicted with a high PAI-1, using a cut-off value of > 12 ng/mg[75].

Cytogenetics In RCC, consistent genetic alterations and their impact on prognosis have not yet been fully defined, but underlying genetic alterations are thought to be responsible for the development and progression of RCC. Previous cytogenetic studies have shown common genetic abnormalities in RCC, particularly deletions of part of chromosome 3. In a normal chromosome there are two copies of a gene; inactivation of both is mandatory to alter the gene function. The first copy is usually lost through deletion, detected as a loss of heterozygosity (LOH), while the second copy is inactivated by mutation or hypermethylation[76]. Several reports of RCC describe LOH involving additional chromosomal arms, including chromosomes 5, 6, 8, 9, 10, 11, 13, 14, 17, 18 and 19[77–83]. Generally, additional deletions are associated with higher-grade and -stage tumors, and these events may result in progression. In an earlier series, the prognostic significance of cytogenetic findings in 50 RCC patients was evaluated. Patients with more than five chromosomal alterations had a significantly worse prognosis than patients with fewer changes[84]. Although patients with deletions (8p)/−8, +12 and +20 had a significantly worse prognosis, grade was the most reliable independent prognosticator for RCC[84]. In a more recent study, patients who had tumors with LOH on chromosomes 8p and 9p were found to be at high risk for disease recurrence, and that genetic information was superior to tumor grade for predicting outcome[77]. None the less, the prognostic significance of karyotype analysis in RCC is still poorly understood and further studies are needed.

Other investigational markers Numerous other molecular markers have been clinically investigated to indicate some level of usefulness, and in an attempt to improve prognostication of RCC. The transcript levels of differentiation markers of proximal renal tubular cells, such as aquaporin-1 and carbonic anhydrase, were recently investigated in RCC[85]. A low level of aquaporin-1 and decreased carbonic anhydrase gene were associated with poor survival in RCC patients[85].

Clusterin has a powerful antiapoptotic activity, and has been regarded as a marker of cell death[86]. In recent study, high expression levels of clusterin mRNA were an independent predictor of tumor recurrence and overall survival[86].

Multidrug resistance-1 (MDR-1) mRNA is elevated in most RCCs, and encodes the membrane protein p-glycoprotein. Immunohisto-chemically detected lower levels of MDR-1 expression were correlated with poor prognosis in one study[87].

Metallothioneins (MTs) play a central role in trace-metal metabolism, and were recently suggested as a potential prognostic marker in RCC because of their developmental profile. MTs are overexpressed in early stages of development and repressed during adulthood, and subsequently re-expressed in malignant states. MT overexpression in RCC was found to be associated with malignant characteristics and poor prognosis of RCC in a recent study[88].

Patient-related factors

The demographic characteristics of patients such as age, gender, race and socioeconomic status have all been demonstrated not to influence survival in RCC.

Presentation

Several studies have demonstrated the growing incidence of RCC diagnosed incidentally with the advent of modern imaging. Patients presenting with late-stage disease often have symptomatic RCC. It was thought that earlier detection should have a significant impact on patient prognosis. In a recent study, presenting symptoms of 661 patients were analyzed and patients divided into three groups: incidental, classic triad (flank pain, hematuria and abdominal mass) and constitutional symptoms (weight loss, fever, anorexia, malaise). The median survival for patients with incidental, triad-associated and constitutional symptom tumors was 117, 56 and 29 months, respectively ($p < 0.05$)[89]. In two recent series, incidentally detected tumors had a lower pathological stage and grade, and patients with incidentally detected tumors also had a significantly higher 5-year cancer-specific survival rate compared with those with symptomatic lesions (85.3% vs. 62.5%)[89,90]. Subsequently, incidental lesions were associated with lower recurrence and metastatic rate[90].

Performance status (PS) is used to define a patient's general well-being according to symptoms related to underlying malignancy and comorbid conditions. In most studies, a PS ≥ 2 was independently associated with a decreased overall survival, and such patients responded less well to treatment[39].

Serum markers

Various laboratory results may be adversely related to prognosis. Inflammatory parameters are commonly elevated in RCC patients with and without distant metastases. In this regard, the significance of serum acute-phase reactants such as erythrocyte sedimentation rate (ESR), C-reactive protein, haptoglobin, ferritin, orosomucoid and α_1-antitrypsin have been studied in RCC[91-93]. All these parameters were correlated with survival, but ESR was the only independent prognostic parameter for survival. Hemoglobin less than 10 mg/dl and the presence of thrombocytosis have also been shown to have a prognostic importance in some studies[35,94]. Serum levels of γ-enolase, alkaline phosphatase, γ-glutamyl transpeptidase, iron, interleukin-10, amyloid A, CA-125, erythropoietin, vascular endothelial growth factor and calcium have all shown correlation with prognosis, and utilization of these markers has been suggested to be useful as an adjunct in the prediction of outcome of RCC patients[95–102]. Analysis of these serum studies might be an additional help in both treatment strategies and prognostication of RCC patients; none the less, the majority of the above should be considered as investigational before widespread acceptance.

Prognostic indices and nomograms

Accurate prediction of long-term disease-free survival immediately after resection of clinically localized RCC would be valuable for counselling, scheduling follow-up visits and identifying poor-risk cases potentially appropriate for adjuvant therapy protocols. An extension to the multiple regression approach for the statistical analysis of prognostic factors can generate patient-specific prognostic indices and nomograms. These take the form of a 'score' derived from a formula that combines a patient's values of several known prognostic factors. In two recent studies including relatively large numbers of patients with extended follow-up, it was attempted to develop accurate prognostic nomograms for RCC[103,104]. Kattan and colleagues modelled the pathological data and disease follow-up of 601 patients who were treated with radical nephrectomy. Predictor variables were patient symptoms, histology, tumor size and TNM 1997 pathological stage[103]. According to that nomogram, the probability

that the patient would not encounter RCC for the next 5 years was calculated with statistical validation. Zisman and associates proposed a classification scheme capable of accurately defining the patient's individual probability for survival. Several parameters, such as Fuhrman grade, TNM 1997 stage, number of symptoms and performance status were implanted into an exponential Nadas equation. The expected survival predicted by use of Nadas equations described the actual survival based on Kaplan–Meier curves[104]. The authors suggested that their resulting formulae were capable of tailoring survival estimates for a specific patient, and were based on widely accepted clinical prognostic variables[103]. However, all these promising attempts are premature at the present time; but, in the future, such probability estimates may be useful for clinicians to plan treatment, provide patient consultation and stratify randomized control trials of new therapies.

Conclusions

The investigation for potential prognostic factors in RCC is still ongoing, but unfortunately no ideal prognostic marker has yet been established. Pathological stage and nuclear grade are still the most powerful predictors of disease outcome. Although the reviewed literature contains numerous promising clinical, anatomical, histological and biomolecular parameters, these should be regarded as investigational. However, the future of RCC prognosis lies not in more precise definition of the anatomical extent of the disease but in incorporation of other biological factors in relation to the host or tumor, which will aid in more accurate prediction of the natural history of the disease. Further studies must continue to explore existing factors and discover novel characteristics.

References

1. Kirkali Z, Tuzel E, Mungan MU. Recent advances in kidney cancer and metastatic disease. *BJU Int* 2001;88:818–24
2. Pantuck AJ, Zisman A, Belldegrun AS. The changing natural history of renal cell carcinoma. *J Urol* 2001;166:1611–23
3. Strigley JR, Hutter RVP, Gelb AB, *et al.* Current prognostic factors – renal cell carcinoma. *Cancer* 1997;80:994–6
4. Belldegrun A, deKernion JB. Renal tumors. In Walsh PC, Retik AB, Vaughan ED Jr, Wein AJ, eds. Campbell's Urology, 7th edn. Philadelphia: WB Saunders, 1998;3:2283–326
5. Thrasher JB, Paulson DF. Prognostic factors in renal cancer. *Urol Clin North Am* 1993;20:247–62
6. Bonsib SM. Risk and prognosis in renal neoplasms. *Urol Clin North Am* 1999;26:643–60
7. Javidan J, Stricker HJ, Tamboli P, *et al.* Prognostic significance of TNM 1997 classification of renal cell carcinoma. *J Urol* 1999;162:1277–81
8. Tsui KH, Shvarts O, Smith RB, *et al.* Prognostic indicators for renal cell carcinoma: a multivariate analysis of 643 patients using the revised 1997 TNM staging criteria. *J Urol* 2000;163:1090–5
9. Kinouchi T, Saiki S, Meguro N, *et al.* Impact of tumor size on the clinical outcomes of patients with Robson stage I renal cell carcinoma. *Cancer* 1999;61:1689–95
10. Stein JP, Esrig D, Eastham J, *et al.* The surgical management of renal cell carcinoma: long term results in a large group of patients. *J Urol* 1998;(Suppl)159:192(abstr)
11. Guinan P, Frank W, Saffrin R, *et al.* Staging and survival of patients with renal cell carcinoma. *Semin Surg Oncol* 1994;10:47–50
12. Licht MR, Novick AC, Goormasric M, *et al.* Nephron sparing surgery in incidental versus suspected renal cell carcinoma. *J Urol* 1994;152:39–42
13. Fergany AF, Hafez KS, Novick AC, *et al.* Long term results of nephron sparing surgery for localized renal cell carcinoma: 10 year follow-up. *J Urol* 2000;163:442–5
14. Skinner DG, Colvin RB, Vermillion CD, *et al.* Diagnosis and management of renal cell carcinoma. A clinical and pathologic study of 309 cases. *Cancer* 1971;28:1165–77
15. Mederios LJ, Gelb AB, Weiss LM, *et al.* Renal cell carcinoma: prognostic significance of morphologic prarameters in 121 cases. *Cancer* 1988;61:1639–51
16. Fuhrman SA, Lasky LC, Limas C, *et al.* Prognostic significance of morphologic parameters in renal cell carcinoma. *Am J Surg Pathol* 1982;6:655–63
17. Selli C, Hinshaw WM, Woodard BH, *et al.* Stratification of risk factors in renal cell carcinoma. *Cancer* 1983;52:899–903
18. Medeiros LJ, Jones EC, Aizawa S, *et al.* Grading of renal cell carcinoma. *Cancer* 1997;80:990–1
19. Goldstein NS. The current state of renal cell carcinoma grading. *Cancer* 1997;80:977–80
20. Störkel S, Eble JN, Adhakha K, *et al.* Classification of renal cell carcinoma. *Cancer* 1997; 80:987–9
21. Gelb AB. Renal cell carcinoma: current prognostic factors. *Cancer* 1997;80:981–6
22. Kirkali Z, Celebi I, Akan G, *et al.* Bellini duct (collecting duct) carcinoma of the kidney. *Urology* 1996;47:921–3
23. Crotty TB, Farrow GM, Lieber MM. Chromophobe cell renal carcinoma. Clinicopathological features of 50 cases. *J Urol* 1995;154:964–67
24. Renshaw AA, Corless CL. Papillary renal cell carcinoma: histology and immunohistochemistry. *Am J Surg Pathol* 1995;19:842–9
25. Lau WK, Cheville JC, Blute ML. Prognostic features of pathologic stage T_1 renal cell carcinoma after radical nephrectomy. *Urology* 2002;59:532–7
26. Ro JY, Ayala AG, Sella A. Sarcomatoid renal cell carcinoma: a clinicopathologic study of 42 cases. *Cancer* 1987;59:516–26
27. Van Poppel H, Vandendriessche H, Boel K, *et al.* Microscopic vascular invasion is the most relevant prognosticator after radical nephrectomy for clinically nonmetastatic renal cell carcinoma. *J Urol* 1997;158:45–9
28. Sevinc M, Kirkali Z, Yorukoglu K, *et al.* Prognostic significance of microvascular invasion in localized renal cell carcinoma. *Eur Urol* 2000;38:728–33
29. de la Taille A, Buttyan R, Katz AE, *et al.* Biomarkers of renal cell carcinoma. Past and future considerations. *Urol Oncol* 2000;5:139–48
30. Lanigan D, McLean PA, Murphy DM, *et al.* Ploidy and prognosis in renal carcinoma. *Br J Urol* 1993;71:21–4
31. Gelb AB, Sudilovsky D, Wu CD, *et al.* Appraisal of intratumoral microvessel density, MIB-1 score, DNA content, and p53 protein expression as prognostic indicators in patients with locally confined renal cell carcinoma. *Cancer* 1997;80:1768–75
32. Ruiz-Cerda JL, Hernandez M, Gomis F, *et al.* Value of deoxyribonucleic acid ploidy and nuclear morphometry for prediction of disease

progression in renal cell carcinoma. *J Urol* 1996;155:459–65

33. Di Silverio F, Casale P, Cotella D, *et al.* Independent value of tumor size and DNA ploidy for the prediction of disease progression in patients with organ-confined renal cell carcinoma. *Cancer* 2000;88:835–43

34. Abou-Rebyeh H, Borgmann V, Nagel R, *et al.* DNA ploidy is a valuable predictor for prognosis of patients with resected renal cell carcinoma. *Cancer* 2001;92:2280–5

35. Yasunaga Y, Shin M, Miki T, *et al.* Prognostic factors of renal cell carcinoma: a multivariate analysis. *J Surg Oncol* 1998;68:11–18

36. Tannapfel A, Hahn HA, Katalinic A, *et al.* Prognostic value of ploidy and proliferation markers in renal cell carcinoma. *Cancer* 1996; 77:164–71

37. Delahunt B, Bethwaite PB, Nacey JN, *et al.* Proliferating cell nuclear antigen (PCNA) expression as a prognostic indicator for renal cell carcinoma: comparison for tumor grade, mitotic index and silver staining nucleolar organizer region numbers. *J Pathol* 1993;170: 471–7

38. Hofmockel G, Tsatalpas P, Muller H, *et al.* Significance of conventional and new prognostic factors for locally confined renal cell carcinoma. *Cancer* 1995;76:296–306

39. Rini BI, Vogelzang NJ. Prognostic factors in renal carcinoma. *Semin Oncol* 2000;27:213–20

40. Yokogi H. Flow cytometric quantitation of the proliferation-associated nuclear antigen p105 and DNA content in patients with renal cell carcinoma. *Cancer* 1996;78:819–26

41. Jochum W, Schroder S, Al-Taha R, *et al.* Prognostic significance of nuclear DNA content and proliferative activity in renal cell carcinoma. *Cancer* 1996;77:514

42. Eskelinen M, Lipponen P, Aitto-Oja L, *et al.* The value of histoquantitative measurements in prognostic assessment of renal adenocarcinoma. *Int J Cancer* 1993;55:547–54

43. Rioux-Leclercq N, Turlin B, Bansard JY, *et al.* Value of immunohistochemical Ki-67 and p53 determinations as predictive factors of outcome in renal cell carcinoma. *Urology* 2000;55:501–5

44. Aaltomaa S, Lipponen P, Ala-Opas M, *et al.* Prognostic value of Ki-67 expression in renal cell carcinomas. *Eur Urol* 1997;31:350–5

45. Ozer E, Yorukoglu K, Sagol O, *et al.* Prognostic significance of nuclear morphometry in renal cell carcinoma. *BJU Int* 2002;90:20–5

46. Kirkali Z, Yorukoglu K, Ozkara E, *et al.* Proliferative activity, angiogenesis and nuclear morphometry in renal cell carcinoma. *Int J Urol* 2001;8:697–703

47. Takashi A, Sasaki H, Kim SJ, *et al.* Markedly increased amounts of messenger RNAs for vascular endothelial growth factor and placental growth factor in renal cell carcinoma associated with angiogenesis. *Cancer Res* 1994; 54:4233–7

48. Nativ O, Sabo E, Reiss A, *et al.* Clinical significance of tumor angiogenesis in patients with localized renal cell carcinoma. *Urology* 1998;51:693–6

49. MacLennan G, Bostwick D. Microvessel density in renal cell carcinoma: lack of prognostic significance. *Urology* 1995;46:27–30

50. Guitterrez JL, Val-Bernal JF, Garijo MF, *et al.* Nuclear morphometry in prognosis of renal adenocarcinoma. *Urology* 1992;39:130–4

51. Ruiz JL, Hernandez M, Martinez J, *et al.* Value of morphometry as an independent prognostic factor in renal cell carcinoma. *Eur Urol* 1995; 27:54–7

52. Nativ O, Sabo E, Raviv G, *et al.* The role of nuclear morphometry for predicting disease outcome in patients with localized renal cell carcinoma. *Cancer* 1995;76:1440–4

53. Kanamaru H, Akino H, Suzuki Y, *et al.* Prognostic value of nuclear area index in combination with the World Health Organization grading system for patients with renal cell carcinoma. *Urology* 2001;57:257–61

54. Yorukoglu K, Aktas S, Guler C, *et al.* Volume weighted mean nuclear volume in renal cell carcinoma. *Urology* 1998;52:44–7

55. Kanamaru H, Sasaki M, Miwa Y, *et al.* Prognostic value of sarcomatoid histology and volume weighted mean nuclear volume in renal cell carcinoma. *BJU Int* 1999;83:222–6

56. Greenblatt MS, Bennett WP, Hollstein M, *et al.* Mutations with *p53* tumor suppressor gene: clues to cancer etiology and molecular pathogenesis. *Cancer Res* 1994;54:4855–78

57. Haitel A, Wiener HG, Blaschitz U, *et al.* Biologic behavior of and p53 overexpression in multifocal renal cell carcinoma of clear cell type. *Cancer* 1999;85:1593–8

58. Vasavada SP, Novick AC, Williams BG. P53, bcl-2 and Bax expression in renal cell carcinoma. *Urology* 1998;51:1057–61

59. Uchida T, Gao JP, Wang C, *et al.* Clinical significance of p53, mdm2, and bcl-2 proteins in renal cell carcinoma. *Urology* 2002;59:615–20

60. Sejima T, Miyagawa I. Expression of Bcl-2, p53 oncoprotein and proliferating cell nuclear antigen in renal cell carcinoma. *Eur Urol* 1998;35:242–8

61. Bot FJ, Godschalk JCJ, Krishnadath KK, *et al.* Prognostic factors in renal cell carcinoma: immunohistochemical detection of p53 protein versus clinico-pathological parameters. *Int J Cancer* 1994;57:634–7

62. Kuczyk MA, Serth J, Bokemeyer C, *et al.* Detection of *p53* gene alteration in renal cell

cancer by micropreparation techniques of tumor specimens. *Int J Cancer* 1995;64:399–406

63. Papadopoulos I, Rudolph P, Weichert-Jacobsen K. Value of p53 expression, cellular proliferation, and DNA content as prognostic indicators in renal cell carcinoma. *Eur Urol* 1997;32:110–17

64. Momand J, Wu H-H, Dasgupta G. Mdm2 – master regulator of the *p53* tumor suppressor gene. *Gene* 2000;242:15–29

65. Aaltomaa S, Lipponen P, Ala-Opas M, *et al.* Expression of cyclin A and D and p21 proteins in renal cell cancer and their relation to clinicopathological variables and patient survival. *Br J Cancer* 1999;80:2001–7

66. Haitel A, Wiener HG, Neudert B, *et al.* Expression of the cell cycle proteins p21, p27 and pRb in clear renal cell carcinoma and their prognostic significance. *Urology* 2001;58:477–81

67. Lanigan D, McLean PA, Murphy DM, *et al.* c-*myc* expression in renal cell carcinoma: correlation with clinical parameters. *Br J Urol* 1993;72:143–7

68. Peter S. Oncogene and growth factors in renal cell carcinoma. *Urol Int* 1991;47:199

69. Nanus DM, Mentle IR, Motzer RJ, *et al.* Infrequent *ras* oncogene point mutations in renal cell carcinoma. *J Urol* 1990;143:175–8

70. Yoshida K, Tosaka A, Takeuchi S, *et al.* Epidermal growth factor receptor content in human renal cell carcinomas. *Cancer* 1994;73:1913–18

71. Paradis V, Ferlicot S, Ghannam E, *et al.* CD44 is an independent prognostic factor in conventional renal cell carcinomas. *J Urol* 1999;161:1984–7

72. Gilcrease MZ, Guzman-Paz M, Niehans G, *et al.* Correlation of CD44S expression in renal clear cell carcinomas with subsequent tumor progression or recurrence. *Cancer* 1999;86:2320–6

73. Katagiri A, Watanabe R, Tomita Y, *et al.* E-cadherin expression in renal cell cancer and its significance in metastasis and survival. *Br J Cancer* 1995;71:376–9

74. Shimazui T, Bringuier PP, van Berkel H, *et al.* Decreased expression of α-catenins associated with poor prognosis with localized renal cell carcinoma. *Int J Cancer* 1997;74:523–8

75. Hoffman R, Lehmer A, Buresch M, *et al.* Clinical relevance of urokinase plasminogen activator, its receptor and its inhibitor in patients with renal cell carcinoma. *Cancer* 1996;78:487–92

76. Jacqmin D, van Poppel H, Kirkali Z, *et al.* Renal cancer. *Eur Urol* 2001;39:361–9

77. Presti JC, Wilhelm M, Reuter V, *et al.* Allelic loss on chromosomes 8 and 9 correlates with clinical outcome in locally advanced clear cell carcinoma of the kidney. *J Urol* 2002;167:1464–8

78. Anglard P, Tory K, Brauch H, *et al.* Molecular analysis of genetic changes in the origin and development of renal cell carcinoma. *Cancer Res* 1991;51:1071–7

79. Presti JC, Rao PH, Chen Q, *et al.* Histopathological, cytogenetic and molecular characterization of renal cortical tumors. *Cancer Res* 1991;51:1544–52

80. Morita R, Ishikawa J, Tsutsumi M, *et al.* Alleotype of renal cell carcinoma. *Cancer Res* 1991;51:820–3

81. Bergerheim U, Nordenskjold M, Collins P. Deletion mapping in human renal cell carcinoma. *Cancer Res* 1989;49:1390–6

82. Cairns P, Tokino K, Eby Y, *et al.* Localization of tumor suppressor loci on chromosome 9 in primary human renal cell carcinomas. *Cancer Res* 1995;55:224–7

83. Wu SQ, Hafez GR, Xing W, *et al.* The correlation between loss of chromosome 14q with histologic tumor grade, pathologic stage, and outcome of patients with nonpapillary renal cell carcinoma. *Cancer* 1996;77:1154–60

84. Elfving P, Mandahl N, Lundgren R, *et al.* Prognostic implications of cytogenetic findings in kidney cancer. *Br J Urol* 1997;80:698–706

85. Takenawa J, Kaneko Y, Kishishita M, *et al.* Transcript levels of aquaporin I and carbonic anhydrase IV as predictive indicators for prognosis of renal cell carcinoma patients after nephrectomy. *Int J Cancer* 1998;79:1–7

86. Miyake H, Hara S, Arakawa S, *et al.* Overexpression of clusterin as an independent prognostic factor for nonpapillary renal cell carcinoma. *J Urol* 2002;167:703–6

87. Hofmockel G, Bassukas ID, Wittman A, *et al.* Is the expression of multidrug resistance gene product a prognostic indicator for the clinical outcome of patients with renal cancer? *Br J Urol* 1997;80:11–17

88. Tuzel E, Kirkali Z, Yorukoglu K, *et al.* Metallothionein expression in renal cell carcinoma: subcellular localization and prognostic significance. *J Urol* 2001;165:1710–13

89. Pantuck AJ, Zisman A, Rauch MK, *et al.* Incidental renal tumors. *Urology* 2000;56:190–6

90. Tsui KH, Shvarts O, Smith RB, *et al.* Renal cell carcinoma: prognostic significance of incidentally detected tumors. *J Urol* 2000;163:426–30

91. Ljunberg B, Grankvist K, Rasmuson T, *et al.* Serum acute phase reactants and prognosis in renal cell carcinoma. *Cancer* 1995;76:1435–9

92. Miyata Y, Koga S, Nishikido M, *et al.* Predictive values of serum acute phase reactants, basic fetoprotein, and immunosuppressive acidic protein for staging and survival in renal cell carcinoma. *Urology* 2001;58:161–4

93. Kirkali Z, Guzelsoy M, Mungan MU, *et al.* Serum ferritin as a clinical marker for renal cell

carcinoma: influence of tumor size and volume. *Urol Int* 1999;62:21–5

94. Symbas NP, Townsend MF, El-Galley R, *et al.* Poor prognosis associated with thrombocytosis in patients with renal cell carcinoma. *BJU Int* 2000;86:203–7

95. Rasmuson T, Grankvist K, Ljungberg B. Serum γ-enolase and prognosis of patients with renal cell carcinoma. *Cancer* 1993;72:1324–8

96. Sandock DS, Seftel AD, Resnick MI. The role of γ-glutamyl transpeptidase in the preoperative metastatic evaluation of renal cell carcinoma. *J Urol* 1997;157:798–9

97. Yu CC, Chen KK, Chen MT, *et al.* Serum iron as a marker in renal cell carcinoma. *Eur Urol* 1991;19:54–8

98. Wittke F, Hoffmann R, Dallmann I, *et al.* Interleukin 10 (IL-10): an immunosuppressive factor and independent predictor in patients with metastatic renal cell carcinoma. *Br J Cancer* 1999;79:1182–4

99. Kimura M, Tomita Y, Imai T, *et al.* Significance of serum amyloid A on the prognosis in patients with renal cell carcinoma. *Cancer* 2001;92:2072–5

100. Grankvist K, Ljungberg B, Rasmuson T. Evaluation of five glycoprotein tumour markers (CEA, CA-50, CA-19-9, CA-125, CA-15-3) for the prognosis of renal cell carcinoma. *Int J Cancer* 1997;74:233–6

101. Ljungberg B, Rasmuson T, Grankvist K. Erythropoietin in renal cell carcinoma: evaluation of its usefulness as a tumor marker. *Eur Urol* 1992;21:160–3

102. Jacopsen J, Rasmuson T, Grankvist K, *et al.* Vascular endothelial growth factor as prognostic factor in renal cell carcinoma. *J Urol* 2000;163:343–7

103. Kattan MW, Reuter V, Motzer RJ, *et al.* A postoperative nomogram for renal cell carcinoma. *J Urol* 2001;166:63–7

104. Zisman A, Pantuck AJ, Dorey F, *et al.* Mathematical model to predict individual survival for patients with renal cell carcinoma. *J Clin Oncol* 2002;20:1368–74

High-tech diagnostic procedures in renal cell carcinoma: promise and practice

36

G. P. Krestin and F. Cademartiri

Introduction

Renal cell carcinoma (RCC) accounts for 2% of all cancers, with a world-wide annual increase of 1.5–5.9%[1,2]. Mean age at time of diagnosis is about 70 years, and there is a predominance of men over women in the range of 1.5–3.1-fold. Mortality from RCC is increasing in parallel with trends in incidence[1]. At present, 25–30% of patients with RCC have overt metastases at initial presentation and, in addition, a substantial fraction of patients have subclinical metastases at that time, explaining the hitherto unsatisfactory outcome of treatment[3,4].

A slight to moderate improvement in survival has been observed in most countries. Survival is closely related to the initial stage and therefore to early diagnosis; 5-year survival is 50–90% for localized disease, decreasing to 0–13% for metastatic disease[3].

The increased incidence of RCC is primarily due to enhanced detection of tumors by expanded use of imaging techniques such as ultrasound and computed tomography (CT)[1].

Clinical symptoms of RCC, such as hematuria, palpable tumor and flank pain, are becoming less frequent. Asymptomatic tumors are more commonly detected[5]. Clinical examination has a limited role in diagnosing RCC, but it may be valuable in assessing comorbidity[5]. In the case of hematuria, additional tumors of the genitourinary tract should be excluded[6]. The most commonly assessed laboratory parameters are: hemoglobin and erythrocyte sedimentation rate (prognosis); creatinine (overall kidney function); and alkaline phosphatase (liver and bone metastases). Serum calcium is frequently included in the preoperative assessment because of its association with paraneoplastic manifestations, which may have clinical implications[7].

The majority of tumors are detected incidentally with ultrasound, performed for various reasons. A standard radiological staging procedure is an abdominal CT scan with and without the intravenous administration of contrast material. It serves to document the diagnosis of RCC and provides information on the function and morphology of the contralateral kidney[8]. Additional diagnostic procedures such as magnetic resonance imaging (MRI), digital subtraction angiography (DSA) or fine-needle aspiration biopsy (FNAB) have a very limited role, but may be considered in selected cases[9].

Techniques

After the first imaging study, which is generally an ultrasound scan performed for different reasons, guidelines on the following diagnostic steps are similar to those for many other applications in oncology. An abdominal CT scan demonstrates primary tumor extension, and provides information on venous involvement and metastatic spread to loco-regional lymph nodes, adrenal glands, contralateral kidney or liver[8]. A chest X-ray is performed to assess pulmonary spread. If indicated by signs and symptoms, other diagnostic procedures may be applied, such as a bone scan, brain CT or chest CT[5].

Ultrasound

Ultrasound represents the first tool with which renal masses are usually detected. Recent improvements in ultrasound imaging allow detection of smaller parenchymal alterations and additional evaluation of vascular abnormalities (e.g. color Doppler and power Doppler techniques with or without administration of an ultrasound contrast agent). These tools sometimes provide sufficient information to define lesions as benign (e.g. cyst), without the need for any further diagnostic procedures. However, patients with suspected renal masses are generally referred to CT and less often to MRI for final classification and staging, and particularly for determining therapeutic choice.

Computed tomography

Spiral CT (SCT) has to a large extent overcome the limitations of previous generations of scanners. SCT has played a central role in most applications related to diagnosis and follow-up of renal diseases since its introduction in 1993.

The *single detector* generation of SCT scanners provided a slice thickness of 3 mm or more (for CT angiographic purposes), and a temporal resolution of 0.75–1 s per slice. In 1998 a *multidetector* CT (MDCT) generation of scanners was introduced, offering higher spatial and temporal resolution. The slice thickness (i.e. spatial resolution) was reduced to 1–1.25 mm and acquisition times decreased to 500 ms per slice, with the possibility of scanning four slices simultaneously. An eight-fold increase in overall speed was gained over the previous generation of SCT scanners, with the possibility of reducing the contrast material dosage (~80–100 ml of non-ionic 320 mgI/ml contrast material) for optimal parenchymal and vascular opacification. These improvements resulted in more accurate visualization of vascular structures as well as optimal depiction of small parenchymal irregularities due to compression, thrombosis and neovascularization[10].

Moreover, high-speed image acquisition allows repeated imaging after administration of the contrast material. In this way, one can visualize arterial opacification (together with cortical enhancement), the equilibrium or nephrographic phase, and finally the excretory phase. The vascular supply of the mass is optimally appreciated in a double-phase study, and the pattern of enhancement in several cases is typical of the disease. The detection of renal masses proved optimal in the equilibrium or late phase of enhancement[11]. In the case of RCC, enhancement progressively increases from the corticomedullary phase to the nephrographic phase[11]. This is the reason why a complete CT study for the detection and staging of RCC should be performed with a double-phase protocol: arterial enhancement and equilibrium phase.

In 2002, a new generation of MDCT scanners was introduced with a 16-slice configuration (Figure 1). Further increase of spatial resolution at even higher speed is now available. The thin collimation acquisition provides almost isotropic voxels of the whole imaged volume. Data post-processing offer visualization in any desired plane, or in three dimensions with unprecedented high resolution. Even if validation studies are still to be performed, it is expected that this new generation of MDCT scanners will replace conventional angiographic studies for diagnostic purposes.

Magnetic resonance imaging

Experience with MRI in the diagnosis and staging of RCC is still limited by the optimal results provided by CT. Indications for MRI remain concentrated in cases of contraindication to CT, and in cases with massive involvement of neighboring organs[12-15]. Magnetic resonance examinations of the kidneys are rendered difficult by artifacts owing to respiratory motion and pulsations of the neighboring abdominal vessels. Moreover, most pathological lesions of the kidneys display the same signal intensity (SI) as the surrounding unaffected structures, leading to decreased soft tissue contrast in unenhanced examinations.

In order to provide morphological information that may compete with the results of CT and ultrasound, special techniques such as artifact

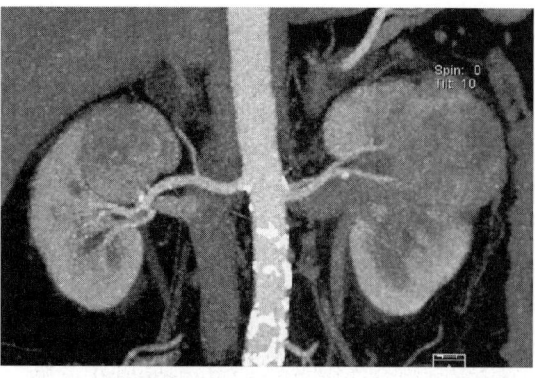 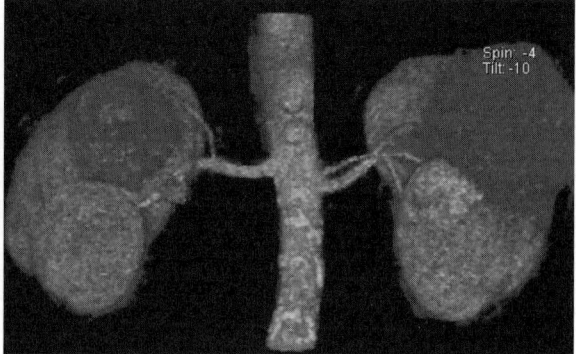

Figure 1 Computed tomography (CT) angiography study with 16-slice multidetector CT in a case with bilateral renal cell carcinoma. In the left image a coronal MIP (multiple intensity projection) reconstruction, and in the right image a frontal direct VR (volume rendering) reconstruction, are shown. The vascular configuration is clearly displayed. On the left kidney side there are two renal arteries

compensation and fast imaging have to be employed. Additional use of a renally eliminated gadolinium-containing paramagnetic contrast agent permits the assessment of different states of perfusion and visualization of the passage of the contrast medium, providing information about hyper- or hypoperfused lesions and about the excretory function of the kidneys. State-of-the-art MRI with optimal technical skills allows delineation of even small lesions with a diameter of approximately 1 cm.

The recent development of fat-suppression techniques, fast-spin-echo sequences and ultra-fast imaging have further expanded the list of potential applications of MRI in the kidneys[16,17]. These techniques can provide further improvement of lesion detection allowing demonstration of small cysts or hypoperfused solid masses with diameters of less than 1 cm; however, there are only a very restricted number of cases in which lesions visible on MRI are not previously detected using CT or ultrasound.

Differentiation of renal tumors

Unenhanced and especially contrast-enhanced CT or MRI can help in differentiating renal and pararenal lesions. A non-enhancing mass with low attenuation values or low SI on the T1-weighted magnetic resonance image, and marked signal increase on T2-weighted scans, represents a simple cyst in the majority of cases. However, for this classification, MRI is needed only if the patient has a contraindication for the use of iodinated contrast agents. Although MRI is highly sensitive in demonstrating hemorrhage, infected cysts with a high protein content cannot be differentiated from hemorrhagic cysts. Hemorrhagic cysts and cystic tumors with hemorrhage are also difficult to differentiate with any modality. However, MRI seems to be superior to CT in this respect, owing to the high contrast between renal parenchyma and usually hypoperfused solid lesions.

Among solid tumors of the kidney, CT as well as MRI allows accurate diagnosis only of fat-containing angiomyolipomas. Other solid lesions, such as oncocytoma, renal cell adenoma or RCC, show very similar SI and enhancement patterns. However, dynamic MRI performed by repeated imaging in the same position at short time intervals, after administration of a gadolinium chelate, allows optimal delineation of the normally functioning renal parenchyma and good visualization of the corticomedullary junction. Using such sequences, renal and extrarenal masses can be differentiated accurately. Additional imaging planes may help in differentiating retroperitoneal masses, which are only displacing and compressing the renal parenchyma[16,17]. This is available using direct acquisition in these planes with MRI, or by reformating CT data acquired with thin collimation and almost isotropic voxels.

Staging of renal cell carcinoma

The most important issues that arise during preoperative staging of RCC are evaluation of intra- and extrarenal extent of the tumor, and involvement of perirenal fat, of renal veins and inferior vena cava, and of regional lymph nodes. Most of these problems can be solved using CT, but MRI seems to provide better results in evaluation of perirenal and vascular involvement.

Biphasic CT or dynamic magnetic resonance studies are also useful for delineation of the intrarenal extent of primary renal malignancies. Although this does not help in terms of correct staging of the tumor, it may allow planning of a partial resection if indicated. A differentiation between stage T2 and T3a is very important, since tumors that are not confined to the kidney lead to a decrease in 5-year survival of more than 50%.

Invasion of perinephric fat may be well visualized with gradient-echo (GRE) MRI using adequate echo times. When fat and water protons are out of phase, a signal loss marks the presence of tumor cells in perirenal fat. However, similar alterations can be observed that are simply due to lymphatic or venous edema around the kidneys. In such cases, detection of perirenal invasion can be improved using fat-suppressed contrast-enhanced images. Enhancement of previously dark areas in perirenal tissue is indicative of extrarenal tumor invasion[16,18–20].

Magnetic resonance imaging is the best non-invasive method for assessment of tumor thrombi in the renal veins or the inferior vena cava (Figure 2). This MRI technique provides the same information as venography. Gradient-echo images allow even delineation of thrombi in non-dilated veins, owing to the lack of high SI of flowing blood. Using GRE images, retroperitoneal lymphadenopathy may be detected as accurately as with CT or ultrasound. However, as with those methods, the only criterion for diagnosis of malignant involvement remains the measurement of lymph node size[19,20].

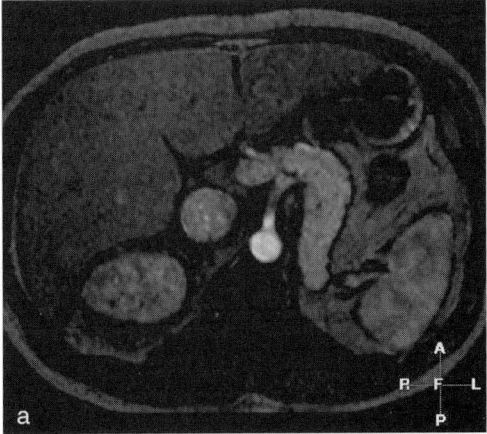

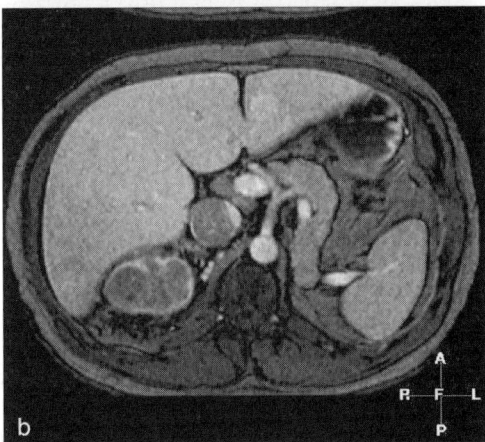

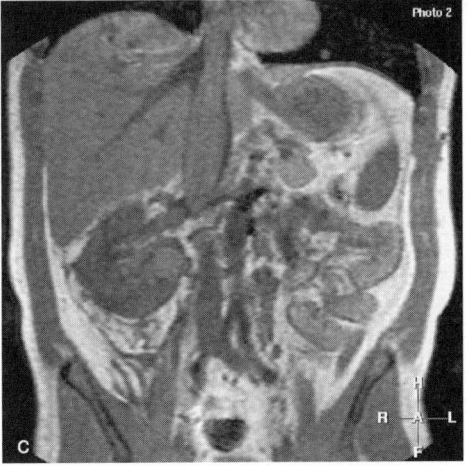

Figure 2 Magnetic resonance imaging (MRI) of stage T3b renal cell carcinoma showing tumor thrombus in the inferior vena cava on flow sensitive (a) and contrast-enhanced (b) axial slices, while the coronal image (c) demonstrates the extent of the thrombus

Conclusions

The kidney has a very unique and well-defined parenchymal and vascular configuration. Therefore, our main aim with diagnostic tools must be the detection of vascular/perfusional modifications. Especially because of the increased number of small lesions detected by ultrasound, accuracy and spatial resolution must be high. The ability to characterize cystic mass lesions has improved, reducing the diagnosis of indeterminate masses and thus facilitating better therapeutic management.

When planning nephron-sparing surgery, three-dimensional display of the renal tumor helps to determine the resectability of the mass, depicting its relationship to renal vessels and the renal collecting system[21].

The diagnosis of RCC has been improved owing to increased sensitivity in detecting small RCC, and increased specificity in the diagnosis of neoplastic lesions. Improved staging of RCC is the result of accurate assessment of extra-capsular tumor spread and of venous extension.

Multiphasic MDCT studies are the corner-stone of RCC diagnosis and follow-up. They provide accurate assessment of abnormal vascular perfusion and impaired tubule transit of contrast material. MRI can be used whenever there is a contraindication for CT (radiation during pregnancy or reduced tolerance to iodinated contrast agents) and in indeterminate cases.

References

1. McCredie M. Bladder and kidney cancers. *Cancer Surv* 1994;20:343–68
2. Parkin DM, Pisani P, Ferlay J. Estimates of the worldwide incidence of eighteen major cancers in 1985. *Int J Cancer* 1993;54:594–606
3. Motzer RJ, Bander NH, Nanus DM. Renal-cell carcinoma. *N Engl J Med* 1996;335:865–75
4. Johnsen JA, Hellsten S. Lymphatogenous spread of renal cell carcinoma: an autopsy study. *J Urol* 1997;157:450–3
5. Mickisch G, Carballido J, Hellsten S, Schulze H, Mensink H. Guidelines on renal cell cancer. *Eur Urol* 2001;40:252–5
6. Messing EM, Young TB, Hunt VB, Emoto SE, Wehbie JM. The significance of asymptomatic microhematuria in men 50 or more years old: findings of a home screening study using urinary dipsticks. *J Urol* 1987;137:919–22
7. Sufrin G, Chasan S, Golio A, Murphy GP. Paraneoplastic and serologic syndromes of renal adenocarcinoma. *Semin Urol* 1989;7:158–71
8. Bechtold RE, Zagoria RJ. Imaging approach to staging of renal cell carcinoma. *Urol Clin North Am* 1997;24:507–22
9. Newhouse JH. The radiologic evaluation of the patient with renal cancer. *Urol Clin North Am* 1993;20:231–46
10. Sheth S, Scatarige JC, Horton KM, Corl FM, Fishman EK. Current concepts in the diagnosis and management of renal cell carcinoma: role of multidetector CT and three-dimensional CT. *Radiographics* 2001;21:S237–54
11. Birnbaum BA, Jacobs JE, Ramchandani P. Multiphasic renal CT: comparison of renal mass enhancement during the corticomedullary and nephrographic phases. *Radiology* 1996;200:753–8
12. Oto A, Herts BR, Remer EM, Novick AC. Inferior vena cava tumor thrombus in renal cell carcinoma: staging by MR imaging and impact on surgical treatment. *Am J Roentgenol* 1998;171:1619–24
13. Cornud F, Bris C, Distefano D, *et al.* [Magnetic resonance imaging and preoperative evaluation of cancer of the kidney. The results apropos of 60 cases.] *Ann Urol (Paris)* 1991;25:11–17
14. Amendola MA, King LR, Pollack HM, Gefter W, Kressel HY, Wein AJ. Staging of renal carcinoma using magnetic resonance imaging at 1.5 tesla. *Cancer* 1990;66:40–4
15. Straton CS, Libertino JA, Larsen CR. Is magnetic resonance imaging alone accurate enough in staging renal cell carcinoma? *Urology* 1992;40:351–3

16. Krestin GP. *Morphologic and Functional MR of the Kidneys and Adrenal Glands.* Philadelphia: Field and Wood, 1990

17. Semelka RC, Shoenut JP, Kroeker MA, MacMahon RG, Greenberg HM. Renal lesions: controlled comparison between CT and 1.5-T MR imaging with nonenhanced and gadolinium-enhanced fat-suppressed spin-echo and breath-hold FLASH techniques. *Radiology* 1992;182: 425–30

18. von Schulthess GK. *Morphology and Function in MRI.* Berlin: Springer, 1989

19. Eilenberg SS, Lee JK, Brown J, Mirowitz SA, Tartar VM. Renal masses: evaluation with gradient-echo Gd-DTPA-enhanced dynamic MR imaging. *Radiology* 1990;176:333–8

20. Hricak H, Thoeni RF, Carroll PR, Demas BE, Marotti M, Tanagho EA. Detection and staging of renal neoplasms: a reassessment of MR imaging. *Radiology* 1988;166:643–9

21. Novick AC. Nephron-sparing surgery for renal cell carcinoma. *Br J Urol* 1998;82:321–4

Technical and surgical progress in organ-sparing approaches for renal cell carcinoma

37

J. Hoang-Böam and P. Alken

Surgical standard

Organ-sparing approaches for renal cell carcinoma (RCC) are the treatment of choice when the incidence of localized RCC is bilateral, or in a solitary functioning kidney. In such patients, nephron-sparing surgery allows complete surgical excision of the primary tumor while sufficient renal parenchyma is preserved to avoid renal replacement therapy[1,2]. The indications for partial nephrectomy have been expanded to include the patient with localized RCC and a functioning opposite kidney, when that kidney is involved with a disorder that might cause progressive renal functional impairment in the future.

A variety of surgical techniques are available for performing partial nephrectomy in patients with malignancy:

(1) Simple enucleation;

(2) Polar segmental nephrectomy with primary ligation of the appropriate renal arterial branch;

(3) Wedge resection;

(4) (Major) transverse resection;

(5) Extracorporeal partial nephrectomy with renal autotransplantation.

The basics of nephron-sparing surgery are:

(1) Early vascular control;

(2) Avoidance of ischemic renal damage;

(3) Complete tumor excision with free margins;

(4) Precise closure of the collecting system;

(5) Careful hemostasis;

(6) Closure or coverage of the renal defect.

In the majority of cases, it is possible to perform nephron-sparing surgery *in situ* by the choice of a surgical approach that optimizes exposure of the kidney. The kidney is mobilized inside Gerota's fascia and the perirenal fat around the tumor is left undisturbed. Temporary occlusion of the renal artery can become unnecessary for small polar or peripheral tumors by combining meticulous surgical technique with an understanding of the renal vascular anatomy in relation to the tumor. Arterial occlusion not only inhibits intraoperative bleeding (main cause for conversion to nephrectomy), but also improves access to intrarenal structures by reducing renal tissue turgor.

Renal ischemia

Because renal metabolic activities are predominantly aerobic, the kidney is very susceptible to damage from warm ischemia. The extent of renal damage following normothermic arterial occlusion depends on the duration of the ischemic insult. Canine studies have shown that warm ischemic intervals of up to 30 min can be sustained with eventual full recovery of renal function[3]. For periods of warm ischemia beyond 30 min there is generally significant immediate functional loss. Late recovery of renal function is either incomplete or absent. The duration of arterial occlusion may surpass 30 min, thus demanding additional protective measures against postischemic renal injury: local hypothermia (20–25°C) is the most efficacious commonly employed method.

Local hypothermia can be achieved with external surface cooling (simple, more widely used), or with perfusion of the kidney with a cold solution instilled in the renal artery (invasive, requires direct entry to the renal artery). Either method is equally effective.

Important standards for nephron-sparing surgery, to limit postischemic renal injury by ensuring optimal perfusion with absence of cortical vasospasm at the time of arterial occlusion, are:

(1) Pre- and intraoperative hydration;

(2) Prevention of hypotension during the period of anesthesia;

(3) Avoidance of unnecessary manipulation of or traction on the renal artery;

(4) Intraoperative administration of mannitol 5–15 min prior to arterial occlusion.

Tissue protection

Pharmacological agents for *in situ* renal preservation are a further popular alternative. Experimental studies have revealed that several such agents could possibly contribute to the prevention of postischemic renal failure. Nephron protection may be achieved by additional pharmacological therapy. Agents that have been tested include:

(1) Vasoactive drugs;

(2) Membrane-stabilizing drugs;

(3) Calcium channel blockers;

(4) Others that act to preserve or replenish intracellular levels of adenosine triphosphate (ATP).

However, so far, no pharmacological option has been as effective as local hypothermia for ischemic intervals of 2 h or more. In the past 3 years, relevant investigations have been carried out in several trials on rats. The protective effect of allopurinol, with or without prostaglandin E₁[4–6], and of the nitric oxide donor molsidomine[7] in ischemia–reperfusion

injury of the rat renal function has been demonstrated by various groups.

Rhoden and co-authors[4] evaluated the effect of allopurinol (an inhibitor of xanthine oxidase) on oxidative stress, renal dysfunction and histological alterations during renal ischemia–reperfusion in 120 uninephrectomized rats. Renal malondialdehyde and serum creatinine levels were significantly increased after renal ischemia–reperfusion. However, pretreatment with allopurinol demonstrated a protector effect in these parameters. Renal ischemia–reperfusion provoked significant renal damage in the operated group. Tubular atrophy and interstitial fibrosis were attenuated by allopurinol when given prior to surgery. These authors were able to show that allopurinol had a strong tendency to exert a beneficial effect during renal ischemia–reperfusion in uninephrectomized rats, implying that patients could be given one dose of allopurinol 300 mg the day before surgery.

Gupta and co-authors[5] studied the effect of allopurinol (50 mg/kg) and prostaglandin E₁ (PGE₁, 20 µg/kg) on renal ischemia–reperfusion injury. They induced left renal ischemia (right nephrectomy) for 1 h and reperfusion in 50 Sprague–Dawley rats (five groups). Group AP received allopurinol and PGE₁, group A allopurinol and group P PGE₁, group C was the control and group S was the sham group. Serum creatinine values were lower in the treatment groups compared with controls on days 1–3 and 7 ($p < 0.05$). Blood urea nitrogen values showed a similar trend. Maximum histological damage was seen in group C, followed by groups A, P and AP, in that order. The authors concluded that allopurinol and PGE₁ attenuate renal ischemia–reperfusion injury in rats. A specific urological indication may be represented by renal transplantation.

Öztürk and his group[7] verified the protective effect of molsidomine on renal function and structural modifications in the ischemia–reperfusion rat kidney. The rats were right nephrectomized and the left renal artery was occluded for 60 min. Molsidomine (orally 30 mg/kg per day for 48 h, 2 days before ischemia–reperfusion)-treated ischemic rats showed a rapid return to normal serum creatinine and blood urea nitrogen values on postoperative days 1, 2, 3 and 4. The values obtained in untreated ischemic rats were significantly lower. The findings of these authors suggest that the administration of molsidomine may vanquish the pernicious effects of warm ischemia on kidney structure and function. They see indications for therapy with molsidomine in ischemia-induced renal failure, as well as pretreatment of the kidney donor and post-transplant treatment of the kidney recipient.

Surgical techniques

A variety of surgical techniques are available for partial nephrectomy in patients with malignancy. Open procedures include enucleation, polar segmental nephrectomy, wedge resection, extracorporeal surgery with autotransplantation, etc. The basic principles of early vascular control should be adhered to for all of these techniques.

A technique with 'selective renal parenchymal clamping'[8] was described by Mejean and colleagues in 2002: a technical maneuver that facilitates nephron-sparing surgery without pedicle dissection and clamping for renal peripheral or pole tumors, using a large curved DeBakey aortic clamp placed around and sufficiently far from the tumor.

Method

(1) Kidney freed from the fatty tissue except around the tumor (standard);

(2) Selective renal parenchymal clamping circumscribing the tumor by using a large curved DeBakey aortic clamp;

(3) Clamping pressure controlled by a surgical loop tied by Kocher forceps to avoid crushing the kidney;

(4) Wedge resection performed.

Results

(1) Successful in 10/10 patients (eight elective, two imperative);

(2) Three tumors at the renal pole, seven peripheral;

(3) Mean tumor size 32 mm (range 19–52 mm);

(4) Insignificant blood loss;

(5) Operative time 81 min (range 61–125 min)

(6) No perioperative or postoperative complications.

They were successful in 10/10 patients. The big advantage was that time was not limited since the artery was not clamped. They concluded that selective renal parenchymal clamping is a simple and efficient technical maneuver for facilitating nephron-sparing surgery without pedicle dissection and clamping for renal peripheral or pole tumors. Limiting factors of this technique are neoplasm location and size.

Laparoscopic partial nephrectomy

In recent years, most reports relating to technical aspects have dealt with the laparoscopic approach in relation to shortening the operating and ischemia time and also preventing bleeding and minimizing blood loss.

Technique of Gill and colleagues

Gill and colleagues[9] successfully duplicated open surgical techniques in 50 patients, and concluded that laparoscopic partial nephrectomy is a viable alternative for selected patients with a renal tumor.

Method The following steps were taken:

(1) Ureteral catheterization;

(2) Laparoscopic renal ultrasonography;

(3) Transient atraumatic clamping of renal artery and vein;

(4) Tumor excision (0.5-cm margin) using cold Endoshears and/or J-hook electrocautery;

(5) Pelvicaliceal suture repair ($n = 18$);

(6) Suture repair of the renal parenchymal defect over surgical bolsters (Surgicel®);

(7) All suturing and knot tying with free-hand intracorporeal laparoscopic techniques.

Results   The study gave the following results:

(1) Operation time 3 h (0.75–5.8 h), no open conversion;

(2) Mean blood loss 270.4 ml (40–1500 ml);

(3) Mean warm ischemia time 23 min (9.8–40 min), slush ice in one patient;

(4) Average hospital stay 2.2 days (1–9 days);

(5) Major complications in three patients (6%): intraoperative hemorrhage in one, delayed hemorrhage (and nephrectomy) in one, urine leak in one, and during a mean follow-up of 7.2 months (range 1–17 months) no patient had local or port site recurrence or metastatic disease.

Selective use of hand assistance

Other authors preferred the selective use of hand assistance[10,11]. They investigated whether hand-assisted techniques may facilitate the procedure in selected cases while maintaining the benefits of minimally invasive surgery to shorten the operating and ischemia time and also to prevent bleeding.

In 2000, Wolf and colleagues[10] compared their initial ten laparoscopic nephron-sparing procedures for suspected malignancy with 11 consecutive open surgical procedures for similar indications, prospectively (mean lesion diameter 2.4 cm in each group). They obtained recovery data using self-administered questionnaires. Although mean operative time was 24% greater in the laparoscopic group, recovery was more favorable than in the open-surgical group, as evidenced by 62% less parenteral narcotic use, 43% shorter hospital stay, 64% more rapid return to normal non-strenuous activity, and improved pain and physical health scores 2 and 6 weeks postoperatively. There were no conversions to open surgery and no major

complications in the laparoscopic group. They concluded that laparoscopic nephron-sparing surgery appears to have an advantage over open surgery in terms of patient recovery, and facilitation by hand assistance may make laparoscopic nephron-sparing surgery a more widely available, minimally invasive alternative to open surgery for small, favorably located renal tumors.

Nelson and Wolf[11] compared 16 standard and 22 hand-assisted laparoscopic radical nephrectomies for suspected RCC, prospectively. They also concluded that hand-assisted laparoscopic radical nephrectomy offers recovery, morbidity and cost comparable to those of standard laparoscopy. The benefits of the technique include shorter operative times, no need for specimen morcellation and direct manual control of the operative field. In their opinion, it is particularly useful early in surgeon experience, for large specimens or when patient comorbidities require a rapid procedure.

Method   Operative and recovery data were collected prospectively. Patients completed pain, activity and the 12-item short form health-related quality-of-life surveys preoperatively and postoperatively.

Results   The detailed results of the study showed that:

(1) Hand-assisted laparoscopic nephrectomied tumors were larger (greater corrected mean specimen weight) and the patients had a greater medical comorbidity;

(2) Significantly shorter mean operative time was recorded for hand-assisted laparoscopic procedures;

(3) With experience mean operative time decreased for standard but not for hand-assisted laparoscopy;

(4) Only significant predictors of operative time were procedure type, surgeon experience and adrenal sparing;

(5) No difference in terms of complication rate, hospital cost or stay, return to activity, overall pain score, or in difference in pre-operative and postoperative 12-item short form scores;

(6) Hand-assisted laparoscopic nephrectomy tended to be associated with more abdominal pain early in convalescence and more wound complications (not significant).

Other techniques

Other minimal invasive laparoscopic methods such as cryoablation[12,13] and the microwave tissue coagulator[14] have also been described.

In 2000, Gill and colleagues[12] presented their evolving experience of a total of 32 patients (34 tumors, mean tumor size 2.3 cm) treated with laparoscopic renal cryoablation. They used real-time ultrasound monitoring, and a double freeze–thaw cycle was routinely performed. Sequential magnetic resonance imaging scans demonstrated a gradual contraction in the mean diameter of the cryolesions. Among 20 patients who underwent a 1-year follow-up magnetic resonance imaging scan, the cryo-ablated tumor was no longer visible in five (25%). Despite its significant potential for false-negative results, it is encouraging that the follow-up computed tomography-directed needle biopsies at 3–6 months were negative for cancer in all 23 patients. The authors concluded that critical long-term data regarding laparo-scopic renal cryoablation, a developmental technique, are awaited. However, their initial experience was cautiously optimistic:

(1) Mean surgical time 2.9 h;

(2) Cryoablation time 15.1 min;

(3) Blood loss 66.8 ml;

(4) Mean cryolesion size 3.2 cm for an intraoperative ultrasonographic tumor size of 2 cm;

(5) Hospital stay less than 23 h in 22/32 (69%) patients;

(6) Twenty-three patients underwent a 3–6-month follow-up computed tomography-directed biopsy of the cryoablated tumor site, which was negative for cancer in all 23 patients;

(7) No evidence of local or port site recurrence was found during a mean follow-up of 16.2 months.

Laparoscopic partial nephrectomy is a challenging procedure owing to the risk of excessive bleeding. The usefulness of a microwave tissue coagulator during laparoscopic partial nephrectomy for a small renal tumor is another minimal invasive laparoscopic method without renal pedicle clamping or surface cooling. Tanaka and co-workers[15] described the first patient in 2000 and Yoshimura and associates[14] a larger series of six patients in 2001:

(1) Six patients;

(2) Tumor diameter 11–25 mm (January–July 2000);

(3) No renal pedicle clamping;

(4) Mean operating time 186 min (131–239 min);

(5) Minimal blood loss;

(6) No significant deterioration of renal function.

The authors concluded that laparoscopic partial nephrectomy with a microwave tissue coagulator may be a useful and less invasive method for treatment of selected small renal tumors. Initial experience gained with these techniques is cautiously optimistic. A long-term patient follow-up is warranted to determine the potential for cancer control with these methods.

Animal trials

Great interest exists with respect to intra-operative bleeding. The effectiveness of various methods was investigated in a number of animal trials: Endoloop[16], hydrojet cutting[17] and cable-tie compression[18]. All authors proclaimed their method to be safe and effective.

Corvin and associates[17] evaluated whether a laparoscopic hydrojet device can provide a safe and effective partial nephrectomy. In open surgery, hydrojet resection is used to cut the renal parenchyma selectively, avoiding damage to the vascular structures or collecting system. The following method was used:

(1) Five pigs under general anesthesia;

(2) Laparoscopic wedge, as well as pole, resections of the kidney;

(3) Exposure of the kidney, incision of the renal capsule (electrocautery), use of the hydrojet to dissect the renal parenchyma;

(4) In pole resections, the use of Endo-GIA to divide the collecting system and central vessels;

(5) By electrocoagulation or clips for hemostasis; the dissection time and intraoperative complications were evaluated.

The results of the study showed:

(1) Successful in all animals without temporary ischemia;

(2) Hydrojet generator allowed precise and effective tissue dissection without significant hemorrhage;

(3) Selective coagulation of the parenchymal vessels;

(4) Collecting system and central vessels remained intact, could be divided after application of the Endo-GIA;

(5) Mean dissection time for wedge resections 42 ± 6 min, 54 ± 8 min for pole resections.

Cadeddu and colleagues[18] investigated a technique of laparoscopic reversible, regional hypoperfusion using cable-tie compression to minimize blood loss and optimize exposure in ten domestic pigs. In the porcine model, cable-tie-assisted laparascopic partial nephrectomy provided an almost bloodless surgical field that facilitated rapid resection of large renal segments and hemostasis during a short ischemic period. The authors anticipated that this technique would broaden the clinical application of laparascopic partial nephrectomy. The method used involved:

(1) Securing a cable-tie around one pole of the kidney, tightening it until the distal parenchymal surface blanched completely;

(2) Eight large amputations involving the collecting system and eight smaller amputations excluding the collecting system (laparoscopic scissors);

(3) Application of fibrin glue to seal the cut surface prior to cable-tie removal;

(4) Four pigs (four large and four small amputations) killed immediately and retrograde injection of methylene blue into the ureter to identify collecting system leaks;

(5) Six pigs (four large and four small amputations) killed 4 weeks later, retrograde urograms to assess collecting system integrity.

The study results demonstrated:

(1) Median cable-tie ischemia time 15 min (7–48 min);

(2) Median blood loss 30 ml (10–300 ml);

(3) Hemostasis was attained with fibrin glue in each case;

(4) Survival group: all four small amputations healed with a fibrotic scar; in the large amputation group, one animal died from urinary extravasation on postoperative day 4.

In 2002, Beck and co-authors[16] described a similar method, the Endoloop-assisted laparoscopic partial nephrectomy. In 12 female Yucatan mini-pigs they performed a lower-pole nephrectomy following cinching of a 1-0 Vicryl suture loop (Endoloop) proximal to the resected lower pole until ischemic discoloration was achieved. The ischemic lower pole was excised with Endo-scissors and the lower pole removed using a laparoscopic bag. They were successful in all procedures. In two cases, the Endoloop slipped off the retained parenchyma. Both problems were corrected immediately with no sequelae. At sacrifice, all upper-pole renal segments functioned, as shown by urography, and no urinomas or abscesses were found. In one pig mild extravasation was demonstrated on the retrograde pyelogram.

All authors concluded that their experimental results demonstrated the suitability of their method for safe laparoscopic partial nephrectomy without temporary ischemia to the kidney. Further investigations and modifications may allow clinical application of these methods.

Barret and his group[19] investigated three different hemostasis techniques to control intraoperative bleeding. The aim of their study was to compare the efficacy and morbidity of three renal parenchymal hemostasis techniques: high-frequency bipolar electrical current, high-frequency unipolar spray electrical current and ultrasound performed in pigs without vascular control. The criteria evaluated were intraoperative and postoperative complications, blood loss, renal function and thickness of the parenchymal lesions induced. Their results showed that ultrasound achieved more superior inhibition of blood loss than either high-frequency bipolar or high-frequency unipolar spray electrical current, but no improved preservation of renal parenchyma was observed.

Indications

The range of indications for renal-sparing surgery has been extended to include patients with localized sporadic RCC smaller than 4 cm and a functioning second kidney[20,21], as nephron-sparing surgery showed a similar outcome to that of radical nephrectomy for low-grade, low-stage RCCs of 4 cm or smaller.

Hafez and colleagues[20] reviewed the postoperative outcome of 485 patients following nephron-sparing surgery for localized sporadic RCC. Cancer-free survival was significantly better in patients with tumors 4 cm or less, compared with those with larger tumors.

Lerner and associates[21] retrospectively investigated the outcome of nephron-sparing surgery in 185 patients with low-grade and low-stage (Robson stage II or less) RCC. Some 209 nephrectomized patients were matched for patient age and sex, and tumor stage and grade. They found no significant difference with respect to progression-free, crude or cancer-specific survival between the nephron-sparing surgery and radical nephrectomy groups. Less than 5% of the patients treated with conservative nephron-sparing surgery had local recurrence. Tumor size was a strong independent predictor of outcome, whereas Robson stage was not. Patients treated with radical nephrectomy had a significant cancer-specific and progression-free survival advantage when controlling for tumor diameter and grade. However, no difference was observed in patients with primary tumor diameters of 4 cm or less.

The risk of local recurrence depends on the multifocality of RCC and tumor-free margins. Relating survival to tumor size, Filipas and colleagues also found no significant difference in patients with a tumor size larger or smaller than 4 cm[22]. This emphasizes the importance of tumor grading rather than tumor size. This supposition has been confirmed by a large series of 14 793 autopsies. The number of tumors with G1 RCC decreased with increasing tumor diameter, whereas this was just the opposite for G3 tumors, and significantly more multifocal malignant RCC was observed in tumors between 21 and 40 mm compared with those 20 mm or less in diameter[23]. In another series[24], preoperative imaging studies and surgical specimens in 44 patients suitable for partial nephrectomy but undergoing radical nephrectomy were prospectively reviewed. Some 25% of the RCCs were pathologically multifocal, 91% in primary tumors < 5 cm. Tumor multifocality was independent of the size of the primary renal tumor but occurred with a slightly higher frequency in tumors of stage T3a or larger, even when the primary tumor was small. This group stated that partial nephrectomy in patients with unilateral renal cancer should be approached with caution, and should not be performed simply because it is technically feasible. However, long-term results with low local recurrence rates seem to contradict this.

An imperative aspect associated with the intraoperative procedure is the at least 1-cm tumor-free margin to prevent the recurrence of RCC after nephron-sparing surgery. All patients with negative margins of more than 1 mm had no recurrence of disease, but 5/7 with positive margins and 9/11 patients with negative margins less than 1 mm[25] had recurrence. The results of a further study by Sutherland and colleagues including 44 patients revealed that none of their patients with negative parenchymal margins after nephron-sparing surgery for stages T1–2N0M0 RCC had local recurrence at the resection site. Margin size was irrelevant[26]. This group declared that only a minimal margin of normal renal parenchyma of less than 5 mm needs to be removed during partial nephrectomy for localized RCC. This underlines the necessitiy of intraoperative frozen section evaluation to confirm complete tumor excision.

References

1. Novick AC. Partial nephrectomy for renal cell carcinoma. *Urol Clin North Am* 1987;14:419–33
2. Fergany AF, Hafez KS, Novick AC. Long-term results of nephron sparing surgery for localized renal cell carcinoma: 10-year followup. *J Urol* 2000;163:442–5
3. Ward JP. Determination of the optimum temperature for regional renal hypothermia during temporary renal ischaemia. *Br J Urol* 1975;47:17–24
4. Rhoden E, Teloken C, Lucas M, *et al*. Protective effect of allopurinol in the renal ischemia–reperfusion in uninephrectomized rats. *Gen Pharmacol* 2000;35:189–93
5. Gupta PC, Matsushita M, Oda K, Nishikimi N, Sakurai T, Nimura Y. Attenuation of renal ischemia–reperfusion injury in rats by allopurinol and prostaglandin E$_1$. *Eur Surg Res* 1998;30:102–7
6. Chatterjee SN, Berne TV. Protective effect of allopurinol in renal ischemia. *Am J Surg* 1976;131:658–9
7. Öztürk H, Aldemir M, Buyukbayram H, Dokucu AI, Otcu S. The effects of the nitric oxide donor molsidomine prevent in warm ischemia–reperfusion injury of the rat renal – a functional and histopathological study. *Int Urol Nephrol* 2001;32:601–7
8. Mejean A, Vot B, Cazin S, Balian C, Poisson JF, Dufour B. Nephron sparing surgery for renal cell carcinoma using selective renal parenchymal clamping. *J Urol* 2002;167:234–5
9. Gill IS, Desai MM, Kaouk JH, *et al*. Laparoscopic partial nephrectomy for renal tumor: duplicating open surgical techniques. *J Urol* 2002;167:469–7, discussion 475–6
10. Wolf JS Jr, Seifman BD, Montie JE. Nephron sparing surgery for suspected malignancy: open surgery compared to laparoscopy with selective use of hand assistance. *J Urol* 2000;163:1659–64
11. Nelson CP, Wolf JS Jr. Comparison of hand assisted versus standard laparoscopic radical nephrectomy for suspected renal cell carcinoma. *J Urol* 2002;167:1989–94
12. Gill IS, Novick AC, Meraney AM, *et al*. Laparoscopic renal cryoablation in 32 patients. *Urology* 2000;56:748–53
13. Johnson DB, Nakada SY. Laparoscopic cryoablation for renal-cell cancer. *J Endourol* 2000;14:873–8
14. Yoshimura K, Okubo K, Ichioka K, Terada N, Matsuta Y, Arai Y. Laparoscopic partial nephrectomy with a microwave tissue coagulator for small renal tumor. *J Urol* 2001;165:1893–6
15. Tanaka M, Kai N, Naito S. Retroperitoneal laparoscopic wedge resection for small renal tumor using microwave tissue coagulator. *J Endourol* 2000;14:569–72
16. Beck SD, Lifshitz DA, Cheng L, Lingeman JE, Shalhav AL. Endoloop-assisted laparoscopic partial nephrectomy. *J Endourol* 2002;16:175–7
17. Corvin S, Oberneder R, Adam C, *et al*. Use of hydro-jet cutting for laparoscopic partial nephrectomy in a porcine model. *Urology* 2001;58:1070–3
18. Cadeddu JA, Corwin TS, Traxer O, Collick C, Saboorian HH, Pearle MS. Hemostatic laparoscopic partial nephrectomy: cable-tie compression. *Urology* 2001;57:562–6
19. Barret E, Guillonneau B, Cathelineau X, Validire P, Vallancien G. Laparoscopic partial nephrectomy in the pig: comparison of three hemostasis techniques. *J Endourol* 2001;15:307–12
20. Hafez KS, Fergany AF, Novick AC. Nephron sparing surgery for localized renal cell carcinoma: impact of tumor size on patient

survival, tumor recurrence and TNM staging. *J Urol* 1999;162:1930–3

21. Lerner SE, Hawkins CA, Blute ML, *et al.* Disease outcome in patients with low stage renal cell carcinoma treated with nephron sparing or radical surgery. *J Urol* 1996;155:1868–73

22. Filipas D, Fichtner J, Spix C, *et al.* Nephron-sparing surgery of renal cell carcinoma with a normal opposite kidney: long-term outcome in 180 patients. *Urology* 2000;56:387–92

23. Wunderlich H, Reichelt O, Schumann S, *et al.* Nephron sparing surgery for renal cell carcinoma 4 cm or less in diameter: indicated or under treated? *J Urol* 1998;159:1465–9

24. Whang M, O'Toole K, Bixon R, *et al.* The incidence of multifocal renal cell carcinoma in patients who are candidates for partial nephrectomy. *J Urol* 1995;154:968–70

25. Piper NY, Bishoff JT, Magee C, *et al.* Is a 1-cm margin necessary during nephron-sparing surgery for renal cell carcinoma? *Urology* 2001;58:849–52

26. Sutherland SE, Resnick MI, Maclennan GT, Goldman HB. Does the size of the surgical margin in partial nephrectomy for renal cell cancer really matter? *J Urol* 2002;167:61–4

Surgery for renal cell carcinoma: the case for open surgery

38

D. Jacqmin

Introduction

Since articles by Robson were published in 1963 and 1969[1,2], radical nephrectomy has been the gold standard treatment for renal cell carcinoma (RCC). In the following years, nephron-sparing surgery (NSS) was developed as a treatment in cases of imperative indications (solitary kidney, bilateral tumors, von Hippel–Lindau disease, etc.). During the past decade, because of the increasing number of incidentally discovered tumors, NSS has also been advocated in certain elective indications (for example small tumors, easily resectable, with a normal controlateral kidney). At the end of the last century, laparoscopic surgery was proposed by some authors for radical nephrectomy and even for NSS.

To be used instead of the gold standard (open radical nephrectomy), all the above techniques should give results at least equivalent in terms of cancer survival and operative mortality and morbidity.

Radical nephrectomy

Open radical nephrectomy

This procedure became a standard because of clinical results obtained in the 1960s, although there are no validated comparative scientific data.

The principles of this technique are primary access to the vessels, and ligation of the artery and vein, followed by *en bloc* removal of the kidney, the surrounding fat tissue, the adrenal gland and some lymph nodes. The surgical approach generally used is transperitoneal, which allows good access to the vessels and a good view of the abdominal organs.

The open technique can be used safely in all cases, whatever the size, location and extension of the tumor. Survival, mortality and morbidity are well documented: the 10-year survival was 82% in cases of pT_{1-2}, 61% in stage pT_{3a}, 40% in pT_{3B} and less than 10% in pT_4 ($n = 3347$)[3]. The perioperative mortality was less than 2%, generally observed in metastatic patients. The perioperative morbidity was around 30%, the most common cause being splenic injury (12.4%) followed by vascular injuries and bleeding[4].

Laparoscopic radical nephrectomy

This technique was proposed in the early 1990s. To date, only short series have been published, including 100 patients or fewer. There are no prospective comparative data. However, laparoscopy allows good primary access to the vessels on both right and left sides, and also allows *en bloc* removal and inspection of the abdominal organs and lymph nodes.

Long-term oncological results are lacking, but short-term cancer survival seems similar to that with open surgery: 85% at 35.6 months ($n = 67$)[5], and 95% at 4 years ($n = 103$)[6].

Mortality and morbidity rates in the published series are comparable to those of open surgery at 0–1.3% and 8–37.7%, respectively. With laparoscopy the use of analgesic is less and the hospital stay is shorter, but in published series the hospital stay varies from 1.6 to 7 days. This is the consequence of differences between health systems in various countries.

Some problems are specific to the laparoscopic technique. The risk of port-site cancer recurrence exists, particularly in cases of tumor morcellation using an endobag[7]. Laparoscopy also has cardiopulmonary effects. It increases atrial filling pressures and systemic vascular resistance, and decreases venous return and cardiac output. There is also a reduction of stroke intensity and a risk of pulmonary embolism. Laparoscopy can also alter renal function. It decreases urine output, and compresses the renal vein, the ureter and the renal parenchyma. It also exerts systemic hormonal effects by increasing serum cathecholamine and endothelin levels[8].

Conclusion

Although not yet validated, laparoscopic radical nephrectomy seems an acceptable option. Appropriate cases are probably T_1 tumors more than 4 cm in diameter, or small tumors not easily accessible to NSS. We cannot recommend laparoscopy in large tumors, or in those with macroscopic lymph node or vascular involvement that are at risk of vascular complications and need a large incision for removal.

Prospective controlled comparative studies are mandatory, with a duration of 10 years' follow-up and a large number of patients to detect an influence on survival, because these patients have a good prognosis.

Nephron-sparing surgery

Nephron-sparing surgery has been used in cases of imperative indications for some decades. The rationale behind this is the poor quality of life and the poor survival of patients under hemodialysis. The definition of an imperative indication is the need to preserve a functioning renal parenchyma as in bilateral RCC, RCC in a solitary functioning kidney, chronic renal failure not necessitating hemodialysis, or unilateral RCC and a functioning opposite kidney at risk of failure because of arterial disease or diabetes mellitus, for example. An elective indication is the presence of a small tumor, easily removable, with a normal controlateral kidney.

Open surgery

This was first used in cases of imperative indications, with good results in terms of survival and recurrence rate. The recurrence rate is usually under 7%, and the 5-year cancer-specific survival around 90%[9–11]. In cases of elective indications the results of historical series are convincing, but validated scientific data are still lacking[12].

The main risk of NSS is overlooking a multifocal tumor. Multifocality is observed in approximately 14% of cases[13], and even in tumors with a small diameter[14]. The risk can be limited by the use of peroperative ultrasound after a complete dissection of the kidney.

The operative risks are mainly bleeding and urinary fistula. Bleeding can be controlled by clamping of the artery, with or without cooling, or by manual parenchymal compression. All these maneuvers can be easily performed during open surgery, generally within less than 20 min. Mobilization of the kidney around its pedicle facilitates hemostasis of the parenchymal cut surface. In the same way, an opening in the urinary tract can be easily detected and treated with an absorbable suture. If necessary, a double-J stent can be inserted. Various tools can be used in open surgery to facilitate hemostasis. Electrocautery, an argon coagulator, a harmonic scalpel, a water-jet device, a radio-frequency probe, lasers and biological glues have been employed for this purpose. The free movements of the kidney and the instruments allow good exposure.

Finally, in some operative indications such as a centrally located tumor, bench surgery is the procedure of choice.

Laparoscopic surgery

In the past few years, the development of laparoscopy in urology has urged some experts to perform NSS by this means. They have proved that it is technically feasible in some circumstances. However, the questions arising are: is it safe and efficient? and are the oncological results as good as in open surgery?

Table 1 Results of laparascopic nephron-sparing surgery. Values are expressed as mean (range)

Authors	n	Tumor size (cm)	Operating time (min)	Blood loss (ml)	Complications (%)
Janetschek et al.[15], 2000	25	1.9 (1–5)	163.5 (90–300)	287 (20–800)	12
Rassweiler et al.[16], 2000	53	2.3 (1.1–5)	190.9 (90–320)	725 (20–1500)	32
Gill et al.[17], 2002	50	3 (1.4–7)	180 (45–315)	270.4 (40–1500)	12

The main limitation of laparoscopic surgery is fixation of the trocars, which limits the movement of instruments as is the case for ultrasound probes.

Hemostasis is a key issue in NSS, the limitation of movement and the difficulty of endosuturing prolonging the time of hemostasis. This implies a need to clamp the renal vessels, which, if prolonged, can induce an alteration of renal function. In published series, the associated blood loss is high for the ablation of such small tumors (Table 1)[15–17].

Cooling and manual parenchymal compression are not suitable.

The tools employed in open surgery are not all adapted to laparoscopic surgery, and their use is limited by access through a trocar.

Finally, bench surgery is not reasonably feasible by means of the laparoscopic technique.

In conclusion, laparoscopic surgery in NSS is not validated, and the development of new devices or major technique modifications are needed. Long-term oncological results are not available.

Conclusion

Open surgery is validated and adapted for the treatment of RCC in all cases.

Laparoscopic procedures are proposed by some experts. The acceptable indications to date are small tumors that are not candidates for NSS. Large or advanced tumors are not suitable cases for this approach. However, even the results of laparoscopy published by experts are not convincing, which means that this procedure should not be recommended in NSS.

References

1. Robson CJ. Radical nephrectomy for renal cell carcinoma. *J Urol* 1963;89:37
2. Robson CJ, Churchill BM, Andersen W. The results of radical nephrectomy for renal cell carcinoma. *J Urol* 1969;101:297–301
3. American Cancer Society. *Results in treating cancer*. Report no. 12. *Kidney cancer*. Chicago: American Cancer Society, 1989
4. Swanson DA, Borges PM. Complications of transabdominal radical nephrectomy for renal cell carcinoma. *J Urol* 1983;129:704–7
5. Chan DY, Cadeddu JA, Jarrett TW, *et al.* Laparoscopic radical nephrectomy: cancer control for renal cell carcinoma. *J Urol* 2001;166:2095–100
6. Ono Y, Kinukawa T, Hattori R, *et al.* The long-term outcome of laparoscopic radical nephrectomy for small renal cell carcinoma. *J Urol* 2001;165:1867–70
7. Castilho LN, Fugita OEH, Mitre AI, *et al.* Port site tumor recurrences of renal cell carcinoma after videolaparoscopic radical nephrectomy. *J Urol* 2001;165:519
8. Dunn MD, McDougall EM. Renal physiology. Laparoscopic considerations. *Urol Clin North Am* 2000;27:609–14
9. Morgan WR, Zincke H. Progression and survival after renal conserving surgery for renal cell carcinoma: experience in 104 patients and extended follow-up. *J Urol* 1990;144:852–8
10. Steinbach F, Stockle M, Muller SC, *et al.* Conservative surgery of renal cell tumors in 140

patients: 21 years' experience. *J Urol* 1992;148: 24–9

11. Licht MR, Novick AC, Goormastic M. Nephron sparing surgery in incidental versus suspected renal cell carcinoma. *J Urol* 1994;152:39–42

12. Novick AC. Partial nephrectomy for renal cell carcinoma. *Urology* 1995;46:149–52

13. Jacqmin D, Saussine C, Roca D, *et al*. Multiple tumors in the same kidney: incidence and therapeutic implications. *Eur Urol* 1992;21:32–34

14. Eschwege P, Saussine C, Steichen G, *et al*. Radical nephrectomy for renal cell carcinoma smaller or equal to 30 mm: long term followup results. *J Urol* 1996;155:1196–9

15. Janetschek G, Jeschke K, Peschel R, *et al*. Laparoscopic surgery for stage T1 renal cell carcinoma: radical nephrectomy and wedge resection. *Eur Urol* 2000;38:131–8

16. Rassweiler JJ, Abbou C, Janetschek G, *et al*. Laparoscopic partial nephrectomy. The European Experience. *Urol Clin North Am* 2000;27: 721–36

17. Gill IS, Desai MM, Kaouk JH, *et al*. Laparoscopic partial nephrectomy for renal tumor: duplicating open surgical techniques. *J Urol* 2002; 167:469–76

Laparoscopic partial nephrectomy

39

J. Rassweiler and S. K. H. Yip

Introduction

In developed countries up to 40% of renal tumors are detected incidentally[1,2]. The majority of these lesions are amenable to partial nephrectomy, i.e. nephron-sparing surgery, where functional nephrons are preserved[3]. However, while laparoscopic total nephrectomy has been successfully introduced as an acceptable surgical option[4], widespread application of laparoscopic partial nephrectomy (LPN) has been limited by the lack of reliable methods for hemostasis upon tumor excision[5]. Time and again, clinicians face the dilemma of whether these small incidental renal lesions should be removed by conventional open methods or should a minimally invasive procedure be attempted.

Laboratory work and innovative approaches

To date, hemostatic modalities including argon beam coagulation, electrocautery, ultrasound dissection and hydrojet dissection, as well as devices such as the cable tie, have been evaluated in various animal models[6–14]. These animal studies are interesting and pave the way for actual performance in the clinical setting (Table 1). For instance, Barret and associates[13] recently compared the use of bipolar energy, argon beam coagulator and ultrasonic dissector in 27 domestic pigs. They found that the latter had the advantage of limitation of blood loss, and may prove to be more useful in clinical LPN. Newer technologies are now being developed, including the Ligasure device (Tyco, Germany)

Table 1 Summary of animal studies and innovative approaches to achieve hemostasis in laparoscopic partial nephrectomy

Devices	*Significance and remarks*
Argon beam coagulator[6*,8,9,13]	caution for excessive pressure from high gas flow, this modality appears to be inferior to bipolar diathermy and ultrasonic dissection[13]
Harmonic scalpel[10,13]	comparative study by Barret and associates[13] shows superiority of device over other coagulation devices
Tourniquet, cable tie[12,15]	the Cleveland group[12] has largely switched to routine arterial clamping[33] in view of the inadequacy of the device
Hydrojet[11,14]	original application reported in hepatic surgery, useful in parenchymal dissection and exposure of vessels that need to be coagulated separately
Microwave[17], radiofrequency coagulation[23,24]	taking advantage of the coagulation effect, tissue transection rendered 'bloodless', architecture of lesions treated apparently still preserved for histological diagnosis
Topical agents: fibrin glue[7*,37], Tachcomb[31], Surgicel[33,37]	taking advantage of the coagulation effect, tissue transection rendered 'bloodless', architecture of lesions treated apparently still preserved for histological diagnosis

* Not laparoscopic work

and the Plasma Kinetic system (Gyrus). Both are bipolar energy delivery systems, which work through a computer that continuously adjusts the output according to impedance across the tissue to be coagulated, thus achieving a better hemostatic effect. The Ligasure system claims to be able to secure hemostasis by sealing vessels up to 7 mm in diameter. While these innovations are fascinating, formal studies to confirm their efficacy are awaited. Obviously, much caution needs to be exercised when trying to adopt laboratory findings in the clinical setting. In fact, there have been numerous small-scale trials of new devices in the human setting, with or without preceding animal studies. These have included the use of tourniquet or cable tie[15,16], and microwave tissue coagulator[17]. Many of these proposed approaches are very innovative, and cutting-edge technology is often employed. While many of the findings are preliminary, there is great potential for them to become the modality of choice; it is hoped that the efficacy of these modalities to control vigorous bleeding can be firmly established in larger scale studies. At this stage, it is sufficient to say that techniques and technologies employed continue to evolve even in major centers. For example, Gill and co-workers[15] initially reported the use of the tourniquet device for circumferential compression, but there were numerous practical shortcomings, which included possible slipping of the device and crushing of tissue at the level of compression. The device was not applicable for mid-pole tumors, and the compression distorted the calyceal configuration and reconstruction was rendered difficult.

Alternative treatment modalities and adopted technologies

In view of all these technical difficulties associated with LPN, investigators have reported the use of radiofrequency coagulation (RFC) techniques as definitive in *in situ* management of selected renal lesions[18–22]. However, since tumors are left *in situ* after treatment with interstitial ablation, the effectiveness of treatment on the target lesion and the cost of radiographic

follow-up cannot be ignored. In fact, follow-up studies of RFC-treated lesions have demonstrated the presence of viable tumors, raising concerns regarding the efficacy of the treatment[21]. From an oncological standpoint, tumors should continue to be excised, examined and staged properly.

During assessment of experimental lesions created by RFC, it was noted that parenchymal thrombosis and coagulation occurred shortly after treatment. Taking advantage of this secondary phenomenon, a bloodless field is created where dissection can be performed with improved visualization, and hemostasis can be secured reliably. There will be no need for arterial clamping or cooling if the target lesion is pre-treated adequately by the RFC. This combination of RFC followed by LPN has been reported only recently[23,24]. Gettman and associates[24] utilized this RFC-assisted LPN in ten patients, and noted that there was minimal bleeding, and rapid and controlled tumor resection was deemed possible. In addition, the architecture of the RFC-treated lesion was preserved; thus accurate histological diagnosis was not compromised by this modality.

Clinical experience

To date, LPN has been successfully completed as the definitive treatment of predominantly small exophytic renal lesions. Clinical series reported thus far are relatively small in number[25–32]. A fairly high conversion rate and long hospital stay were noted in earlier series[26,27]. Uncontrolled bleeding led to conversion to open surgery, while prolonged hospital stay was generally caused by postoperative urinary leakage. However, later series carried much higher success rates[28–32], presumably in relation to the accumulation of experience, especially in terms of control of bleeding even in the absence of vascular pedicle control. The true advantage of reduced hospital stay, decreased analgesic requirements and shorter convalescence became evident.

To date, there are few reports that consist of 50 or more patients[31–33]. Rassweiler and colleagues[31] conducted a multicenter trial using data from France, Germany and Austria. Jeschke and associates[32] reported an updated series from the two participating centers in Austria involved in the earlier multicenter report. (Some 25 patients' data could have overlapped in the two reports.) The latest series by Gill and co-workers[33] remains the largest single institute experience of LPN (Tables 2 and 3).

There is continuing interest in re-examining the feasibility of performing LPN in a similar manner to open surgery. The key steps of open partial nephrectomy are vascular control, ice cooling, excision of tumor, coagulation/ ligation of the bleeding vessels, repair of the pelvocalyceal system and closure of the parenchymal defect by suturing[3,34]. Many of the above steps would be very demanding if performed laparoscopically. However, major centers have shown that many of these techniques can be acquired through persistent and dedicated training. Of course, it is debatable whether 30 min of warm ischemia should be allowed during a LPN. However, the technique described by the group bears close resemblance to the open surgical technique, and their series is by far the world's biggest single institute experience[33].

Warm ischemia or cold ischemia?

The major hurdle remaining to enable LPN to be performed in a manner similar to the open procedure is the creation of cold ischemia. To the best of our knowledge, none of the leading centers have produced a reliable and reproducible method of rendering complete cold ischemia laparoscopically, although ice sludge was used successfully on one occasion[33]. However, with temporary arterial occlusion and appropriate hydration, the 'window of ischemia' is usually adequate even for the laparoscopic excision and closure of defect without significant renal damage. This approach has the closest resemblance to the open procedure, and entirely employs well-established surgical principles and techniques. There has been much discussion on the recent report where routine arterial clamping was employed[33,35], and we believe that arterial clamping should be employed in a selective manner. For small, predominantly exophytic lesions in a favorable location, arterial clamping may not be routinely required. On the other hand, for lesions with substantial intra-renal extension, or centrally located tumors, arterial clamping should be

Table 2 Recent major series on laparoscopic partial nephrectomy

Authors	Number of patients	Mean tumor size (cm) (range)	Selection criteria	Approach	Hilar control	Main modality for hemostasis
Rassweiler et al., 2000[31] (four centers from Europe)*	53	2.3 (1.1–5)	exophytic lesions	retroperitoneal (n = 38) transperitoneal (n = 15)	no no	bipolar coagulation
Jeschke et al., 2001[32] (two centers from Austria)*	51	2 (1–5)	favorable peripheral locations, normal contralateral kidneys	retroperitoneal (n = 32) transperitoneal (n = 19)		ultracision, bipolar coagulation
Gill et al., 2002[33] (single institute)	50	3 (1.4–7)	included 24 (48%) patients with compromised contralateral kidneys	retroperitoneal (n = 22) transperitoneal (n = 28)	artery only (n = 4), artery and vein (n = 46), 1 case with additional ice sludge; mean warm ischemia 23 min	monopolar J-hook, 'figure of 8' sutures, parenchymal stitches over surgicel bolsters

*Overlap of data presented

Table 3 Recent major series on laparoscopic partial nephrectomy: perioperative parameters

Authors	Mean operating time (min)	Mean blood loss (ml)	Conversion (%)	Complications	Open re-intervention rate (%)	Postoperative hospital stay (days)
Rassweiler et al., 2000[31] (four centers from Europe)*	191 (90–320)	725 (20–1500)	8	intra-operative hemorrhage (n = 4), delayed hemorrhage (n = 1), urine leakage (n = 5)	6	5.4 (3–28)
Jeschke et al., 2001[32] (two centres from Austria)*	132 (70–300)	282 (20–800)	0	delayed hemorrhage (n = 1), urinary leakage (n = 3)	4	5.8 (3–12)
Gill et al., 2002[33] (single institute)	180 (45–345)	270 (40–1500)	0	intra-operative hemorrhage (n = 1), delayed hemorrhage and nephrectomy (n = 1), urine leak (n = 1)	2	2.2 (1–9)

* Overlap of data presented

considered (Table 4). A delicate balance between the availability of surgical expertise to complete secure hemostasis and the tight time window in which to perform the procedure remains. If there is reasonable concern that the warm ischemia could extend well beyond 30 min, conventional open surgery may still be considered as the primary treatment at this stage of development of LPN techniques. We eagerly await the development of a reliable means to induce ice sludge-based cold ischemia.

Surgical technique

Transperitoneal or retroperitoneal approach?

Obviously, different authors have their preferred approaches[31–33] (Table 2). However, it may be advisable to be familiar with both to provide some degree of flexibility. The Innsbruck group, for instance, preferred the transperitoneal route for anterior tumors, but had to 'rotate' the kidney for posterior tumors[36]. A reasonable guide could be retroperitoneal for posterior tumors and transperitoneal for anterior tumours. However,

there is no hard and fast rule, and there is little if any evidence to prove that one approach is superior to the other.

The authors prefer the retroperitoneal approach, the surgical technique of which is described in detail below. A 2-cm incision is made in the lumbar triangle between the 12th rib and the iliac crest, at a point along the posterior axillary line (corresponding to the posterior axillary line). A tunnel down to the retroperitoneal space is created by blunt dissection using Kocher forceps. This tunnel is dilated until an index finger can be introduced to push the peritoneum forward, creating a retroperitoneal space. Further opening up of the space between the lumbar aponeurosis and the Gerota's fascia is performed exclusively with the index finger. In general, we do not use balloon dilators, but disposable balloons are available commercially. Alternatively, a home-made balloon can be obtained simply by tying securely the thumb portion of a glove to the end of the suction catheter, this can easily take up 500–800 ml of saline injected to create the retroperitoneal space. The space can then be assessed by introducing the camera through the

Table 4 Selection of patients and recommended approach

Description of lesion	Suggested approach
Small (e.g. < 2 cm), exophytic lesion in easily accessible location	wedge excision *without* arterial clamping, bipolar coagulation for hemostasis and sealing of surface by Tachcomb, Surgicel and/or fibrin glue
Central location, medium-size tumor (e.g. 2–3.5 cm)	wedge excision *with* arterial clamping, bipolar coagulation for hemostasis and sealing of surface by Tachcomb, Surgicel and/or fibrin glue, suture closure of defect
Big lesion (e.g. > 3.5 cm), significant intrarenal extension	partial nephrectomy *with* arterial clamping, bipolar coagulation for hemostasis and sealing of surface by Tachcomb, Surgicel and/or fibrin glue, careful closure of breached pelvocalyceal system, (consider preoperative ureteral catheterization or intra-operative stenting), suture closure of surgical defect, *reconsider indication for laparoscopic partial nephrectomy*

primary incision, and placement of additional ports can be performed under direct vision. We prefer to place the two secondary trocars (port II, 10 mm for the surgeon's dominant hand; port III, 5 mm for the non-dominant hand) under guidance of the index finger placed in the retroperitoneal space. These secondary ports being placed in front of the primary incision are arranged in a triangular manner. Port II is for various dissecting instruments including a 10-mm clip applicator. The initial wound is used for placement of the camera port (12 mm) and subsequent specimen retrieval; application of mattress sutures around the port helps to minimize air leakage. At this stage, pneumo-retroperitoneum can be established to a pressure of about 12–15 mmHg, residue minor adhesion can be removed easily. The psoas muscle, which represents the most important anatomical landmark of retroperitoneoscopy, is exposed to the level of the diaphragm by blunt and sharp dissection. Additional 5-mm trocars can be inserted under endoscopic guidance to help retraction where necessary. Occasionally, when excessive retroperitoneal fat hangs down and obscures the view, it is helpful to simply trim off the fat to ensure an unhindered camera view of the retroperitoneal space. Partial tear of the peritoneum and gas distention of the perito-neal cavity can be a nuisance; extending the 'incision' of the peritoneum to convert the procedure to 'transperitoneal' is a simple way out. The pressure will quickly 'equalize' and a

good view of the retroperitoneal structures can be maintained.

It is important to incise the Gerota's fascia completely. The wide longitudinal incision allows retraction of the peritoneum and exposes the kidneys, the upper ureter and renal hilum. Medial retraction (or lifting upward) of the kidney by instruments controlled by the surgeon's non-dominant hand will help to expose the hilum. The renal artery is the first structure to be identified! Irrespective of whether hilar clamping is planned, it is advisable to expose the hilum, especially the renal artery, in the event that temporary clamping is required to help to control unexpected major bleeding during the parenchymal resection. Additional entry ports would be required to accommodate a different configuration of commercially available vascu-lar clamps. We use a home-made right-angled dissector with elastic tubing over the jaws for 'cushioning' as the arterial clamp. The clamp is applied when the tumor has been adequately exposed and is ready for resection. To expose the lesion, the perinephric fat is dissected from the renal surface until the renal tumor is identified. The immediate fat overlying the tumor can be left attached to the tumor pro-vided there is clear identification of the boundary of the renal tumor, with respect to the renal surface. If the overlying tissue obscures the view to the tumor, it is advisable to dissect the tissue and send it off as a separate specimen. Laparoscopic ultrasonography, if available, may be valuable to help determine the nature of indeterminate lesions, and to map out the extent of the lesion, especially its inner margin.

The principle of wedge resection is similar to the open technique, apart from the absence of arterial clamping. However, for practical and oncological considerations, wedge resection should be restricted to lesions < 2.5 cm in size, and predominantly exophytic lesions. Wedge resection should incorporate a 5-mm margin on all sides.

Wedge resection without ischemia

A monopolar J hook can be used to map out the boundary of resection. It should be limited to the level of the renal capsule, as monopolar coagulation is not very secure once paren-chymal bleeding starts. The authors use almost exclusively bipolar coagulation forceps for simultaneous dissection and hemostasis. Other modalities that can be employed include harmonic scalpel, which can be used in con-junction with the bipolar device. Jeschke and colleagues[32] recommended the use of Ultra-cision scalpel (Ethicon, Norderstedt, Germany) for parenchymal incision to reduce bleeding to a minimum. Bleeding from larger vessels, how-ever, should be treated by bipolar coagulation. While bipolar coagulation is highly efficient, delayed fistula formation has been attributed to excessive use, which could lead to tissue necrosis. It may be advisable, therefore, to employ the Ultracision especially for dissection of the central portion of the wedge, and to mini-mize the use of bipolar diathermy at this point. The exposure of the undersurface of the tumor can be enhanced by 'lifting' up the tumor speci-men and simultaneous suction of the blood using the irrigation suction device. Sharp dis-section can be achieved using the endoshear. It is important to maintain the three-dimensional orientation of the tumor to avoid cutting into the tumor as dissection proceeds. Once dissected free, the tumor is entrapped in a specimen retrieval bag to reduce any chance of 'seeding' .The delivery of the specimen is left until towards the end of the procedure.

Sealing the cut surface

Cauterization of the cut surface with an argon beam coagulator promotes further hemostasis. However, animal studies and clinical impression did not particularly support its use[13]. If the device is to be utilized, caution is required to avoid excessive pressure as a result of the high gas flow from the argon beam coagulator. Whether other forms of laser energies, e.g. Holmium laser, are useful has not yet been evaluated. We prefer to apply a piece of fibrin-coated hemostyptic gauze (Tachcomb, Munich, Germany) which sticks to the resected surface and stops bleeding effectively. Other authors apply oxidized regenerated cellulose or Surgicel (Ethicon) under pressure, in combina-tion with fibrin glue, which has been found to control major bleeding effectively. Stifelman and co-workers[37] have a special 'recipe' for the application of the fibrin glue. They use fibrinogen-soaked Gelfoam (Upjohn, Germany) to press onto the resection defect, then thrombin spray (delivered via a needle inserted percutaneously) is utilized to activate the fibrinogen and pressure is maintained for 10 min. While hemostasis is generally satisfac-tory, they prefer to place three or four addi-tional pledget sutures where necessary. Others disagree with additional sutures over the paren-chyma, which might reduce the functioning parenchyma owing to scar formation caused by the sutures[32]. It is noteworthy that the fibrin glue preparation comes in small vials, a special sequence of preparing the glue must be followed and it is very expensive.

Practical consideration

Patient preparation

Mechanical bowel preparation using saline solutions is advisable, whether a transperitoneal or retroperitoneal approach is planned. Sub-cutaneous heparin is given perioperatively until full ambulation. Pressure stockings are prescribed. Preoperatively, it is prudent to explain fully to the patient and relatives the oncological as well as the technical aspects of

LPN. Special mention needs to be made regarding the possibility of open conversion, secondary intervention and the remote possibility of total nephrectomy.

Patient selection

Surgical experience and laparoscopic expertise dictate how 'aggressively' laparoscopic surgery should be offered as the primary modality. Initially, careful selection of small, exophytic tumors is advisable (Table 4).

Management of postoperative complications

Even in the best hands, there may be complications whether the surgery is performed in an open manner or laparoscopically. Specific complications of partial nephrectomy include postoperative hemorrhage and urinary leakage. When significant postoperative bleeding is encountered, open exploration should be proceeded to promptly. On the other hand, urinary leakage can often be managed conservatively, either by endoscopic or percutaneous diversion, provided infection is under control.

Augmented techniques

Hand assistance using various access devices has been utilized for laparoscopic nephrectomy[38]. The arguments for this include that the same incision would be required for subsequent specimen retrieval anyway, and that placement of the hand would render much 'assistance'. Similarly, there have been arguments for hand-assisted LPN[37,39]. In LPN, the hand can squeeze the kidney to control bleeding, and to facilitate hemostasis and suturing. Wolf and colleagues[39] reported improved convalescence after laparoscopic surgery with selective use of hand assistance when compared with open surgery. Similarly, Stifelman and associates[37] noted very minimal analgesia requirements and short hospital stay for 11 patients with an average tumor size of 1.9 cm. However, as tumor size in most of the LPN group is consistently

small, the 'beauty' of a true keyhole minimally invasive surgery is 'lost', to some extent, by utilizing hand assistance. There has also been concern that the intermittent 'squeeze and perfusion' to the renal parenchyma may induce some form of 're-perfusion' injury, although this has not been studied specifically. The use of hand-assisted devices also increases the cost to the entire surgery (US dollar 400–800 depending on the product) and this should be considered. In the unlikely event that significant bleeding complicates a hand-assisted procedure, an additional incision may be required for open conversion, which is different from the hand-assisted entry wound. In the authors' opinion, hand-assisted LPN may not be ideal as a primary procedure, but may be considered as a 'salvage' approach before full conversion to open surgery when a significant amount of bleeding occurs during a standard laparoscopic LPN. In this scenario, some form of compression may prove useful. Obviously, the surgeon needs to decide whether the situation warrants immediate open conversion, or is likely to be completed with hand assistance.

Conclusion

We are faced with the challenge of providing minimally invasive surgery in a safe manner. To date, many average-sized, non-academic units are performing adrenalectomy, ablative total nephrectomy and live donor nephrectomy laparoscopically[40,41]. For example, in Yip's (co-author) unit, > 70% of total nephrectomies, but < 5% of partial nephrectomies, are performed laparoscopically. It can be expected that the majority of partial nephrectomies will be performed laparoscopically should the technique of securing the hemostasis continue to improve. Innovative approaches including use of tissue glue are fascinating. In the foreseeable future, the final barrier to a complete spectrum of laparoscopic renal and adrenal surgery may be overcome.

On the other hand, the follow-up data of patients who have undergone LPN are very limited at this stage. The longest follow-up reported to date was from Jeschke and associates[32], with a mean follow-up of 34 months (range 3–78 months); no local, port site or distant metastasis has been documented. We await longer-term follow-up data to confirm its efficacy as a proven oncological modality. Based on recent major series of long-term follow-up on nephron-sparing surgery, and that we are following exactly the same surgical principle as in open surgery, we believe that we should be able to achieve a similar degree of cancer control.

References

1. Aso Y, Homma Y. A survey on incidental renal cell carcinoma in Japan. *J Urol* 1992;147:340–4
2. Siow WY, Yip SKH, Tan PH, *et al.* Incidental renal cell carcinoma: clinical and pathological staging. *J R Coll Surg Edinb* 2000;45:291–5
3. Hafez KS, Fergany AF, Novick AC. Nephron sparing surgery for localised renal cell carcinoma: impact of tumour size on patient survival, tumour recurrence and TNM staging. *J Urol* 1999;162:1930–3
4. Rassweiler J, Fornara P, Weber M, *et al.* Laparoscopic nephrectomy: the experience of the laparoscopic working group of the German Urological Association. *J Urol* 1998;160:18–21
5. Tierney AC, Nakada SY. Laparoscopic radical and partial nephrectomy. *World J Urol* 2000;18: 249–56
6. Hernandez AD, Smith JA Jr, Jeppson KG, *et al.* A controlled study of the argon beam coagulator for partial nephrectomy. *J Urol* 1990;143:1062–5
7. Levinson AK, Swanson DA, Johnson DE, *et al.* Fibrin glue for partial nephrectomy. *Urology* 1991;38:314–16
8. McDougall SM, Clayman RV, Chandhoke PS, *et al.* Laparoscopic partial nephrectomy in the pig model. *J Urol* 1993;149:1633–6
9. Kletscher BA, Lauvetz RW, Segura JW. Nephron sparing laparoscopic surgery: techniques to control the renal pedicle and manage parenchymal bleeding. *J Endourol* 1995;9:23–30
10. Jackman SV, Cadeddu JA, Chen RN, *et al.* Utility of the Harmonic scalpel for laparoscopic partial nephrectomy. *J Endourol* 1998;12:441–4
11. Shekarriz H, Shekarriz B, Upadhyay J, *et al.* Hydrojet assisted laparoscopic partial nephrectomy: initial experience in a porcine model. *J Urol* 2000;163:1005–8
12. Cadeddu JA, Corwin TS, Traxer O, *et al.* Hemostatic laparoscopic partial nephrectomy: cable tie compression. *Urology* 2001;57:562–6
13. Barret E, Guillonneau B, Cathelineau X, Validire P, Vallencien G. Laparoscopic partial nephrectomy in the pig: comparison of three hemostasis techniques. *J Endourol* 2001;15:307–12
14. Corvin S, Oberneder R, Adam C, *et al.* Use of hydro-jet cutting for laparoscopic partial nephrectomy in a porcine model. *Urology* 2001;58:1070–3
15. Gill IS, Munch LC, Clayman RV, *et al.* A new renal tourniquet for open and laparoscopic partial nephrectomy. *J Urol* 1995;154:1113–16
16. Cadeddu JA, Corwin TS. Cable tie compression to facilitate laparoscopic partial nephrectomy. *J Urol* 2001;165:177–8
17. Yoshimura K, Okubo K, Ichioka K, *et al.* Laparoscopic partial nephrectomy with a microwave tissue coagulator for small renal tumor. *J Urol* 2001;165:1893–6
18. Zlotta AR, Wildschutz T, Raviv G, *et al.* Radiofrequency interstitial tumour ablation (RITA) is a possible new modality for treatment of renal cancer: *ex vivo* and *in vivo* experience. *J Endourol* 1997;11:251–8
19. Hsu THS, Fidler ME, Gill IS. Radiofrequency ablation of the kidney: acute and chronic histology in porcine model. *Urology* 2000;56: 872–5
20. Gill IS, Hsu THS, Fox RL, *et al.* Laparoscopic and percutaneous radiofrequency ablation of the kidney: acute and chronic porcine study. *Urology* 2000;56:197–200
21. Rendon RA, Kachura JR, Sweet JM, *et al.* The uncertainty of radiofrequency treatment of renal cell carcinoma: findings at immediate and delayed nephrectomy. *J Urol* 2002;167:1587–92
22. de Vaere T, Kuoch V, Smayra T, *et al.* Radiofrequency ablation of renal cell carcinoma. *J Urol* 2002;167:1961–4

23. Corwin TS, Cadeddu JA. Radiofrequency coagulation to facilitate laparoscopic partial nephrectomy. *J Urol* 2001;165:175–6
24. Gettman MT, Bishoff JT, Su LM, *et al.* Hemostatic laparoscopic partial nephrectomy: initial experience with the radiofrequency coagulation-assisted technique. *Urology* 2001;58:8–11
25. Winfield HN, Donovan JF, Godet AS, *et al.* Human laparoscopic partial nephrectomy. *J Endourol* 1992;6:559
26. Winfield HN, Donovan JF, Lund GO, *et al.* Laparoscopic partial nephrectomy: initial experience and comparison to the open surgical approach. *J Urol* 1995;153:1409–14
27. McDougall EM, Elbahnasy AM, Clayman RV. Laparoscopic wedge resection and partial nephrectomy – the Washington University experience and review of the literature. *J Soc Lap Surg* 1998;2:15–23
28. Janetschek G, Daffner P, Peschel R, *et al.* Laparoscopic nephron sparing surgery for small renal cell carcinoma. *J Urol* 1998;159:1152–5
29. Hoznek A, Salomon L, Antiphon P, *et al.* Partial nephrectomy with retroperitoneal laparoscopy. *J Urol* 1999;162:1922–6
30. Harmon WJ, Kavoussi LR, Bishoff JT. Laparoscopic nephron-sparing surgery for solid renal masses. *Urology* 2000;56:754–9
31. Rassweiler JJ, Abbou C, Janetschek G, *et al.* Laparoscopic partial nephrectomy, the European experience. *Urol Clin N Am* 2000;27:721–36
32. Jeschke K, Peschel R, Wakonig L, *et al.* Laparoscopic nephron-sparing surgery for renal tumors. *Urology* 2001;58:688–92
33. Gill IS, Desai MM, Kaouk JH, *et al.* Laparoscopic partial nephrectomy for renal tumour: duplicating open surgical techniques *J Urol* 2002;167:469–76
34. Yip SKH, Cheng WS, Tan BS, *et al.* Partial nephrectomy for renal tumours: the Singapore General Hospital experience. *J R Coll Surg Edinb* 1999;44:156–61
35. Wolf JS Jr. Laparoscopic partial nephrectomy [Editorial]. *J Urol* 2002;167:475–6
36. Janetschek G, Jeschke K, Peschel R, *et al.* Laparoscopic surgery for low stage renal cell carcinoma: radical nephrectomy and wedge excision. *Eur Urol* 2000;38:131–8
37. Stifelman MD, Sosa RE, Nakada SY, *et al.* Hand assisted laparoscopic partial nephrectomy. *J Endourol* 2001;15:161–4
38. Wolf JS Jr, Mood TD, Nakada SY. Hand assisted laparoscopic nephrectomy: comparison to standard laparoscopic nephrectomy. *J Urol* 1998;162:806–7
39. Wolf JS, Seifman BD, Montie JE. Nephron sparing surgery for suspected malignancy: open surgery compared to laparoscopy with selective use of hand assistance. *J Urol* 2000;163:1659–64
40. Yip SKH, Tan YH, Cheng WS. Hand assisted laparoscopic nephrectomy: comparison to open radical nephrectomy [Letter]. *Urology* 2002;59:632–3
41. Tan YH, Yip SKH, Cheng WS. Laparoscopic versus open adrenalectomy, the Singapore General Hospital Experience. *Asian J Surgery*; in press

Laparoscopic radical nephrectomy   40

D. Teber, V. Moraga, S. Yip, Y. Dekel, T. Frede, O. Seemann and J. Rassweiler

Introduction

At the beginning of the decade, Clayman and associates[1] pioneered laparoscopic nephrectomy, when they removed a renal oncocytoma in 1990. Almost 1 year later, Coptcoat and co-workers[2] used the same technique for a radical exstirpation of a T2 renal cell carcinoma. In 1992, Chiu and associates[3] reported on laparoscopic nephroureterectomy for malignant disease. This technique has become one of the most innovative and successful challenges to the conventional, and traditionally gold standard, open approach, and currently this option is the surgery of choice in many urology centers all over the world, particularly focused towards T1 tumors[4].

Numerous experiences world-wide have demonstrated very good surgical and perioperative results, at least comparable to, if not better than, open surgery in many aspects[5], and a few published series with long-term follow-up show similar oncological results to the open procedure[5]. The technique, however, still demands adequate laparoscopic urological surgical skills and its development continues to grow, as does the number of urologists adequately trained in this area.

The basic oncological surgical principles applied to open surgery are exactly the same as for laparoscopic surgery, as are the criteria used for diagnostic staging, follow-up and general management. Thus, the objective of this communication is to focus more on the technical aspects of the surgery than on the disease aspects, presenting a review of the current state of the art of laparoscopic radical nephrectomy and a description of the surgical technique. On the other hand, we want to present and review long-term follow-up data.

Technique

Principally, there are two approaches for laparoscopic radical nephrectomy, the transperitoneal and the retroperitoneal techniques.

Transperitoneal laparoscopic radical nephrectomy

Patient preparation

All patients receive similar preoperative preparation to that performed prior to open surgery (including informed consent and bowel preparation with 10 mg bisacodyl orally). Prior to the procedure, a nasogastric tube and a bladder catheter are inserted. Under general anesthesia, the patient is placed in the lateral traditional flank position with the table broken to extend the uppermost flank, the table is then turned to a more oblique position.

Trocar placement

After pneumoperitoneum is attained, with the inserted Veress needle placed lateral to the rectus abdominis muscle on the line with the umbilicus, trocars are inserted through the ventral abdominal wall. Port I is located 10 mm periumbilical (lateral edge of muscularis rectus abdominis); port II is located 12 mm subcostal (mammillary line) for the right kidney, 5 mm for the left side; and port III is located 12 mm above the spina iliaca superior (mammillary line) for the left kidney, 5 mm for the right side.

The laparoscope is passed through port I and used intra-abdominally to inspect the trocar insertion for ports II and III. The ports are 'secured' with sterile adhesive tape and sutured to the skin. After complete inspection of the intra-abdominal situs, either the ascending (right kidney) or descending (left kidney) colon is mobilized by laterocolic incision of the peritoneum (line of Toldt). Since the respective colon is free to fall off medially, one or two further ports can be inserted through the newly exposed retroperitoneum. Port IV is located 5 mm along the lateral abdominal wall parallel to port II and port V is located 5 mm along the lateral abdominal wall parallel to port III. These two ports are mainly used to grasp the kidney during dissection and for kidney retrieval[4,6].

Clipping the ureter

The ovarian/spermatic vein is identified in proximity to the sacral promontory, clipped and dissected, as is the ureter thereafter. Retraction of the ureter can be established with an Endo-bowel-clamp inserted through port IV or V and may be helpful during dissection of the renal hilum. The lower pole of the kidney is isolated, including the fatty capsule.

Renal vessel clipping

The main renal artery and vein are stapled with the Endo GIA 30, while smaller vessels can be clipped in typical fashion. For cost reduction, the main renal artery may be dissected between large double clips at each side; however, the main renal vein should be stapled in almost every situation. Dissection of the renal vessels is carried out bi-manually with Endo-shears, Endo-dissector and Endo-right-angle-clamp, quite similarly to open surgery.

Organ retrieval

The upper pole of the kidney, including the fatty capsule, is then dissected free of the respective adrenal gland and the relevant peritoneum. Next, the organ is grasped in the hilar region and moved down into the pelvic area, preventing any interference with intra-abdominal introduction of the organ bag. In selected cases (i.e. upper pole renal cell carcinoma), we have additionally taken out the adrenal gland by use of clips or the Endo-GIA-stapler. The Lapsac is twirled around on a 4.5-mm converter-reduced Endo-Grasp and previously passed through port III. The organ bag unfolds intra-abdominally and is held open by three Endo-clamps (via port II , IV and V), while the kidney is maneuvered into the LapSac® (Cook-Europe)[7].

Digital fragmentation

After the Endo-dissector pulls the drawstring, thereby closing the bag, the trocar sleeve is removed and the neck of the bag is pulled out over the surface of the abdomen (subcostal port II for the right kidney, suprailiacal port for the left side). The port wound is further incised (20 mm) making possible forceps removal of fatty tissue and digital fragmentation of the kidney in three to five pieces. This is done very carefully to distinguish between fatty capsule, normal renal tissue and renal tumor, which are sent for separate histopathological analysis. We never use a mechanical liquidizer, aspirator or morcellator device[1,8].

Complete organ removal

In some cases, we have used a 8–10-cm muscle-splitting lower abdominal incision for complete organ removal[9,10]. This access was also used for a hand-assisted laparoscopic approach towards the end of the procedure.

Before all trocar sleeves were removed under direct vision, the nephrectomy situs was inspected to rule out any active bleeding. Similar to open surgery, a drainage tube was placed routinely through port IV or V. This permits drainage of blood and irrigation fluid and may reveal postoperative bleeding. The enlarged incision(s) were closed with fascia and skin suture. All other port incisions were sutured intracutaneously or covered with adhesive strips.

Retroperitoneal laparoscopic radical nephrectomy

Patient preparation

All patients receive similar preoperative preparation to that performed prior to open surgery or transperitoneal laparoscopic nephrectomy.

Access to the retroperitoneum

Under general anesthesia, the patient is placed in the typical kidney position. Trendelenburg position is not necessary. A 15–18 mm incision is then made in the 'muscle-free' triangle between the 12th rib and the anterior iliac spine (between the lateral edges of the musculus latissimus dorsi and musculus obliquus externus). A canal down to the retroperitoneal space is then created by blunt dissection with an Overhold-forceps. The canal is then dilated such that the index finger can be introduced to push forward the peritoneum, thus creating a retroperitoneal cavity for correct placement of the secondary trocars.

Placement of secondary tocars

We then place the next two secondary trocars directly under palpation lateral to the index finger introduced via the primary access[11]. To avoid any injury to the surgeon's finger, the canal needs to be dilated using forceps: port II (10/11 mm) for the right hand of the surgeon (use of Endo-shears and Endo-clip-applicator, port III (5 mm) for the left hand of the surgeon (use of Endo-dissect). Then the trocar wound is closed around the sheath to avoid gas leakage (matress suture) and the trocar is connected to the CO_2-insufflator to establish a pneumoretroperitoneum (15 mmHg, 3.5 l/min) and retroperitoneoscopy is performed.

Finally, if necessary, medially to the rim of the peritoneum, another 5-mm trocar is inserted (port IV), under endoscopic view, serving for retraction of the kidney during the dissection. After placement of all trocars, the maximal insufflation pressure is decreased to 12 mmHg. As in the open procedure, the surgeon and the camera assistant stand on the dorsal side of the patient.

Patients

Since 1992, we have performed laparoscopic radical nephrectomy in 53 patients (36 male, 16 female) with localized renal cell carcinoma of the kidney. Stage and grade of the tumors are listed on Table 1; the majority were pT1 tumors,

Table 1 Pathological classification in 53 patients with laparoscopic radical nephrectomy

Tumor	Stage	n
Renal cell carcinoma	pT1	38
	pT2	10
	pT3a	3
	pT3b	2
Oncocytoma		2
Total		55

and there were two bilateral renal cell carcinomas in patients under dialysis. All relevant perioperative data have been recorded, concerning operative time, complications, conversion and reintervention rate, as well as hospital stay. The follow-up time averaged 75 months (range 7–105 months). We focused on local recurrence, regional progression, development of metastases and disease-specific survival.

Results

Laparoscopic radical nephrectomy

Perioperative data

The operating time averaged 153 min (range 90–410 min); there was no difference whether a transperitoneal ($n = 18$) or retroperitoneal ($n = 35$) approach was used (Table 2). In 18 cases, the specimen was entrapped in an organ bag (LapSac) and retrieved after digital morcellation, whereas in 37 instances the intact organ was removed via a 6–8-cm incision in the lower abdomen. This incision was used for manual assistance during the procedure. The mean estimated blood loss was 120 ml (range 100–700 ml). There was no conversion to open surgery. We observed one bleeding from the surface of the spleen which was managed by laparoscopic tamponading using a hemostyptic gauze (Tachotamp®, Ethicon, Norderstedt). Another patient developed bleeding from one of the trocar sites 6 h after the operation, which was controlled by a transcutaneous suture. Two months later, the same patient suffered from ileus due to a stenosis of the terminal ileum, most probably induced by the aforementioned suture. The patient was successfully treated by a

Table 2 Perioperative data on laparoscopic radical nephrectomy for renal cell carcinoma

Criteria	Nephrectomy
Total number	55
Access	
transperitoneal	18
retroperitoneal	37
Specimen retrieval	
morcellation	18
by incision	37
Mean operating time (min)	153
Mean blood loss (ml)	120
Conversion to open surgery	0
Complications (%)	5.5
bleeding	1
pulmonary embolism	1
ileal stenosis	1
Reintervention	1
Hospital stay (days)	7
Back to normal activity (days)	21

Table 3 Follow-up data for laparoscopic radical nephrectomy for renal cell carcinoma

Criteria	Radical nephrectomy
Total number	55
Mean observation time (months)	60
Dead of disease	2
Dead of other causes	—
Overall survival (%)	91
Disease-free survival (5 years) (%)	
overall	91
pT1/pT2	96
pT3	82

segmental ileal resection. One patient had a pulmonary embolism which was managed conservatively. The mean postoperative hospital stay was 7 days (range 4–16 days).

Pathology

The tumor was right-sided in 20 (37%) patients, left-sided in 31 (56%) patients, and bilateral in two (7%) patients. The tumor was located at the upper pole in 14 (25%), at the central area in 28 (48%) and at the lower pole in 13 (26%) of the cases. Mean tumor size was 4.1 cm (range 0.5–8 cm). The pathological examination revealed renal cell carcinoma in 53 (96.4%) and an Onkocytoma in two (3.6%) specimens. In the renal cell carcinoma group, the tumor stage was pT1 in 38 (69.1%), pT2 in ten (18.2%), pT3a in three (5.5%) and pT3b in two (3.6%) of the specimens. The surgical margins were negative in all cases.

Follow-up data

The mean observation time was 60 months (range 36–80 months) (Table 3). There was no recurrence at the site of the trocars. One patient with a pT2G2 tumor developed a local recurrence and bone metastases 4 years after laparoscopic radical nephrectomy. He died 56 months after the procedure. Another patient with a pT2G3 tumor developed pulmonary and bone metastases 31 months after the procedure and died 34 months after surgery. The cumulative overall disease-free survival rate after 5 years is 91%; however, it was 96% for pT1/pT2 and 82% for pT3 tumors.

Discussion

Since the first laparoscopic nephrectomy reported by Clayman and colleagues in 1991[1], experience with laparoscopy in urology, especially in laparoscopic nephrectomy, has increased. The role of laparoscopic radical nephrectomy in patients with malignancies of the kidney and ureter still remains a subject of debate. Primary concerns have centered around the safety of the procedure, the reproducibility of the open technique by laparoscopy, the risk of tumor cell spillage, and port site metastases. Further concerns have been related to cost-effectiveness and the steep learning curve of the procedure. Finally, until now, no long-term follow-up was available.

In the meantime, more than 10 years after its first description, the technique of trans-peritoneal laparoscopic radical nephrectomy has been standardized, fulfilling the principles of non-touch uro-oncological surgery. Various series have proposed a retroperitoneal approach[12], advocating the advantage of earlier control of the renal artery and the reduced need for dissection (i.e. deflection of the colon). However, we feel that, as in open surgery, the access should be only of secondary interest. Nevertheless, the reproducibility of the procedure has been documented in multicenter studies[13,14], as well as in a review of the literature (Table 4). The complication rate is acceptable and still decreasing; the operative time exceeds that of open surgery (140–150 min) by about 60–100 min. The retrieval of the specimen is accomplished mostly by a small incision after entrapment in an organ bag, rather than by morcellation.

Some authors have used this incision earlier during the procedure to perform hand-assisted laparoscopy. They emphasize that this would speed up the procedure and reduce the learning curve[6,9,10,15]. According to our own early experience, we could reduce the operative time by about 60 min[9,10]; however, standardization of the use of the hand proved to be very difficult, particularly because the surgeon has to insert different hands for left- and right-sided radical nephrectomies. Particularly, with the interest of a standard training program for laparoscopy and retroperitoneoscopy in urology, we feel that hand assistance should be limited to management of problematic situations. In contrast to this, the increasing expertise of first-generation laparoscopists offers a variety of dissecting techniques; the following generations are performing the operation much easier and with fewer complications than the pioneers[11,13]. Subsequently, our own operating times have dropped significantly and are now in the same range as those for open surgery (Table 2).

Concerning the cost–benefit analysis of laparoscopic radical nephrectomy, the situation in the United States differs significantly from that in Europe. The operating times reported by the different groups are mostly longer, the charges for the theater are higher, and the postoperative hospital stay is shorter for both open and laparoscopic surgery than in Europe[6,16,17]. Therefore, the higher perioperative costs of laparoscopy cannot be completely compensated by the reduction in hospital stay. At our center, we have exchanged almost all of our disposable instruments for a re-usable armamentarium (i.e. metal trocars, endo-shears, endo-graspers, clip-appliers). The operative time in these centers is still 60 min longer for laparoscopy; however, these costs can be mostly compensated by the reduced postoperative hospital stay. Based on this, a significant benefit for the social security system can be obtained by the shorter convalescence time of about 2–3 weeks, compared to open surgery[16–18].

In summary, despite some technical modifications by the different groups, laparoscopic radical nephrectomy can be regarded as a standardized and safe procedure, which allows the transmission and reproduction of the surgical principles of the open procedure. Additionally, the perioperative morbidity of the patients can be reduced significantly by use of laparoscopy.

Much more important than the technical feasibility of laparoscopic radical nephrectomy is the long-term outcome. In the meantime, there are some studies available (Table 4). It has to be noted that all authors limited their range

Table 4 Review of the literature on laparoscopic radical nephrectomy

Author	n	Method of specimen removal	pT stage	Surgical margin	Follow-up (months)	Relapse trocar/local/ distant (%)	5-year survival
Janetschek, 2001	73	intact	T1–T3a	negative	13.3	0/0/0	n.a.
Abbou, 2000	41	intact	T1–T3b	negative	24.7	0/2/0	n.a.
Ono, 2001	103	morcellated & intact	—	—	29	0/1/3	92%
Chan, 2001	67	morcellated & intact	T1–T3b	negative	35.7	0/0/3	n.a.
Gill, 2001	100	intact	T1–T3b	negative	16.1	0/0/2	n.a.
Portis, 2002	64	morcellated & intact	T1–T3b	negative	54	0/1/2	n.a.
Rassweller, 2002	55	morcellated & intact	T1–T3b	negative	60	0/2/4	91%

n.a., not available

of indications to small-sized renal tumors (3–6 cm), according to clinical stage T1. However, like in our series, histopathology evidenced also pT3 tumors among the treated cases[14,16,17]. This has to be taken into consideration when discussing the long-term results. The overall 5-year disease-free survival rates are excellent, ranging between 89 and 96%. The recently published long-term follow-up by Portis and colleagues in 2002 (mean follow-up 5 years) reports equivalent long-term results to the traditional open technique[5]. Our own 10-year experience confirms these results (Table 3).

Even after open surgery of clinical T1 tumors, local recurrence as well as distant metastases have been observed[20–22]. It must be emphasized that, until now after more than 2000 documented cases, three port-site metastases have been documented (all related to advanced diseases) following laparoscopic radical nephrectomy for renal cell cancer. The role of an intact specimen removal in still discussed controversely, although there is no difference in morbidity and oncological outcome, as reported recently[24]. Despite the risk of understaging the tumor on preoperative CT scan, morcellation can be safely done without compromising survival[25]. There is no effective adjunctive therapy for cases with high-stage renal cancers.

In conclusion, despite some technical modifications concerning the access, laparoscopic radical nephrectomy has become a well-standardized and thus reproducible, but technically demanding, procedure. We are now able to perform an oncologically adequate procedure, with negative tumor margins achieved in all cases. Ideal indications are small tumors (T1) that are not candidates for nephron-sparing surgery. The complication rates are acceptable and still decreasing. The long-term results are excellent and are equivalent to the results of open surgery.

References

1. Clayman RV, Kavoussi LR, Soper NJ, et al. Laparoscopic nephrectomy: initial case report. *J Urol* 1991;146:278–82
2. Coptcoat MJ, Rassweiler J, Wickham JEA, Joyce A. Laparoscopic nephrectomy for renal cell carcinoma. Proceedings of *Third International Congress for Minimal Invasive Therapy*, Boston, 10–12 November 1991, Abstr D-66
3. Chiu AW, Chen MT, Huang WJS, Juang GD, Lu SH, Chang LS. Laparoscopic nephroureterectomy and endoscopic incision of bladder cuff. *Min Inv Ther* 1992;1:299–303
4. Abbou CC, Cicco A, Gasman D, et al. Retroperitoneal laparoscopy versus open radical nephrectomy. *J Urol* 1999;161:1776–80
5. Portis AJ, Yan Y, Landman J, et al. Long-term followup after laparoscopic radical nephrectomy. *J Urol* 2002;167:1257–62
6. Wolf S, Moon TD, Madisom WI, Nakada SY. Hand-assisted laparoscopic nephrectomy: comparison to standard laparoscopic nephrectomy. *J Urol* 1998;160:22–7
7. Rassweiler J, Stock C, Frede T, Seemann O, Alken P. Organ retrieval systems for endoscopic nephrectomy: a comparative study. *J Endourol* 1998;12:325–33
8. Coptcoat MJ, Ison KT, Wickham JEA. Endoscopic tissue liquidization and surgical aspiration. *J Endourol* 1988;2:321–9
9. Tschada RK, Henkel TO, Seemann O, Rassweiler JJ, Alken P. First experiences with laparoscopic radical nephrectomy. *J Endourol* 1994;8:S80 (Abstr P1–68)
10. Tschada RK, Rassweiler JJ, Schmeller N, Theodorakis J. Laparoscopic radical nephrectomy – the German experience. *J Urol* 1995;153:479 A (Abstr 1003)
11. Rassweiler JJ, Seemann O, Frede T, Henkel TO, Alken P. Retroperitoneoscopy: experience with 200 cases. *J Urol* 1999;160:1265–9
12. Gill IS, Grune MT, Munch LC. Access technique for retroperitoneoscopy. *J Urol* 1996;156:1120
13. Rassweiler J, Fornara P, Weber M, et al. Laparoscopic nephrectomy: the experience of the

laparoscopic working group of the German Urological Association. *J Urol* 1998;160:18–21

14. Cadeddu JA, Moore RG, Nelson JB, *et al.* Laparoscopic nephrectomy for renal cell cancer: a multi-center evaluation of efficacy. *J Urol* 1998;159:147 A (Abstr 557)

15. Barrett PH, Fentie DD, Taranger LA, *et al.* Laparoscopic assisted nephroureterectomy (TCC). *J Endourol* 1998;12:S103 (Abstr F 1–3)

16. McDougall EM, Clayman RV, Elashry OM. Laparoscopic nephroureterectomy for upper tract transitional cell cancer: Washington University experience. *J Urol* 1995;154:975–80

17. McDougall EM, Clayman RV, Elashry OM. Laparoscopic radical nephrectomy for renal tumor: the Washington University experience. *J Urol* 1996;155:1180–5

18. Rassweiler J, Coptcoat MJ. Laparoscopic surgery of the kidney and adrenal gland. In Janetschek G, Rassweiler J, Griffith D, eds. *Laparoscopic Surgery in Urology*. New York: Thieme, 1996:139–55

19. Ono Y, Kinukawa T, Hattori R, Yamada S, Nishiyama N, Ohshima S. Long-term result of

laparoscopic radical nephrectomy. *J Endourol* 1998;12:S103 (Abstr F 1–2)

20. Levy DA, Slaton JW, Swanson DA, Dinney CPN. Stage specific guidelines for survival after radical nephrectomy for local renal cell carcinoma. *J Urol* 1998;159:1163–7

21. Mickisch G, Tschada R, Rassweiler J, Löbelenz M, Alken P. Das lokale Rezidiv nach Nierentumoroperation. *Akt Urol* 1990;21:77–81

22. Moch H, Gasser TC, Urrejola C, Sauter G, Torhorst J, Mihatsch MJ. Metastatic behaviour of renal cell cancer: an analysis of 871 autopsies. *J Urol* 1997;157:66 A (Abstr 254)

23. Gettman MT, Napper C, Spark-Corwin T, Cadeddu J. Laparoscopic radical nephrectomy: prospective assessment of impact of intact versus fragmented specimen removal on postoperatve quality of life. *J Endourol* 2002;1:23–5

24. Landman J, Lento P, Hassen W, Unger P, Waterhouse R. Feasibility of pathological evaluation of morcellated kidneys after radical nephrectomy. *J Urol* 2001;164:2086–9

Clinical research avenues in metastatic renal cell carcinoma

41

G. H. J. Mickisch

Introduction

Approximately 2–3% of all malignant tumors in adults develop in the kidney. In 85% of them, the tumor originates from cells of the proximal tubules and is known as Grawitz tumor, hypernephroma or renal cell carcinoma (RCC). In The Netherlands, the annual incidence of this, since recently, second most common urological tumor is about 11 per 100 000 inhabitants. Men are twice as often afflicted as women, usually in the 5th–7th decades of life. The incidence of RCC has gradually increased over the years, and 5-year survival rates in contemporary series reach 60%. However, for patients with metastatic disease, the 2-year survival rate is between 0 and 20%[1].

At the time of diagnosis, about 20% of patients have disseminated disease and another 25% have locally advanced disease. Since approximately one-third of all patients with a tumor limited to the kidney at the time of diagnosis will subsequently develop metastatic disease postoperatively, about 50% of all patients with RCC will, sooner or later, require complex treatment decisions. With the advent of modern immunotherapeutic strategies, albeit with limited efficacy, including cyto-reductive surgery in the multimodality setting, the time may have come to re-valuate critically our standard approach to metastatic disease.

Despite an increasing number of patients with an objective response to immunotherapy, long-term survival usually ranges between 4 and 5%. Patient selection still appears to have a higher impact on prognosis than actual therapeutic strategies, and the demonstrated survival benefit with interferon-α (IFN-α) therapy in large randomized protocols[2,3] is modest, but reproducible. Clearly, there is a need for more effective therapies in metastatic renal cell carcinoma (MRCC), and the question arises which control arm to select for randomized comparison, to demonstrate any improvement realistically. This is the topic of the present chapter.

Regulatory affairs: the registration study

For many years, there was no scientifically accepted or even registered therapy for MRCC. This changed slowly some 10 years ago, when prospective randomized trials in relation to MRCC were published.

IFN-α plus vinblastine versus IFN-α alone, phase III trial[4]

A total of 178 patients with MRCC were randomized to receive IFN-α$_{2a}$ or IFN-α$_{2a}$ plus vinblastine (VBL). IFN-α$_{2a}$ was injected intramuscularly at a dose of 18 MU three times a week, and VBL was given intravenously at a dose of 0.1 mg/kg once every 3 weeks. The response rate was 11% for patients on monotherapy and 24% for those on combination treatment. The 5-year survival for 145 eligible patients was 9%, independent of treatment arm. The performance status was significantly related to long-term prognosis, and 13% of patients with performance status 0 were alive at 5 years, compared with 6% and 0% for patients with a World Health Organization (WHO) grade of 1 and 2, respectively. The most frequent adverse events in both treatment arms were flu-like symptoms (95%), fatigue (70%) and gastrointestinal disturbances (68%). Leukopenia was observed more frequently with combination treatment (53%) than with IFN-α_{2a} alone (30%). It was concluded that IFN-α_{2a} monotherapy at this dose and schedule has modest antitumor activity in MRCC. The combination of IFN-α_{2a} plus VBL resulted in a doubling of the response rate, but this does not translate into prolonged survival. Toxicity (except leukopenia) and tolerance were similar in both treatment arms.

IFN-α treatment in MRCC consistently produces objective response rates between 10 and 20%, which is confirmed by the mono-therapy arm of the above-mentioned study. There is a trend of a possible dose–response relationship for interferon therapy in MRCC, with lower doses resulting in a less than 10% objective response, whereas higher doses can generate objective response rates beyond 20%. The combination of IFN-α with VBL has resulted in an increase of the objective response rate in several phase II studies with response rates between 16 and 36%. The prospective randomized study confirmed previous data by demonstrating a two-fold increase in the response rate to 24%. This higher response rate with the combination therapy in the above study was due to an increase in partial responses, while the complete response rate remained below the 5% level. This may explain why the higher response rate in the combination arm did not translate into a prolongation of median survival compared with IFN-α_{2a} monotherapy. On the other hand, a median survival of 12 months in both treatment groups in the above trial com-pares favorably with other published data, where only the best prognostic subgroup (e.g. excellent performance status, time from initial diagnosis > 1 year, maximally one metastatic site, no prior chemotherapy and no recent weight loss) showed a similar median survival.

Scientific evidence after registration

IFN-α plus VBL versus VBL alone, phase III trial[2]

The combination of IFN-α_{2a} plus VBL induces objective tumor responses in patients with advanced RCC. However, no prospective randomized trial has shown that this treatment prolongs overall survival. In this study, overall survival after treatment with IFN-α_{2a} plus VBL versus VBL alone in patients with advanced RCC was compared.

The authors prospectively randomized 160 patients with locally advanced RCC or MRCC to receive either VBL alone or IFN-α_{2a} plus VBL for 12 months or until progression of disease. In both groups, VBL was administered intra-venously at 0.1 mg/kg every 3 weeks, and in the combination group IFN-α_{2a} was administered subcutaneously at 3 MU three times a week for 1 week, and 18 MU three times a week there-after for the second and subsequent weeks. For patients unable to tolerate IFN-α_{2a} at 18 MU per injection, the dose was reduced to 9 MU.

Median survival was 67.6 weeks for the 79 patients receiving IFN-α_{2a} plus VBL and 37.8 weeks for the 81 patients treated with VBL alone ($p = 0.0049$). Overall response rates were 16.5% for patients treated with IFN-α_{2a} plus VBL and 2.5% for patients treated with VBL alone ($p = 0.0025$). Treatment with the combination was associated with constitutional symptoms and abnormalities in laboratory parameters, but no toxic deaths were reported.

It was concluded that the combination of IFN-α_{2a} plus VBL is superior to VBL alone in the treatment of patients with locally advanced or MRCC. This is the first study to demonstrate that survival can be prolonged by using IFN-α_{2a} for these patients.

This prospective randomized trial indicates that overall survival is significantly prolonged in patients with advanced RCC when IFN-α_{2a} is used in combination with a palliative regimen of VBL, in comparison with survival with VBL therapy alone. The increase in median survival from 37.8 to 67.6 weeks was statistically and clinically significant, and long-term survivors who remained in remission after 4–5 years were noted. Survival was prolonged in the overall patient population, even in the subset of patients who did not have objective tumor responses. Also, a similar survival advantage was observed in patients who required a reduction of their IFN-α_{2a} dose from 18 MU to 9 MU per injection to improve tolerability. The combination was also associated with higher response rates, a larger number of complete responses, and prolonged time to progression. The gain in survival was achieved without toxic deaths or substantial serious toxicity. Treatment was generally well tolerated and easily administered in an ambulatory setting, although most patients treated with the combination experienced adverse events commonly associated with IFN-α therapy such as fatigue, fever, flu-like symptoms or reversible granulocytopenia.

In conclusion, beyond reasonable doubt, IFN-α is the effective ingredient for combination therapy. VBL has no place in the management of MRCC. This trial confirmed a previous phase II observation of the European Organization for Radiation Therapy in Cancer (EORTC 30882), in which VBL as a mono-therapy was considered ineffective for MRCC[5].

IFN-α with or without cis-retinoic acid, phase III trial[6]

A randomized phase III trial was conducted to determine whether combination therapy with 13-*cis*-retinoic acid (13-CRA) plus IFN-α_{2a} is superior to IFN-α_{2a} alone in patients with advanced RCC.

Two hundred and eighty-four patients were randomized to treatment with IFN-α_{2a} plus 13-CRA or treatment with IFN-α_{2a} alone. IFN-α_{2a} was given daily subcutaneously, starting at a dose of 3 MU. The dose was escalated every 7 days from 3 to 9 MU (by increments of 3 MU), unless grade 2 toxicity occurred, in which case dose escalation was stopped. Patients randomized to combination therapy were given oral 13-CRA 1 mg/kg/day plus IFN-α_{2a}. Quality of life (QoL) was assessed.

Complete or partial responses were achieved by 12% of patients treated with IFN-α_{2a} plus 13-CRA and 6% of patients treated with IFN-α_{2a} ($p = 0.14$). Median duration of response (complete and partial combined) in the group treated with the combination was 33 months (range 9–50 months), versus 22 months (range 5–38 months) for the second group ($p = 0.03$). Nineteen per cent of patients treated with IFN-α_{2a} plus 13-CRA were progression-free at

24 months, compared with 10% of patients treated with IFN-α_{2a} alone ($p = 0.05$). Median survival time for all patients was 15 months, with no difference in survival between the two treatment arms ($p = 0.26$). QoL decreased during the first 8 weeks of treatment, and a partial recovery followed. Lower scores were associated with the combination therapy.

It was concluded that improvement in response proportion and survival was not significant when 13-CRA was added to IFN-α_{2a} therapy in patients with advanced RCC. The response proportion for patients treated with IFN-α_{2a} plus 13-CRA was greater than that for patients treated with IFN-α_{2a}, with more complete responses in the combination therapy arm. Moreover, the duration of response for patients who achieved a complete or partial response was longer after treatment with IFN-α_{2a} plus 13-CRA than after treatment with IFN-α_{2a} alone. However, the overall response proportion for all patients treated on the trial was low (9%), with no significant difference in major response proportion (complete and partial combined) between arms. 13-CRA may lengthen response to IFN-α_{2a} therapy in patients with IFN-α_{2a}-sensitive tumors. Treatment, particularly the combination therapy, was associated with a decrease in QoL.

Interleukin-2-based regimens

There is no standard treatment for MRCC, but many patients with this condition receive interleukin-2 (IL-2) or IFN-α outside the setting of a therapeutic trial. These cytokines are the only drugs that have been shown to induce tumor regression in some patients. There are, however, no data to indicate which patients are most likely to benefit from such treatment and which cytokine regimen is the most active.

Response proportions in individual phase II trials involving patients with advanced RCC ranged from 0 to 30% for single-agent IFN-α therapy, 0 to 37% for combinations of IFN-α_{2a} plus IL-2 and 0 to 37% for the three-drug combination of IFN-α, IL-2 plus fluorouracil. Responsible factors include differences in treatment schedules, sample size and patient selection. The impact of IFN-α_{2a} treatment on survival is controversial, but the two larger phase III trials found IFN-α_{2a} therapy to be associated with longer survival than VBL or medroxy-progesterone therapy[2,3]. In contrast, no randomized phase III trial has shown a survival benefit for combination therapy compared with treatment with IFN-α_{2a} or IL-2 alone in patients with advanced RCC. Each combination therapy showed promise in phase II trials but lacked survival benefit, compared with monotherapy, in the randomized trial. The outcome of these trials reaffirms the necessity to conduct phase III trials to evaluate the efficacy of combination therapies, compared with treatment with IFN-α_{2a} or IL-2 *alone* in patients with MRCC.

IFN-α versus IL-2 versus IFN-α plus IL-2, phase III trial[7]

Recombinant human IL-2 and recombinant human IFN-α can induce notable tumor regression in a limited number of patients with MRCC. The authors conducted a multicenter, randomized trial to determine the effect of each cytokine independently and in combination, and to identify patients who are best suited to this treatment.

Four hundred and twenty-five patients with MRCC were randomly assigned to receive either a continuous intravenous infusion of IL-2, sub-cutaneous injections of IFN-α_{2a} or both. The main outcome measure was the response rate; secondary outcomes were the rates of event-free and overall survival. Predictive factors for response and rapid progression were identified by multivariate analysis.

Response rates were 6.5%, 7.5% and 18.6% ($p < 0.01$) for the groups receiving IL-2, IFN-α_{2a} and IL-2 plus IFN-α_{2a}, respectively. At 1 year, the event-free survival rates were 15%, 12% and 20%, respectively ($p = 0.01$). There was no significant difference in overall survival among the three groups. Toxic effects of therapy were more common in patients receiving IL-2 than in those receiving IFN-α_{2a}. Response to treatment was associated with having metastasis to a single organ and with receiving the combined treatment. The probability of rapid progression of

disease was at least 70% for patients with at least two metastatic sites, liver metastases and a period of less than 1 year between diagnosis of the primary tumor and the appearance of metastases.

It was concluded that cytokines are active in a few patients with MRCC. The higher response rate and longer event-free survival obtained with a combination of cytokines must be balanced against the toxicity of such treatment.

These results confirm that clinically relevant tumor regression occurs in a minority of cytokine-treated patients. Moreover, mono-therapy with IFN-α_{2a} or IL-2 gave very low response rates (7.5% and 6.5%, respectively, at 10 weeks). The group treated with both cytokines had a response rate of 18.6% and significantly longer event-free survival. However, since there was no significant difference in overall survival among the three groups, it *cannot* be concluded that the combined treatment provided a significant advantage.

In this study, the toxicity of the regimens containing IL-2 was, as expected, dramatically higher than the toxicity of IFN-α_{2a} alone. Indeed, the severity of the toxic reactions to IL-2 limits the use of regimens based on this cytokine. The toxic effects frequently observed with combined therapy emphasize the need for careful selection of patients. It is usually recommended that cytokine treatment be restricted to patients who are ambulatory and have no major organ failure.

IFN-α plus IL-2 with or without 5-fluorouracil, phase III trial[8]

Subcutaneous recombinant IL-2 and recom-binant IFN-α have been used extensively in the treatment of MRCC. Most results, coming from non-controlled phase II trials, showed inconsistent rates of response. More recently, the addition of fluorouracil (FU) was proposed to improve the efficacy of these regimens.

The role of a subcutaneous combination of IL-2 and IFN-α_{2a} with or without FU was investigated. Patients were randomly assigned to receive a combination of IL-2 and IFN-α_{2a} at weeks 1, 3, 5 and 7, or the same combination together with a continuous infusion of FU at weeks 1 and 5. The major end-points of this multicenter, randomized trial were progression-free survival, response rate and toxicity. Overall survival was a secondary end-point. Tumor responses were reviewed by an independent committee. Analysis of the results was performed on an intention-to-treat basis.

One hundred and thirty-one patients were enrolled. There was no difference in toxicity between the arms, and no toxic death was observed. One partial response was observed in arm A and five in arm B. Progression-free survival did not differ between the arms, and rates at 1 year were 12% and 15% in arms A and B, respectively. No statistically significant differences were detected in any end-point.

It was concluded that the subcutaneous combination of IL-2 and IFN-α_{2a} with or without FU does not benefit patients with metastatic renal carcinoma. Neither of these regimens can be recommended as standard treatment. The results of the subcutaneous cytokine regimen seem disappointing.

Survival benefit analysis

For the compound IL-2, multivariate retrospective analysis seemed to support a life-prolonging effect of IL-2 monotherapy[9]. Scientifically more appropriate data are currently available for IFN-α. An initial Finnish study[2] in which a regimen containing IFN-α resulted in a modest but significant survival benefit over VBL set the tone; other evaluations followed.

IFN-α versus medroxyprogesterone acetate, phase III trial[3]

MRCC has a 2-year survival of maximally 20%, and is largely resistant to chemotherapy. The use of interferons in the treatment of MRCC remains controversial. Although non-randomized studies suggest that biological therapy with interferons induces a small number of tumor responses, most clinicians judge such treatment to be ineffective. The

authors have investigated the effect of treatment with IFN-α on survival in patients with MRCC.

In a multicenter, randomized trial, patients with MRCC were randomly assigned to subcutaneous IFN-α (three doses – 5 MU, 5 MU, 10 MU – for the first week, then 10 MU three times per week for a further 11 weeks; $n = 174$) or oral medroxyprogesterone acetate (MPA; 300 mg once daily for 12 weeks; $n = 176$). The primary end-point was overall survival. Analysis was by intention to treat. The trial used a triangular sequential design for early termination as soon as results were conclusive. The trial was stopped in November 1997, when data were available for 335 patients (167 IFN-α, 168 MPA).

A total of 111 patients has died in the interferon group, and 125 patients have died in the MPA group. There was a 28% reduction in the risk of death in the IFN-α group (hazard ratio 0.72 (95% confidence interval 0.55–0.94), $p = 0.017$). IFN-α gave an improvement in 1-year survival of 12% (MPA 31% survival, IFN-α 43%), and an improvement in median survival of 2.5 months (MPA 6 months, IFN-α 8.5 months).

It was concluded that the benefit of treatment with IFN-α should be weighed against the drug's toxic effects. Combination regimens of biological therapy and chemotherapy should now be compared with interferon monotherapy in randomized controlled trials.

As yet, this analysis has not shown good evidence of a greater effect of IFN-α in any particular subgroup. However, the numbers in these subgroups were small, and tests for such interactions are not very powerful. In particular, few patients had performance status 0 and single metastases, and therefore this study lacked power to detect interactions between these factors and treatment. Further follow-up may provide more information and increase the power of the study.

Memorial Sloan Kettering Cancer Center retrospective analysis[10]

Further analysis was performed to evaluate the relationship between treatment with cytokine therapy and survival, investigate the effect of nephrectomy on survival and identify long-term survivors among a cohort of 670 patients with advanced RCC.

A total of 670 patients with advanced RCC treated in 24 clinical trials of systemic chemotherapy or cytokine therapy were the subjects of this retrospective analysis. Treatment was categorized as cytokine (containing IFN-α and/or IL-2) in 396 patients (59%) and as chemotherapy (cytotoxic or hormonal therapy) in 274 (41%). Among the 670 patients, those with survival times of greater than 5 years were identified as long-term survivors.

Patients treated with cytokine therapy had a longer survival time than did those treated with chemotherapy, regardless of the year of treatment or risk category based on pretreatment features. The median survival times for favorable-, intermediate- and poor-risk patients were 27, 12 and 6 months for those treated with cytokines and 15, 7 and 3 months for those treated with chemotherapy, respectively. The magnitude of difference in median survival was greater in the favorable- and intermediate-risk groups. The median survival time was less than 6 months in the poor-risk group for both treatment programs. Median survival time was 14 months among patients with prior nephrectomy plus time from diagnosis to treatment greater than 1 year versus 8 months among those with time from diagnosis to treatment less than 1 year, regardless of pretreatment nephrectomy status. Thirty patients (4.5%) among the 670 patients were identified as long-term survivors; 12 were free of disease after nephrectomy and treatment with IFN-α, IL-2 or surgical resection of metastasis.

It was concluded that the low proportion of patients with advanced RCC who achieved long-term survival emphasizes the need for clinical investigation to identify more effective therapy.

The role of cytokine therapy with IL-2 and/or IFN-α in prolonging survival for patients with MRCC remains controversial. Selection factors influence treatment outcome, and phase III randomized trials are required for definitive comparison of treatment programs. Several randomized trials failed to show benefit, but the two largest trials showed that INF-α resulted in a modest prolongation in survival compared with medroxyprogesterone or VBL[2,3]. Factors that could influence the outcome for these randomized trials include differences in sample size, prognostic clinical features of the patient population and treatment programs.

In this retrospective study, patients treated with cytokine therapy experienced longer survival compared with patients treated with chemotherapy. When survival after cytokine or chemotherapy treatment was considered according to pretreatment risk status, the difference in median survival was greater in the group with the more favorable prognostic features, characterized by the fewest number of risk factors. In contrast, survival for patients with poor-risk features was short, with a median survival time of less than 6 months, regardless of treatment type. These observations suggest that patients with favorable prognostic features may derive therapeutic benefit from cytokine therapy. Prospective identification of patients who are more likely to benefit from cytokine therapy could be used as a stratification factor in phase III trials and in risk-directed therapy.

Triple-drug therapy (IFN-α, IL-2 and 5FU) versus tamoxifen, phase III trial[11]

The authors conducted a prospectively randomized clinical trial to compare the efficacy and safety of subcutaneous IFN-α_{2a}, subcutaneous IL-2 and intravenous 5-fluorouracil as outpatient therapy against oral tamoxifen in 78 patients with progressive MRCC. Treatment courses consisted of IFN-α_{2a} 5 MU/m^2, day 1 weeks 1 and 4, days 1, 3, 5 weeks 2 and 3; 10 MU/m^2, days 1, 3, 5 weeks 5–8; IL-2 10 MU/m^2, twice daily days 3–5 weeks 1 and 4; 5 MU/m^2, days 1, 3, 5 weeks 2 and 3; and 5-fluorouracil 1000 mg/m^2, day 1 weeks 5–8. The tamoxifen group received tamoxifen 80 mg twice daily over 8 weeks. Among 41 patients treated with IL-2, IFN-α_{2a} and 5-fluorouracil there were seven complete (17.1%) and nine partial responders (21.9%), with an overall objective response rate of 39.1% (95% confidence interval 24.2–55.5%). An additional 15 patients (36.6%) were stable throughout therapy. The overall survival was 24 months (range 5–76+). In 37 patients receiving tamoxifen no objective remissions occurred. Thirteen patients (35.1%) had stable disease and 24 patients (64.9%) showed continued disease progression. The overall survival was 13 months (range 3–73+). The authors concluded that this home-based therapy regimen of IFN-α$_{2a}$, IL-2 and 5-fluorouracil demonstrated significant therapeutic efficacy in patients with progressive RCC, when compared with hormonal therapy.

Weighing the small numbers of patients and the unexplained randomization imbalance (41 vs. 37 patients) as well as the unusually high response rate (39.1%) leading to an impressive 24-month median survival in the treatment arm, these results should be interpreted with some caution. Patient selection as well as other yet undefined patterns may have contributed to this outcome. By no means should these data be construed as proving a survival benefit over monotherapies such as IFN-α or IL-2. Nevertheless, triple-drug therapy is apparently superior to ineffective therapy such as tamoxifen.

Improving on IFN-α monotherapy

Surgery plus IFN-α versus IFN-α alone, EORTC phase III trial[12]

Surgery is the main treatment for localized RCC, but use of radical nephrectomy for metastatic disease is highly controversial. The authors aimed to establish whether radical nephrectomy performed before IFN-α-based immunotherapy improved time to progression and overall survival (primary end-points), compared with IFN-α alone.

The EORTC trial included 85 patients from June 1995 to July 1998, and two (one per group) were ineligible; 42 of the participants were randomly assigned to combined treatment (study group) and 43 to immunotherapy alone (controls). All patients had MRCC that had been histologically confirmed and was progressive at entry. In study patients, surgery was

performed within 4 weeks of randomization, and immunotherapy (5×10^6 IU/m^2 subcutaneously three times per week) started 2–4 weeks later. In controls, immunotherapy was started within one working day of randomization. Follow-up visits were monthly. All analyses were by intention to treat.

Forty (53%) of 75 patients received at least 16 weeks of IFN-α treatment, which was also the median duration of treatment. Time to progression (5 vs. 3 months, hazard ratio 0.60, 95% confidence interval 0.36–0.97) and median duration of survival were significantly better in study patients than in controls (17 vs. 7 months, 0.54, 0.31–0.94). Five patients responded completely to combined treatment, and one to IFN-α alone. Dose modification was necessary in 32% of patients, most commonly because of non-hematological side-effects.

It was concluded that radical nephrectomy before interferon-based immunotherapy might substantially delay time to progression and improve survival of patients with MRCC who present with good performance status.

These results clearly show an important survival benefit for nephrectomized patients presenting with a good performance score, whose primary tumor has been assessed to be surgically operable and who are good candidates for subsequent immunotherapy.

On the basis of the results of this study and the preliminary report of South West Oncology Group (SWOG) 8949, the EORTC recommended tumor nephrectomy before immunotherapy as a standard treatment for MRCC patients who are suitable for this approach.

Surgery plus IFN-α versus IFN-α alone, SWOG phase III trial[13]

The value of nephrectomy in MRCC has long been debated. Several non-randomized studies suggest a higher rate of response to systemic therapy and longer survival in patients who have undergone nephrectomy.

The authors randomly assigned patients with MRCC who were acceptable candidates for nephrectomy to undergo radical nephrectomy followed by therapy with IFN-α_{2b} or to receive IFN-α therapy alone. The primary end-point of survival in 120 eligible patients assigned to surgery followed by interferon was 11.1 months, and among the 121 eligible patients assigned to interferon alone it was 8.1 months ($p = 0.05$). The difference in median survival between the two groups was independent of performance status, metastatic site and the presence or absence of a measurable metastatic lesion.

It was concluded that nephrectomy followed by interferon therapy results in longer survival among patients with MRCC than does interferon therapy alone.

Most patients who die of cancer die because of metastatic disease, and therefore removal of the primary tumor in patients who already have evidence of metastasis seems illogical, at least in the absence of symptoms caused by the primary tumor. Many oncologists have asked, 'What is the point of closing the barn door once the horse has bolted?' They reason that subjecting patients with incurable disease to the risks involved in unnecessary surgery is a poor medical decision.

This idea is challenged by EORTC and SWOG, who report the results of a randomized trial that suggests that nephrectomy benefits selected patients with MRCC. The authors recruited 246 patients with high performance status from 80 institutions, and found that survival was better in those who were randomly assigned to undergo removal of the kidney containing the primary tumor before treatment with IFN-α than in those who were assigned to undergo treatment with IFN-α alone. Trials of this design are much more difficult to undertake than trials in which the effects of two drugs are compared, and both groups are to be commended for addressing an important issue.

Although the evidence of improved survival in association with nephrectomy provided by any of these studies in statistically not very strong, that the results of these trials are consistent with each other supports the validity of these results.

IFN-α comparative arm, retrospective analysis of Memorial Sloan Kettering Cancer Center[14]

Four hundred and sixty-three patients with advanced RCC, administered IFN-α as first-line systemic therapy in six prospective clinical trials, were the subjects of this retrospective analysis. Three risk categories for predicting survival were identified on the basis of five pretreatment clinical features by a stratified Cox proportional hazards model.

The median overall survival time was 13 months. The median time to progression was 4.7 months. Five variables were used as risk factors for short survival: low Karnofsky performance status, high lactate dehydrogenase, low serum hemoglobin, high corrected serum calcium and time from initial RCC diagnosis to start of IFN-α therapy of less than 1 year. Each patient was assigned to one of three risk groups: those with zero risk factors (favorable risk), those with one or two (intermediate risk) and those with three or more (poor risk). The median time to death of patients deemed at favorable risk was 30 months. Median survival time in the intermediate-risk group was 14 months. In contrast, the poor-risk group had a median survival time of 5 months.

It was concluded that progression-free and overall survival with IFN-α treatment can be compared with new therapies in phase II and III clinical investigations. The prognostic model is suitable for risk stratification of phase III trials using IFN-α as the comparative treatment arm.

IFN-α and IL-2 show a low degree of antitumor effect against RCC. Outcome data from either cytokine may be considered in clinical trial design and interpretation of new therapies. Patients treated with high-dose bolus IL-2 have been reported to achieve durable responses. However, treatment-related toxicity can be severe, mandating stringent patient selection, intensive supportive care and specialized treatment centers; therefore, its use as the comparative treatment arm in phase III trials limits both center and patient participation. Also, the patient population selected to tolerate the intensive therapy may differ from those deemed appropriate for the investigational therapy. In contrast, IFN-α is administered as out-patient therapy and can be used in a less-restricted patient population. Several recently reported phase III trials in advanced RCC used IFN-α as the compared treatment arm[2,3,12,13].

In summary, the low proportion of patients with advanced RCC achieving long-term survival emphasizes the need for clinical investigation to identify more effective therapy. Progression-free and overall survival for IFN-α treatment can be used as a baseline for assessment of new therapies in phase II and III clinical investigations. The prognostic model is suitable for risk stratification of phase III trials using IFN-α as the comparative treatment arm, and single-arm phase II trials to study progression-free survival or overall survival as an end-point.

An overview of all randomized trials with survival as an end-point in MRCC is presented in Table 1.

Conclusion

When considering the rational selection of a suitable control arm to be used in randomized trials evaluating investigational agents, one has to take into account the present regulatory status, the scientific evidence and the practical use of available agents.

IFN-α is registered at a dose of 18×10^6 IU, three times per week, and VBL 0.1 mg/kg once every 3 weeks[4]. Both the dose of IFN-α and the addition of VBL have become unusual contemporarily, because scientific scrutiny applied since registration has led to different concepts.

The registration study itself[4] has not shown a survival advantage for the combined treatment arm; merely the number of responses increased. The EORTC 30882 trial revealed that VBL monotherapy is ineffective[5] for MRCC. Randomized investigation confirmed beyond reasonable doubt that IFN-α is the active ingredient of the combined treatment arm and that VBL alone has no place in MRCC[2]. In consequence, the use of VBL in MRCC has stopped, at least in randomized trials. Lately, the addition of other compounds, such as *cis*-retinoic acid, has also been shown not to be superior to IFN-α monotherapy in MRCC[6].

Furthermore, when comparing the efficacy of registered cytokines such as IFN-α or IL-2, or the combination thereof, the randomized trial demonstrated similar response rates for either drug. The combination induced more responses, but failed to translate into any improved survival[7].

Moreover, when evaluating the addition of 5-fluorouracil to IFN-α plus IL-2, efficacy assessment discarded the triple-drug combination[8]. Subsequently, the comparative use of accepted monotherapies such as IFN-α or IL-2 prevailed in randomized trials.

Finally, any prolongation of life achieved under such cytokine monotherapies became an important research topic. For the compound IL-2, a multivariate retrospective analysis seemed to support a positive answer[9]. Scientifically more appropriate data are currently available for IFN-α: the two largest randomized trials[2,3] concluded invariably in favor of IFN-α, providing a modest, but reproducible, survival

Table 1 Randomized trials in metastatic renal cell carcinoma (MRCC) using survival as an end-point

Trial design	Number of patients	Response rate (CR, PR) (%)	Survival benefit (months)	Reference
IFN-α + VBL vs. VBL	79/81	16.5/2.5	6.9	2
IFN-α vs. MPA	174/176	14/2	2.5	3
Surgery + IFN-α vs. IFN-α	42/43	19/12	10	12
Surgery + IFN-α vs. IFN-α	120/121	*	3.0	13
IFN-α, IL-2 and 5FU vs. tamoxifen	41/37	39.1/0	11.0	11

*Available in only a minority of patients; IFN-α, interferon-α; VBL, vinblastine; MPA, medroxyprogesterone acetate; IL-2, interleukin-2; 5FU, 5-fluorouracil; CR, PR, complete or partial response

benefit over VBL or medroxyprogesterone acetate, respectively.

Last but not least, the randomized phase III trials of EORTC[12] and SWOG[13] demonstrated an additional and significant survival benefit in MRCC when cytoreductive tumor nephrectomy is combined with IFN-α monotherapy, compared with IFN-α alone, in patients presenting with a good performance status. Thus, both organizations decided to apply *tumor nephrectomy plus IFN-α* as the *curent standard therapy* for MRCC. The Memorial Sloan Kettering Cancer Centre Genitourinary Group joined in with this recommendation based on a separate analysis of their patient material[14].

For a variety of reasons, IFN-α monotherapy administered subcutaneously has become a widespread therapy for MRCC. It has an appealing safety profile, allowing for an out-patient setting. This contributes to a favorable risk–benefit analysis, and the majority of patients with MRCC can be included in such treatment regimens. In addition, this therapy can be given by anyone with adequate experience in the administration and follow-up of cytokine therapy; no highly specialized oncology units including intensive care are needed. However, dosing and administrative intervals have evolved differently from the original registration study[4]. Large contemporary studies[3,6,12–14] used doses of 9×10^6 IU or 5×10^6 IU/m^2, respectively, which for most patients are comparable. Again, the intervals vary from three times weekly to five times weekly to seven times weekly, but are usually better tolerated by more patients than 18×10^6 IU three times weekly, which was originally described. Subsequently, three times 18×10^6 IU is no longer a widely used regimen. In general, it is believed that oncological efficacy is similar with adapted dosing and intervals, as long as weekly total doses between 25 and 45×10^6 IU are guaranteed, no matter how single doses and intervals are prescribed.

In summary, given the need for more effective therapies in MRCC, randomized trials are mandatory. In these trials, the current standard of tumor nephrectomy plus interferon-α monotherapy should serve as the standard arm. Dosing and intervals of IFN-α monotherapy should be applied at the discretion of the individual trial management, as long as accepted minimum doses are delivered.

References

1. Mickisch G, Carballido J, Hellsten S, Schulze H, Mensink H. Guidelines on renal cell cancer. *Eur Urol* 2001;140:252–5
2. Pyrhönen S, Salminen E, Ruutu M, *et al.* Prospective randomized trial of interferon-α$_{2a}$ plus vinblastine versus vinblastine alone in patients with advanced renal cell carcinoma. *J Clin Oncol* 1999;17:2859–70
3. Medical Research Council Renal Cancer Collaborators. Interferon-α and survival in metastatic renal carcinoma: early results of a randomised controlled trial. *Lancet* 1999;353:14–17
4. Fossa S, Martinelli G, Otto U, *et al.* Recombinant interferon α-2a with or without vinblastine in metastatic renal cell carcinoma: results of a European multicenter phase III study. *Ann Oncol* 1992;3:301–5
5. Fossa S, Droz JP, Pavone-Macaluso M, Debruyne F, Vermeylen K, Sylvester R and members of the EORTC-GU group. Vinblastine in metastatic renal cell carcinoma: EORTC phase III trial 30882. *Eur J Cancer* 1992;28a:878–80
6. Motzer R, Murphy B, Bacik J, *et al.* Phase III trial of interferon α-2a with or without 13-*cis*-retinoic acid for patients with advanced renal cell carcinoma. *J Clin Oncol* 2000;18:2972–80
7. Negrier S, Escudier B, Lasset C, *et al.* Recombinant human interleukin-2, recombinant human interferon α-2a, or both in metastatic renal-cell carcinoma. *N Engl J Med* 2000;338:1272–8
8. Negrier S, Caty A, Lesimple T, Douillard J, Escudier B, Rossi J. Treatment of patients with metastatic renal carcinoma with a combination of subcutaneous interleukin-2 and interferon α

with or without fluorouracil. *J Clin Oncol* 2000; 18:4009–15

9. Jones M, Selby P, Frances C. The impact of interleukin-2 on survival in renal cancer: a multivariate analysis. *Cancer Biother* 1993;8:275–82

10. Motzer R, Mazumdar M, Bacik J, Russo P, Berg W, Metz E. Effect of cytokine therapy on survival for patients with advanced renal cell carcinoma. *J Clin Oncol* 2000;18:1928–35

11. Atzpodien J, Kirchner H, Illiger HJ, *et al*. IL-2 in combination with IFN-α and 5-FU versus tamoxifen in metastatic renal cell carcinoma: long-term results of a controlled randomized clinical trial. *Br J Cancer* 2001;85:1130–6

12. Mickisch G, Garin A, Van Poppel H, De Prijck L, Sylvester R. Radical nephrectomy plus interferon-α-based immunotherapy compared with interferon α alone in metastatic renal cell carcinoma: a randomised trial. *Lancet* 2001;358: 966–70

13. Flanigan R, Salmon S, Blumenstein B, *et al*. Nephrectomy followed by interferon α-2b compared with interferon α-2b alone for metastatic renal cell cancer. *N Engl J Med* 2001;345:1655–9

14. Motzer R, Bacik J, Murphy B, Russo P, Mazumdar M. Interferon-α as a comparative treatment for clinical trials of new therapies against advanced renal cell carcinoma. *J Clin Oncol* 2002;20:289–96

Diet and prostate cancer

42

K. Griffiths, L. J. Denis and A. Turkes

Introduction

In the 60 years since Charles Huggins established the scientific basis for the treatment of advanced prostate cancer by androgen ablative therapy, the urological community has concentrated on refining the means of restraining the influence of testosterone on the gland. Androgens were seen as the predominant growth promoter. During this time, it was recognized that prostate cancer is a disease of the middle-aged man, involving a slowly growing tumor that takes 25 or more years to develop from a focal lesion to the malignant aggressive phenotype. But recent years have witnessed a revolution in medical science, with men now presenting with early cancer, small enough to be removable by surgery or treated with radiotherapy. The urologist can now cure prostate cancer.

However, prevention is better than cure. Today, interest centers on whether prostate cancer can be prevented or at least restrained in its latent, indolent form, so prevalent in men of all ethnic groups world-wide. The Prostate Cancer Prevention Trial[1] will soon provide information on the preventive value of finasteride, and the potential of particular dietary factors to influence the pathogenesis of prostate cancer now exercises the minds of many researchers. There is compelling evidence[2] that certain phyto-constituents, isoflavonoids, flavonoids and lignans, for example, protect against prostate cancer. Some are weak estrogens, and the recent recognition of estrogen receptor β (ERβ) in prostate tissue[3–5] now demands a reassessment of the role of 17β-estradiol in growth-regulatory mechanisms and the influence that such phytoestrogens could exercise on these events. There seems little doubt that 17β-estradiol may be more important than

hitherto has been believed. Apart from the phytoestrogens, however, many other dietary factors are currently seen to be of interest and deserve consideration.

Noteworthy with regard to progress are comments made by Huggins[6] in 1962 highlighting unresolved problems, one being the geographical variation in prostate cancer incidence world-wide. The disease is prevalent in developed Western countries but rare in Asia, with other countries such as those surrounding the Mediterranean occupying an intermediary position (Figure 1). These regional differences in cancer incidence rates are most probably due to the influence of dietary components on carcinogenesis, either 'causative or protective'[7]. Invariably, emphasis has centered on factors that might cause cancer in the West, with the high-fat diet often seen as the 'root of all dietary evil'. Expressed simply, a 'Western diet' is one in which fat and animal protein consumption is high and 'fiber' intake low. In contrast, the caloric intake related to fat in the vegetarian-style Asian diet is low, whereas the fiber, fruit and vegetable intake is high. The marked geographical diversity of dietary patterns reflects traditional life-styles, culture and evolved preferences that often relate to their regional economic status. High-fiber, low-fat diets dominate in Asia, as well as in South America and Africa, with more than 50% of the total caloric intake associated with particular cereals, rice, maize and wheat. In Northern Europe and in North America, up to 40% of the intake is often related to fat consumption. These differences are reflected in geographical patterns of the incidence of prostate cancer. The highest mortality rate is seen in the Afro-American population of the USA, twice that of their white

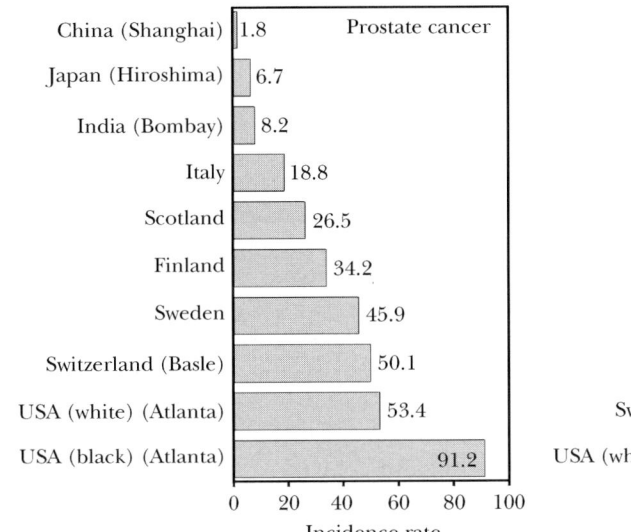
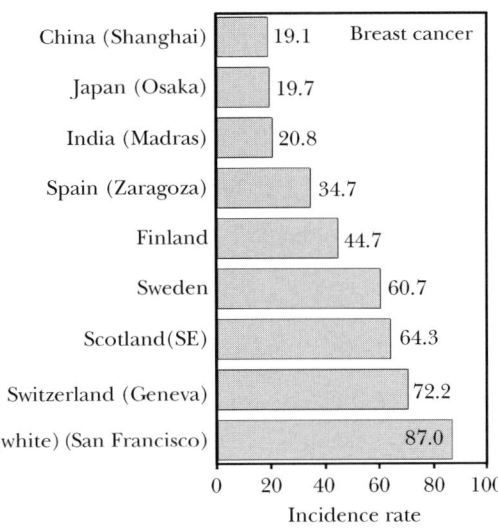

Figure 1 Differences in the age-adjusted incidence rates for cancers of breast and prostate in countries from East and West. Numbers represent incidence per 100 000 population per annum

counterparts. Relative to this high rate, the incidence is about 120 times less in Shanghai in China and 30-fold less in Osaka, Japan.

More pragmatic, however, is the concept promulgated by Adlercreutz and Mazur[8] that phyto-constituents of the Asian diet could prevent disease. Changes in dietary practice by reducing fat intake, but increasing vegetable and fruit consumption, have long been seen as beneficial[7,9]. Controversy has surrounded the relationship between fat intake and cancer risk, particularly of the breast, and the question whether fat does constitute a cancer risk remains unresolved. Despite this, epidemiologists have most effectively directed attention towards the important relationship between diet and cancer, thereby provoking interest in preventive approaches to better health care through changes in dietary intake.

Does diet influence cancer risk?

Objective evidence suggests, therefore, that particular dietary constituents would seem to be protective against Western diseases. Support for the concept comes from studies of migrants who move from a country with a low risk for particular cancers to one where the risk is higher. This is well illustrated by data[10,11] on the migration of people from Japan and China to Hawaii and to mainland USA, where the incidence of prostate and breast cancer rises closer to that of the existing population. Noteworthy, however, is that continuing regular intake of soy-protein products, a major component of the Asian diet, protects against breast cancer. Clearly, supplementation of the Western diet by such natural Eastern 'protective factors' could provide a certain degree of health benefit, and isoflavonoids derived from soy-protein[2,12], as well as the lignans and flavonoids, demand attention.

As weak estrogens, they can act as estrogen antagonists or as agonists, and could influence prostate growth-regulatory processes in which estrogens are implicated. Also important is that these dietary constituents exhibit many other interesting properties[2,12] that could readily be seen to interfere with the pathogenesis of prostate cancer (Table 1). The concept that dietary constituents may influence the biological effects of 17β-estradiol in the male is especially of interest. Although the male or female phenotype is determined to a large extent by differences in the concentrations of steroid hormones in plasma, there is no sexual

Table 1 Range of biological activities of isoflavonoids and lignans

Agonist and antagonistic estrogenic effects
Inhibition of the 5α-reductase enzyme system
Inhibition of 17β-hydroxysteroid dehydrogenase
Inhibition of the aromatase enzyme system
Inhibition of the tyrosine-specific protein kinase enzyme
Inhibition of angiogenesis
Influence on sex hormone-binding globulin (SHBG) synthesis
Certain phytoestrogens are antioxidants
Some phytoestrogens affect the topoisomerases
Many phytoestrogens inhibit the growth of experimental tumors

specificity with regard to any particular hormone. There are substantial levels of estrogens in the human male and males of other species. Particularly striking are the urinary levels of estrogenic steroids in the stallion, that epitome of male sexuality[13]. Despite this, our understanding of the precise part played by estrogens in the physiology of the human male and in growth-regulatory mechanisms within the prostate is less than might be expected.

Despite the prevalence of prostate cancer in the West, an enigmatic issue is that the incidence of the latent, slow-growing indolent cancer of the prostate is similar in men worldwide, irrespective of ethnic origins, although it may be that, in the West, the growth rate is a little higher[14]. Any effect of dietary factors would appear to be directed more towards the progression of latent cancer to the aggressive, malignant phenotype than towards cancer initiation. It is now established that precancerous lesions are recognized in the prostate soon after puberty, when the gland has attained its maximal size. Latent cancer presumably develops and then grows over a period of 25 years. Mid-life endocrine changes associated with the andropause would then appear to influence progression[2,15]. The concept that Asian dietary factors influence cancer progression offers a real challenge.

Also noteworthy is that even within a country differences in dietary patterns would seem to influence cancer risk. In a 17-year Japanese study[16] of 265 118 adults aged over 40 years, a daily consumption of green–yellow vegetables, often in soy-bean soup, was reported to be a protective factor against not only prostate and breast cancer, but also liver cirrhosis, ischemic heart disease and atherosclerosis. Green and yellow vegetables included spinach, pumpkin, green asparagus, green lettuce and carrots. The benefits of daily soy-bean soup intake were seen despite frequent smoking of more than 25 cigarettes each day (Figure 2). It was suggested that constituents of the vegetables, possibly β-carotene, or a component of the soy-protein exercised this protective effect.

Any health benefit, or cancer-preventive action, is most likely due to the multifactorial influence of a lifelong intake of various dietary constituents, and the isoflavonoids, flavonoids and lignans constitute one such important group. There are many others (Figure 3) for which eminent protagonists proffer support, but the accumulation and evaluation of all information on such dietary components[7] are important.

Isoflavonoids, lignans and flavonoids: the phytoestrogens

The presence in plants of substances with estrogenic activity has long been recognized[2,17], and Adlercreutz is the 'father figure' who suggested that specific phytoestrogens may influence steroid metabolism and action, such that the overall effect is protective against endocrine cancer[8]. The Leguminosae family, which includes soya, is a major source of isoflavonoids. Lignans and flavonoids are non-nutrient components of vegetables, fruit and whole-grain products. High concentrations of isoflavonoids are found in the plasma (Figure 4) of Asian people. Soy-protein contains glycoside conjugates of genistein and daidzein, which together with their methylated derivatives, biochanin A and formononetin, can be metabolized by the enzymes of the normal microflora of the gut to produce the phytoestrogens genistein and daidzein (Figure 5). They are then absorbed, and appear in blood and body fluids before being excreted in urine. The weakly

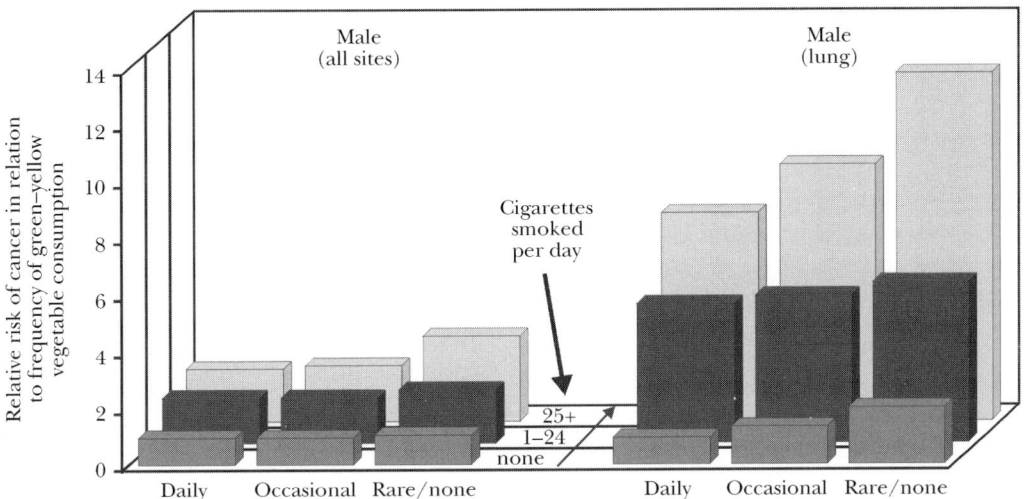

Figure 2 Relative risks of cancer in relation to the frequency of green–yellow vegetable consumption and the numbers of cigarettes smoked each day[16]

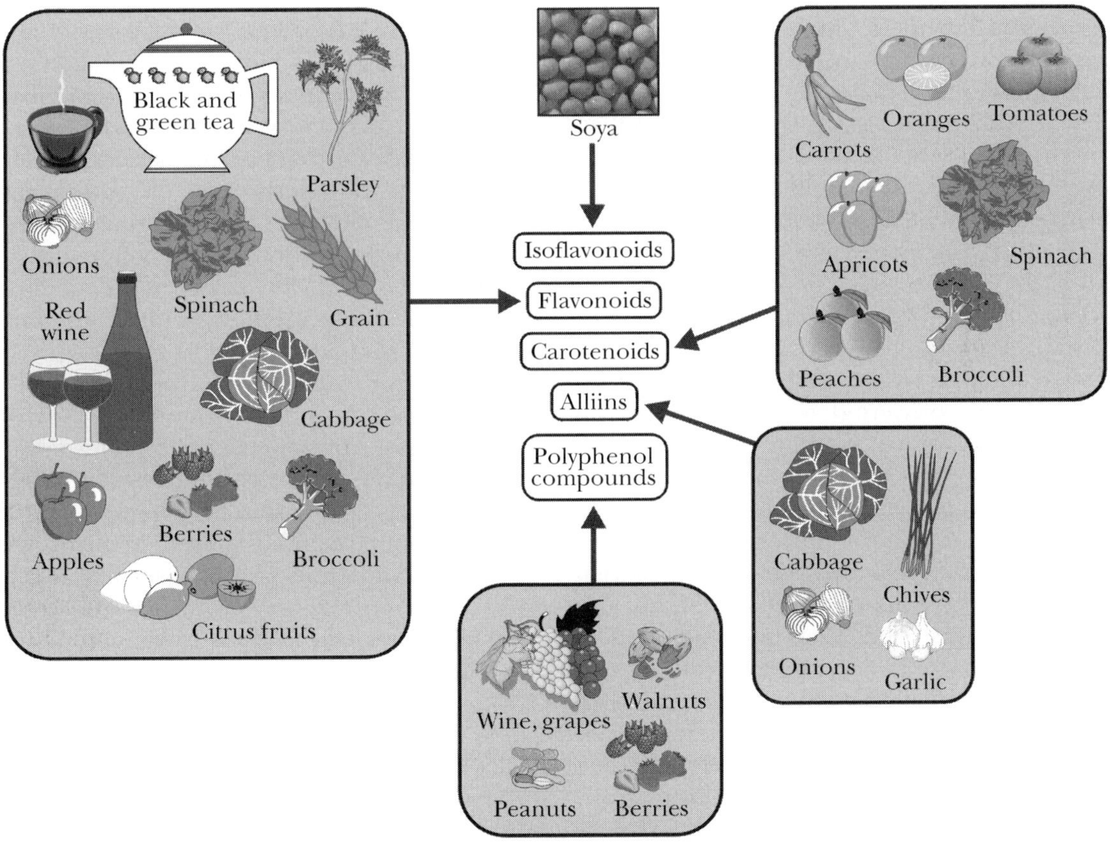

Figure 3 Particular foodstuffs as sources of important nutritional factors

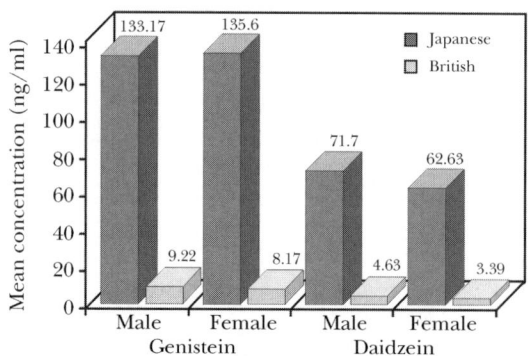

Figure 4 Comparative mean concentrations of genistein and daidzein in Japanese and British male and female plasma samples. Data from the Tenovus Cancer Research Centre, Cardiff, UK

estrogenic isoflavonoid, equol, is formed from daidzein in the gut, but interestingly, only in a proportion of people. Soy bean is a staple dietary constituent in China and Japan, in the form of bean curd (tofu), soy-bean milk, miso and tempeh, and there are many traditional diets of Asia, India, Africa, the Mediterranean countries and South America which have a high legume content, associated particularly with beans, soy-protein, lentils and chick peas.

The two principal, weakly estrogenic lignans are enterolactone and enterodiol[12,18], formed from precursors in foodstuffs, matairesinol and secoisolariciresinol, respectively, which again are metabolized by gut microflora (Figure 5). Enterodiol is converted to enterolactone in the colon[12]. More recently[12], pinoresinol, lariciresinol and syringaresinol have been recognized in cereals and whole-grain rye food-stuffs, as precursors of enterolactone. Linseed, or flaxseed, berries and fruits provide a rich source of these compounds, but they are also present in other seeds such as sesame and in cereals, whole-grain foodstuffs, rye bran and vegetables. The concentration of lignans is high in the biological fluids of vegetarians and people from the Mediterranean countries.

Another geographical variable must logically be the microflora content of the gut and its inherent enzymic activity directed towards the metabolism of these phyto-constituents. Anti-

biotics will therefore suppress their plasma levels[19].

For many years, the vitamins and trace elements attracted the interest of nutritional scientists. Of late, interest in the isoflavonoids and lignans and their extensive range of biological activities (Table 1) has acquired special attention, whereas potential benefits of the polyphenolic compounds referred to as the flavonoids have tended to be less appreciated. Unlike the isoflavonoids, the flavonoids (Figure 6) are ubiquitous in nature, contributing to the color and flavor of fruits and vegetables. Their chemistry has been well studied[20,21], and their pharmacological effects would suggest that their influence on human health could be quite profound. They make up a vast and complex group of plant constituents that are further classified as flavones, flavonols, flavanones, catechins and anthocyanidins. Flavonoids were once considered by the eminent Hungarian Nobel Laureate, Professor Szent-Gyorgyi[22], and his group to have the biological characteristics of vitamins, and certain flavonoids from citrus fruits were referred to as vitamin P. Some major sources of flavonoids are onions, apples, tea, red wine and certain herbs such as thyme and parsley. Since ancient times, herbs and plants have been used as forms of medicine, cruciferous vegetables, garlic, celery and cucumber being well recognized. Several commonly occurring flavonoids, apigenin and kaempferol (Figure 6), for example, also have weak estrogenic activity[23]. Apigenin is found in the leaves, seeds and fruits of flowering plants and makes up to 7% of the dry weight of leafy vegetables. Tea leaves are a major source of apigenin. Little is known about flavonoids present in the plasma or tissues of different groups of people worldwide. Until recently, any protective role would have been ascribed to their capacity to act as antioxidants.

Why are phytoestrogens estrogenic?

17β-Estradiol is the natural estrogenic hormone seen generally in relation to the female reproductive system. It is also synthesized in the male, and is implicated in many biological processes

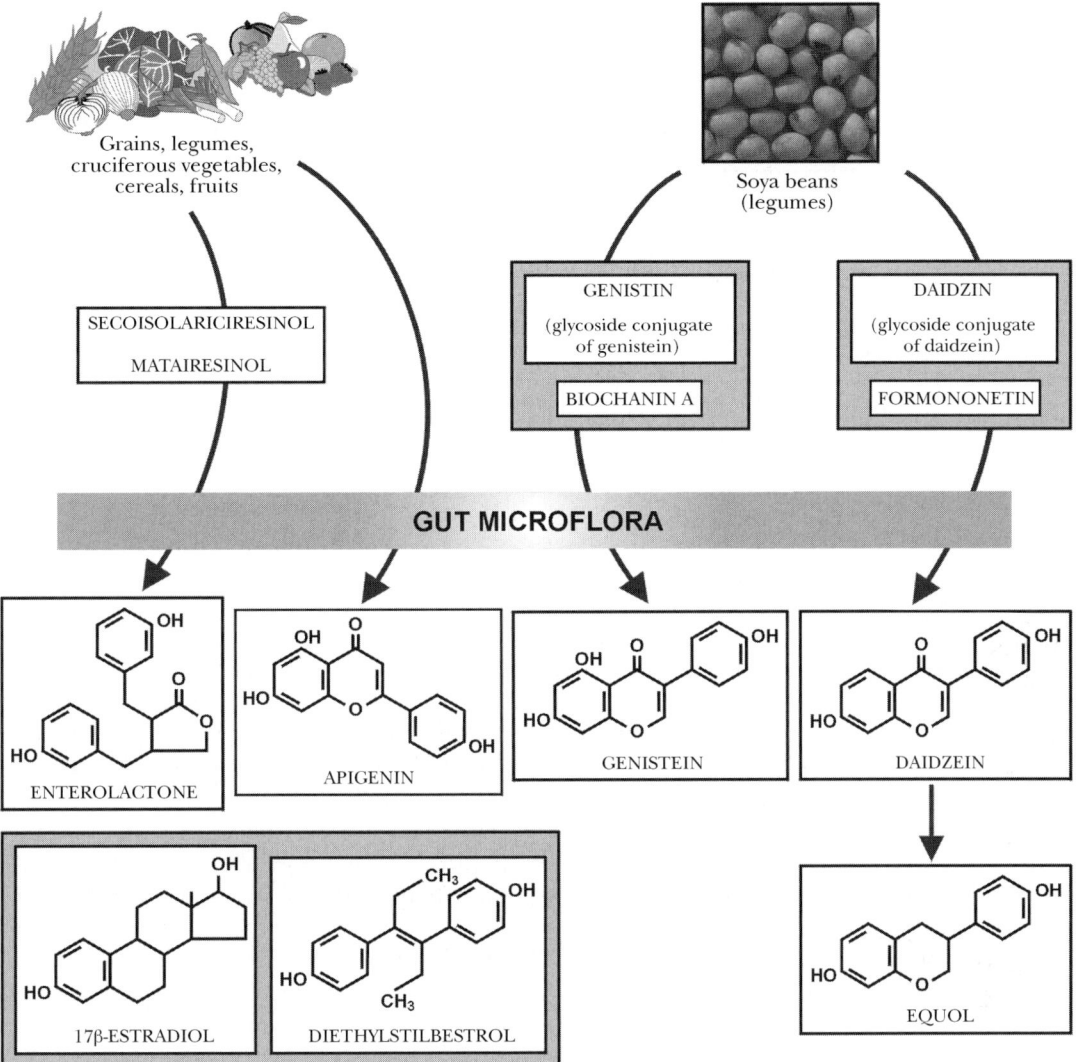

Figure 5 Production of the phytoestrogens, illustrating the role of the gut microflora and some chemical structures. The structures of 17β-estradiol and diethylstilbestrol are shown for comparison

including those of the prostate, the vascular system and bone. Within particular target sites, 17β-estradiol specifically and avidly binds to estrogen receptor (ER) proteins, and it is the estradiol–ER complex that directly modulates gene expression through its association with the genome. The spatial arrangement of the molecule, with the OH groups approximately 10.3 Å apart (Figure 5), allows it to associate with the receptor and thereby promote an estrogenic response. Similarly, diethylstilbestrol (DES), the first synthetic estrogen to be used orally for the treatment of cancer, has two OH groups spatially separated by the same distance. The spatial geometry of certain of the phytoestrogens also shows some structural similarity to the 17β-estradiol molecule, thereby conferring some degree of weak estrogenicity. Certain of the phytoestrogens bind most avidly to ERβ[5].

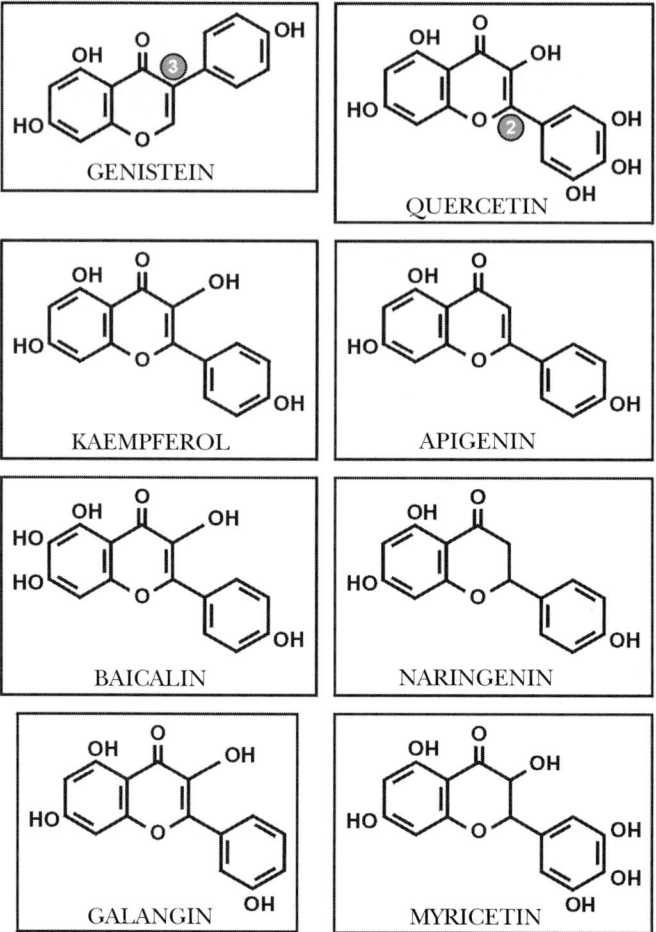

Figure 6 Chemical structures of some of the flavonoids, illustrating differences from the isoflavonoids represented by genistein

Preventive therapy for prostate disease

Phytoestrogens may therefore protect against cancer, and it is not unreasonable to assume that their agonistic and antagonistic action as weak estrogens could help to prevent cancers of the breast, ovary and uterus. But why should such weak estrogens influence the androgen-promoted growth that is characteristic of prostate cancer? Any putative restraint on cancer of the prostate could simply be due to the antioxidant properties of isoflavonoids and flavonoids, rather than to any estrogenic influence. The classical effects of androgens on prostate disease are well recognized, but do the natural estrogens influence these growth-

regulatory mechanisms, and if so, can phyto-estrogens disturb this relationship? Any prevention concept must also encompass, however, the additional and possibly more important biological characteristics of the phyto-constituents, other than their action as estrogen agonists or antagonists (Table 1). This is quite an imposing list of properties, and one might be excused for speculating on what could be seen as the properties of the 'magic cancer bullet'. With regard to the regional differences in pros-tate cancer incidence, it may also be that the bio-logical influence of these phyto-constituents is effected at birth, adolescence, puberty or, indeed, throughout life. The influence in all

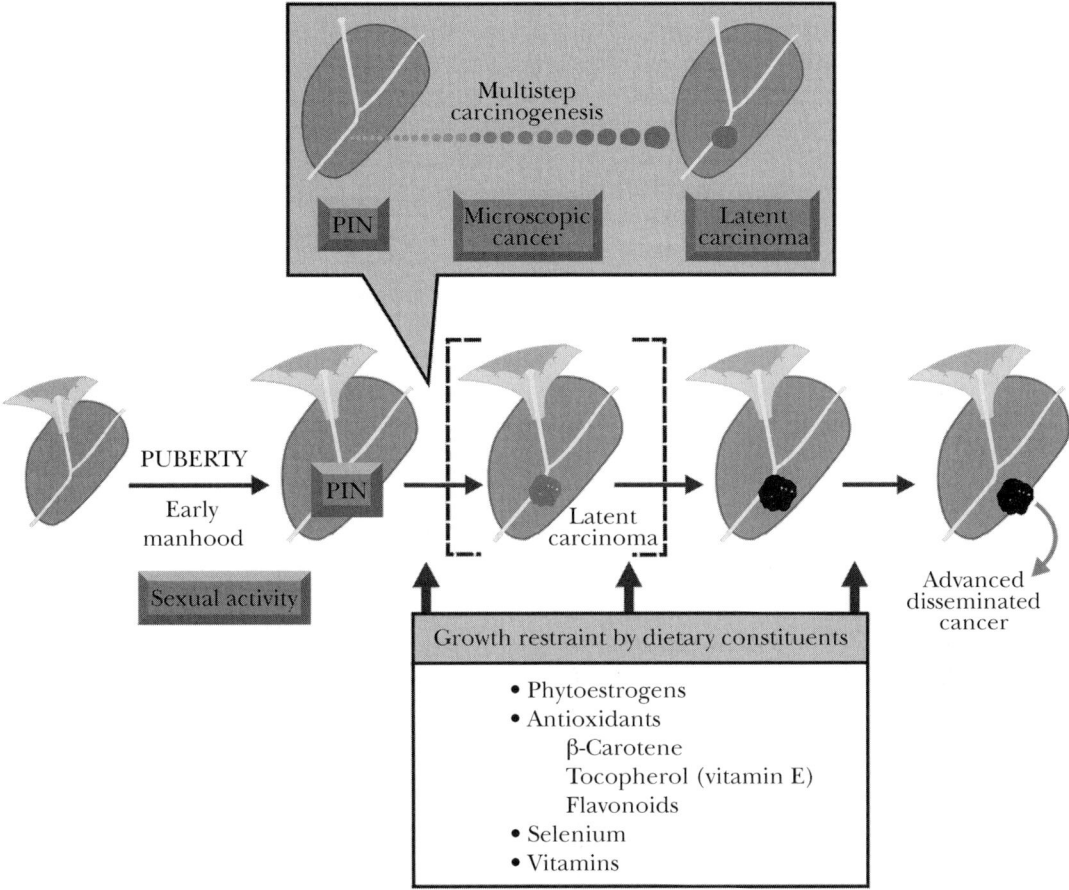

Figure 7 A simple representation of the natural history of prostate cancer and some possible dietary factors that may influence cancer progression. The figure illustrates prostate cancer initiation soon after puberty and the attainment of maximal prostate size. PIN, prostatic intraepithelial neoplasia

probability is multifactorial, with the constituents eliciting their range of effects at varying times throughout life. The antioxidant properties may be of paramount importance at some precise time; other investigators may be convinced by the protective effects of such micronutrients as protease inhibitors. Any health benefits ascribed to the disparate dietary patterns will eventually be seen as the result of the combined effects of many agents. Accordingly, the personal prejudices of individual researchers must be encouraged, in order to gain a greater understanding of these complex inter-relationships.

As preventive measures, government agencies have recommended prudent diets. If such guidelines were accepted and adopted by people of the developed countries, together with the realization that smoking is dangerous, then the incidence of cancer and cardiovascular disease would fall quite precipitously. Unfortunately, since the incidence rates do not markedly change, it must be concluded that the benefits of such dietary patterns are not sufficiently appreciated. It seems less easy to change dietary habits than has been believed and, moreover, the younger generation of those populations who, through the years, have benefited from 'healthy diets' now seem intent on discarding their traditional foods with associated protective factors, for the acquisition of 'Western eating habits'. Should medical science be more assertive about the benefits of certain dietary constituents, for example the phytoestrogens? Moreover, rather than dietary change, can dietary supplementation be specifically recommended, on the basis of data accumulated to date?

Some older classical viewpoints on estrogens and cancer

Estrogens were probably the first natural compounds to be implicated as a possible cause of cancer[24] in various tissues, not only in the female. Moreover, they suppressed cancer growth. The viewpoint was not that a sudden 'overabundance' of estrogen was important, but a long-term, prolonged supply of relatively small amounts of the hormone. Males were generally thought to be 'more reactive' to estrogens than females. The general theme, even in the 1930s, was that there was a long interval between the 'cause' and the clinical manifestation of cancer. Multistep carcinogenesis was recognized: hyperplasia, followed by the development of an 'innocent tumor' during the early years of reproductive life, from which there is the gradual transition to malignancy[25]. Prostate cancer would appear to be similar, with growth dysregulation occurring immediately after the period of puberty and during the earlier phases of sexual activity. It was recognized in the 1930s that physiological doses of estrogens enhanced the biological effects of androgens, and it is interesting that, in 1935, before Doisy and colleagues[26] had isolated and characterized 17β-estradiol, De Jongh[27] believed that benign prostatic hyperplasia (BPH) resulted from an excess of estrogen, relative to androgen. Noteworthy in this regard are consensus viewpoints[28], prepared some 60 years later, that prostate enlargement causing bladder outlet obstruction would seem to be due to a decreased concentration of plasma testosterone as a result of decreased testicular function with increasing age, relative to a level of plasma 17β-estradiol that is sustained at normal physiological concentrations, despite aging: essentially, therefore, an androgen–estrogen imbalance.

The impact of phytoestrogens on prostate cancer restraint appears to be exercised at this period of endocrine change beyond 50 years of age, when the biological role of the estrogens may become more important. They constitute one group of many dietary constituents (Figure 7) that are currently seen to offer potential benefit. Professor Bill Fair describes prostate cancer as an enigma[29], a common cause of death, yet a cancer that appears to progress at a particularly slow rate of growth. Although initiated in the earlier phases of a male's post-pubertal years, it remains asymptomatic and dormant until well beyond the age of 50. Can dietary change, or appropriate supplementation, extend the time during which the cancer slowly develops through this latent, although not 'innocent', asymptomatic stage? Data from Boyle and colleagues[14] suggest that this is possible.

Latent cancer refers to cancer found at autopsy but hitherto unsuspected, and Rich in 1935[30] reported that up to 30% of 'Western' men by 50 years of age had an intraprostatic microscopic focus of cancer. It was subsequently reported[31] to be just as common in Japanese males, and more recent studies support this. A study[32] of 1327 prostates, removed at autopsy from men over 45 years of age and from East and West, revealed small foci of latent cancer in 12% of all men, a prevalence that did not vary with age. The prevalence of larger foci of latent cancer showed a geographical variation, similar to that observed for clinical cancer, with a higher prevalence in the West. This and a similar study[33] confirmed that the incidence of small foci of well-differentiated latent carcinoma does not relate to race, geography or age, but occurs with equal prevalence in about 12% of males, over the age of 40, world-wide. The prevalence of larger, less well-differentiated foci of latent cancer is lower in Asian men[14]. Sakr and co-workers[34–36] reported that microfoci of prostate cancer were present in men between 30 and 40 years of age. Cancer is present in the earlier years of life, as portrayed in Figure 7. The rate of prostate cancer initiation appears to be the same in all males, world-wide, but geographical differences in the incidence of clinical cancer seem to relate primarily to the subsequent rate of growth of the latent cancer and to progression to the malignant phenotype.

Also important are the classical studies of Coffey and colleagues[37,38] indicating that 'microscopic BPH', essentially microscopic foci of epithelial hyperplasia, can be recognized in young men as early as 25–30 years of age, not long after the gland has reached its mature, adult size. This 'microscopic BPH' can be identified in the prostates of men from the East and the West, both Asian and Caucasian. The process again represents early dysfunctional growth regulation, an imbalance between cell proliferation and apoptosis. It is interesting that

Japanese prostate glands, overall, are smaller[39] than their Western counterparts (Figure 8). What, then, are the biological effects that phyto-nutrients could impose on these events?

Phytoestrogens: effects on endocrinology and growth regulation

Estrogenic activity

Phytoestrogens can act as estrogen agonists or as antagonists[2], depending on the target tissue. If estrogens have a significant role in the prostate growth-signalling network, then phytoestrogens may be expected to influence these processes. For 30 years, it was accepted that there was one

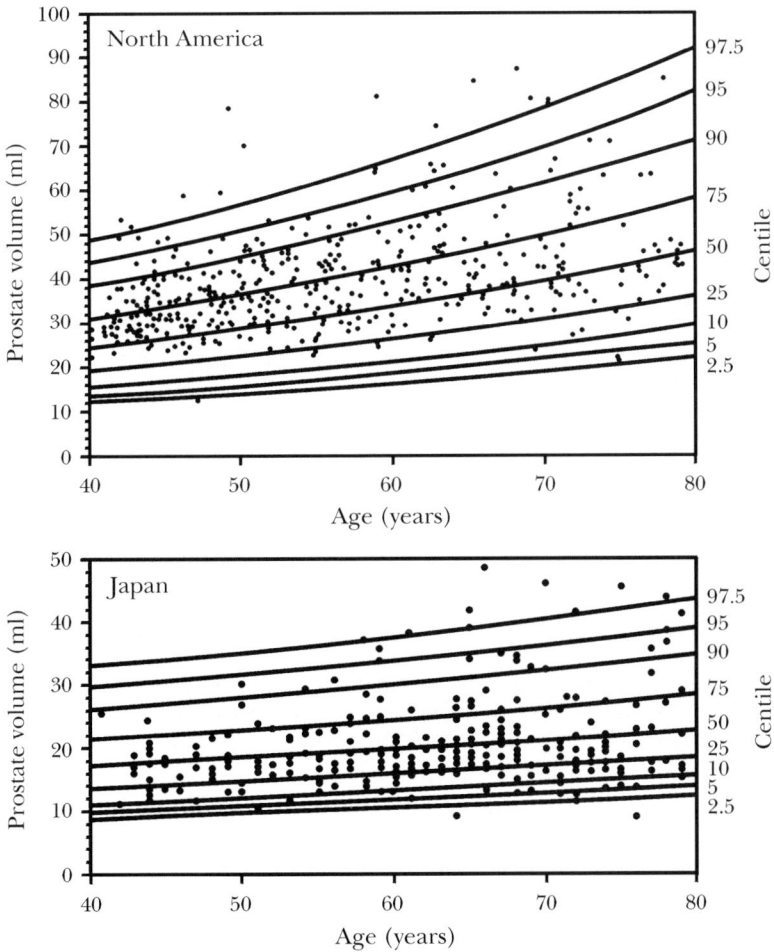

Figure 8   Distribution of prostate volume by age in studies from Japan and North America

'classical' estrogen receptor, ERα. In the prostate, it was localized in the smooth muscle cells of the stromal compartment. Stromal hyperplasia is promoted by estrogen, suggesting that 17β-estradiol, as well as dihydrotestosterone (DHT), may be synergistically implicated in promoting stromal growth[2,28]. Like ERα, the new, distinct ERβ[3–5] also has a high affinity for 17β-estradiol and is the principal prostate estrogen receptor, localized in the epithelial cells. 17β-Estradiol may therefore mediate signalling pathways through ERβ[4], and interest centers on the biological action of ERβ relative to that of ERα. Their roles may be quite distinct, complementary or antagonistic[2], and, moreover[5], certain phytoestrogens, such as genistein, bind preferentially to ERβ.

The similar amino acid sequences in both DNA- and estrogen-binding domains of ERα and ERβ suggest that they would associate with the same recognition sites on the genome (Figure 9). The N-terminal A/B regions and related transcription activation functions (TAF-1) are, however, different. Cross-talk between signalling pathways involving steroid receptors and those promoted by growth-stimulatory factors, and the synergistic functional interaction between the ERs and other cell-specific coactivators and -repressors in juxtaposition on the genome of the prostate cells, could be different for ERβ relative to ERα[40–42]. The hormone response elements could specifically interact with a ERα–ERβ heterodimer rather than ERα or ERβ homodimers. These investigations have decidedly revitalized interest in the molecular events in which estrogens are involved within the human prostate gland, with the inter-relationship between androgens, estrogens and phytoestrogens very relevant.

Whether the estrogenic function of the phytoestrogens allows them to influence significantly man's endocrine status during the various periods of life must remain, at present, somewhat controversial. Their influence on the developing fetus, on the neonate, through

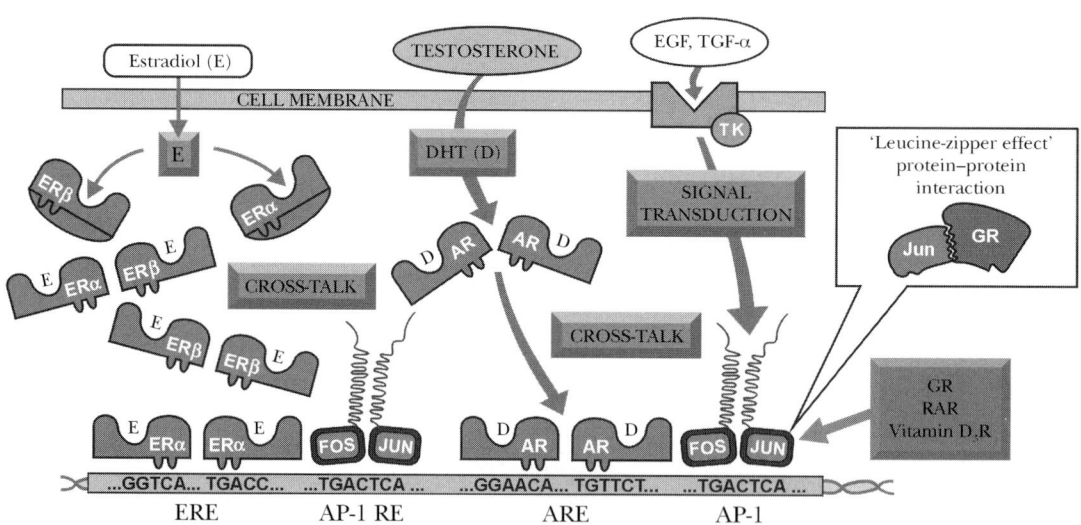

Figure 9 A simple representation of steroid- and growth factor-mediated intracellular signalling and the relationship to recognition sites on the genome. Cross-talk is shown and the potential complexity of estrogen signalling. The possible influence of retinoic acid, vitamin D_3 and progesterone on these signalling mechanisms is suggested. ER, estrogen receptor; DHT, dihydrotestosterone; AR, androgen receptor; EGF, epidermal growth factor; TGF, transforming growth factor; TK, tyrosine-specific protein kinase; ERE, estrogen response element; AP-1 RE, activation protein-1 response element; ARE, androgen response element; GR, gestagen receptor; RAR, retinoic acid receptor; vitamin D_3R, vitamin D_3 receptor

adrenarche and puberty and at the andropause will be determined over the next few years[2]. In a study of Japanese women[43], substantial soy-protein intake during adolescence decreased the subsequent risk of breast cancer.

The isoflavonoids daidzein, genistein, coumestrol and equol and the flavonoids apigenin, kaempferol and phloretin all possess weak estrogenic activity. As weak estrogens, they may influence 17β-estradiol binding sites.

Estrogens, together with insulin and the thyroid hormones, participate in the control of sex hormone-binding globulin (SHBG) synthesis by the liver, and genistein and entero-lactone also stimulate the synthesis of SHBG by human liver cells[8,12]. Vegetarians and Asian men have higher plasma levels of SHBG and lower free testosterone than Western omnivores, and in Japanese women high soy-protein intake relates to lower levels of plasma estrogens[44]. An increased intake of soy-protein, vegetables, fruit, berries, cereals and products like whole-grain rye bread enhances plasma SHBG levels, thereby influencing the levels of free biologically active steroid in plasma.

Inhibition of the 5α-reductase enzyme

Isoflavonoids and lignans inhibit both 5α-reductase and 17β-hydroxysteroid dehydrogenase enzyme systems[45], the latter regulating the interconversion of 17β-hydroxy and 17-oxo steroids (Figure 10). Such an effect, in vivo, could markedly influence the metabolism of both androgens and estrogens. 5α-Reductase is important for prostate growth, the gland failing to grow in the absence of DHT[46].

As well as affecting steroid hormone metabolism, the phytoestrogens could influence androgen-mediated signalling pathways within the prostate. Possibly related, although more probably of genetic origin, is the report of lower levels of 5α-reductase activity in young Japanese men in comparison with their Western counterparts[47]. It is, however, interesting to speculate whether this is a consequence of long-term consumption of substantial amounts of iso-flavonoids, rather than of genetic origin. Finasteride, used in the treatment of obstructive BPH, is currently being evaluated as to its effectiveness in the prevention of early prostate cancer[1].

Inhibition of tyrosine-specific protein kinases

The tyrosine-specific protein kinases (TK enzymes) are intimately involved in the transmission of signals induced by the association of various growth factors such as epidermal growth factor (EGF) with their specific transmembrane receptors (Figure 9). In addition, many oncogenes such as src, abl, fps, yes, fes and cas all encode TK enzymes. Tyrosine phosphorylation and activation of the TK enzymes play a major role in the control of cell proliferation and growth-regulatory events. Currently, various TK-specific inhibitors are being evaluated as anticancer agents[48].

Genistein is a specific inhibitor of TK activity[49], and the flavonoids, apigenin and kaempferol, reverse the transformed phenotypes of v-H-ras NIH3T3 cells, an effect mediated by the inhibition of TK enzymes[50]. Equally important are the inhibitory effects of phyto-constituents on TK enzymes associated with angiogenesis[51,52]. Any putative growth restraint imposed on latent cancer may be related to the control of angiogenesis, the neovascularization required for cancer to progress beyond 2 mm in size (Figure 11). As well as the angiogenic action of both vascular endothelial growth factor (VEGF) and fibroblast growth factor-2 (FGF-2), 17β-estradiol, nitric oxide and insulin-like growth factor-I (IGF-I) are all intimately concerned in the promotion of neovascularization[2]. The TK-inhibiting action of genistein suppresses angiogenesis, and the estrogen-related agonistic or antagonistic effects of the phytoestrogens may also be implicated. Their effect on the estrogen-promoted activity of NO synthase and NO production may be of interest.

The potential difficulties of using specific TK inhibitors as anticancer agents in relation to the compensatory response of the cells have been recognized[53], and the basis of an alternative strategy developed, essentially the means to deliver a non-specific TK inhibitor selectively to

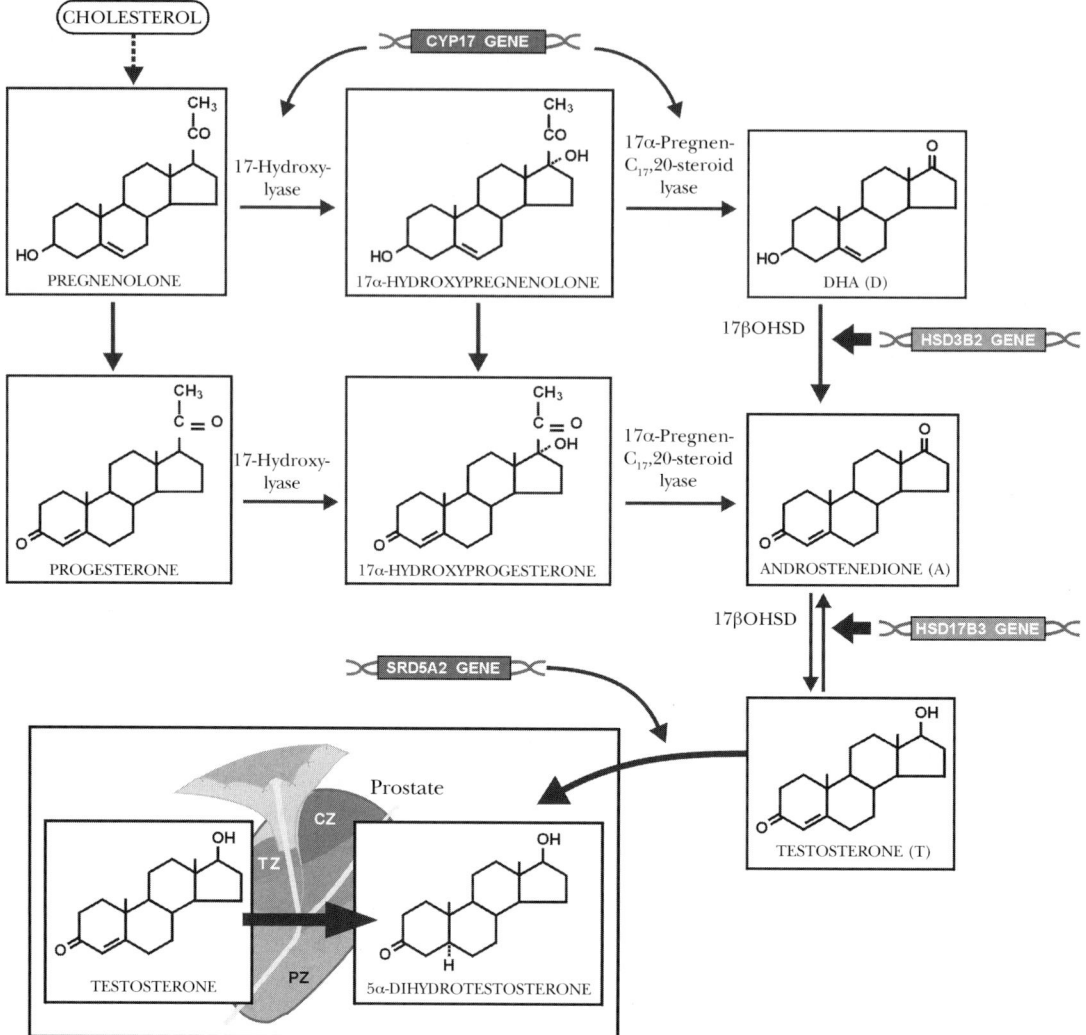

Figure 10 Pathways for steroid synthesis and certain genes which encode enzymes concerned in the production of testosterone and its conversion to dihydrotestosterone (DHT). DHA, dihydroalanine; 17βOHSD, 17β-hydroxysteroid dehydrogenase; CZ, central zone; PZ, peripheral zone; TZ, transition zone

target cancer cells. B-cell precursor leukemic cells express a cell surface receptor, CD19, which is absent from related normal cells and which is functionally and structurally associated with the transmembrane receptor TKs and their signalling pathways. CD19 can be internalized by a specific monoclonal antibody, B43, which was raised against CD19. Treatment of these leukemic cells in an immunodeficient mouse model system, by an immunoconjugate of genistein bound to the B43 antibody, selectively inhibited CD19-related TK enzyme systems and

induced rapid apoptosis. A dose ten-fold less than that maximally tolerated induced a 99.999% cell kill and 100% long-term, event-free survival. Moreover, a recent study[54] has drawn attention to the anticancer activity of a related EGF–genistein conjugate.

Experimental animal cancer model systems

Soy-bean preparations inhibited experimental carcinogenesis in a wide variety of systems[55]. Of 26 animal studies in which diets containing soy

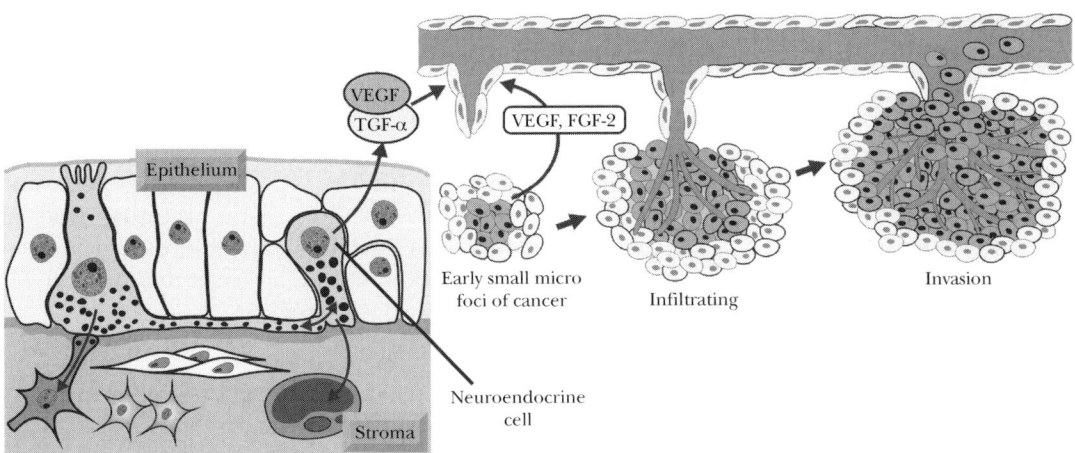

Figure 11 Diagrammatic representation of the processes of angiogenesis and the action of vascular endothelial growth factor (VEGF) and fibroblast growth factor-2 (FGF-2) on the proliferation of vascular endothelial cells. The figure portrays the neuroendocrine cells as the source of VEGF. TGF-α, transforming growth factor-α

or soy-bean isoflavonoids were employed, 17 (65%) reported protective effects. None of the studies stated that soy intake increased tumor development. Moreover, the studies with no evidence of tumor inhibition used soya protein isolate, a preparation treated with alkali which causes a five-fold reduction in isoflavonoid levels. Genistein also inhibits the growth of androgen-dependent and androgen-independent cultured prostate cancer cells[56,57].

Inhibition of DNA topoisomerases

Genistein inhibits DNA topoisomerases[58], enzymes that alter the conformation of DNA and, crucial to cell division, untangle supercoiled DNA. The flavonoids, quercetin, fisetin and morin, also inhibit DNA topoisomerases I and II, while kaempferol inhibits only DNA topoisomerase II[59]. The inhibition of topoisomerases is also a target for the design of new anticancer drugs.

Inhibition of the aromatase enzyme system

Approximately 40% of plasma estrogens in the human male are secreted by the testes, the remainder being derived from the peripheral conversion of adrenal androgens to estrogens by the aromatase enzyme system in adipose and muscle tissue. As a man ages, declining testicular activity and increasing aromatization sustain the plasma 17β-estradiol concentration relative to the falling level of free testosterone. This enhanced mid-life 'estrogenic stimulus' has been considered responsible for the increased level of plasma SHBG at this time, and, furthermore, this change in the estrogen–androgen balance has been implicated as a predominant factor in the induction of stromal hyperplasia of the prostate[28]. The possibility that estrogens have a role at the andropause in influencing the progression of latent cancer to the malignant phenotype has also been considered[2,15,60]. Enterolactone is a reasonable inhibitor of the aromatase enzyme[8,12]. The issue centers on whether phytoestrogens suppress stromal hyperplasia, inhibiting the peripheral aromatization of adrenal androgens. Second, is there a significant effect of the phytoestrogens on the promotion of SHBG synthesis by the liver, such that the estrogen–androgen balance is positively affected?

Some other biological effects of interest

Certain biological effects, sometimes recognized in systems other than the prostate gland, may have relevance. The antioxidant properties of the phyto-constituents may be important with regard to men's health[2,61], influencing glutathione peroxidase and superoxide dismutase. Genistein is also cytostatic, arresting cell cycle progression in G_2–M, and it induces apoptosis in immature human thymocytes by inhibiting DNA topoisomerase II. Rye bran and soy-protein enhanced apoptosis in LNCaP (lymph node cancer of the prostate) cells in nude mice[62]. Genistein and apigenin induce morphological differentiation and G_2–M arrest in rat neuronal cells, and glycosylated quercetin is a selective inhibitor of topoisomerase IV. In addition, isoflavonoids and flavonoids can inhibit the bioactivation of potent chemical carcinogens[63], the genistein precursor, bio-chanin A, as well as quercetin and kaempferol, inhibit the activation of the mutagen, benzo[a]pyrene, and the flavonoid catechins, constituents of green and black tea, inhibit the activation of the potent tobacco carcinogen 4-(methylnitrosoamino)-1-(3-pyridyl)-1-butano ne (NNK) and subsequent lung tumorigenesis in A/J mice[64]. Apigenin and tangeretin, a citrus flavonoid, influence mono-oxygenase activity, the enhancement of gap-junction intercellular communication between liver epithelial cells and, possibly, tumor promotion. Moreover, tangeretin is reported to inhibit the growth of leukemic HL-60 cells by the induction of apoptosis. TPA (12-O-tetradecanoyl-phorbol-13-acetate), a cancer promoter, activates protein kinase C (PKC) and induces proto-oncogene expression. Apigenin and curcumin inhibit PKC by competing with adenosine triphosphate (ATP) and blocking the enhanced TPA-induction of c-fos and c-jun expression. Apigenin, quercetin and myricetin inhibit phosphatidylinositol 3-kinase activity and associated intracellular signal transduction systems.

Tangeretin and the catechins derived from tea (Figure 12), also inhibit the invasive capacity of murine sarcoma cells, suppressing cell motility, an effect mediated through the E-cadherin–catenin complex. Cadherins are important in cancer dissemination, the capacity of tumor cells to invade being enhanced by disruption in cell–cell adhesion. Cadherins, mediators of epithelial cell adhesion, relate to cancer of the prostate, with poorly differentiated cancers reported to have decreased E-cadherin content[65]. Little is known about cadherin expression, although in the mouse ovary and uterus 17β-estradiol has been implicated. Tamoxifen, IGF-I, retinoic acid and the citrus flavonoid tangeretin all increase the aggregation of cancer cells and inhibit their invasive capacity in vitro.

Estrogens, phytoestrogens, imprinting and prostate cancer

There is much to learn about the pathogenesis of prostate cancer. Certain risk factors have been recognized[14]: androgenic status, age, ethnicity and family history, with the role of male estrogenic status now a controversial issue. The close relationship of prostate cancer initiation to puberty, when an 'endocrine shock', massive hormonal changes, are 'inflicted' on 'young' men, is interesting. A link between sexual awareness, sexual activity and prostate disease has inevitably been considered[66]. Do men who develop prostate cancer have a greater sex drive and enhanced libido? Delayed onset of sexuality in the late adolescent period, and early suppression of a male's sexual activity, have been discussed in relation to etiology. Is ejaculation and the clearing of prostate secretion important? Prostate cancer mortality is related to marital status, but with a greater prevalence in widowed and divorced men than in married or single men. Does a greater libido and enhanced sexual activity relate to a relatively higher 'androgenic status' and a lesser risk of prostate cancer? It would seem important normally to sustain a relatively high level of plasma testosterone, and would, for example, inguinal hernia result in a disruption of testosterone output from the testis and a greater risk of prostate cancer? Inguinal hernia in relation to estrogen metabolism in East African men has been reported[67], and data from the British Prostate Group's investigation into hormone levels in relation to prostate cancer suggested to Dr Maureen Harper (unpublished observation) a greater prevalence

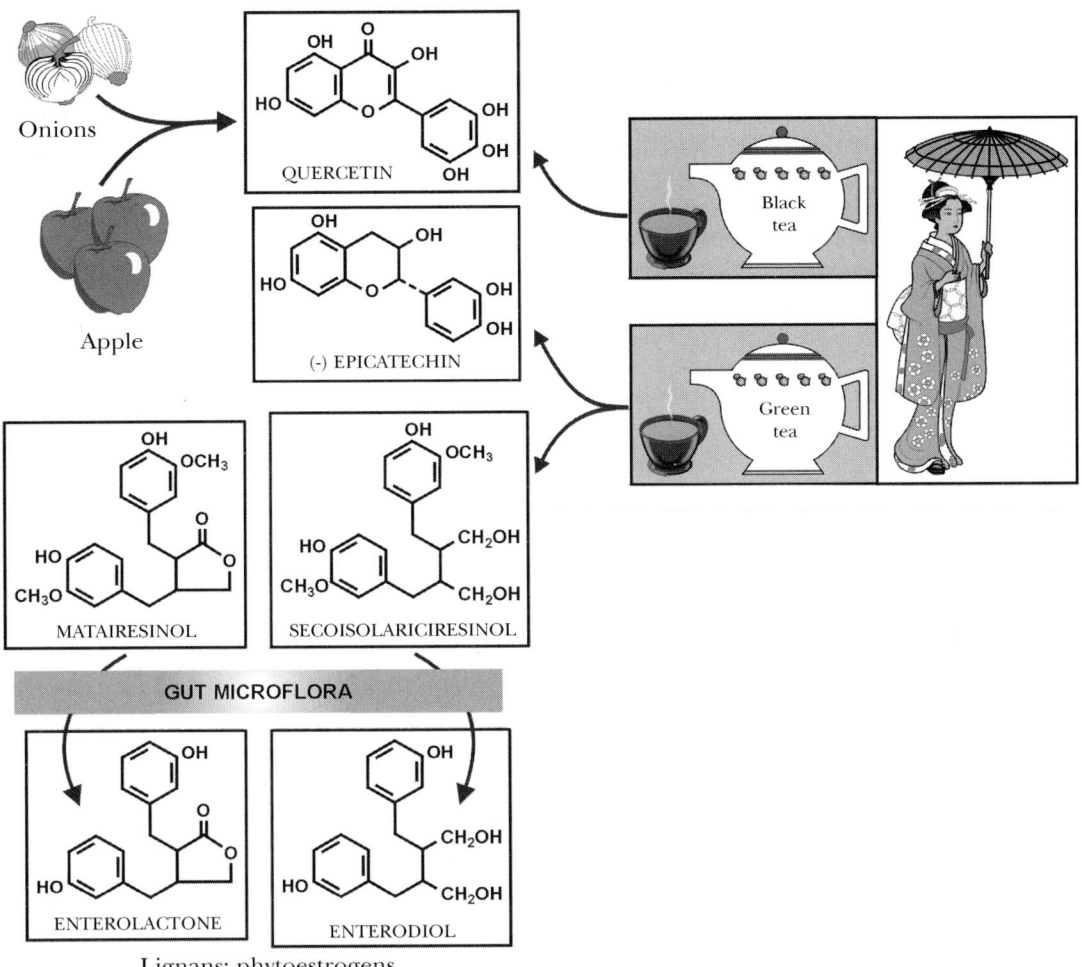

Figure 12 Some potential health benefits from tea

of inguinal hernia in men who subsequently developed cancer of the prostate. Can phytoestrogens influence the fine androgen–estrogen balance that is created during early adolescence and puberty, and thereby affect prostate function? In rodent model systems, the protective influence of soy-protein on cancer was seen if administered during early puberty[68].

In this regard, the process of 'imprinting', by which certain endocrine-mediated molecular signals can be induced into the DNA during embryogenesis, may impinge on this endocrine balance. These genomic 'signals', which are generated in a tissue *in utero*, result in a greater propensity to develop cancer in the tissue, later

in life. In the prostate, this could be in relation to the changing endocrine status at puberty[2]. The high prevalence of prostate cancer in the North American black male could be related to the process of 'imprinting'.

DES, administered for threatened abortion, generates a message in embryonic vaginal tissue that can result in clear cell carcinoma 20 years later[69]. The issue centers on whether estradiol can similarly 'speak' to the embryonic prostate gland, inducing a genomic signal that can be recognized during puberty which induces post-pubertal dysfunctional growth regulation in the prostate and cellular proliferation.

An imprinted gene is inactive or 'silent'. Within the normal diploid mammalian cell, it is generally assumed that most genes are expressed in both alleles. In genetics, this is illustrated by reference to the gametic contribution of the maternal and paternal genomes to the development of the preimplantation blastocyst, which are not functionally identical[70]. These differences are imposed during gametogenesis when certain genes are 'imprinted'. After implantation of the blastocyst, the IGF-II gene is exclusively expressed in most mouse fetal tissues by the paternal allele, whereas the corresponding maternal allele is silent. The biallelic expression of the IGF-II gene is manifested only later in development. Imprinting relates to the methylation of specific cytosine residues on the DNA, an event exercised through specific DNA methyltransferases, with gene inactivation being at the level of transcription. The imprint is retained within the parental chromosomes during cell division and is therefore heritable. DNA methylation represses a gene and, correspondingly, demethylation results in reactivation of gene transcription.

Dysfunctional growth of the adult male reproductive tract has been reported after prenatal or neonatal exposure to estrogens[71]. Important is that a 50% physiological increase in the serum 17β-estradiol concentration, within the male mouse fetus, resulted in an enlarged adult prostate gland, with a six-fold higher level of androgen receptor, relative to controls. A five-fold pharmacological increase produced a smaller adult gland. In relation to the higher incidence of prostate cancer in the Afro-American male is the report[72] that their mothers may have up to 40% higher concentrations of plasma 17β-estradiol than white mothers.

Can 17β-estradiol 'speak' to the fetal prostate, subsequently impinging on endocrine events of male puberty? Since the IGF network is particularly concerned with imprinting, it may be that the IGF family of growth factors is associated with these events and dysfunctional growth regulation. The biallelic expression of imprinted genes in human embryonic cancers such as the Wilms' tumor, or neuroblastoma, is considered by Wilkins[73] to result from the removal of an imprint, or an inability to respond to it. It was suggested that imprinting was implicated in the early stages of carcinogenesis, following the recognition that, in Wilms' tumor, the tumor-specific alteration of human chromosome 11, the location of the imprinted IGF-II gene, with loss of heterozygosity, invariably involved the loss of the 11p maternal allele. Similar events were reported for neuroblastomas and rhabdosarcomas. Dysfunctional IGF-II imprinting has also been recognized in relation to cancer of the lung. The time- and tissue-specific reprogramming of mono- and biallelic expression of the genes of the IGF-family, and the availability of particular growth and transcription factors at critical periods in tissue development, could be implicated in early molecular events of prostate cancer.

If prenatal imprinting induces a predisposition to prostate cancer, a complex multifactorial picture emerges, centered on estrogen-mediated events (Figure 13). Estrogens promote growth hormone output, which relates to IGF-I release and the normal induction and progression of puberty, including luteinizing hormone-releasing hormone secretion[2,15,60]. Estrogens regulate expression of the growth hormone receptor in the liver and IGF-I secretion. IGF-I is a necessary survival factor, promoting cellular proliferation and transformation, its action modulated by the relative affinity of IGF-I for its receptor, IGF-IR and for its circulating plasma binding protein, IGFBP-3. The overriding influence of the dietary phytoestrogens on these events could be important.

These are interesting facets of human biology. Abnormal epididymides have been identified after prenatal exposure to DES[74], as well as dysfunctional seminal vesicles, which express ERα and an estrogen-induced protein, lactoferrin, that would normally be a product of the uterus but not of the male seminal vesicles. Chang and colleagues[75,76] have also emphasized that estrogen-mediated imprinting induces dysfunctional prostate growth, with transforming

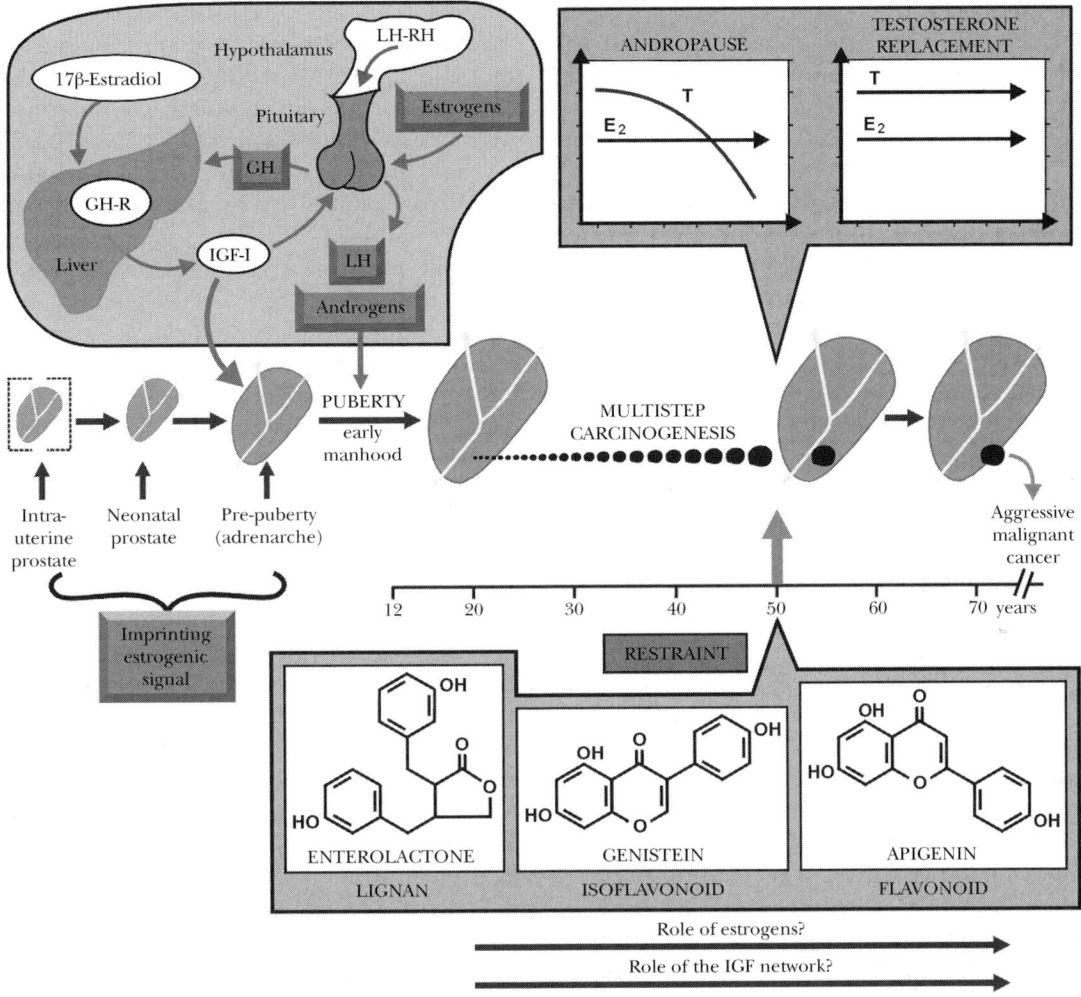

Figure 13 Natural history of prostate cancer highlighting the possible influence of imprinting *in utero* or prior to puberty, and the role of estrogens in the endocrine events associated with puberty. The potential regulatory action of the insulin-like growth factor (IGF) network is illustrated. LH-RH, luteinizing hormone-releasing hormone; GH, growth hormone; LH, luteinizing hormone; GH-R, growth hormone receptor; E_2, estradiol; T, testosterone

growth factor-β (TGF-β) signalling perturbed such that epithelial cell differentiation was inhibited, with enhanced proliferation of periductal fibroblasts. Expression of TGF-β1, localized to the periductal smooth muscle cells, was enhanced, whereas TGF-β2 and TGF-β3 expression, located in differentiating epithelial cells in developing prostates, was restrained. They proposed that a layer of periductal fibroblasts causes a physical barrier that constrains branching morphogenesis. ERα is located in the

fibroblasts, and 17β-estradiol promotes their proliferation. The 'fibroblast barrier' would restrain normal paracrine signalling between stromal and epithelial compartments. The TGF-β1R levels were also repressed in epithelial cells. The cyclin-dependent kinase inhibitor, p21 (cip-1/waf-1), which is induced by TGF-β1 in the prostate, was also influenced by neonatal estrogenization. Cellular hyperplasia is promoted by either the effects of the growth-stimulatory factors, or dysfunctional growth restraint by factors such as TGF-β. Available evidence indicates that the expression of TGF-β1 is regulated by estrogens and, hence, may be influenced by phytoestrogens.

Molecular events which ultimately control the expression of androgen receptor in the epithelial cells of the adult prostate may therefore be programmed early in life, possibly not genetically and probably before birth. Professor Leland Chung[77] emphasizes that these early programming events and imprinting actions are irreversible. Professor Don Coffey[78], long interested in steroid 'imprinting' and its influence on enhanced responsiveness to steroid-mediated signalling pathways in later life, has emphasized that it may even occur just prior to adolescence when the protective influence of phytoestrogens may invoke their maximal influence.

Some other dietary factors that may influence prostate cancer

Throughout this chapter, there may be a somewhat biased approach to the potential protective value of isoflavonoids, flavonoids and lignans. But a much wider range of dietary factors could equally exercise cancer restraint, and a concerted research endeavor is now dedicated to the identification of the many and varied constituents of foodstuffs that may have a biological role in cancer prevention, the keyword for the 2000s.

The concept of prevention is not new. During the 1980s, Wattenberg[79] described a wide range of dietary constituents which were believed to be protective against cancer, including various indoles, dithiolthiones, indole-3-carbinol and aromatic isothiocyanates, products of cruciferous vegetables such as cabbage, cauliflower, Brussels sprouts and broccoli. It was considered that they prevented genotoxic agents reaching their target sites. Such compounds were also believed to influence the metabolism of estrogens[80,81], especially 2- and 16-hydroxylated estrogens. Simply stated, 16α-hydroxylation of estrone (E_1) was related to increased risk of spontaneous mammary cancer, 16α-OHE$_1$ promoting *wnt*-1 oncogene expression in mammary

epithelium, and 16-hydroxylation being elevated after exposure of mammary tissue to the carcinogen dimethylbenz(a)anthracene (DMBA). Moreover, 16α-OHE$_1$ induced c-*ras*, *erb*-B2, c-*myc* and c-*jun* proto-oncogene activity and enhanced cell proliferation. Essentially, 16-hydroxylation of estrogens relates to cancer initiation, whereas 2-hydroxylation is associated with suppression[80,81]. Indole-3-carbinol, a constituent of cruciferous vegetables, is a potent inducer of C2-hydroxylase. Moreover, 2-methoxyestradiol, like genistein, inhibits angiogenesis, and people who produce equol (Figure 5) have a higher 2-OHE$_1$/16-OHE$_1$ ratio in urine[82]. As Bradlow and colleagues state[82], '2-OHE$_1$ is the good estrogen'!

Other dietary constituents promote interest. Certain organosulfur constituents of the allium vegetables, garlic, chives, leeks and onion oils (Figure 14), such as alliin, or the diallyl sulfides, have been reported to inhibit carcinogenesis, but more specifically, cancer of the colon. Noteworthy also is that garlic and chives contain substantial levels of secoisolariciresinol, precursor of the lignan enterodiol.

Certain components of tea inhibit tumorigenesis, with extracts of green or black tea in drinking water suppressing the development of lung cancer in experimental animals to which the potent tobacco carcinogen, 4-(methylnitrosamino)-1-(3-pyridyl)-1-butanone (NNK) had been administered[83]. The polyphenols, epigallocatechin and epigallocatechin-3-gallate (Figure 12), in tea are effective antioxidants. Black tea also has a high content of quercetin, which constitutes 75% of the daily 20 mg total flavonoid intake of Dutch people. There are other polyphenols in tea, including phenolic acids, theaflavins and thearubigens, and infusion of green tea with hot water also liberates substantial amounts of secoisolariciresinol and matairesinol, plant precursors of enterolactone.

Peto and colleagues[84] believed that the protective role of β-carotene relates to its antioxidant capacity to 'scavenge for free radicals'. The normal processing of molecular oxygen can give rise to the free radical, superoxide, which can damage DNA. Cancer can be

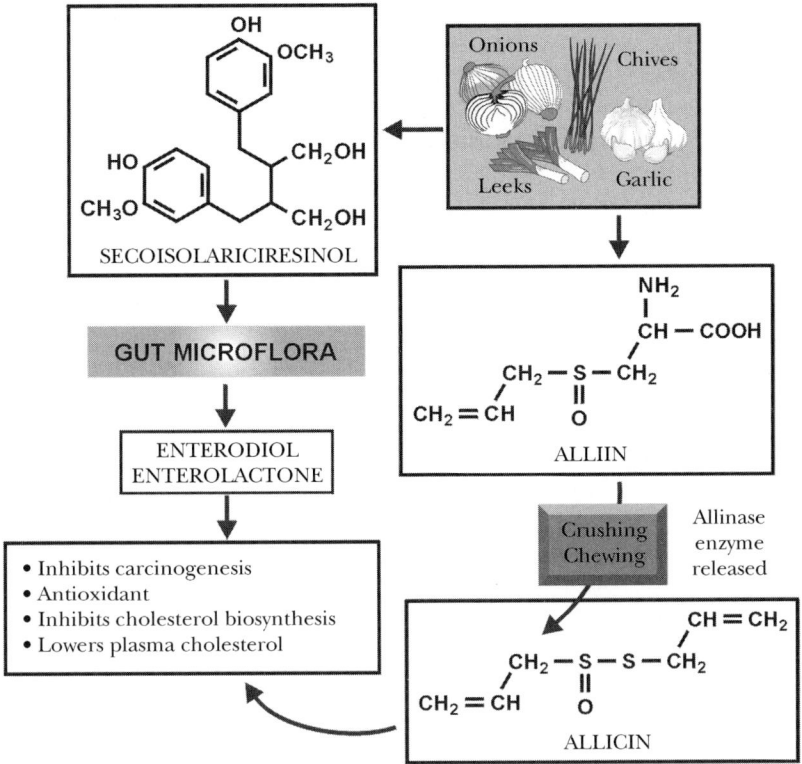

Figure 14 Organosulfur constituents of allium vegetables

inhibited[61] by antioxidants, which prevent the formation of free radicals. Selenium acts as a catalyst in the glutathione peroxidase- and catalase-regulated reactions involved in removing from tissues the hydrogen peroxide that is formed as part of the protective effect of antioxidants[2]. A recent study[85] indicated that men with high body levels of selenium were at lower risk of developing prostate cancer. A daily intake of 86 μg was seen as being in the lower range of selenium intake, and 159 μg each day as being in the higher range. Selenium, an essential trace element found principally in fish, meat and grains, enters the food chain from soil to plants. The possibility that selenium may be protective against cancer was suggested more than 30 years ago[86], but subsequent epidemiological studies failed to provide unequivocal support. More recent investigations[87] have now established a protective effect on the risk of prostate cancer following selenium supple-

mentation. In the UK, it is suggested that the daily intake may be as low as 30–40 μg. However, interest centers on the USA and a trial to evaluate the protective effect on prostate cancer risk of a daily 200-μg selenium supplementation to the diet[88].

Dietary vitamins

Epidemiological studies directed towards the protective value of dietary vitamins have been fraught with difficulties, and the data are somewhat equivocal. For example, in a meta-analysis[89] of the results from case–control studies on the risk of breast cancer and the consumption of major nutrients, a consistent protective effect was found for 'fruit and vegetable intake'. Vitamin C was recognized as the most consistent and statistically significant factor. Conversely, another review[90] concluded that the association between vitamin C and breast cancer risk was limited and inconsistent, but, none the less, a modest, protective effect of vitamin A was recognized. To compound the inconsistency, however, results from the US Nurses' Health Study[91] found no association between the intake of vitamin C, vitamin E or β-carotene and cancer risk. From this study, however, a protective effect of vitamin A was identified.

Boyle and colleagues[92] urge caution regarding conclusions derived from vitamin supplementation studies, an attitude well supported by recent data suggesting that prostate cancer incidence increases with increasing intake of β-carotene[93]. The diet of 29 133 Finnish male smokers was supplemented with vitamin antioxidants, essentially vitamin E and β-carotene (Figure 15). The administration of β-carotene

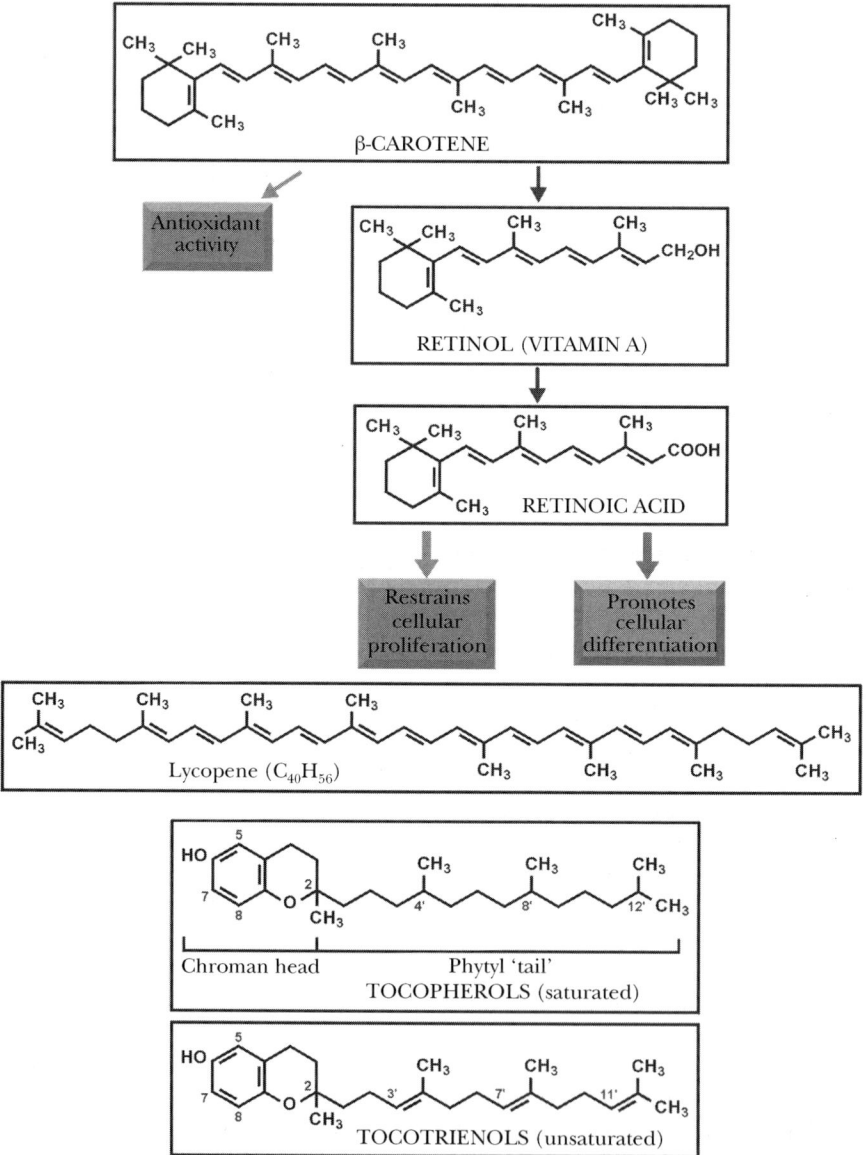

Figure 15 Chemical structures of some of the potentially important vitamin constituents of diet

revealed 138 cases of prostate cancer relative to 112 in the placebo group, whereas conversely, among men receiving α-tocopherol, vitamin E, 99 cases of prostate cancer were reported compared with 151 in men receiving placebo. The study suggests that vitamin E would appear to be protective against prostate cancer, but β-carotene not so.

Vitamin A, retinoids and retinoic acid

Vitamin A is essential for normal cellular growth and differentiation, essentially restraining cell proliferation and promoting differentiation. The synthetic analogs, the retinoids, manifest similar characteristics and have potential as anticancer agents. It is the β-carotene from vegetables and fruits that is generally recognized as the major human source of vitamin A (Figure 15). Schroeder's group[94] have described an increased prostate cancer risk associated with a decreased serum vitamin A concentration. Recent interest has centered on lycopene, another retinoid (Figure 15) that is found in tomatoes and is responsible for the red coloration. Lycopene is released by cooking and subsequent processing of tomatoes, whereas uncooked raw tomatoes are a poorer source. Lycopene is now recognized as one of the potentially valuable antioxidants that would also confer significant protection against free-radical tissue damage[95].

Roberts and Sporn[96] reviewed the evidence for the influence of retinoids and retinoic acid receptors (RARs) on physiological processes. The retinoic acid–RAR complex would appear to antagonize the biological actions of the Fos–Jun heterodimer by protein–protein interactions (Figure 9). These subtle protein–protein interactions provide another insight into the complexity of growth regulation, the cross-talk between the signalling pathways is clearly of importance with regard to the fine-tuning of growth control. Retinoic acid inhibits the expression of ER-responsive genes, down-regulating TGF-β1 expression by antagonizing Fos–Jun dimer (AP-1) activity (Figure 9).

Vitamin D and endocrine cancer

Vitamin D intake relates to prostate cancer risk[97]. A study considered relevant by Boyle and colleagues[14] involved a cohort of 250 000 men, among whom 90 cases of prostate cancer were identified in African–American men and a similar number in Caucasians. Levels of 1,25-dihydroxyvitamin D_3 (1,25-diOH-VitD$_3$) in stored serum were compared with those in control samples. The levels were reported to be a significant 1.81 pg/ml lower than in controls. Although prostate cancer risk decreased with higher levels of the vitamin, it was noteworthy that the risk factor related to palpable tumors, not incidental cancer identified at prostatectomy.

The skin is the only source of vitamin D_3, where 7-dehydrocholesterol is converted by solar UV radiation to the provitamin D_3 (Figure 16). Thermal isomerization of the provitamin D_3 to vitamin D_3 occurs in the epidermis, from where the vitamin enters the blood. In the liver, vitamin D_3 is 25-hydroxylated and this molecule is then converted, primarily in the kidney, to 1,25-diOH-VitD$_3$, the biologically potent metabolite. Its biological effects, mediated[98] through its receptor protein (VDR), involve the suppression of cell proliferation by inhibition of the c-*myc* proto-oncogene, actions similar to those described for retinoic acid (Figure 9). Both VDR and RAR can also regulate transcription by association with genomic recognition sites, essentially nucleotide sequences composed of estrogen response element (ERE) half sites, an -AGGTCA-sequence repeated along the nucleotide chain.

Red wine, flavonoids and disease prevention

Campaigns directed towards cancer prevention can tend to focus attention on the gloomy aspects of life, but on a brighter note is the evidence that a moderate 'alcohol' intake provides health gain. Although possibly an anathema to many who promote the benefits of a healthy diet devoted to seven helpings of

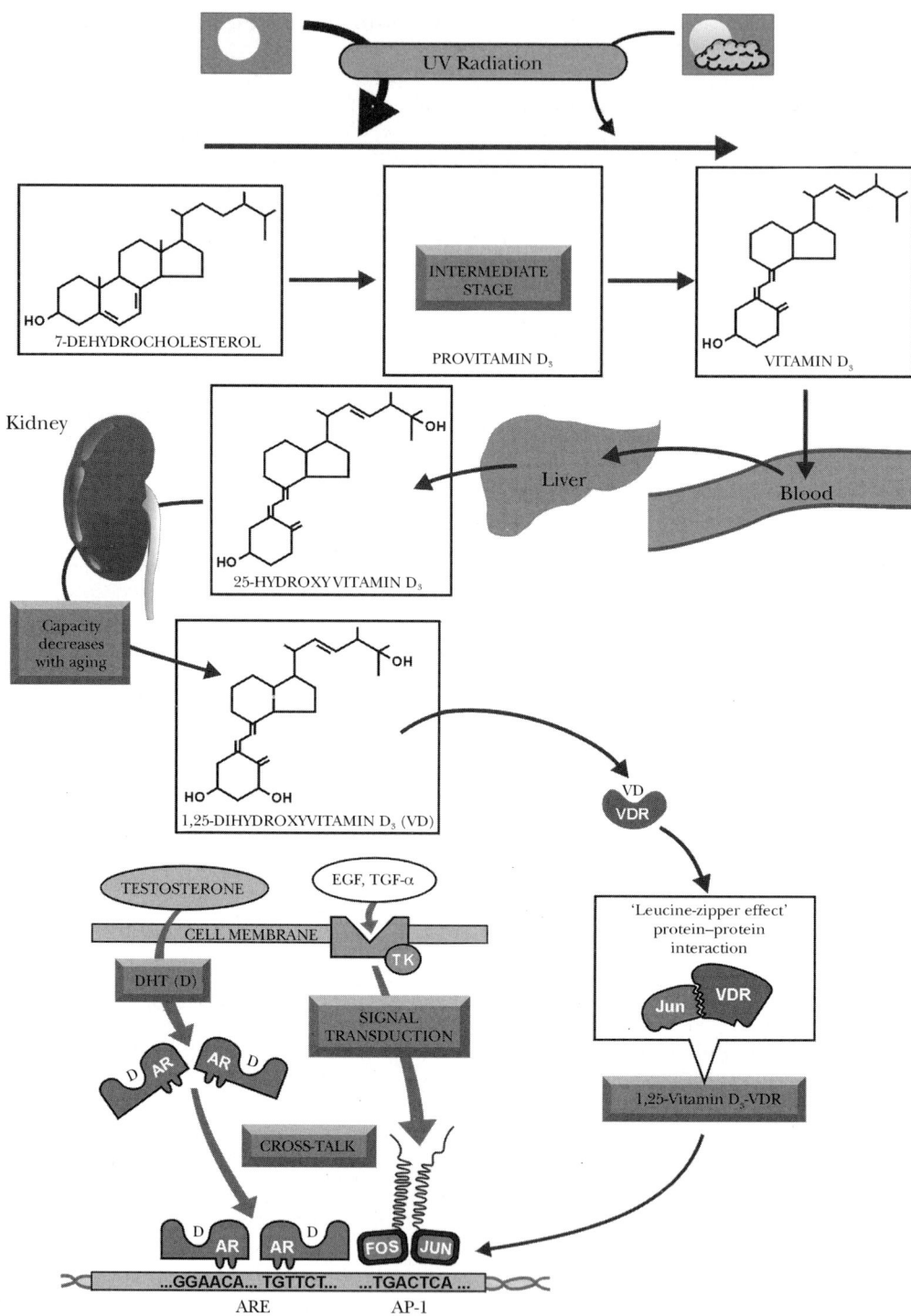

Figure 16 Stages in the production of the biologically active 1,25-dihydroxyvitamin D_3. EGF, epidermal growth factor; TGF, transforming growth factor; TK, tyrosine-specific protein kinase; DHT, dihydrotestosterone; AR, androgen receptor; VDR, vitamin D receptor; ARE, androgen response element; AP-1, activation protein-1

vegetables each day, adequate fruit, little red meat and much exercise, some evidence has accrued[99] supporting the value of a moderate daily amount of 'alcohol', particularly with regard to coronary heart disease. It is known that red wine, for example, contains substantial levels of polyphenolic flavonoids. Consumption of red wine, with its inherent antioxidant activity, has classically been given the credit for the paradoxical relationship between the high fat intake of many regions of France, particularly the Dordogne region, and a remarkably low incidence of coronary heart disease, certainly no greater than that in the British Isles. This 'French paradox' has been related to the antioxidants of red wine, certain flavonoids which inhibit low-density lipoprotein (LDL) peroxidation.

Controversy surrounds the benefits of red wine and its constituents, but a recent, comprehensive and fascinating treatise on the subject has done much to rectify the problem, and the review[100] provides an appraisal of 'wine as a biological fluid'. It indicates that wine has played an integral part in man's cultural life since ancient times, a dietary constituent that prevented disease and extended the span of life.

Catechins are the most common flavonoids in red wine (Figure 12), as well as quercetin, kaempferol and myricetin and the anthocyanins, constituents relating to the quality of wine, that are derived from skins, seeds and stems of the fruit. Also important are the proanthocyanidins, proven antioxidants, probably up to 30-fold better than vitamins E and C. Interest also centers on a stilbene molecule in wine, referred to as resveratrol (Figure 17). In plant biology, resveratrol prevents fungal infections. In man, it inhibits LDL peroxidation, has anti-inflammatory effects, prevents platelet aggregation, suppresses certain animal model cancers and, moreover, blocks the binding of estradiol to the ER, and suppresses the transcription of estrogen-responsive reporter genes in human breast cancer cells.

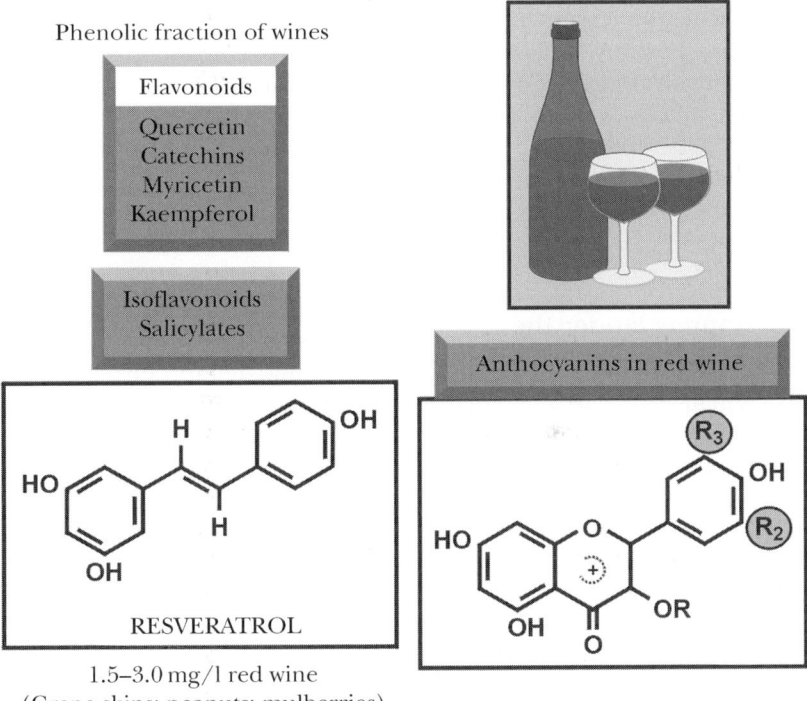

Figure 17 Some potentially valuable constituents of red wine

Although somewhat controversial, it seems that wine also contains a high content of salicylic acid and its metabolites[2], an amount equivalent per liter that is twice the daily dose of aspirin (30 mg/day) frequently recommended these days to sustain cardiovascular patency. It may be that the synergistic effects of both salicylic acid and the flavonoids of wine play an effective role in human health. There are sound arguments against elderly folk drinking alcohol, with fractures caused by falling and the promotion of hemorrhagic stroke generally being put forward. A recent report[101], however, emphasizes possible benefits of wine for the prevention of age-related vision loss, or macular degeneration, based on the antioxidant's influence on 'platelet aggregability'. Well accepted, however, is the U-shaped relationship between alcohol and mortality, with heavy drinkers and abstainers having higher mortality rates than moderate drinkers. The moderate drinker seems to have better health. Some would confidently assert that two glasses of red wine each day will provide approximately 40% of the total antioxidant content of a healthy diet, together with resveratrol, which is not present in fruit and vegetables. Possibly only English 'tea-time' can offer the advantages provided by wine, although coffee increases plasma enterolactone levels[102] and Adlercreutz and Mazur[12] reveal that certain beers contain significant amounts of biologically active isoflavonoids.

The process of isoprenylation: the tocotrienols

Reference has been made to the health benefits of fruit. One particular constituent of citrus fruit oils, d-limonene, has a protective effect against cancer. It inhibits both 3-hydroxymethylglutaryl coenzyme A (HMG-CoA) reductase[103], an enzyme involved in mevalonic acid and cholesterol synthesis (Figure 18), as well as enzymes concerned with the isoprenylation of the p21 Ras oncogene protein. Isoprenylation is important with regard to Ras guanosine triphosphate (GTP)ase signalling and intracellular trafficking, with the p21 Ras proteins involved in the transfer of isoprene residues,

either C15-farnesyl or C20-geranylgeranyl units, to cystein 186 of the COOH-terminal region of the protein, increasing its lipophobic nature. Ras mutations are implicated in many cancers, and signalling cross-talk involving the Rho proteins and cytoskeletal structure is associated with cell adhesion and motility, and, like Ras, Rho proteins, part of the GTPase family, are isoprenylated.

Inhibition of isoprenylation offers a new approach to the management of cancer. Transfection of the p21 mutated Ras oncogene protein into mouse fibroblasts in the presence of insulin and IGF-I promotes transformation and enhanced cell proliferation. Of interest with regard to isoprenylation is the recent report[104] of a new type of phytoestrogen, the prenyl-flavonoids, in particular isopentenyl-naringenin, which acts as an estrogen agonist. Certain isoprenoid constituents of fruits, vegetables and cereal grains, various tocotrienols (Figure 15), suppress the growth of experimental melanomas. Tocotrienols[105] are natural analogs of tocopherol and, as with statins, the inhibitory action of these isoprenoids is directed towards HMG-CoA reductase. The tocotrienols induce apoptosis and inhibit DNA synthesis. Again, the information focuses attention on the potential health benefits of the diverse range of constituents of fruits, vegetables and grains.

There can be little doubt that the potential health benefits of the various dietary factors and their potential protective role against cancer now provides a unique challenge. The relationship is complex, and information in the media proffering dietary advice is immense. Amidst the 'euphoria' that this promotes, the pragmatic scientific approach must first endeavor to identify and measure the potentially important constituents in biological tissues and fluids. Second, the precise biological role that such constituents exercise must be determined. This will require some time, and it is interesting that in recent weeks a Danish group[106] has stated that 'neither amount nor type of alcohol is associated with the risk of prostate cancer', whereas an American study[107] has indicated that resveratrol, but not DES, induced caspase-mediated apoptosis!

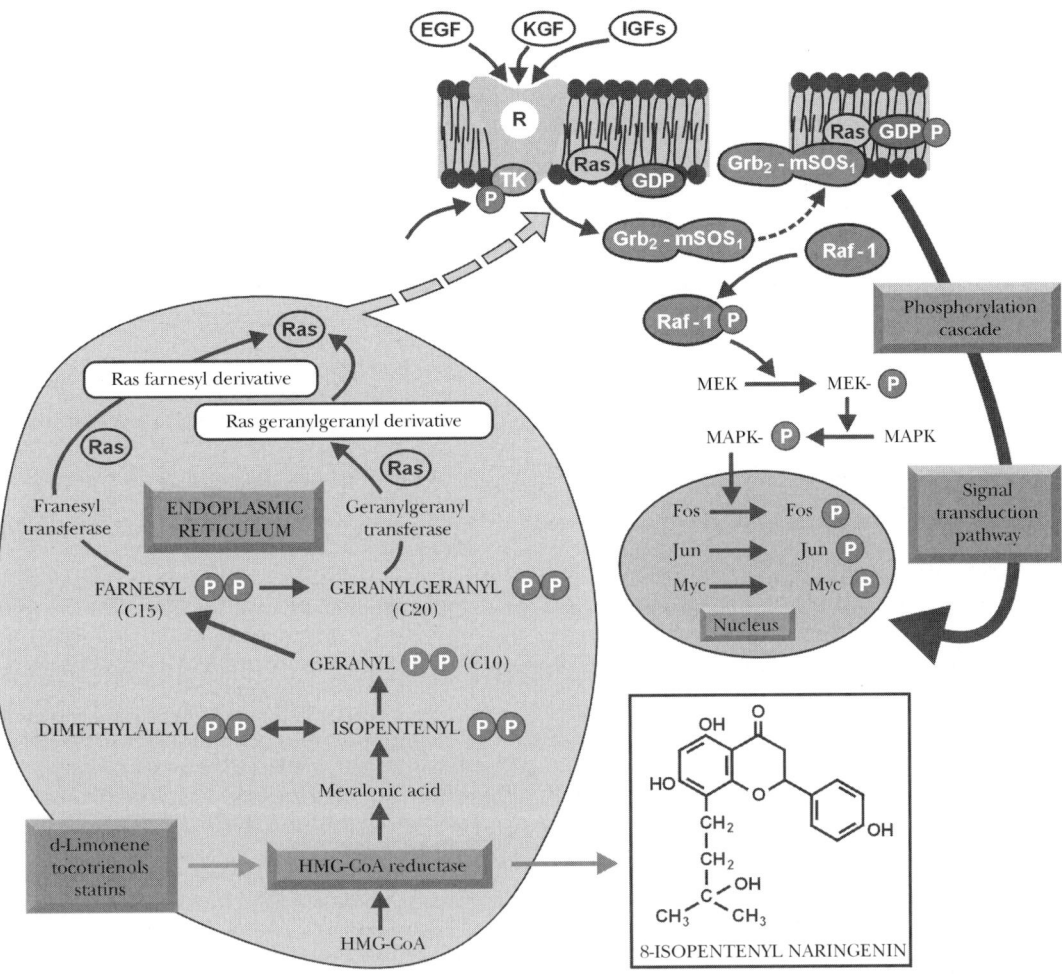

8-ISOPENTENYL NARINGENIN

Figure 18 Isoprenylation of the Ras protein with products originating from hydroxymethylglutaryl coenzyme A (HMG-CoA) and mevalonic acid. These pathways, involving 5-C isoprenyl units, are also concerned with cholesterol synthesis. The inhibition of HMG-CoA reductase is illustrated, as is the isoprenylation of the flavonoid, naringenin. The complex intracellular signalling pathways and the phosphorylation cascade are also shown. EGF, epidermal growth factor; KGF, keratinocyte growth factor; IGF, insulin-like growth factor; R, receptor; TK, tyrosine-specific protein kinase; P, phosphorylation; ATP, adenosine triphosphate; GDP, guanosine diphosphate; MAPK, mitogen-activated protein kinase; Grb$_2$, growth factor receptor bound protein; mSOS, mammalian son-of-sevenless; MEK, mitogen activated protein signal-regulated kinase kinase; Raf-1, serine/threonin kinase

Acknowledgements

The authors wish to thank David Griffiths (CompGraphics Services, Cardiff, UK) for permission to use the illustrations presented in this review, some of which have appeared in a previous review[2], *Oestrogens, Phyto-oestrogens and the Pathogenesis of Prostatic Disease*, Martin Dunitz, London, 2002.

References

1. Coltman CA Jr, Thompson IM, Feigl P. Prostate Cancer Prevention Trial (PCPT) update. *Eur Urol* 1999;35:544–7
2. Griffiths K, Denis LJ, Turkes A. *Oestrogens, Phyto-oestrogens and the Pathogenesis of Prostatic Disease.* London: Martin Dunitz, 2002
3. Kuiper GGJM, Enmark E, Pelto-Huikko M, *et al.* Cloning of a novel estrogen receptor expressed in rat prostate and ovary. *Proc Natl Acad Sci USA* 1996;93:5925–30
4. Pettersson K, Gustafsson JA. Role of estrogen receptor β in estrogen action. *Annu Rev Physiol* 2001;63:165–92
5. Kuiper GGJM, Carlsson B, Grandien J, *et al.* Comparison of the ligand binding specificity and transcript tissue distribution of estrogen receptors α and β. *Endocrinology* 1997;138:863–70
6. Huggins C. Introduction. In Vollmer EP, Kauffmann G, eds. *Biology of the Prostate and Related Tissues.* Monograph 12, National Cancer Institute. Washington: US Department of Health, Education and Welfare, 1963:xi–xii
7. World Cancer Research Fund. *Food, Nutrition and the Prevention of Cancer: A Global Perspective.* Manasha, USA: Banta Book Group,1997
8. Adlercreutz H, Mazur W. Phyto-oestrogens and western diseases. *Ann Med* 1997;29:95–120
9. Potter JD, Steinmetz K. Vegetables, fruit and phytoestrogens as preventive agents. In Stewart BW, McGregor D, Kleihues P, eds. *Principles of Chemoprevention.* Lyon: IARC Scientific Publications, 1996:61–90
10. Kolonel LN, Nomura AMY, Hinds MW, *et al.* Role of diet in cancer incidence in Hawaii. *Cancer Res* 1983;43(Suppl):2397s–402s
11. Wu AH, Ziegler RG, Horn-Ross PL, *et al.* Tofu and risk of breast cancer in Asian–Americans. *Cancer Epidemiol Biomarkers Prev* 1995;5:901–6
12. Adlercreutz H. Phyto-oestrogens and cancer. *Lancet Oncology* 2002;3:364–73
13. Zondek B. Mass excretion of oestrogenic hormone in the urine of the stallion. *Nature (London)* 1934;133:209–11
14. Boyle P, Napalkov P, Barry MJ, *et al.* Epidemiology and natural history of prostate cancer. In Murphy G, Denis L, Chatelain C, *et al.*, eds. *First International Consultation on Prostate Cancer.* Paris: SCI, 1997:1–29
15. Griffiths K. Estrogens and prostatic disease. International Prostate Health Council Study Group. *Prostate* 2000;45:87–100
16. Hirayama T. A large scale cohort study on cancer risks by diet – with special reference to the risk reducing effects of green–yellow vegetable consumption. In Hayashi Y, Nagano M, Sigimura T, eds. *Diet, Nutrition and Cancer.* Tokyo/Utrecht: Japan Science Society Press/ VNU Science Press, 1986:41–53
17. Shutt DA, Cox RI. Steroid and phyto-oestrogen binding to sheep uterine receptors *in vitro*. *J Endocrinol* 1972;52:299–310
18. Rao CBS, ed. *The Chemistry of Lignans.* Waltair, India: Andra University Press and Publications, 1978
19. Kilkkinen A, Pietinen P, Klaukka T, *et al.* Use of oral antmicrobials decreases serum enterolactone concentration. *Am J Epidemiol* 2002;155:472–3
20. Kuhnau J. The flavonoids. A class of semi-essential food components: their role in human nutrition. *World Rev Nutr Diet* 1976;24:117–91
21. Waladkhani A, Clemens MR. Effect of dietary phytochemicals on cancer development [Review]. *Int J Mol Med* 1998;1:747–53
22. Bentsath A, Rusznyak S, Szent-Gyorgyi A. Vitamin P. *Nature (London)* 1937;139:326–7
23. Miksicek RJ. Estrogenic flavonoids: structural requirements for biological activity. *Proc Soc Exp Biol Med* 1995;208:440–50
24. Burrows H, Horning ES, eds. *Oestrogens and Neoplasia.* Oxford: Blackwell Scientific Publications, 1952
25. Burrows H. The influence of oestrogens on tissue growth. In Burrows H, Horning ES, eds. *Oestrogens and Neoplasia.* Oxford: Blackwell Scientific Publications, 1952:26–42
26. Doisy EA, Eler CD, Thayer SA. Preparation of the crystalline ovarian hormone from the urine of pregnant women. *J Biol Chem* 1931;24:499–509
27. De Jongh SE. Der Einfluss von Geschlechtshormonen auf die Prostata und ihre Umgebung bei der Maus. *Acta Brev Neerl* 1935;5:28
28. Griffiths K, Cockett ATK, Coffey DS, *et al.* Regulation of prostate growth. In Denis LJ, Cockett ATK, Chatelain C, *et al.*, eds. *The 4th International Consultation on BPH.* Paris: SCI, 1998:85–128
29. McGuire MS, Fair WR. Prostate cancer and diet: investigations, interventions and future considerations. *Mol Urol* 1997;1:3–9
30. Rich AR. On frequency of occurrence of occult carcinoma of the prostate. *J Urol* 1935;33:215–23
31. Oota K, Misu Y. A study of latent carcinoma of the prostate in Japanese. *J Urol* 1958;50:680–710

32. Breslow N, Chan CE, Dhom G, *et al.* Latent carcinoma of the prostate at autopsy in seven areas. *Int J Cancer* 1977;20:680–8

33. Yatani R, Shiraishi T, Akazaki K, *et al.* Incidental prostatic carcinoma: morphometry correlated with histological grade. *Virchow's Arch A Pathol Anat Histopathol* 1986;409:395–405

34. Sakr WA, Grignon DJ, Haas GP, *et al.* Age and racial distribution of prostatic intraepithelial neoplasia. *Eur Urol* 1996;30:138–44

35. Sakr WA. Prostatic intraepithelial neoplasia: a marker for high-risk groups and a potential target for chemoprevention. In Schulman CC, Kelloff GJ, eds. *Strategies for the Chemoprevention of Prostate Cancer.* Basel: Karger, 1999:474–8

36. Sakr WA, Haas GP, Cassin BF, *et al.* The frequency of carcinoma and intraepithelial neoplasia of the prostate in young male patients. *J Urol* 1993;150:379–85

37. Berry SJ, Coffey DS, Walsh PC, *et al.* The development of human benign prostatic hyperplasia with age. *J Urol* 1984;132:474–9

38. Isaacs JT, Coffey DS. Etiology and disease process of benign prostatic hyperplasia. *Prostate* 1989;2(Suppl):33–50

39. McNeal JE. Origin and evolution of benign prostatic enlargement. *Invest Urol* 1978;15:340–5

40. Tzukerman MT, Esty A, Santiso-Mere D, *et al.* Human estrogen receptor transactivational capacity is determined by both cellular and promoter content and mediated by two functionally distinct intramolecular regions. *Mol Endocrinol* 1994;8:21–30

41. Kraus WL, McInerny EM, Katzenellenbogen BS. Ligand-dependent, transcriptionally productive association of the amino- and carboxy-terminal regions of a steroid hormone nuclear receptor. *Proc Natl Acad Sci USA* 1995;92:12314–18

42. Tzukeman MT, Esty A, Santiso-Mere D, *et al.* Human estrogen receptor transcriptional capacity is determined by both cellular and promoter context and mediated by functionally distict intramolecular regions. *Mol Endocrinol* 1994;8:21–30

43. Shu XO, Jin F, Dai Q, *et al.* Soyfood intake during adolescence and subsequent risk of breast cancer among Chinese women. *Cancer Epidemiol Biomarkers Prev* 2001;10:483–8

44. Nagata C, Kabuto M, Kurisu Y, *et al.* Decreased serum estradiol concentration associated with high dietary intake of soya products in premenopausal Japanese women. *Nutr Cancer* 1997;29:228–33

45. Evans BAJ, Griffiths K, Morton MS. Inhibition of 5α-reductase and 17β-hydroxysteroid dehydrogenase in genital skin fibroblasts by dietary lignans and isoflavonoids. *J Endocrinol* 1995;147:295–302

46. Imperato-McGinley J, Guerrero L, Gautier T, *et al.* Steroid 5α-reductase deficiency in man: an inherited form of male pseudohermaphroditism. *Science* 1974;186:1213–15

47. Ross RK, Bernstein L, Lobo RA, *et al.* 5-α-Reductase activity and risk of prostate cancer among Japanese and US white and black males. *Lancet* 1992;339:887–9

48. Woodburn JR, Morris CQ, Kelly H, *et al.* EGF receptor tyrosine kinase inhibitors as anti-cancer agents: preclinical and early clinical profile of ZD1839. *Cell Mol Biol Lett* 1998;3:348–9

49. Akiyama T, Ishida J, Nakagawa S, *et al.* Genistein, a specific inhibitor of tyrosine-specific protein kinases. *J Biol Chem* 1987;262:5592–5

50. Kuo ML, Lin JK, Huang TS, *et al.* Reversion of the transformed phenotypes of v-H-*ras* NIH3T3 cells by flavonoids through attenuating the content of phosphotyrosine. *Cancer Lett* 1994;87:91–7

51. Hanagan D, Folkman J. Patterns and emerging mechanisms of the angiogenic switch during tumorigenesis. *Cell* 1996;86:801–10

52. Fotsis T, Pepper MS, Montesano R, *et al.* Phyto-estrogens and inhibition of angio-genesis. *Baillière's Clin Endocrinol Metab* 1996;12:649–66

53. Uckun FM, Evans WE, Forsyth CJ, *et al.* Biotherapy of B-cell precursor leukaemia by targeting genistein to CD19-associated tyrosine kinases. *Science* 1995;267:886–91

54. Uckun FM, Naria RK, Zeren T, *et al. In vivo* toxicity, pharmacokinetics and anticancer activity of genistein linked to recombinant human epidermal growth factor. *Clin Cancer Res* 1998;4:1125–34

55. Anderson JJB, Anthony M, Messina M, *et al.* Effects of phyto-oestrogens on tissues. *Nutr Res Rev* 1999;12:75–116

56. Hempstock J, Kavanagh JP, George NJ. Growth inhibition of prostate cell lines *in vitro* by phyto-oestrogens. *Br J Urol* 1998;82:560–3

57. Geller J, Sionit L, Partido C, *et al.* Genistein inhibits the growth of human patient BPH and prostate cancer in histoculture. *Prostate* 1998;34:75–9

58. McCabe MJ Jr, Orrenius S. Genistein induces apoptosis in immature human thymocytes by inhibiting topoisomerase-II. *Biochem Biophys Res Commun* 1993;194:944–50

59. Constantinou A, Mehta R, Runyan C, *et al.* Flavonoids as DNA topoisomerase antagonists and poisons: structure–activity relationships. *J Nat Prod* 1995;58:217–25

60. Griffiths K, Turkes A, Denis LJ. Oestrogens and the prostate gland. In Menchini Fabris GF, ed. *The Human Testis: Its Role in Reproduction and Sexuality.* Bologna: Monduzzi Editore, 1999: 163–72

61. Halliwell B, Cross CE, Gutteridge JMC. Free radicals, antioxidants and human disease: where are we now? *J Lab Clin Med* 1992; 119:598–620

62. Bylund A, Zhang JX, Bergh A, *et al.* Rye bran and soy protein delay growth and increase apoptosis of human LNCaP prostate adenocarcinoma in nude mice. *Prostate* 2000;42:304–14

63. Conney AH, Buening MK, Pantuck EJ, *et al.* Regulation of human drug metabolism by dietary factors. *Ciba Found Symp* 1980;76:147–67

64. Shi ST, Wang ZY, Smith TJ, *et al.* Effects of green tea and black tea on 4-(methylnitrosoamino)-1-(3-pyridyl)-1-butanone bioactivation, DNA methylation and lung tumorigenesis in A/J mice. *Cancer Res* 1994;54:4641–7

65. Giroldi LA, Schalken JA. Decreased expression of the intercellular adhesion molecule E-cadherin in prostate cancer: biological significance and clinical implications. *Cancer Metastasis Rev* 1993;12:29–37

66. Rotkin ID. Epidemiology of benign prostatic hypertrophy: review and speculations. In Grayhack JT, Wilson JD, Saherbenske MJ, eds. *Benign Prostatic Hyperplasia.* DHEW Publications No. (NIH) 76–1113. Washington: US Department of Health, Education and Welfare, 1976:105–17

67. Connell WK. Hernia in Africans. *Br J Surg* 1930;18:16–19

68. Lamartiniere CA. Protection against breast cancer with genistein: a component of soy. *Am J Clin Nutr* 2000;71:1705S–7S

69. Herbst AL, Poskanzer DC, Robboy SJ, *et al.* Prenatal exposure to stilboestrol: a prospective comparison of exposed female offspring with unexposed controls. *N Engl J Med* 1975;292: 334–9

70. DeChiara TM, Robertson EJ, Efstratiadis A. Parental imprinting of the mouse insulin-like growth factor II gene. *Cell* 1991;64:849–59

71. Newbold RR, McLauchlan JA. Diethylstilbo-estrol-associated defects in murine genital tract development. In McLauchlan JA, ed. *Estrogens in the Environment: Influences on Development.* New York: Elsevier, North-Holland, 1985:288–318

72. Henderson BE, Bernstein L, Ross RK, *et al.* The early *in utero* oestrogen and testosterone environment of blacks and whites: potential effects on male offspring. *Br J Cancer* 1988;57: 216–18

73. Wilkins RJ. Genomic imprinting and carcinogenesis. *Lancet* 1988;1:329–31

74. Newbold RR, Pentecost BT, Yamashita S, *et al.* Female gene expression in the seminal vesicle of mice after prenatal exposure to diethylstilboestrol. *Endocrinology* 1989;124:2568–74

75. Chang WY, Birch L, Woodham C, *et al.* Neonatal estrogen exposure alters the transforming growth factor-β signaling system in the developing rat prostate and blocks the transient p21 (cip1/waf1) expression associated with epithelial differentiation. *Endocrinology* 1999; 140:2801–13

76. Chang WY, Wilson MJ, Birch L, *et al.* Neonatal estrogen stimulates proliferation of periductal fibroblasts and alters the extracellular matrix composition in the rat prostate. *Endocrinology* 1999;140:405–15

77. Chung LWK, MacFadden DK. Sex steroids imprinting and prostatic growth. *Invest Urol* 1980;17:337–42

78. Naslund M, Coffey D. The differential effects of neonatal androgen, estrogen and progesterone on adult rat prostate growth. *J Urol* 1986; 136:1136–40

79. Wattenberg LW. Inhibition of neoplasia by minor dietary constituents. *Cancer Res* 1983;43: 2448s–53s

80. Telang NT, Suto A, Wong GY, *et al.* Induction by estrogen metabolite 16α-hydroxyestrone of genotoxic damage and aberrant proliferation in mouse mammary epithelial cells. *J Natl Cancer Inst* 1992;84:634–6

81. Fotsis T, Zhang Y, Pepper MS, *et al.* The endogenous oestrogen metabolite 2-methoxyo-estradiol inhibits angiogenesis and suppresses tumour growth. *Nature (London)* 1994;368: 237–9

82. Bradlow HI, Telang NT, Sepkovic DW, *et al.* 2-Hydroxyoestrone: the good estrogen. *J Endocrinol* 1996;150(Suppl):S259–65

83. Yang CS, Hong J-Y, Wang Z-Y. Inhibition of nitrosamine-induced tumorigenesis by diallyl sulphide and tea. In Waldron KW, Johnson IT, Fenwick GR, eds. *Food and Cancer Prevention: Chemical and Biological Aspects.* Letchworth, UK: Royal Society of Chemistry, 1993:247–52

84. Peto R, Doll R, Buckley JD, *et al.* Can dietary β-carotene materially reduce human cancer rates? *Nature (London)* 1981;290:201–8

85. Yoshizawa K, Willett WC, Morris SJ, *et al.* Study of prediagnostic selenium levels in toenails and the risk of advanced prostate cancer. *J Natl Cancer Inst* 1998;90:1219–24

86. Shamberger RJ, Frost DV. Possible protective effect of selenium against human cancer. *Can Med Assoc J* 1969;100:682

87. Clark LC, Dalkin B, Krongrad A, *et al.* Decreased incidence of prostate cancer with selenium supplementation: results of a double-blind cancer prevention trial. *Br J Urol* 1998;81:730–4

88. Klein EA, Thompson IM, Lippman SM, *et al.* SELECT: the next prostate cancer prevention trial. Selenium and Vitamin E Cancer Prevention Trial. *J Urol* 2001;166:1311–15

89. Howe GR, Hirohata T, Hislop TG, *et al.* Dietary fat and risk of breast cancer: combined analysis of 12 case–control studies. *J Natl Cancer Inst* 1990;82:561–9

90. Garland M, Willett WC, Manson JE, *et al.* Antioxidant micronutrients and breast cancer. *J Am Coll Nutr* 1993;12:400–11

91. Hunter DJ, Manson J, Colditz GA, *et al.* A prospective study of the intake of vitamins C, E, and A and the risk of breast cancer. *N Engl J Med* 1993;329:234–40

92. Boyle P, Maisonneuve P, Evstififeeva T, *et al.* What is the significance of trends in prostate cancer? In Murphy GP, Khoury S, Chatelain C, *et al.*, eds. *Fourth International Symposium on Recent Advances in Urological Cancer, Diagnosis and Treatment.* Paris: SCI, 1995:51–65

93. Albanes D, Heinonen OP, Huttunen JK, *et al.* Effects of α-tocopherol and β-carotene supplements on cancer incidence in the Alpha-Tocopherol Beta-Carotene Cancer Prevention Study. *Am J Clin Nutr* 1995;62(Suppl): 1427S–30S

94. Hayes RB, Bogdanovicz JFAT, Schroeder FH, *et al.* Serum retinol and prostatic cancer. *Cancer* 1988;62:2021–6

95. Kohimeier L, Kark JD, Gomez-Gracia E, *et al.* Lycopene and myocardial infarction risk in the EURAMIC Study. *Am J Epidemiol* 1997;146: 618–26

96. Roberts AB, Sporn MB. Cellular biology and biochemistry of the retinoids. In Sporn MB, Roberts AB, Goodman DS, eds. *The Retinoids.* Orlando, FL: Academic Press, 1984:209–86

97. Schwartz GG, Hulka BS. Is vitamin D deficiency a risk factor for prostate cancer? *Anticancer Res* 1990;10:1307–11

98. Pike JW. Vitamin D_3 receptors: structure and function in transcription. *Annu Rev Nutr* 1991;11:189–216

99. Kannel WB, Ellison RC. Alcohol and coronary heart disease: the evidence for a protective effect. *Clin Chim Acta* 1996;246:59–76

100. Soleas GJ, Diamandis EP, Goldberg DM. Wine as a biological fluid: history, production and role in disease prevention. *J Clin Lab Anal* 1997;11:287–313

101. Obisesan TO, Hirsch R, Kosoko O, *et al.* Moderate wine consumption is associated with decreased odds of developing age-related macular degeneration in NHANES-1. *J Am Geriatr Soc* 1998;46:1–7

102. Horner NK, Kristal AR, Prunty J, *et al.* Dietary determinants of plasma enterolactone. *Cancer Epidemiol Biomarkers Prev* 2000;11:121–6

103. Crowell PL, Chang RR, Ren Z, *et al.* Selective inhibition of isoprenylation of 21/26 kDa proteins by the anti-carcinogenic *d*-limonene and its metabolites. *J Biol Chem* 1991;266:176–9

104. Miyamoto M, Matsushita Y, Kiyokawa A, *et al.* Prenylflavonoids: a new class of non-steroidal phytoestrogen (Part 2). Estrogenic effects of 8-isopentenylnaringenin on bone metabolism. *Planta Med* 1998;64:516–19

105. Theriault A, Chao JT, Wang Q, *et al.* Tocotrienol: a review of its therapeutic potential. *Clin Biochem* 1999;32:309–19

106. Albertsen K, Gronbaek M. Does amount or type of alcohol influence the risk of prostate cancer? *Prostate* 2002;52:297–304

107. Elliott MS, Beebe SJ. Resveratrol induces apoptosis in LNCaP cells and requires hydroxyl groups to decrease viability in LNCaP and DU145 cells. *Prostate* 2002;52:319–29

Determinants of prostate cancer-specific survival following radiation therapy for patients with clinically localized prostate cancer

43

A. V. D'Amico

Introduction

Prostate-specific antigen (PSA) failure following either radical prostatectomy (RP)[1] or external beam radiation therapy (RT)[2] for patients with clinically localized prostate cancer occurs in approximately 30–50% of cases within 10 years following treatment, and is a great source of anxiety for both patients and physicians. Therefore, in an attempt to identify patients at high risk of failure following RP or RT, investigators have developed pretreatment risk groups[3] and nomograms[4] based on the relative values of time to post-treatment PSA failure following RP or RT. Yet, for whom PSA failure predicts death from prostate cancer remains unanswered. The inability to answer this question has been attributed to inadequate power in databases because of relatively short follow-up and the protracted clinical course of prostate cancer, as well as the competing causes of mortality in this patient population[5].

A second issue related to PSA failure following RT that has had significant ramifications on the patient's quality of life and the overall cost to the health-care system is whether survival is prolonged when salvage hormonal therapy is initiated at, or following, PSA failure at a time when the bone scan is negative as opposed to positive. Unfortunately, owing to patient and physician views on this matter, a randomized trial of early versus delayed hormonal therapy following PSA failure has not been successfully completed.

Therefore, the present study had two goals. The first was to determine whether pretreatment risk groups[3], that have been shown to stratify patients by time to post-treatment PSA failure, could also stratify patients by time to post-treatment prostate cancer-specific death (PCSD). The second was to evaluate whether post-treatment factors could predict time to PCSD following PSA failure. Realizing that previous investigators have shown that both the time interval to PSA failure following RP[6] and the PSA doubling time following RP[6] or RT[7] were predictors of time to distal failure, these factors in addition to the timing of salvage hormonal therapy were included in our analysis.

Patients and methods

Patient selection

Three hundred and eighty-one patients with a diagnosis of clinically localized prostate cancer and treated with external beam RT by a single physician group at a Harvard-associated community-outreach facility (St Anne's Hospital, Fall River, MA) from 1987 to 2000 constituted the study cohort. The median (range) age of the patient population at the time of initial therapy was 73 (49–86) years. The pretreatment clinical characteristics of the entire study cohort and the 94 patients (25%) who sustained PSA failure are listed in Table 1.

Staging, treatment and follow-up

In all cases, staging evaluation involved a history and physical examination including digital rectal examination (DRE), serum PSA and transrectal ultrasound-guided (TRUS) needle biopsy of the prostate, with Gleason score histological grading[8]. The prostate biopsy was performed using an 18-gauge Tru-Cut® needle (Travenol Laboratories, Deerfield, IL) via a transrectal approach. All biopsy material was reviewed and assigned a primary and secondary Gleason grade by a single genitourinary pathologist (Dr A. A. Renshaw, Brigham and Women's Hospital, Boston, USA). Prior to 1996, all patients had a computed tomographic scan of the pelvis and a bone scan. After 1996, patients with both a pretreatment PSA level less than 10 ng/ml and a biopsy Gleason score of 6 or less did not undergo radiological staging owing to the < 1% chance that these studies would reveal metastatic disease[9]. Clinical stage was obtained from DRE findings using the 1992 American Joint Commission on Cancer (AJCC) staging system[10]. Radiological and biopsy information was not used to determine clinical stage. The PSA was obtained on an ambulatory basis within 6 weeks of the start of RT and prior to radiological studies and biopsy. All PSA measurements were made using the Hybritech (San Diego, CA), Tosoh (Foster City, CA) or Abbott (Chicago, IL) assay. PSA values prior to

Table 1 Pretreatment clinical characteristics of the 381 study patients and 94 patients who experienced prostate-specific antigen (PSA) failure

All study patients (*n* = 381)		*Patients with PSA failure* (*n* = 94)	
Low-risk (*n* = 90)		*Low-risk* (*n* = 10)	
PSA ≤ 4 ng/ml	18 (20%)	PSA ≤ 4 ng/ml	0 (0%)
PSA > 4–10 ng/ml	72 (80%)	PSA > 4–10 ng/ml	10 (100%)
Biopsy Gleason 5–6	90 (100%)	Biopsy Gleason 5–6	10 (100%)
1992 Category T1c	50 (56%)	1992 Category T1c	6 (60%)
1992 Category T2a	40 (44%)	1992 Category T2a	4 (40%)
Intermediate-risk (*n* = 173)		*Intermediate-risk* (*n* = 29)	
PSA ≤ 4 ng/ml	11 (6%)	PSA ≤ 4 ng/ml	1 (3%)
PSA > 4–10 ng/ml	72 (42%)	PSA > 4–10 ng/ml	8 (28%)
PSA > 10–20 ng/ml	90 (52%)	PSA > 10–20 ng/ml	20 (69%)
Biopsy Gleason 5–6	43 (25%)*	Biopsy Gleason 5–6	13 (45%)
Biopsy Gleason 7	129 (75%)	Biopsy Gleason 7	16 (55%)
1992 Category T1c	80 (46%)	1992 Category T1c	12 (41%)
1992 Category T2a	51 (30%)	1992 Category T2a	8 (28%)
1992 Category T2b	42 (24%)	1992 Category T2b	9 (31%)
High-risk (*n* = 118)		*High-risk* (*n* = 55)	
PSA ≤ 4 ng/ml	4 (3%)	PSA ≤ 4 ng/ml	0 (0%)
PSA > 4–10 ng/ml	29 (25%)	PSA > 4–10 ng/ml	8 (15%)
PSA > 10–20 ng/ml	25 (21%)	PSA > 10–20 ng/ml	15 (27%)
PSA > 20 ng/ml	60 (51%)	PSA > 20 ng/ml	32 (58%)
Biopsy Gleason 5–6	36 (31%)	Biopsy Gleason 5–6	14 (25%)
Biopsy Gleason 7	40 (34%)	Biopsy Gleason 7	19 (35%)
Biopsy Gleason ≥ 8	42 (35%)	Biopsy Gleason ≥ 8	22 (40%)
1992 Category T1c	26 (22%)	1992 Category T1c	6 (11%)
1992 Category T2a	14 (12%)	1992 Category T2a	7 (13%)
1992 Category T2b	24 (20%)	1992 Category T2b	15 (27%)
1992 Category T2c	54 (46%)	1992 Category T2c	27 (49%)

*One intermediate-risk patient had a biopsy Gleason score of 4; low-risk, PSA ≤ 10 ng/ml and biopsy Gleason score ≤ 6 and 1992 American Joint Commission on Cancer (AJCC) clinical T category T1c or T2a; intermediate-risk, PSA > 10 ng/ml and ≤ 20 ng/ml or biopsy Gleason score 7 or 1992 AJCC clinical T category T2b; high-risk, PSA > 20 ng/ml or biopsy Gleason score ≥ 8 or 1992 AJCC clinical T category T2c

1989 were obtained as part of an American Cancer Society-sponsored screening program.

The treatment was conformal RT starting in 1994; conventional RT was performed prior to 1994. However, a randomized trial of conventional versus conformal RT[11] has not shown a difference in cancer control outcomes. The total median dose (range) delivered to the prostate was 70.4 Gy (69.3–70.4 Gy) after using a 95% normalization. A first course of RT to the prostate and seminal vesicles was prescribed for patients with either a PSA > 10 ng/ml or a biopsy Gleason score of 7 or higher, and the median dose (range) was 45.0 Gy (45.0–50.4 Gy). No patient received neo-adjuvant, concurrent or adjuvant hormonal therapy.

The median follow-up for the entire study cohort of 381 patients was 4 (0.5–13) years using the first day of RT as time zero. The median time interval (range) from diagnosis to start of RT was 2 (1.5–3.5) months. Prior to PSA failure, which was defined using the American Society for Therapeutic Radiology and Oncology (ASTRO) consensus criteria[12], all patients generally had a serum PSA measurement and DRE performed every 3 months following RT for 2 years, then every 6 months for three additional years, then annually thereafter. Following PSA failure, patients were followed with radiation, medical oncology and urology in rotation on a 3–6-monthly basis until death. The median follow-up defining the date of PSA failure as time zero for the 94 patients who experienced PSA failure was 2.9 (0.5–9.8) years. No patient was lost to follow-up, and there have been 54 deaths, 20 of which were from prostate cancer.

Determination of cause of death

To be considered to have died of prostate cancer, the patient needed to have developed documented (i.e. positive bone scan) metastatic disease and progressed biochemically despite having exhausted all known hormonal manipulations, and was currently undergoing or had previously had cytotoxic chemotherapy. He also had to either have clinical evidence of prostate cancer progression, despite chemotherapy, at the time of death, or be enrolled in a hospice program for end-stage prostate cancer at the time of death. As a result, no patient was scored as dying of prostate cancer unless he had hormone-refractory metastatic prostate cancer.

Salvage hormonal therapy

Given the lack of information regarding whether early, compared with delayed, initiation of salvage hormonal therapy prolongs survival, there was no policy on when to deliver hormonal therapy following PSA failure during the study period. Therefore, this decision was left to the discretion of the treating physician. Of the 94 patients who sustained PSA failure, all had received salvage hormonal therapy at the time of this analysis. The median time from PSA failure to the start of hormonal therapy was 1.5 (0.5–5.1) years. A bone scan was obtained at the time of PSA failure, prior to and within 1 week of the initiation of hormonal therapy or at the time of clinical symptomatic progression. Of the ten patients who received hormones at the time of a positive bone scan, one had a PSA level of 10 ng/ml or less and nine had a PSA level > 10 ng/ml. One of these ten men had back pain that prompted the bone scan. Hormonal therapy consisted of an orchiectomy or at least 2 weeks of a non-steroidal antiandrogen followed by lifelong luteinizing hormone-releasing hormone (LHRH) agonist in two and 92 patients, respectively.

Statistical methods

A Cox regression analysis[13] was used to evaluate the ability of previously defined pretreatment risk groups[3] to predict time to death from prostate cancer for the entire study cohort of 381 patients. Time zero was taken as the first day of RT. A Cox regression multivariable analysis was also used to evaluate the ability of time to PSA failure, post-treatment PSA doubling time and the timing of salvage hormonal therapy to predict time to death from prostate cancer or any cause for the 94 patients who had experienced PSA failure. For this analysis, time zero was taken as the day of PSA failure, which was defined as the mid-point between the PSA nadir and first rise[12]. For all analyses, the assumptions of the Cox model were tested and met.

The pretreatment risk group and the timing of salvage hormonal therapy were treated as categorical variables, whereas the time interval to PSA failure and the PSA doubling time were treated first as continuous and then as categorical variables in separate Cox regression analyses. The categories selected for the time interval to PSA failure and the PSA doubling time were 2 years and 12 months, respectively. These times were selected for the purpose of illustration and because, based on the results of previous studies[6,7,14], these values were suggested to be clinically useful break-points for predicting time to distal failure. The PSA doubling time was calculated assuming first-order kinetics and using a minimum of three PSA values each separated in time by a minimum of 3 months. Timing of salvage hormonal therapy was categorized as being initiated at a PSA level of 10 ng/ml or less and bone scan negative, versus at a PSA level of greater than 10 ng/ml and bone scan negative, versus at any PSA level and bone scan positive. The PSA level of 10 ng/ml was selected as a break-point because all 94 patients scored as PSA failures in this study had sustained PSA failure by that PSA level.

The relative risks of prostate cancer-specific death (PCSD) and all-cause death were calculated for patients based on the coefficients from the Cox regression model, and are reported with 95% confidence intervals (CIs). For the purpose of illustration, estimates of prostate cancer-specific survival (PCSS) and overall survival were determined using the actuarial method of Kaplan and Meier[15], and are graphically displayed. Comparisons of survivorship between groups were made using the log rank test, and an adjustment for multiple comparisons was made using the methodology of Bonferonni[13]. To avoid the potential for overestimating cause-specific death using the method of Kaplan and Meier[15] given the competing causes of mortality in this patient cohort[16], the cumulative incidence method was also applied to calculate this end-point

in cases where PCSD and all-cause death were compared.

Results

Pretreatment prognostic factors

The median age and follow-up for patients in the low-, intermediate- and high-risk groups were 73, 73 and 73 years and 3.9, 3.8 and 4.2 years, respectively. The results of the Cox regression time to PSA failure analysis evaluating the pretreatment risk groups are given in Table 2, and 10-year estimates of PCSS (100% vs. 94% vs. 55%; $p = 0.005$) and overall survival (89% vs. 79% vs. 39%; $p = 0.03$) are illustrated in Figures 1 and 2. The relative risk (RR) (95% CI) of death due to prostate cancer was 6 (2.5–10) for high-risk compared with low- or intermediate-risk patients. There was no significant difference (all pairwise p values > 0.54) in the estimates of non-prostate cancer-specific survival, being 88% vs. 83% vs. 73% at 10 years when stratified by the low-, intermediate- and high-pretreatment-risk groups, respectively, as noted in Figure 3.

Post-treatment prognostic factors

The median age and follow-up beyond PSA failure for patients in the PSA doubling time ≤ 12 vs. > 12 months groups were 73 and 72 years and 2.9 and 2.9 years, respectively. Similarly, the median age and follow-up beyond PSA failure for patients who received salvage hormonal therapy at the time of a negative bone scan and PSA of 10 ng/ml or less or greater than 10 ng/ml versus a positive bone scan were 73, 72 and 72 years and 2.9, 3.2 and 2.9 years, respectively. PSA doubling time as a continuous variable and the initiation of salvage hormonal therapy at the time of a positive bone scan were significant independent predictors of both time to death from prostate cancer and any cause, as indicated in Table 2 and illustrated in Figures 4–7. The lack of significance for the time interval to PSA failure on multivariable analysis can be explained by the high degree of concordance between a short time interval to

Table 2 p Values from Cox regression analyses evaluating the ability of pretreatment risk groups to predict time to prostate cancer-specific death and post-treatment indicators to predict time to prostate cancer-specific and all-cause death

	Time to prostate cancer death		Time to death from any cause	
	Univariable	Multivariable	Univariable	Multivariable
Pretreatment risk group				
Low	baseline group*			
Intermediate	0.03*			
High	0.0007*			
Post-treatment analysis 1**				
Time to PSA failure	0.06	0.77	0.25	0.71
PSA DT	0.0004	0.01	0.005	0.05
Hormone 2[†]	0.002	0.04	0.05	0.39
Hormone 3[†]	< 0.0001	0.001	0.0001	0.0001
Post-treatment analysis 2[‡]				
Time to PSA failure ≤ 2 years	0.25	0.60	0.54	0.67
PSA DT ≤ 12 months	0.003	0.03	0.02	0.05
Hormone 2[†]	0.002	0.02	0.04	0.39
Hormone 3[†]	< 0.0001	0.0006	0.0001	0.0001

*Pretreatment analysis; **time to prostate-specific antigen (PSA) failure and PSA doubling time (DT) are continuous variables; [†]baseline group (hormone 1) is salvage hormonal therapy initiated at a PSA level of 10 ng/ml or less and a negative bone scan, hormone 2 is salvage hormonal therapy initiated at a PSA level of greater than 10 ng/ml and a negative bone scan, hormone 3 is salvage hormonal therapy initiated at any PSA level and a positive bone scan; [‡]time to PSA failure and PSA DT are categorical variables, baseline groups are time to PSA failure > 2 years and PSA DT > 12 months

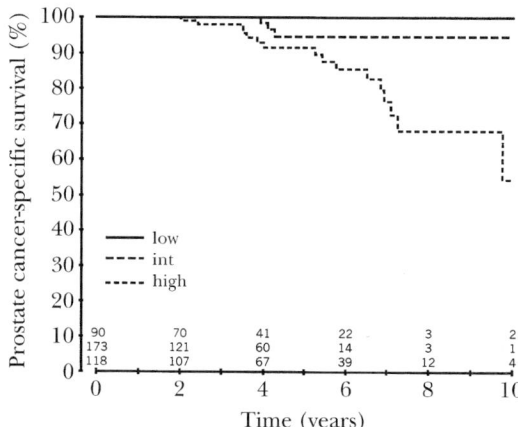

Figure 1 Prostate cancer-specific survival following radiation therapy (RT) stratified by pretreatment risk group: p value overall 0.005, low vs. intermediate (int) 0.06, int vs. high 0.05, low vs. high 0.004

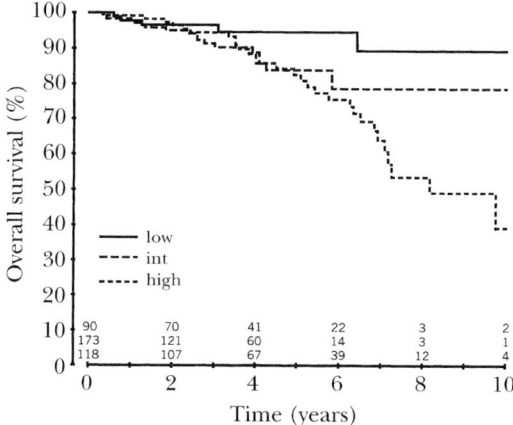

Figure 2 Overall survival following radiation therapy (RT) stratified by pretreatment risk group: p value overall 0.03, low vs. intermediate (int) 0.13, int vs. high 0.52, low vs. high 0.02

PSA failure (2 years or less) and a short PSA doubling time (12 months or less).

Twenty patients (17 high-risk, three intermediate-risk) have died of prostate cancer and five from other causes among the 94 patients who experienced PSA failure. Of the 57 patients with a PSA doubling time ≤ 12 months, 18 have died, 17 (94%) from prostate cancer (15

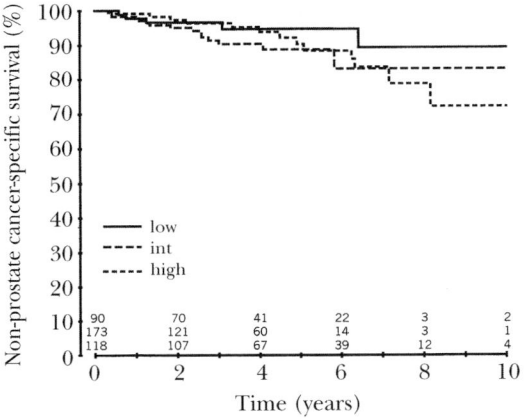

Figure 3 Non-prostate cancer-specific survival following radiation therapy (RT) stratified by pretreatment risk group: *p* value overall 0.57, all pairwise *p* values > 0.54. int, intermediate risk

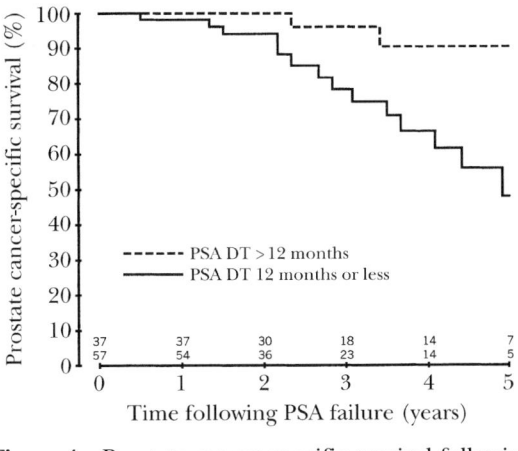

Figure 4 Prostate cancer-specific survival following prostate-specific antigen (PSA) failure stratified by PSA doubling time (DT): *p* value 0.004

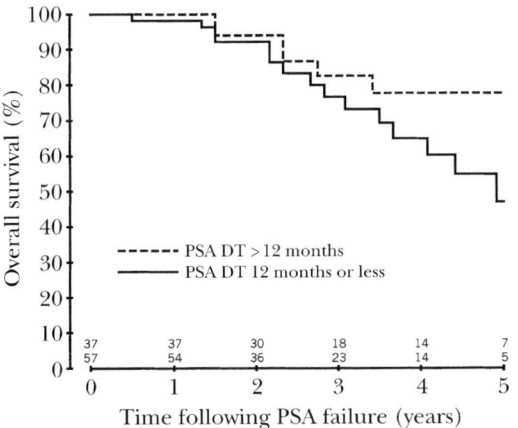

Figure 5 Overall survival following prostate-specific antigen (PSA) failure stratified by PSA doubling time (DT): *p* value 0.04

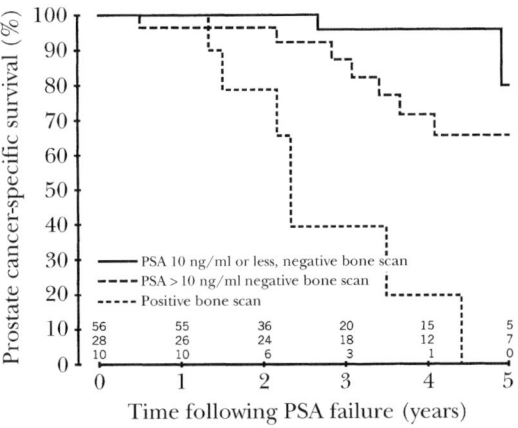

Figure 6 Prostate cancer-specific survival following prostate-specific antigen (PSA) failure stratified by PSA/bone scan (BS) findings at the initiation of salvage hormonal therapy: *p* value overall < 0.0001; PSA ≤ 10 vs. > 10, BS(−) 0.03; PSA ≤ 10, BS(−) vs. BS(+) < 0.0001; PSA > 10, BS(−) vs. BS(+) 0.0006

high-risk, two intermediate-risk); whereas, for the 37 patients with a PSA doubling time > 12 months, seven have died, three (43%) from prostate cancer (two high-risk, one intermediate-risk). For men with a short PSA doubling time (i.e. 12 months or less), estimates of PCSD and all-cause death following PSA failure were nearly identical, as shown in Figures 4 and 5. This similarity in estimates of PCSD and all-cause death remained unchanged when the cumulative incidence method[16] was used to estimate prostate cancer-specific survival in patients with a short PSA doubling time (i.e. 12 months or less). Specifically, the 5-year estimate of PCSD following PSA failure was 52% and 49% using the Kaplan–Meier[15] and cumulative incidence[16] methods, respectively, which both closely approximated the 53% 5-year estimate for all-cause death. The RR (95% CI) of PCSD and all-cause death was 5.1 (2–8.9, *p* = 0.03) and

2.2 (1.2–4, p = 0.05) for patients, respectively, with a PSA doubling time ≤ 12 compared with > 12 months.

Patients who began salvage hormonal therapy when the bone scan was positive versus negative had a RR (95% CI) of 12 (6.2–18,

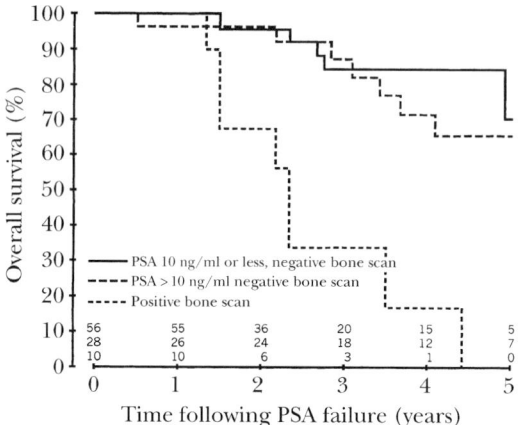

Figure 7 Overall survival following prostate-specific antigen (PSA) failure stratified by PSA/bone scan (BS) findings at the initiation of salvage hormonal therapy: p value overall < 0.0001; PSA ≤ 10 vs. > 10, BS(–) 0.51; PSA ≤ 10, BS(–) vs. BS(+) < 0.0001; PSA > 10, BS(–) vs. BS(+) 0.0001

p = 0.0006) and 9.1 (4–14.3, p = 0.0001) for PCSD and all-cause death, respectively. After correcting for multiple comparisons, there was a near-significant increase in prostate cancer-specific survival (p = 0.03), but not in overall survival (p = 0.51), if salvage hormonal therapy was initiated when the bone scan was negative with a PSA ≤ 10 ng/ml compared with > 10 ng/ml, as noted in Figures 6 and 7. In order to minimize the potential for lead-time bias introduced by defining PSA failure as time zero, this analysis was repeated using the date of initiation of salvage hormonal therapy as time zero. The results using this approach to estimate prostate cancer-specific and all-cause survival were similar to those found using PSA failure as time zero, and are illustrated in Figures 8 and 9.

In order to evaluate whether an imbalance in prognostic factors could have contributed to the survival differences displayed in Figures 6–9, distributions of the known prognostic factors were compared for patients who initiated salvage hormonal therapy when the bone scan was positive, compared with negative. As indicated in Table 3, there were no imbalances noted in the pretreatment risk group (p = 0.97) or the post-treatment PSA doubling time

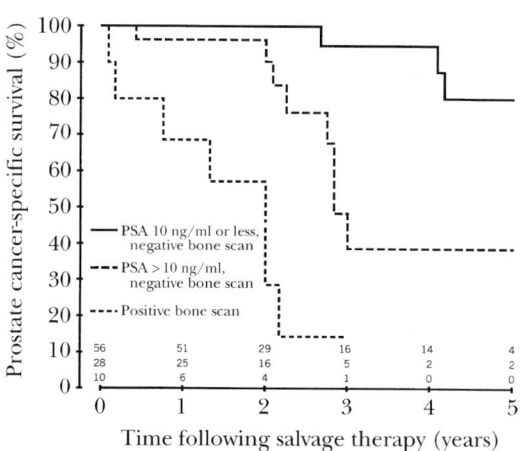

Figure 8 Prostate cancer-specific survival following initiation of salvage hormonal therapy stratified by prostate-specific antigen (PSA)/bone scan (BS) findings: p value overall < 0.0001; PSA ≤ 10 vs. > 10, BS(–) 0.0005; PSA ≤ 10, BS(–) vs. BS(+) < 0.0001; PSA > 10, BS(–) vs. BS(+) 0.002

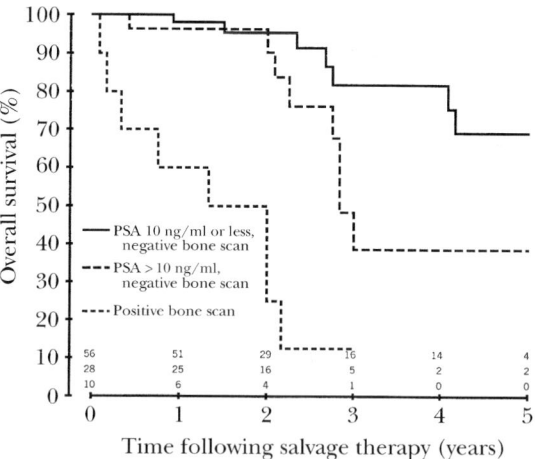

Figure 9 Overall survival following initiation of salvage hormonal therapy stratified by prostate-specific antigen (PSA)/bone scan (BS) findings: p value overall < 0.0001; PSA ≤ 10 vs. > 10, BS(–) 0.02; PSA ≤ 10, BS(–) vs. BS(+) < 0.0001; PSA > 10, BS(–) vs. BS(+) 0.0005

Table 3 Comparison of the proportion of patients within each pretreatment risk group and prostate-specific antigen doubling time (PSA DT) cohort stratified by bone scan findings at the time of initiation of salvage hormonal therapy

Risk group	Bone scan (−)	Bone scan (+)	p Value
Low	9/84 (11%)	1/10 (10%)	0.97
Intermediate	26/84 (31%)	3/10 (30%)	
High	49/84 (58%)	6/10 (60%)	
PSA DT ≤ 12 months	50/84 (60%)	7/10 (70%)	0.73
PSA DT > 12 months	34/84 (40%)	3/10 (30%)	

($p = 0.73$) distributions among patients who received salvage hormonal therapy when the bone scan was positive versus negative.

Discussion

The widespread use of monitoring serum PSA following treatment for patients with clinically localized prostate cancer has been the basis for the generation of pretreatment risk groups[3] and nomograms[4] that provide the probability of being free from PSA failure following RP or RT. These tools have enabled the identification of men at high risk for PSA recurrence based on pretreatment[3,4], post-treatment[17] parameters or both[18]. However, it remains unclear whether patients who sustain PSA failure following primary therapy die of prostate cancer or other causes. Therefore, this study was performed to identify the determinants of PCSD based on pretreatment and post-treatment predictors for men who underwent RT for clinically localized prostate cancer diagnosed during the PSA era.

The results of the study disclose that 45% of patients with high-risk disease were estimated to die of prostate cancer within 10 years following RT, compared with 0% ($p = 0.004$) and 6% ($p = 0.05$) for patients with low- or intermediate-risk disease, respectively. Evaluating this finding in conjunction with Figure 3, where the 10-year estimate of non-prostate cancer-specific death is 27% for patients with high-risk disease, reveals that high-risk prostate cancer was the leading cause of mortality. This observation is particularly important given the competing causes of mortality expected in men whose diagnosis was made at a median age of 73.

Whether the addition of concurrent and adjuvant androgen-suppression therapy to RT for patients with high-risk but clinically localized disease will prolong survival, as has been shown for men with locally advanced prostate cancer[19], awaits further follow-up of completed randomized trials.

The results of the multivariable analysis of post-treatment factors show that the PSA doubling time when evaluated as a continuous variable was a significant predictor of both time to prostate cancer-specific and all-cause death. Specifically, the study reveals that patients with a short PSA doubling time (12 months or less) had estimates of PCSD and all-cause death following PSA failure that were nearly identical, illustrating the prognostic significance of the PSA doubling time. Surgically managed patients are generally younger at diagnosis than the median age in this study (73 years), and also healthier. Therefore, they are less likely to have a non-prostate cancer-specific mortality profile like that shown in Figure 3. As a result, the prognostic significance of a short PSA doubling time following RT may also extend to patients managed surgically, but this remains to be shown.

To support further the potential prognostic significance of the PSA doubling time following primary local therapy, there are now several reports from both surgically managed[6,20,21] and radiation-managed[7,14,22] patients suggesting that a rapid post-treatment PSA doubling time (6–12 months) is a significant predictor of time to distal failure following PSA failure. In addition, one of the radiation studies also found the PSA doubling time to be predictive of time to PCSD[14]. Specifically, these authors estimated the 5-year PCSD to be 52% vs. 10% ($p = 0.007$) for patients with a post-treatment PSA doubling time of approximately 1 year or less compared with greater than 1 year, respectively, similar to the results of the present study. Further follow-up of the published studies associating the post-treatment PSA doubling time with time to distal failure[6,7,14,20–22] will enhance our understanding of the potential prognostic significance of post-treatment PSA doubling time.

To date, no randomized study has evaluated whether a difference in survival exists for the use of early as opposed to delayed salvage hormonal therapy following PSA failure after primary RT. There is evidence, however, from randomized studies that supports a survival benefit of adjuvant as opposed to salvage hormonal therapy in patients with locally advanced[19] and metastatic[23] prostate cancer treated using RT and node-positive[24] prostate cancer managed with RP. While these adjuvant therapy trials did not specifically address the question of salvage hormonal therapy, they provided the basis for the hypothesis that a prolongation in survival may be possible for early as opposed to delayed initiation of salvage hormonal therapy for patients who have experienced PSA failure following primary local therapy. Therefore, in evaluating the determinants of PCSD and all-cause death following PSA failure in the present study, the question of whether the timing of salvage hormonal therapy has an impact on PCSS and overall survival was also addressed.

The final finding in this study was a prolongation in both PCSS and overall survival for early

(any PSA level and a negative bone scan) as opposed to delayed (any PSA level and a positive bone scan) initiation of salvage hormonal therapy for patients who had sustained PSA failure following RT. While these data are retrospective, there were no imbalances measured in the proportion of patients within each pre-treatment risk group and post-treatment PSA doubling time cohort for patients who began salvage hormonal therapy when the bone scan was positive versus negative, as indicated in Table 3. However, a retrospective study cannot control for unknown prognostic factors, and the sample size of patients with a positive bone scan was small ($n = 10$). Therefore, this result awaits validation from a prospective randomized trial. Beyond the timing of initiation of salvage hormonal therapy, other unanswered issues remain regarding salvage hormonal therapy that are not addressed in this study, and include type (LHRH antagonist or orchiectomy with or without a non-steroidal anti-androgen) and duration (intermittent versus continuous).

In summary, despite a median age of 73 years at diagnosis, prostate cancer was a major cause of death during the first decade following radiotherapy for patients with clinically localized but high-risk disease. Moreover, the cause of death in patients with a short PSA doubling time (12 months or less) following radiotherapy was nearly always prostate cancer. While prospective validation utilizing Prentice's criteria[25] is needed, the data in this study provide evidence to propose the hypothesis that a short post-treatment PSA doubling time may serve as a possible surrogate marker for prostate cancer-specific death.

References

1. Han M, Lai S, Partin AW, Epstein JI, Walsh PC. Biochemical (PSA) recurrence probability following radical retropubic prostatectomy for clinically localized prostate cancer. *J Urol* 2001; 165:149(abstr 610)

2. Shipley WU, Thames HD, Sandler HM, *et al.* Radiation therapy for clinically localized prostate cancer: a multi-institutional pooled analysis. *J Am Med Assoc* 1999;281:1598–604

3. D'Amico AV, Whittington R, Malkowicz SB, *et al.* Biochemical outcome after radical prostatectomy, external beam radiation therapy, or interstitial radiation therapy for clinically localized prostate cancer. *J Am Med Assoc* 1998;280: 969–74

4. Kattan MW, Easthan JA, Stapleton AMF, Wheeler TM, Scardino PT. A preoperative nomogram for disease recurrence following radical prostatectomy for prostate cancer. *J Natl Cancer Inst* 1998;90:766–71

5. Albertsen PC, Hanley JA, Gleason DF, Barry MJ. Competing risk analysis of men aged 55 to 74 years at diagnosis managed conservatively for clinically localized prostate cancer. *J Am Med Assoc* 1998;280:975–80

6. Pound CR, Partin AW, Eisenberger MA, *et al.* Natural history of progression after PSA elevation following radical prostatectomy. *J Am Med Assoc* 1999;281:1591–7

7. Lee WR, Hanks GE, Hanlon A. Increasing prostate-specific antigen profile following definitive radiation therapy for localized prostate cancer: clinical observations. *J Clin Oncol* 1997; 15:230–8

8. Gleason DF and the Veterans Administration Cooperative Urological Research Group. Histologic grading and staging of prostatic carcinoma. In Tannenbaum M, ed. *Urologic Pathology.* Philadelphia, PA: Lea & Febiger, 1977:171–87

9. Lee CT, Oesterling JE. Using prostate-specific antigen to eliminate the staging radionuclide bone scan. *Urol Clin North Am* 1997;24:389–94

10. Beahrs OH, Henson DE, Hutter RVP. *American Joint Committee on Cancer, Manual for Staging Cancer,* 4th edn. Philadelphia, PA: JP Lippincott, 1992

11. Dearnaley D, Khoo V, Norman A, *et al.* Comparison of radiation side effects of conformal and conventional radiotherapy in prostate cancer: a randomized trial. *Lancet* 1999;353:267–72

12. Cox JD, for the American Society for Therapeutic Radiology and Oncology Consensus Panel. Consensus statement: guidelines for PSA following radiation therapy. *Int J Radiat Oncol Biol Phys* 1997;37:1035–41

13. Neter J, Kutner M, Nachtstein CJ. Simultaneous inferences and other topics in regression analysis – 1. In Neter J, Wasserman W, Kutner M, eds. *Applied Linear Regression Models,* 1st edn. Homewood, IL: Richard D Irwin, 1983:150–3

14. Sandler HM, Dunn RL, McLaughlin PW, Hayman JA, Sullivan MA, Taylor JM. Overall survival after prostate-specific-antigen-detected recurrence following conformal radiation therapy. *Int J Radiat Oncol Biol Phys* 2000;48: 629–33

15. Kaplan EL, Meier P. Non-parametric estimation from incomplete observations. *J Am Stat Assoc* 1958;53:457–500

16. Gaynor JJ, Feur EJ, Tan CC, *et al.* On the use of cause-specific failure and conditional failure probabilities: examples from clinical oncology data. *J Am Stat Assoc* 1993;88:400–9

17. Kattan MW, Wheeler TM, Scardino PT. Postoperative nomogram for disease recurrence after radical prostatectomy for prostate cancer. *J Clin Oncol* 1999;17:1499–507

18. D'Amico AV, Whittington R, Malkowicz SB, *et al.* Utilizing predictions of early prostate-specific antigen failure to optimize patient selection for adjuvant therapy trials. *J Clin Oncol* 2000;18: 3240–6

19. Bolla M, Gonsalez D, Warde P, *et al.* Improved survival in patients with locally advanced prostate cancer treated with radiotherapy and goserelin. *N Engl J Med* 1997;337:295–300

20. Patel A, Dorey F, Franklin J, deKernion JB. Recurrence patterns after radical retropubic prostatectomy: clinical usefulness of prostate specific antigen doubling times and log slope prostate specific antigen. *J Urol* 1997;158: 1441–5

21. Roberts SG, Blute ML, Bergstralh EJ, Slezak JM, Zincke H. PSA doubling time as a predictor of clinical progression after biochemical failure following radical prostatectomy for prostate cancer. *Mayo Clin Proc* 2001;76:576–81

22. Sartor CI, Strawderman MH, Lin XH, Kish KE, McLaughlin PW, Sandler HM. Rate of PSA rise predicts metastatic versus local recurrence after definitive radiotherapy. *Int J Radiat Oncol Biol Phys* 1997;38:941–7

23. The Medical Research Council Prostate Cancer Working Party Investigators Group. Immediate versus deferred treatment for advanced prostatic cancer: initial results of the Medical Research Council Trial. *Br J Urol* 1997;79:235–46

24. Messing EM, Manola J, Sarosdy M, Wilding G, Crawford ED, Trump D. Immediate hormonal therapy compared with observation after radical prostatectomy and pelvic lymphadenectomy in men with node-positive prostate cancer. *N Engl J Med* 1999;341:1781–8

25. Prentice RL. Surrogate endpoints in clinical trials: definition and operational criteria. *Stat Med* 1989;8:431–40

Use of adjuvant hormonal therapy with radical prostatectomy in lymph node-positive disease: rationale and contribution to outcome

44

*R. P. Myers, E. J. Bergstralh, J. M. Slezak, G. M. Farrow, M. M. Lieber,
M. L. Blute and H. Zincke*

Introduction

In this era of serum prostate-specific antigen (PSA), which has been revolutionary in the early diagnosis of prostate cancer since 1987, the frequency of positive pelvic lymph nodes at radical prostatectomy dropped remarkably from 21% in 1987 to 2% in 1999[1]. The decrease has occurred largely because of stage migration to a greater prevalence of low-stage cancers from the finding at diagnosis of progressively smaller cancers. A minor, unmonitored but possibly contributing factor could be less extensive node dissections as the period ensued. Nevertheless, lymph node-positive disease is now encountered much less often. However, in the course of any radical prostatectomy, the preliminary finding of metastasis to one or more pelvic lymph nodes (N+ disease) is widely recognized to be associated with additional systemic disease[2,3]. At one time, it was reported that 'no patient with pelvic lymph node metastasis has survived free of tumor for > 5 years'[2,4].

Today, many patients with N+ disease can expect to live beyond 5 years, but radical prostatectomy and pelvic lymph node dissection (RP/PLND) as monotherapy rarely cures, with most patients eventually developing postoperative, progressively increasing PSA levels.

Radical prostatectomy and pelvic lymph node dissection in the face of N+ disease is a reasonable endeavor if patients can expect skilful surgery and excellent functional recovery. In this regard, Steinberg and associates stressed 'excellent palliation' of the local lesion with acceptable morbidity[3]. Even if local control of the primary tumor is achieved, recurrence is almost certain; the future for most patients is a decision with respect to the appropriate timing of androgen deprivation by medication or surgery. Whether to introduce such treatment early after the finding of N+ disease or on a delayed basis has been the subject of enormous controversy[1,5–9]. The compelling issue relates to demonstrating a clear benefit of early adjuvant hormonal therapy (AHT) in terms of overall and/or cause (prostate cancer)-specific survival. For many patients, androgen deprivation is associated with significantly reduced health-related quality-of-life issues[8–10], and if early hormonal therapy has no demonstrable benefit, there is every good reason to wait for clearly defined progression and, in some cases, symptoms, either local or systemic.

In the only randomized, prospective study of the Eastern Co-operative Oncology Group (ECOG) comparing immediate hormonal therapy with observation after RP/PLND in men with N+ disease, Messing and associates showed both overall survival ($p = 0.02$) and cause-specific survival ($p = 0.001$) to be significant for the patient cohort receiving immediate androgen deprivation versus those assigned to observation[6].

Previously, in a non-randomized, retrospective, pre-PSA era study of 370 RP/PLND N+ patients from 1966 to 1988, all with DNA ploidy analysis of their primary tumors, Zincke and associates[11] found, with respect to overall survival, no benefit from AHT < 90 days from surgery, but did find significant cause-specific survival ($p = 0.02$) for a DNA diploid subset after 10 years of follow-up. Because that study was of limited follow-up (median 4.1 years for 296 surviving patients) and, on current review, 79 patients had received preoperative hormonal therapy for down-staging, we aimed to re-examine the original cohort with longer follow-up and pure cohorts (AHT versus no AHT) unblemished by preoperative hormonal therapy.

Patients and methods

Of the 370 patients originally reported[11], two refused access to their medical records, and 79 were excluded because they received pre-operative hormonal therapy. For reporting purposes of this new study, hormonal therapy was said to be adjuvant (AHT) if it was given or planned within 90 days postoperatively. Hence, AHT herein means early androgen deprivation. All patients underwent RP/PLND and had N+ disease. Exclusion of the 81 patients provided 289 for analysis (125 last known alive with a mean (standard deviation) follow-up of 15.3 (2.7) years). All patients alive have been actively followed on a yearly basis with respect to status and treatment. When deaths have occurred, they have been assiduously recorded with respect to time and cause of death in an actively maintained Mayo Clinic prostate cancer database overseen by a registered nurse abstractor. The breakdown of the AHT and no-AHT cohorts is given in Table 1.

Ploidy analysis by flow cytometry of the primary tumor specimen was available for all patients. In the original 1992 study of 370 patients[11], all primary tumors were regraded by a single referee pathologist (G.M.F.) using the Mayo grading system of four grades[12]. The same grading for each primary tumor was used for the present study. Mayo grade (G) 1 = Gleason score (GS) 2, 3; G2 = GS 4, 5; G3 = GS 6, 7, 8; G4 = GS 9, 10. Cellular detail (depending primarily on degree of nuclear atypia and prominence of nucleoli) would have placed some Gleason

Table 1 Cohort definitions based on adjuvant therapy

Cohort	n	Type of adjuvant (within 90 days after RP) therapy
AHT	231	adjuvant hormonal therapy: 188 hormonal therapy only 177 bilateral orchiectomy (orch) 11 medication (oral) 6 orch + oral 43 hormonal (42 orch + 1 oral) + radiation
No AHT	58	no adjuvant hormonal therapy: 53 neither hormonal nor radiation therapy 5 radiation therapy only

RP, radical prostatectomy

score 6s in a Mayo grade 2 category (G. M. Farrow, personal communication).

Statistical analysis

For this study, using the Kaplan–Meier method[13], end-points were time to local or systemic progression, overall survival and cause-specific survival. The log-rank test[14] was used for the association of nominal factors with survival. The Cox proportional hazards model[15] was used to generate univariate survival comparisons for continuous or ordinal factors. Multivariate analysis was also performed using the Cox model applied to parameters of age, ploidy, Mayo grade, margin positivity, capsular perforation, maximum tumor dimension and number of positive pelvic lymph nodes. Given the nature of the long-term follow-up of this study, cumulative incidence analysis[16] was also performed to take into account deaths from competing risks. All tests were two-sided, with α level 0.05.

Results

Baseline comparison of treatment groups

In Table 2, groups are compared regarding characteristics of clinical and pathological characteristics. There were no significant differences in age or ploidy distribution between

Table 2 Baseline characteristics of patients receiving adjuvant hormonal therapy (AHT) vs. no AHT

	AHT (n = 231)	No AHT (n = 58)	p value[†]
Mean (SD) age (years)	64 (6)	63 (6)	0.12
Ploidy (%)			0.38
diploid	35.1	44.8	
tetraploid	45.9	39.7	
aneuploid	19.0	15.5	0.006
Mayo pathology grade (%)			
1, 2	38.5	58.6	
3, 4	61.5	41.4	< 0.001
Margin positive (%)	51.9	17.2	0.015
Extraprostatic extension (%)	83.4	69.0	0.002
Maximum tumor dimension (mm)*:	3.4 (2.5, 4.0)	3.0 (2.0, 3.5)	
median (25th, 75th)			0.008
Number of positive lymph nodes (%)			
1	40.6	55.2	
2	24.5	27.6	
3	13.5	8.6	
4+	21.4	8.6	

*Tumor dimension not available for 30 patients (21 AHT, nine no-AHT); [†]AHT vs. no AHT

AHT and no-AHT patients. However, AHT patients generally had more extensive or aggressive disease as seen by significant differences in Mayo grade, margin status, extraprostatic extension, maximum tumor dimension and number of positive nodes.

Univariate predictors of cause-specific survival

Neither age ($p = 0.07$) nor extraprostatic extension ($p = 0.47$) were significant predictors of cause-specific survival. While DNA ploidy did not achieve significance overall ($p = 0.078$, log-rank test with 2 degrees of freedom; Figure 1), when aneuploid patients were compared with non-aneuploid patients, the effect of aneuploidy was significant ($p = 0.03$). Other significant univariate predictors of cause-specific survival included high Mayo grade ($p = 0.007$), margin positivity ($p = 0.02$), maximal tumor dimension ($p = 0.02$) and number of positive lymph nodes ($p = 0.002$ for 1 vs. 2 or more nodes positive; Figure 2). Cause-specific survival at 15 years for patients with 1, 2, 3 or 4 or more positive nodes was 82, 63, 67 and 63%, respectively.

Effects of adjuvant hormonal therapy

In univariate analysis, AHT patients had significantly better progression-free survival, with systemic or local recurrence as end-points, than no-AHT patients ($p < 0.001$; Figure 3, Table 3). Additionally, AHT patients had significantly better cause-specific survival than no-AHT patients ($p = 0.015$; Figure 4, Table 3). Cause-specific survival (CSS) for patients with AHT at 15 and 20 years was 75% and 72%, respectively, compared with 58% and 51% for no-AHT patients. Using the Cox model, the estimated risk ratio (RR) and 95% confidence interval associated with the use of AHT was 0.54 (0.33–0.89). Upon adjustment for age, grade, ploidy (diploid vs. non-diploid), extraprostatic extension, margin status, tumor dimension and positive nodes (1 vs. 2 or more), the RR for AHT remained statistically significant ($p = 0.002$) and suggested an even stronger benefit, RR = 0.38 (0.21–0.69).

With follow-up to 20 years, many patients will die of causes unrelated to prostate cancer. In this setting, using '1 minus cause-specific survival' (1 − CSS) to estimate the proportion dying of prostate cancer will overestimate the

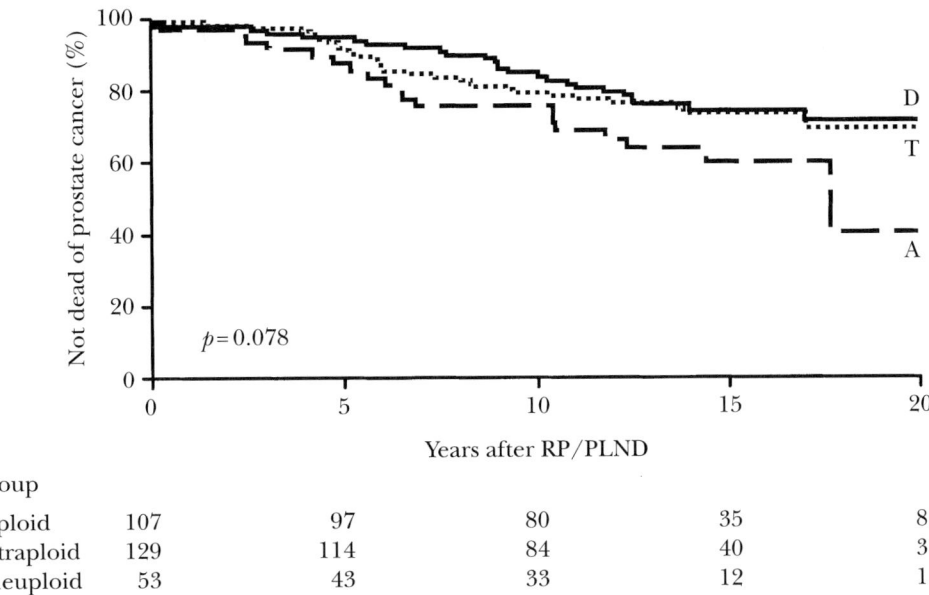

Group				
Diploid	107	97	80	35	8
Tetraploid	129	114	84	40	3
Aneuploid	53	43	33	12	1

Figure 1 Cause-specific survival after radical prostatectomy/pelvic lymph node dissection (RP/PLND) comparing patients with diploid (D), tetraploid (T) and aneuploid (A) primary tumors using flow cytometry

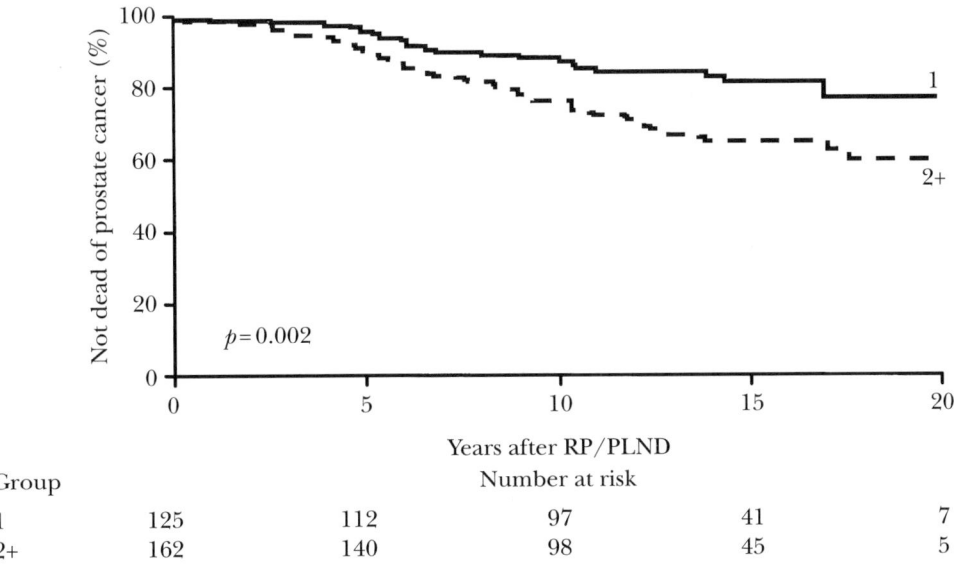

Group	Number at risk			
1	125	112	97	41	7
2+	162	140	98	45	5

Figure 2 Cause-specific survival after radical prostatectomy/pelvic lymph node dissection (RP/PLND) comparing patients with 1 vs. 2 or more positive pelvic lymph nodes

true value, as it assumes that the death rate due to other causes is zero. The cumulative incidence estimator does not make this assumption, and hence gives a fair estimate of the percentage of men who will actually die of prostate cancer in the presence of competing risks. The 20-year cumulative incidence of prostate cancer death was 24% for AHT patients and 39% for patients with no AHT (Table 3). This is in contrast to values of 28% and 49% using '1 – CSS'.

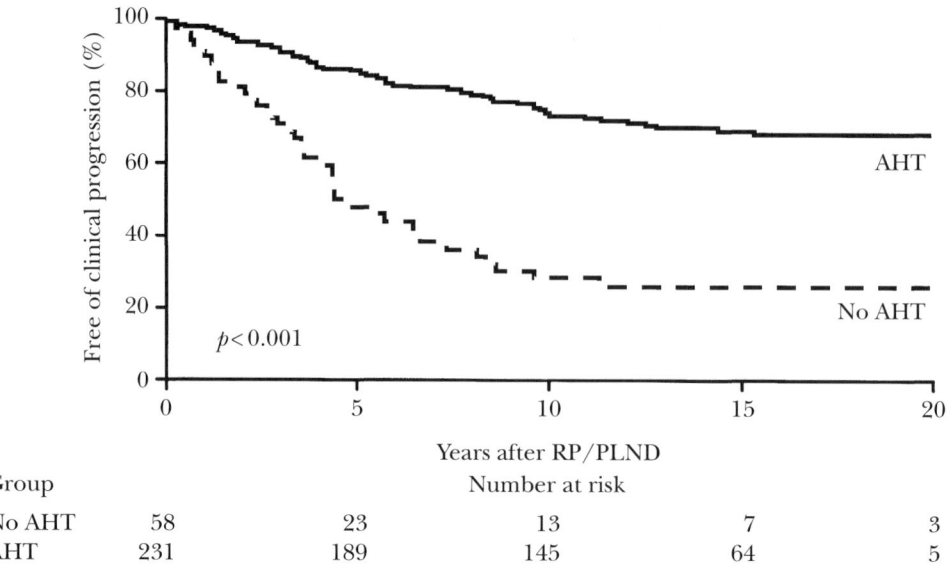

Group		Number at risk		
No AHT	58	23	13	7	3
AHT	231	189	145	64	5

Figure 3 Survival free of either local or systemic progression after radical prostatectomy/pelvic lymph node dissection (RP/PLND) comparing those receiving adjuvant hormonal therapy (AHT) vs. no AHT

Table 3 Long-term outcomes by use of adjuvant hormonal therapy (AHT)

	AHT (n = 231)	No AHT (n = 58)	p Value[†]
Event-free (Kaplan–Meier) rate (% (SE))			
Event: clinical progression			< 0.001
5 years	86 (2)	47 (7)	
10 years	74 (3)	27 (6)	
15 years	69 (3)	24 (6)	
Event: any death			0.085
10 years	70 (3)	64 (6)	
15 years	52 (3)	40 (6)	
20 years	23 (6)	24 (6)	
Event: prostate cancer death			0.015
10 years	83 (3)	77 (6)	
15 years	75 (3)	58 (7)	
20 years	72 (4)	51 (8)	
*Cumulative incidence of death at 20 years (%)**			
Any death	77	76	NA
Prostate cancer death	24	39	NA
Other death	53	37	NA

*Taking into account competing risks; [†]log-rank test; NA, not applicable

Overall survival was not significantly different ($p = 0.085$), even though for many years the curve for AHT patients remained above that for the no-AHT patients (Figure 5).

Shortening the accrual period for cases from 1966 to the end of 1983 results in roughly equal numbers of patients with AHT ($n = 57$) and without AHT ($n = 50$). Consistent with the overall results, within this shorter time period during which AHT was used about half of the time, AHT patients had significantly better cause-specific survival than did the no-AHT patients (75% vs. 52% at 15 years, $p = 0.018$).

Discussion

This retrospective study with long-term follow-up clearly demonstrates, irrespective of ploidy, a significant benefit of AHT in terms of cause-specific survival ($p < 0.001$), but not overall survival ($p = 0.085$). Cumulative incidence analysis was added even though it reduces to some degree the impact of prostate cancer death, but the disparity in prostate cancer death using cumulative incidence methodology for those

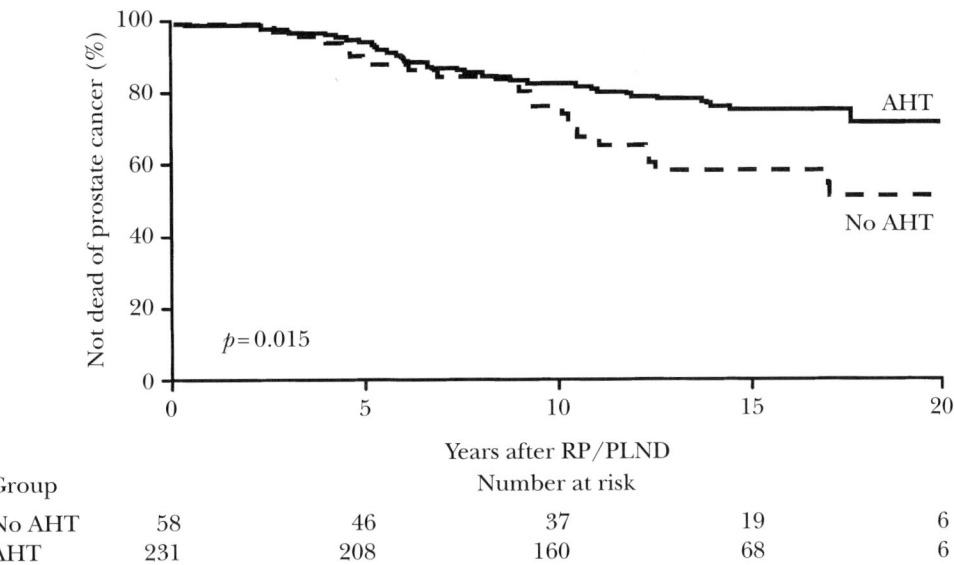

Figure 4 Cause-specific survival after radical prostatectomy/pelvic lymph node dissection (RP/PLND) comparing those receiving adjuvant hormonal therapy (AHT) vs. no AHT

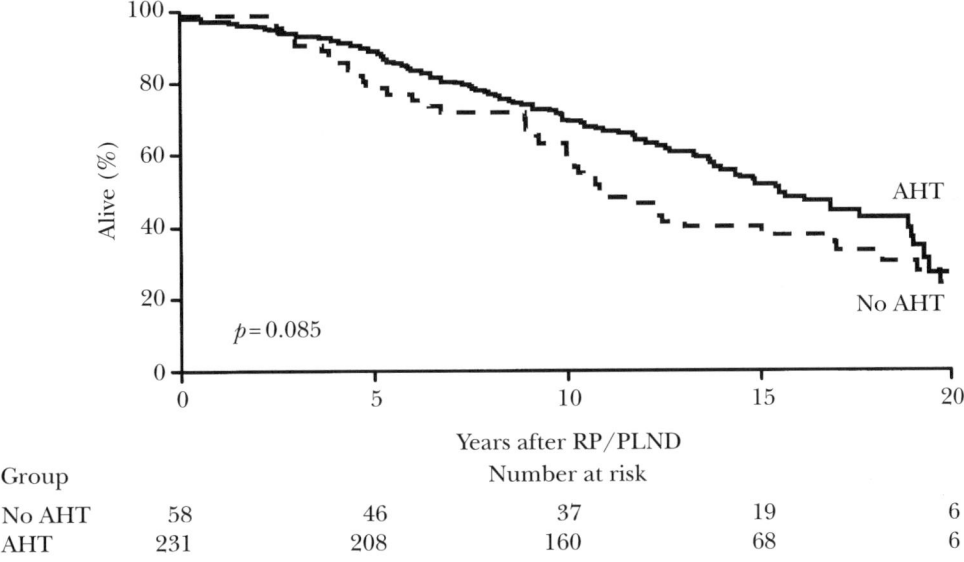

Figure 5 Overall survival after radical prostatectomy/pelvic lymph node dissection (RP/PLND) comparing those receiving adjuvant hormonal therapy (AHT) vs. no AHT

who received AHT and those who did not is still substantial at 20 years. We emphasize that the cohort of 231 patients treated early (AHT) had significantly worse pathological parameters including tumor grade, positive margins, extraprostatic extension, maximum tumor dimension and number of positive nodes. Three times as many patients in the AHT group had tumors of maximal tumor dimension greater than 4 cm. Maximal tumor dimension can be taken as a surrogate of primary tumor volume, which was not directly measured in this study but has been shown to be a significant parameter in prostate cancer[17–21].

This study again confirms, like others[7], the benefit of early hormonal therapy in prolonging time to progression. When patients do not receive AHT, they can expect a much shorter time to treatment of local or systemic disease[22]. However, prolonging the time to symptomatic disease is only one issue; the other two pressing issues are the effects on cause-specific and overall survival.

Our study suggests that RP/PLND N+ patients who receive hormonal therapy on a delayed basis at the time of systemic and/or local progression are more likely to die of prostate cancer. The cohort of 58 patients placed on observation with delayed hormonal therapy at the time of local or systemic progression did worse with respect to cause-specific survival but not overall survival when analyzed at 20 years. Looking at the curves, overall survival appears to be superior for a number of 'middle' years for the AHT group (Figure 5).

Our study has several limitations, the primary one being that patients were not randomized to AHT versus no AHT. Overall, AHT was used in 80% of N+ patients during the study period. Its use was probably more selective initially, with preference given to a few high-risk patients (Table 1). However, the estimated effect of AHT on cause-specific survival remained significant, and was even more pronounced (beneficial estimated risk ratio decreasing from 0.54 to 0.38) upon adjustment for group differences in tumor characteristics using multivariate analysis. Additionally, restricting the analysis to a period in which patients had about a 50/50 chance of receiving AHT, implying perhaps less selectivity, had no effect on the conclusions regarding AHT and cause-specific survival.

At the time of this analysis, 11 patients (3.8%) had not been subjected to the adverse effects of hormonal therapy (47 patients (37 bilateral orchiectomy, ten oral medication) received hormonal therapy on a delayed basis at the time of clinical local or systemic progression). Three of the 11 untreated patients were being followed with progressively increasing PSA, two showing minimal values after many years and one having a PSA of 89 ng/ml. These three patients demonstrate that some prostate cancers metastatic to regional lymph nodes progress slowly in the absence of intervention. The challenge then is to identify those cases with slow PSA doubling times and possibly save those patients from unnecessary androgen deprivation[23]. The adverse consequences of hormonal therapy are not to be taken lightly[8–10]. For many individuals, side-effects include hot flushes, loss of libido, poor concentration, loss of muscle mass and vigor, osteoporosis and pathological fractures. The cumulative incidence of fracture due to bilateral orchiectomy has been shown to be highly significant[24]. Patients on hormonal therapy should be monitored for evidence of osteoporosis and appropriate countermeasures taken. Antiandrogens such as cyproterone acetate may cause fatigue, mood changes and liver toxicity. Bicalutamide may cause breast tenderness and enlargement. In the face of N+ disease there is the obvious need to balance quality of life from lack of disease control versus treatment-related quality of life. Failure to use AHT presents the threat of earlier onset of painful bony metastasis, pathological fracture, spinal cord compression, extraskeletal soft tissue metastasis and urinary obstructive symptoms[5]. Patients who are not treated can expect symptomatic progression sooner than those treated on a delayed basis. They have the choice of living with a potentially increasing PSA level, or being treated and experiencing the adverse side-effects of androgen deprivation (e.g. failure to enjoy normal libido and sexual life) for 9–12 years before developing symptomatic progression[8]. Some patients may want to put off as long as possible the time to first symptoms, but they must be made fully aware of the known treatment-related side-effects mentioned above so that they understand the possible compromise in overall feeling of well-being.

In our study, AHT given within 90 days of surgery delayed symptomatic progression and decreased the likelihood of prostate cancer death irrespective of ploidy, but nevertheless exposed 231 (80%) to the possible adverse side-effects of androgen withdrawal. Historically, treatment considerations for patients with N+ disease have been greatly influenced by the Veterans' Administration Co-operative

Urological Research Group (VACURG), who recommended that hormonal therapy be initiated when patients become so symptomatic that 'they require relief'[25]. Our study certainly counters the VACURG notion, because waiting until symptomatic progression may expose a considerable number of patients to premature death from prostate cancer.

The importance of not dying of prostate cancer as an end-point should be emphasized. In a recently reported, randomized, prospective study of T1–2N0M0 localized prostate cancer patients, Holmberg and colleagues reported that radical prostatectomy significantly reduced prostate cancer mortality ($p = 0.02$)[26]. Because metastatic bone pain and skeletal degradation associated with most cases are horrendous, a valid point (in response to the foregoing study[26]) has been made that not dying of prostate cancer is a worthy goal[27].

Early androgen deprivation may render some patients with positive nodes no worse off than patients with negative nodes. After PLND and radiation therapy for presumably localized prostate cancer, Gervasi and associates concluded that a single pelvic lymph node with metastasis 'markedly worsened the prognosis'[28]. But, in 2001, Cheng and associates showed, in a multivariate analysis with a median follow-up of 6.3 years, that patients with a single positive node did as well in terms of cause-specific survival as patients with negative nodes if treated by RP/PLND and AHT ($p = 0.478$)[29].

One perennially unanswered issue is the actual impact on survival by removing the prostate in the presence of positive pelvic lymph nodes. To date, retrospective studies that attempt to answer the question have produced equivocal results[30–32]. The real answer with respect to the benefit of prostate removal on survival in N+ disease will remain unknown until a proper, prospective, randomized study is completed. Given the current, marked decrease in the frequency of patients with N+ disease at the time of RP/PLND, such a study, from a practical standpoint, may never be successfully completed.

Summary

It is widely acknowledged that the treatment of prostate cancer patients who have node positive (N+) disease at the time of radical prostatectomy and pelvic lymph node dissection (RP/PLND) is controversial. With a median 15.3 years of follow-up, our findings in this retrospective study support, as a primary rationale, adjuvant hormonal therapy (AHT) as an addition to RP/PLND in patients with N+ disease. Cause-specific survival at 15 years was 75% for AHT patients versus 58% for no AHT ($p = 0.015$). Our results are in keeping with those outcomes of both the randomized, prospective ECOG and Medical Research Council (MRC) PR03 trials[5,6] that relate to the use of early endocrine therapy in significantly improving cause-specific survival or not dying of prostate cancer, even with adverse pathological prognostic features as discussed herein.

Our view is that the putative main benefits of prostate removal in the face of N+ disease include local disease control, removal of a potential primary source of cancer cells that could continue to metastasize, and the psychological benefit[3] for the patient to have his cancerous prostate and positive lymph nodes removed. Psychological benefit assumes, of course, that the patient can look forward to satisfactory functional recovery of urinary control and, when feasible, maintenance of potency. No patient should be saddled with crippling quality-of-life after-effects because of surgery. Whether there might be a benefit from prostate removal as an obvious immediate reduction of cancer volume in terms of potentially enhancing host immunity remains to be determined.

In our study, improved overall survival was not demonstrable (similar to the MRC PR03 trial[5,33]), an issue of obvious importance[9]. To date, only the ECOG study has shown a significant improvement in overall survival from immediate hormonal therapy ($p = 0.02$) in RP/PLND N+ patients[6].

Acknowledgement

The authors wish to thank Sandra K. Martin, RN, data analyst, who maintains the Mayo Clinic prostate cancer database with Urology Department Faculty assistance.

References

1. Zincke H, Lau W, Bergstralh E, *et al.* Role of early adjuvant hormonal therapy after radical prostatectomy for prostate cancer. *J Urol* 2001; 166:2208–15

2. Kramer SA, Cline WA Jr, Farnham R, *et al.* Prognosis of patients with stage D1 prostatic adenocarcinoma. *J Urol* 1981;125:817–19

3. Steinberg GD, Epstein JI, Piantadosi S, *et al.* Management of stage D1 adenocarcinoma of the prostate: the Johns Hopkins experience 1974 to 1987. *J Urol* 1990;144:1425–32

4. Whitmore WF Jr, MacKenzie AR. Experiences with different operative procedures for the total excision of prostatic cancer. *Cancer* 1959;12: 396–405

5. Medical Research Council Prostate Cancer Working Party Investigators Group. Immediate versus deferred treatment for advanced prostatic cancer: initial results of the Medical Research Council trial. *Br J Urol* 1997;79:235–46

6. Messing EM, Manola J, Sarosdy M, *et al.* Immediate hormonal therapy compared with observation after radical prostatectomy and pelvic lymphadenectomy in men with node-positive cancer. *N Engl J Med* 1999;341:1781–8

7. DeKernion JB, Neuwirth H, Stein A, *et al.* Prognosis of patients with stage D1 prostate carcinoma following radical prostatectomy with and without early endocrine therapy. *J Urol* 1990;144:700–3

8. Schröder FH. Endocrine treatment of prostate cancer – recent developments and the future. Part 1: maximal androgen blockade, early vs. delayed endocrine treatment and side effects. *BJU Int* 1999;83:161–70

9. Walsh PC, DeWeese TL, Eisenberger MA. A structured debate: immediate versus deferred androgen suppression in prostate cancer – evidence for deferred treatment. *J Urol* 2001; 166:508–16

10. Iversen P. Quality of life issues relating to endocrine treatment options. *Eur Urol* 1999; 39(Suppl 2):20–6

11. Zincke H, Bergstralh EJ, Larson-Keller J, *et al.* Stage D1 prostate cancer treated by radical prostatectomy and adjuvant hormonal therapy. *Cancer* 1992;70:311–23

12. Utz DC, Farrow GM. Pathologic differentiation and prognosis of prostatic carcinoma. *J Am Med Assoc* 1969;209:1701–5

13. Kaplan EL, Meier P. Nonparametric estimation from incomplete observations. *J Am Stat Assoc* 1958;53:457–81

14. Mantel N. Evaluation of survival data and two new rank order statistics arising in its consideration. *Cancer Chemother Rep* 1966;50:163–70

15. Cox DR. Regression models and life-tables. *J R Stat Soc (B)* 1972;34:187–202

16. Cheng SC, Fine JB, Wei LJ. Prediction of cumulative incidence function under the proportional hazards model. *Biometrics* 1998;54:219–28

17. Barzell W, Bean MA, Hilaris BS, *et al.* Prostatic adenocarcinoma: relationship of grade and local extent to the pattern of metastasis. *J Urol* 1977; 118:278–82

18. Smith JA Jr, Middleton RG. Implications of volume of nodal metastasis in patients with adenocarcinoma of the prostate. *J Urol* 1985; 133:617–19

19. McNeal JE, Bostwick DG, Kindrachuk RA, *et al.* Patterns of progression in prostate cancer. *Lancet* 1986;1:60–3

20. Henry JM, Isaacs JT. Relationship between tumor size and the curability of metastatic prostatic cancer by surgery alone or in combination with adjuvant chemotherapy. *J Urol* 1988;139:1119–23

21. Cheng L, Bergstralh EJ, Cheville JC, *et al.* Cancer volume of lymph node metastasis predicts progression in prostate cancer. *Am J Surg Pathol* 1998;22:1491–500

22. Frohmüller HGW, Theiss M, Manseck A, *et al.* Survival and quality of life of patients with stage D1 (T1–3 pN1–2 M0) prostate cancer. *Eur Urol* 1995;27:202–6

23. Roberts SG, Blute ML, Bergstralh EJ, *et al.* PSA doubling time as predictor of clinical

progression after biochemical failure following radical prostatectomy for prostate cancer. *Mayo Clin Proc* 2001;76:576–81

24. Melton LJ, Alothman KI, Khosla S, *et al.* Fracture risk following bilateral orchiectomy. *J Urol* 2003;in press

25. The Veterans' Administration Co-operative Urological Research Group. Treatment and survival of patients with cancer of the prostate. *Surg Gynecol Obstet* 1967;124:1101–7

26. Holmberg L, Bill-Axelson A, Helgesen F, *et al.* A randomized trial comparing radical prostatectomy with watchful waiting in early prostate cancer. *N Engl J Med* 2002;34:781–9

27. Walsh PC. Commentary. In Kolata G. Dilemma on prostate cancer splits experts. *New York Times* Tuesday, September 17, 2002:5

28. Gervasi LA, Mata J, Easley JD, *et al.* Prognostic significance of lymph node metastasis in prostate cancer. *J Urol* 1989;142:332–6

29. Cheng L, Zincke H, Blute ML, *et al.* Risk of prostate carcinoma death in patients with lymph node metastasis. *Cancer* 2001;91:66–73

30. Frazier HA II, Robertson JE, Paulson DF. Does radical prostatectomy in the presence of positive pelvic lymph nodes enhance survival? *World J Urol* 1994;12:308–12

31. Cadeddu JA, Partin AW, Epstein JI, *et al.* Stage D1 (T1–3, N1–3, M0) prostate cancer: a case-controlled comparison of conservative treatment versus radical prostatectomy. *Urology* 1997;50:251–5

32. Ghavamian R, Bergstralh EJ, Blute ML, *et al.* Radical retropubic prostatectomy plus orchiectomy versus orchiectomy alone for pTxN+ prostate cancer: a matched comparison. *J Urol* 1999;161:1223–8

33. Kirk D. Immediate vs. delayed hormone treatment for prostate cancer: how safe is androgen deprivation? *BJU Int* 2000;86(Suppl 3):220

Side-effects of endocrine treatment: role of duration of treatment

45

D. Kirk

Introduction

Endocrine treatment remains the most effective therapy for advanced prostate cancer[1]. Evidence is accruing for benefit from earlier use[2,3]. In patients presenting in the traditional manner with bone metastases or substantial local disease, the main consideration has been immediate toxicity. Now, earlier diagnosis has identified men either at presentation, or following failure of curative treatment, in whom endocrine treatment may be considered when survival for many years is likely[4]. Not only are such patients liable to the immediate side-effects of treatment for longer, they may also be of an age when loss of libido is less tolerable. In addition, if hormone treatment is administered for many years, long-term complications become a significant issue. Alternative methods of hormone treatment may avoid some of the hazards associated with traditional androgen deprivation by medical or surgical castration. There is renewed interest in estrogen therapy as a method of avoiding problems with steroid deficiency[5]. New hormone treatment strategies – treatment escalation and intermittent therapy – are also proposed to avoid toxicity. Optimum treatment remains a balance between survival and the reduction of the adverse effects of the disease, on the one hand, and the quality-of-life deficit from its side-effects, on the other[6].

Effects of endocrine treatment

Androgen deprivation

Orchidectomy and luteinizing hormone-releasing hormone (LH-RH) analog therapy are considered therapeutically equivalent[7]. Orchidectomy involves the insult of, albeit minor, surgery and its potential complications. To what extent psychological problems arise from 'castration' is not clear; this risk is probably reduced with the more commonly performed subcapsular operation[8]. Tumor flare from the initial increase in testosterone with LH-RH analog treatment is avoidable by using an antiandrogen to cover the initial period of treatment[9]. Orchidectomy, once done, is over, while LH-RH analogs require continuing injections. Endocrinologically, orchidectomy will increase levels of luteinizing hormone (LH) and follicle-stimulating hormone (FSH), which will be reduced by LH-RH analog. The extent to which this might have practical effects is not clear. It should also be mentioned that the trials comparing these two treatments were comparatively small and may not be sufficiently powered to reveal small differences. An effect of testosterone deficiency is loss of sexual function, although this is not inevitable[10], and sudden loss of steroid hormones, be they male or female, causes hot flushes, apparently due to the proximity of the thermoregulatory center in the hypothalamus to the synapses involved in LH-RH release[11]. Other immediate effects of the removal of testosterone include weight increase and lack of physical drive. Recently, Gardiner and his colleagues have documented a loss of cognitive function as an additional consequence of androgen deprivation[12]. They have also performed a small randomized study comparing quality of life after orchidectomy, LH-RH analog and cyproterone acetate with no treatment, demonstrating a clear detriment in those receiving hormonal therapy[13]. There was a significant loss of quality of life at 6 and 12 months.

Long-term consequences of androgen deprivation

Testosterone deficiency is now recognized to have consequences as important as those related to lack of estrogen in postmenopausal women. Obesity, loss of muscle mass, anemia and, most critically, osteoporosis can occur[14]. Pathological fractures, incorrectly attributed to the effect of metastases, may be a more frequent effect of long-term treatment than has been recognized[15]. Osteoporosis in old age is not confined to women. Additional loss of bone density probably occurs in men treated for prostate cancer. The extent to which androgen deprivation contributes directly to this is a somewhat complicated issue. In Daniell's series[15], patients undergoing orchidectomy had more risk factors for osteoporosis than the 'control group'. However, there was a cumulative incidence in the orchidectomy group, not seen in the untreated men. Length of treatment, the patient's age and the presence of risk factors (e.g. smoking) are clearly related to the development of osteoporosis[15,16]. More attention should be given to bone density in patents receiving this type of treatment.

Steroidal antiandrogens

Progesterone drugs, usually cyproterone acetate, were at one time the main alternative to orchidectomy, and commonly used in the 1980s. They have a combined action, centrally reducing testosterone release and peripheral competitive antagonism of testosterone[17]. As a steroid hormone, the central effects leading to hot flushes are avoided, and indeed, one of the main uses for cyproterone acetate now is in the treatment of hot flushes. However, the use of cyproterone acetate has been restricted by the serious, and potentially fatal, liver toxicity. This seems to be related to cumulative dose, and has restricted the use of this drug to short-term administration to prevent tumor flare on commencing LH-RH therapy.

Non-steroidal antiandrogens

These preserve, indeed cause an elevation of, testosterone levels[1]. The potential for this to preserve sexual function is one of the main incentives to use these agents. With the older drugs such as flutamide, side-effects, particularly gastrointestinal disturbances[18], restricted their use, and limited dosage to levels mainly appropriate for combined androgen blockade regimens. Bicalutamide can be used in a dose (150 mg) which, at least in locally advanced disease, is therapeutically equivalent to androgen deprivation[19]. The main side-effect of bicalutamide, breast pain and gynecomastia, is troublesome but preventable by radiation therapy to the breast area. Although liver toxicity has been particularly associated with cyproterone acetate, this merely reflects the longer life span of this drug, and monitoring of liver function is recommended with non-steroidal antiandrogens.

Estrogens

Following the recognition that stilbestrol use was associated with an increase in cardiovascular mortality[20], the use of estrogens as a primary hormonal treatment for prostate cancer has largely ceased. The cardiovascular toxicity is multifactorial. Stilbestrol causes fluid retention, changes in plasma lipids, platelet aggregation and reduction of antithrombin III. Gynecomastia is troublesome, and liver toxicity can occur. However, in other respects, as a treatment estrogens have significant advantages. Their action seems to be due to more than simple suppression of testosterone secretion. Increased levels of sex hormone-binding globulin will further reduce androgenic effects[21]. There may in addition be a direct tumor-suppression effect, which can be utilized in treating patients after relapse. Side-effects of steroid hormone deprivation, hot flushes and osteoporosis, are avoided. The side-effects of estrogen treatment are dose related, and the cardiovascular toxicity may be due not to the drug itself, but to metabolites produced in the liver after oral administration. As discussed below, this has led to alternative treatment strategies.

Does hormone treatment cause premature death?

Despite its undoubted efficacy in causing disease remission, the impact of hormonal treatment on overall survival remains less clear (Figure 1). This is to be expected as, at the age of most men with prostate cancer, shortened life expectation owing to conflicting comorbidities will dilute any benefit resulting from improved disease-specific survival. However, could there in addition be a treatment-related mortality counteracting any disease-specific survival benefit? The increased risk of cardiovascular disease with estrogen treatment has been recognized since the Veteran's Administration Co-operative Urological Research Group (VACURG) studies; might it also occur with other forms of hormone treatment? If so, this should be identified in trials comparing immediate versus deferred treatment. Curves for non-prostate cancer deaths in the Medical Research Council (MRC) trial PR03 of immediate versus deferred hormone treatment[2] do not show a significant survival disadvantage (Figure 2). Table 1, in which causes of non-prostate cancer death are recorded, shows there to be *more* deaths from cardiovascular disease in those in whom treatment was *deferred*. In this study an excess of deaths after immediate treatment (albeit not statistically significant) occurred from other forms of cancer[22]. Most of those dying from non-prostate cancer had undergone orchidectomy. It has been suggested that an increase in serum LH with age is a predisposing factor in developing cancer[23]. Does orchidectomy, a rise in LH after which is the main endocrine difference from LH-RH treatment, cause cancer? Data from the Scottish Cancer registry (Brewster, unpublished) show that the relative risk of developing other malignancies is reduced in men with prostate cancer, and is lower in those undergoing orchidectomy

(Table 2). The cancer types leading to non-prostate cancer deaths in PR03 were those characterized by rapid progression, and with deferred treatment their incidence may simply have been masked by earlier death from prostate cancer.

Overall, the possibility of death occurring from the effects of non-estrogen hormone treatments remains arguable.

Strategies to reduce treatment-related morbidity

Choice of drug

The majority of patients are managed by androgen deprivation with LH-RH analog or orchidectomy, either alone or as part of a combined androgen-deprivation regimen. Since the major side-effects of endocrine therapy can be ascribed to the lack of steroid hormones, should alternative drug regimens be considered? Substitution of another steroid hormone is one possibility. Although cyproterone acetate was popular, its long-term use is contraindicated by the risk of liver toxicity, although it remains the main drug for tumor flare prevention, and is useful as treatment for hot flushes.

Non-steroidal antiandrogens preserve or increase levels of serum testosterone. In one study[24], sexual interest was preserved in 64% of patients receiving bicalutamide, compared with 30% treated by androgen deprivation (LH-RH analog or orchidectomy). However, when flutamide was compared with cyproterone acetate, there was a progressive loss of ejaculation, affecting 90% by 2 years, with no difference between the two groups[25]. Bone mineral density appears to be preserved in patients on bicalutamide compared with LH-RH analog treatment[26]. However, in large studies of adjuvant treatment with bicalutamide in early prostate cancer, 25.8% of patients receiving the drug withdrew because of side-effects (mainly gynecomastia or breast pain). Since it is the use of hormone therapy in early disease that causes most concern about

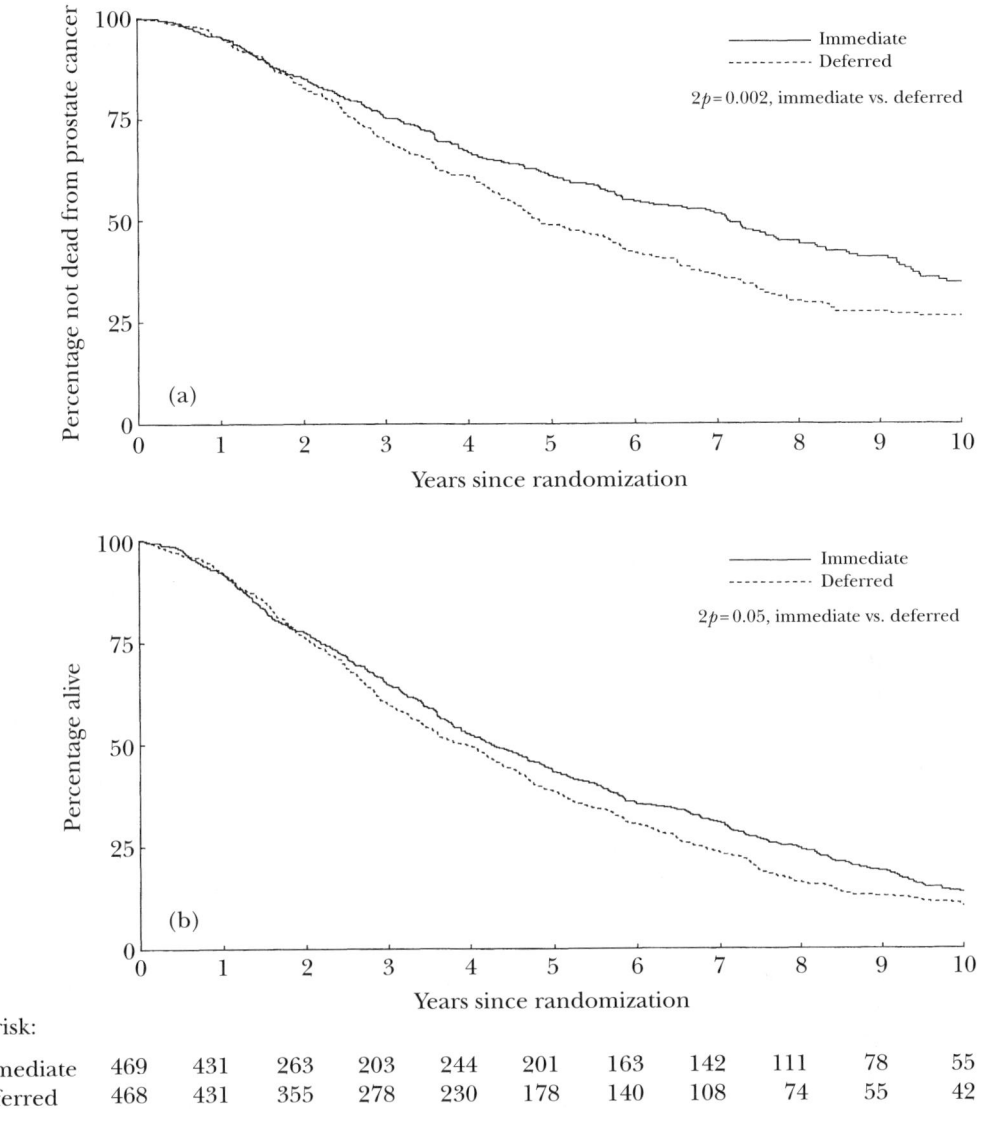

Figure 1 Medical Research Council (MRC) trial PR03: (a) death from prostate cancer, by randomization group; (b) death from all causes, by randomization group. Data to May 2002 (previously unpublished)

long-term side-toxicity, we may still be some way from a urological drug comparable to tamoxifen in breast cancer.

Should estrogens be revisited? Two strategies to reduce the risk of cardiovascular complications have been proposed. The risk is dose related, becoming significant with stilbestrol 3 mg and above. Although lower doses do not fully suppress serum testosterone levels, as a result of other effects of stilbestrol on the tumor this dose may be as efficacious as higher doses[27]. It is proposed that stilbestrol 1 mg prescribed with aspirin may be a safe alternative to other treatments. Parenteral administration, usually by injection (although the use of patches has also been proposed), may be safer as it avoids the liver metabolism which seems to produce the toxic derivatives. The Scandinavian

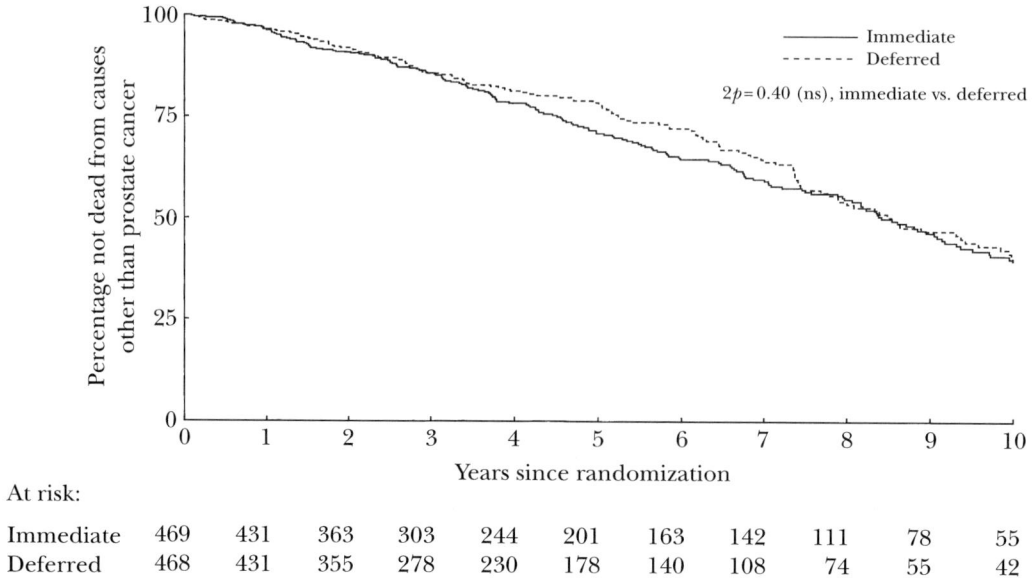

At risk:

Immediate	469	431	363	303	244	201	163	142	111	78	55
Deferred	468	431	355	278	230	178	140	108	74	55	42

Figure 2 Medical Research Council (MRC) trial PRO 3, death from causes other than prostate cancer, by randomization group. Data to May 2002 (previously unpublished)

Table 1 Medical Research Council (MRC) trial PR03: causes of death other than prostate cancer: immediate versus deferred treatment. Data from reference 22

	Immediate (n)	Deferred (n)		
		All	Treated	Untreated
Cardiovascular	77	91	51	40
Cancer (non-prostate)	27	15	10	5
COPD/ respiratory	22	9	5	4
Other	21	14	7	7
Total	147	129	73	56

COPD, chronic obstructive pulmonary disease

Table 2 Relative risk (RR) of developing second malignancy in men with prostate cancer: unpublished data from the Scottish Cancer Registry, with thanks to D. Brewster

	n	RR (95% CI)
Total prostate cancer	23 437	
Prostate first malignancy	22 015	
Treated by orchidectomy	3318	
Second cancer	1148	0.7 (0.6–0.7)
Orchidectomy group		0.6 (0.5–0.7)
Orchidectomy vs. non-orchidectomy		0.84 (0.72–0.97) $p = 0.0166$

CI, confidence interval

Prostatic Cancer Group's study SPCG 5 has compared parenteral estrogen (Estradurin®) with combined androgen deprivation in the treatment of metastatic prostate cancer[28]. Efficacy is equivalent. The incidence of cardiovascular deaths was similar in both groups, although more non-fatal cardiovascular events were noted among the estrogen-treated patients.

Bisphosphonates

The role of these agents in prostate cancer has been explored, both as treatment on relapse and, in two MRC studies, as adjuvant treatment commenced alongside hormone therapy[29]. Their potential to reduce the risk of osteoporosis would provide an incentive for their use on top of any cancer-specific benefit[30].

Strategies for administration

Deferred treatment   When the VACURG studies suggested that delaying treatment might not affect survival[20], it was the avoidance of side-effects that was the main justification for deferring treatment until specific indications occurred. If there was indeed no survival advantage in immediate treatment, there would be every argument in favor of delay[6]. As evidence for a survival advantage emerges, the argument becomes more complicated, and becomes a balance between longevity on the one hand and quality-of-life issues on the other. Potential quality-of-life benefits proposed from the control of disease by immediate treatment[6] have been confirmed in MRC trial PR03[2], where the reduced incidence of serious complications (spinal cord compression, pathological fracture, ureteric obstruction, extraskeletal metastases) and local progression as measured by the transurethral resection of the prostate (TURP) rate in the immediate-treatment group has persisted as data have matured, with over 90% of the patients having now died. On the other hand, Gardiner and colleagues' albeit small study has demonstrated a definite reduction in quality of life in those undergoing immediate hormone treatment, at least during the first 12 months[13]. There remains a need for studies involving modern quality-of-life instruments to determine the true balance of risk and benefit. Meanwhile, the correct treatment has to be determined for each patient on the basis of his priorities: some will wish to achieve maximum longevity while others will accept the risk of a shorter life to preserve their immediate quality of life.

Intermittent treatment is another strategy designed to reduce toxicity, which also may delay the onset of hormone-refractory disease[31]. In those with minimal disease in whom hormone treatment is considered, for example on biochemical relapse after radical curative treatment, *sequential androgen blockade*, commencing with 5α-reductase inhibition, through antiandrogen to LH-RH analog and perhaps combined androgen blockade, as and when further progression occurs, has been proposed[32]. These regimens must still be considered experimental.

Conclusions

Endocrine treatment for prostate cancer has been in use for over 60 years. Discussion of side-effects, and enthusiasm for the development of novel treatments, must not obscure the fact that this remains one of the most effective systemic treatments in oncology. The challenge in the 21st century is to devise treatments which preserve the benefits, but without the side-effects and toxicity. If this were combined with a solution to the problem of hormone-refractory disease, we would enter a new era of therapy for advanced prostate cancer, which would render many other therapies redundant.

References

1. Rabbini F, Gleave ME. Treatment of metastatic prostate cancer: endocrine therapy. In Hamdy FC, Basler JW, Neal DE, Catalona WJ, eds. *Management of Urologic Malignancies*. Edinburgh: Churchill Livingstone, 2002:210–26
2. Medical Research Council Prostate Cancer Working Party Investigators Group. Immediate versus deferred treatment for advanced prostatic cancer: initial results of the Medical Research Council trial. *Br J Urol* 1997;79:235–46
3. Bolla M, Gonzalez D, Ward P, *et al.* Improved survival in patients with locally advanced prostate cancer treated with radiotherapy and goserelin. *N Engl J Med* 1997;337:295–300
4. Mayer FJ, Crawford ED. The role of endocrine therapy in the management of local and distant recurrence of prostate cancer following radical

prostatectomy or radiation therapy. *Urol Clin North Am* 1994;21:707–15

5. Carlstrom K, Stege R, Henriksson P, *et al.* Possible bone-preserving capacity of high dose intramuscular depot oestrogen as compared to orchiectomy in the treatment of patients with prostatic carcinoma. *Prostate* 1997;31:193–7

6. Kirk D. Trials and tribulations in prostatic cancer. *Br J Urol* 1987;59:375–9

7. Kaisary AV, Tyrrell CJ, Peeling WB, *et al.* Comparison of LHRH analogue (Zoladex) versus orchiectomy in patients with metastatic prostate cancer. *Br J Urol* 1991;67:502–8

8. O'Connor VJ, Chiang SP, Grayhack JT. Is subcapsular orchiectomy a definitive procedure? Studies of hormone excretion before and after orchiectomy. *J Urol* 1963;89:236–40

9. Mahler C. Is disease flare a problem? *Cancer* 1993;72:3799–802

10. Ellis WJ, Grayhack JT. Sexual function in aging males after orchiectomy and estrogen therapy. *J Urol* 1963;89:895–9

11. Radlmier A, Bormacher K, Neumann F. Hot flushes: mechanism and prevention. *Prog Clin Biol Res* 1990;359:131–40

12. Gardiner RA, Green H, Yaxley J, *et al.* Cognition and hormonal manipulation in prostate cancer. *BJU Int* 2000;86(Suppl 3):218–19

13. Gardiner RA, Green H, Pakenham K, *et al.* Quality of life effects of hormonal medications for prostate cancer: a randomised controlled trial. *BJU Int* 2000;90(Suppl 2):179

14. Morley JE, Kaiser FE, Hajjar R, Perr HM III. Testosterone and frailty. *Clin Geriatr Med* 1997;13:655–95

15. Daniell HW. Osteoporosis after orchiectomy for prostate cancer. *J Urol* 1997;157:439–44

16. Stein B, Ashok S. Osteoporosis as a complication of androgen deprivation for carcinoma of the prostate. *BJU Int* 2002;90(Suppl 2):180

17. Goldenberg SL, Bruckovsky N. Use of cyproterone acetate in prostate cancer. *Urol Clin North Am* 1991;18:111–22

18. Sogani PC, Vagaiwala MR, Whitmore WF Jr. Experience with flutamide in patients with advanced prostate cancer without prior endocrine therapy. *Cancer* 1984;54:744–50

19. Iversen P, Tyrrell CJ, Kaisary AV, *et al.* Bicalutamide monotherapy compared with castration in patients with nonmetastatic locally advanced prostate cancer: 6.3 years of follow up. *J Urol* 2000;164:1579–82

20. Byar DP. The Veteran's Administration Co-operative Research Group's studies of cancer of the prostate. *Cancer* 1973;32:1126–30

21. Cox RL, Crawford ED. Estrogens in the treatment of prostate cancer. *J Urol* 1995;154:1991–8

22. Kirk D and the Medical Research Council Prostate Cancer Working Party Investigators Group. Does hormonal treatment for prostate cancer cause excess deaths: data from the MRC immediate versus deferred hormone treatment study. *BJU Int* 1999;83(Suppl 4):9

23. Bowles JT. Ageing and evolution. *Med Hypoth* 1998;51:179

24. Anderson JB, Iversen P, Tyrrell CJ, *et al.* The effect on sexual interest of 'Casodex' (bicalutamide) 150 mg compared with castration in patients with advanced prostate cancer. *BJU Int* 2000;86(Suppl 3):220

25. Schröder FH and members of the European Organization for Radiation Therapy in Cancer Genitourinary Group. Prostate cancer treated by antiandrogens – is preservation of sexual function possible? In press

26. Seiber PR, Keiller DL, Kahnoski RJ, *et al.* Bone density is maintained during bicalutamide ('Casodex') treatment. Presented at the *American Society of Clinical Oncology*, Orlando, May 2002

27. Bishop MC. Experience with low-dose oestrogen in the treatment of advanced prostate cancer: a personal view. *Br J Urol* 1996;78:921–8

28. Hedland PO, Ala-Opas M, Brekkan E, *et al.* Parenteral estrogen versus combined androgen deprivation in the treatment of metastatic prostate cancer. *Scand J Urol Nephrol* 2002;in press

29. Dearnaley DP, Sydes MR, on behalf of the Medical Research Council PR05 collaboration. Preliminary evidence that oral clodrinate delays symptomatic progression of bone metastases from prostate cancer: first results of the MRC PR05 trial. *Proc Am Soc Clin Oncol* 2001;20:174a

30. Clarke NW, McClure J, George NJR. The effects of orchidectomy on skeletal metabolism in metastatic prostate cancer. *Scand J Urol Nephrol* 1993;27:475–83

31. Goldenberg SL, Bruchovsky N, Gleave ME, *et al.* Intermittent androgen suppression in the treatment of prostate cancer: a preliminary report. *Urology* 1995;45:839–44

32. Fleshner NE, Trachtenberg J. Sequential androgen blockade: a biological study in the inhibition of prostatic growth. *J Urol* 1992;148:1928–31

Chemotherapy for the treatment of hormone-refractory prostate cancer: evaluating new targets based on apoptotic pathways

46

D. P. Petrylak

Introduction

Androgen ablation was identified as effective for the treatment of metastatic prostate cancer more than 60 years ago. Rapid and dramatic regression of metastatic lesions follow the achievement of castrate testosterone levels; this response generally lasts 18–24 months, with almost all patients experiencing disease progression. Once patients become refractory to androgen blockade, their prognosis is dismal, with a median survival time of 9–12 months. An estimated 31 000 men will die from metastatic disease in the year 2002. Unfortunately, until recently few treatment options were available to men with hormone-refractory prostate cancer (HRPC). Single-agent chemotherapy has been, in the past, viewed as ineffective. A review by Yagoda and Petrylak of single-agent chemotherapeutic trials published between 1988 and 1991 demonstrated a disappointing response rate of 8.7% (95% confidence interval 6.4–9.0%), with median survivals of 9–12 months[1]. This review demonstrated the need for new agents and drug targets.

Currently used chemotherapeutic regimens for androgen-independent prostate cancer

Mitoxantrone combined with corticosteroids

Two randomized trials established the combination of mitoxantrone with a corticosteroid as a palliative standard of care. When combined with prednisone alone, mitoxantrone 12 mg/m^2 (plus prednisone 5 mg) orally, twice a day improves pain but does not improve survival[2]. The Cancer and Leukemia Group B (CALGB) also found similar results in patients treated with mitoxantrone 14 mg/m^2 combined with hydrocortisone[3]. Unfortunately, despite significant pain relief, the median survivals reported by these studies are in the 10–12-month range, which is similar to that for historical controls.

Estramustine–vinblastine chemotherapy

A nor-nitrogen mustard conjugated with estradiol, estramustine phosphate was originally designed to be cleaved to allow the mustard moiety to alkylate DNA. However, estramustine has several other distinct mechanisms, including disruption of cytoplasmic microtubules, inhibition of the assembly of the nuclear matrix and inhibition of *p*-glycoprotein. Estramustine has modest activity in the treatment of prostate cancer as a single agent. Results of *in vitro* studies have demonstrated synergy between estramustine and tubulin-directed agents such as vincalkyloids and taxanes[4–6].

Do these preclinical observations translate into clinical benefit for men with hormone-refractory prostate cancer? A phase III study reported by Hudes and colleagues compared single-agent vinblastine with the combination of estramustine–vinblastine in 201 men with HRPC. The primary end-point was overall survival; secondary end-points were time to disease progression, response of measurable disease, prostate-specific antigen (PSA) level declines and changes in quality of life measures. At first analysis, only a trend towards improved overall survival was observed in patients receiving combination therapy compared with vinblastine alone (11.9 months vs. 9.2 months, $p = 0.08$). However, with further follow-up, this trend became statistically significant ($p = 0.051$). Unfortunately, it is unclear whether this survival difference is real or due to differences in the treatment arms. Although not significant individually, small differences in the distribution of prognostic factors such as serum lactate dehydrogenase, alkaline phosphatase and hemoglobin in favor of the estramustine–vinblastine arm may in part account for the differences in survival. The relatively small number of patients entered in this trial could further magnify the effect of small differences in prognostic factors. The fact that the treatment arm was not found to be significant to survival in a multivariate analysis further supports the contention that the survival difference observed may be due to a more favorable group of patients treated in the estramustine–vinblastine arm[7,8].

Paclitaxel-based chemotherapy

Paclitaxel, either as a single agent or in combination with estramustine, has been evaluated in men with progressive HRPC. As a 24-h infusion every 3 weeks, paclitaxel has only a 4% response rate[9]. Higher PSA decline rates were observed with weekly administration in comparison with the 24-h infusion every 3 weeks[10]. Approximately 25% of patients treated with the 24-h infusion of paclitaxel developed neutropenic fevers, whereas myelosuppression was not nearly as common with the weekly regimen.

Based on preclinical data demonstrating synergy, investigators have also evaluated paclitaxel in combination with estramustine. Response to estramustine–paclitaxel, as measured by PSA declines of > 50%, ranges from 53 to 64%. Responses in bidimensionally measurable disease range from 44 to 58%[11-13].

Docetaxel-based chemotherapy

Single-agent docetaxel produced PSA declines of > 50% in 38–58% and measurable disease response rates ranging from 17 to 33%[14,15]. A similar pattern of increased response rates can be observed when estramustine is combined with docetaxel. At Columba Presbyterian Medical Center, the combination of estramustine (280 mg orally, three times a day, days 1–5) with docetaxel (40–80 mg/m² every 3 weeks) in men with androgen-independent prostate cancer was studied in a phase I trial. The estramustine was administered over a short course to maximize drug interaction while minimizing toxicity[16]. Dexamethasone 20 mg for three doses was administered as pre-medication; a subsequent trial demonstrated that this steroid premedication regimen did not significantly contribute to the response rate[17]. Myelosuppression was dose-limiting, and occurred in 17.6% of patients treated with docetaxel 80 mg/m². Thus, the recommended dose for phase II trials was 70 mg/m² in minimally pretreated patients and 60 mg/m² in extensively pretreated patients. Eight of 15 patients receiving narcotic analgesics for the management of bone pain discontinued use of narcotic analgesics for a median of 6 weeks, with one patient able to reduce his requirement by more than 50%.

Decreases in serum PSA levels of > 50% were observed at all dose levels. Fifty-eight per cent of those who received 40 mg/m² had a ≥ 50% decline in serum PSA post-treatment, whereas all seven patients treated at the 70-mg/m² dose level achieved a 50% or higher decline in PSA. An objective response was observed in 28% of the 18 patients with bidimensionally measurable disease. The median survival time was 23 months, and the 1-year survival rate was 68%. A second phase I trial using a higher dose of estramustine (14 mg/kg/day continuously) also found a similar maximum tolerated dose of 70 mg/m² of docetaxel every 3 weeks[18].

Similar results have been noted in phase II studies where PSA response rates ranged from 45 to 74%[19-21] and response in measurable disease ranged from 11 to 57%. The median survivals have been found to parallel the phase I results; studies by Savarese and colleagues[20] and Petrylak and associates[19] have demonstrated median survivals of 20 months.

Two randomized trials are evaluating whether docetaxel-based therapy is superior to mitoxantrone-based therapy in terms of survival. The Southwest Oncology Group (SWOG) and CALGB are conducting a multicenter randomized trial comparing docetaxel–estramustine with mitoxantrone–prednisone. The primary end-point of this study is survival, and it is powered to detect a 33% difference between the two treatment arms. At the time of preparation of this chapter, the trial is near the accrual goal of 620 eligible patients. A second trial comparing weekly docetaxel–prednisone, every 3 weeks, with mitoxantrone is similarly powered to detect a 33% difference. It has met its accrual goal of 1004 patients, and preliminary survival data should be reported within 1 year.

Strategies for improving the response rate of taxane-based therapy

Bcl-2-targeted therapy

The antiapoptotic protein Bcl-2, originally identified in follicular lymphomas, is expressed in a variety of human tumors, including breast, lung and prostate cancer. In prostate cancer, Bcl-2 appears to be important to the development of the androgen-independent phenotype. Bcl-2 is expressed in approximately 65–90% of specimens obtained from men with androgen-independent prostate cancer, and, in contrast, in approximately 25% of prostate cancer tissue obtained from men with hormone-naive disease. Inhibition of Bcl-2 function can delay the time to androgen resistance in cell lines and animal models[22]. Transfection of Bcl-2 in the androgen-sensitive human prostate cancer cell line LNCaP (lymph node cancer of the prostate) imparts resistance to androgen ablation. Gleave's group demonstrated that administration of an antisense oligonucleotide to Bcl-2 to mice inoculated with the LNCaP prostate cancer cell line at the time of castration decreased the volume of recurrent tumors as well as prolonged survival, when compared with controls treated with castration or a 1- or 2-b mismatch antisense to Bcl-2[23].

Taxanes can phosphorylate Bcl-2 and thus abrogate its ability to induce apoptosis[24]. One strategy of improving the efficacy of taxane-based therapy would be to down-regulate Bcl-2 via specific antisense to Bcl-2. Antisense compounds have been safely combined with weekly docetaxel regimens; studies are now being designed to determine whether this approach leads to increased therapeutic efficacy[25].

NF-κB

The transcription factor nuclear-factor-κB (NF-κB) regulates the expression of genes related to tumor invasion, metastases, immune response, cell proliferation and regulation of apoptotic death[26]. This protein is sequestered, and thus inactivated, by inhibitor of κB (IκB). When released from this complex, NF-κB will translocate to the nucleus and activate gene expression. This process is under the control of growth factors and cytokines. A variety of antiapoptotic genes are regulated by NF-κB, including c-inhibitor of apoptosis, and manganese superoxide dismutase. Regulation of NF-κB may be under hormonal control. In human breast cancer cells, NF-κB is constitutively expressed in estrogen receptor-negative breast cancer and poorly differentiated primary tumors. In the human prostate cancer cell lines PC3 and DU 145, NF-κB is constitutively activated, whereby a significantly lower level of NF-κB can be found in the hormone-sensitive LNCaP line[27]. NF-κB can also enhance PSA expression without androgen, with androgen-independent tissues demonstrating higher binding than androgen-dependent tissues.

The NF-κB pathway may be used as a target for improving the efficacy of taxane-based therapy. However, contradictory preclinical studies demonstrate that NF-κB may enhance or negate the effectiveness of taxane. In human breast cancer cell lines, NF-κB inducable genes protect against paclitaxel-induced cell death[28]. In prostate cancer, NF-κB is associated with increased Bcl-2 expression. In human prostate cancer cell lines, expression of a dominant negative IκB mutant protein significantly enhanced TNF-α-mediated apoptosis; however, overexpression of Bcl-2 abrogated this effect[29]. The constitutive expression of NF-κB has been demonstrated to be related to phosphorylation of IκB through activation of IKK[30,31].

Proteosomes ubiquitinate a variety of proteins, including IκB, and thus are essential to their degradation. PS-341, a boronic acid dipeptide which is highly selective for proteosome inhibition, can inhibit degradation of IκB and thus effectively inhibit NF-κB release. Combinations of proteosome inhibitors with chemotherapeutic agents increase the number of cells undergoing apoptosis *in vitro*. In human colorectal carcinoma cell lines, pretreatment of cells with PS-341 followed by treatment with SN 38, the active metabolite of CPT-11, demonstrated a 64–75% decrease in cell counts. In comparison, treatment with either SN 38 or PS-341 alone resulted in 22–30% and 24–47% growth inhibition, respectively. Since NF-κB expression appears to be associated with taxane resistance, proteosome inhibition may improve the efficacy of either paclitaxel or docetaxel. A phase I/II trial evaluating escalating doses of PS-341 combined with docetaxel is currently accruing patients at Vanderbilt University, the Cleveland Clinic and New York Presbyterian, and will generate preliminary toxicity and efficacy data.

Role of vitamin D

Calcitriol, in human prostate cancer cell models, induces a significant G_0/G_1 arrest and modulates p21 (Waf1/Cip1) and p27 (Kip1), the cyclin-dependent kinase inhibitors. Preclinical synergy has also been noted when paclitaxel is combined with calcitriol[32,33]. Based on this preclinical data, Beer at Oregon State University evaluated 37 men with HRPC treated with weekly docetaxel 36 mg/m² for 6–8 weeks and calcitrol 0.5 μg/kg[34]. Toxicities of treated patients included grade 3 or 4 neutropenia in 41%, with one patient succumbing to pneumonia. Of note, 3% of patients were found to have a deep venous thrombosis, despite the fact that no estramustine was used in the regimen. Of the eligible patients treated, 81% achieved a PSA decline of > 50% confirmed by a second measurement 1 month later, with 53% of patients demonstrating a partial response in measurable disease. The median survival was 19.5 months. The response rates and survival with the Beer regimen appear to be similar to those of phase II estramustine– docetaxel studies reported by Savarese and Petrylak and their groups[19,20].

Role for early chemotherapy

Complete responses are rare when these regimens are administered to patients with advanced disease. Perhaps one reason for the failure of chemotherapy to prolong survival in prostate cancer patients is that these men are treated too late in the course of their disease. In breast and colon cancer, chemotherapeutic agents administered to patients with metastatic disease will improve survival minimally, or not at all. Yet, when these drugs are administered to high-risk colon and breast cancer patients in the adjuvant setting, clear survival differences are observed. Investigators are now evaluating the role of administration of chemotherapy to high-risk prostate cancer patients in conjunction with definitive local therapy. Thus, the hormone-sensitive as well as the hormone-refractory clones are potentially eradicated by this approach.

Current trials evaluating chemotherapy in early disease

Neoadjuvant therapy

Two regimens known to have activity in advanced-disease patients have been evaluated in high-risk men prior to radical prostatectomy. Pettaway and colleagues administered a regimen that alternated the combination of ketoconazole and adriamycin with vinblastine and estramustine in 30 patients[35], while Clark and associates administered oral estramustine– VP-16 to 18 patients[36]. Both regimens are estramustine-based, which can affect androgen ablation, and thus make it difficult to differentiate the effect of chemotherapy from that of hormonal therapy. The results of two small phase II studies appear similar, with the rates of organ-confined disease post-chemotherapy/prostatectomy ranging between 33 and 31%. Most disappointingly, neither study was able to demonstrate a complete pathological response despite normalization of PSA in 50% of patients[37].

Studies have also evaluated the combination of estramustine and vinblastine concomitantly with radiation therapy. Kelly and co-workers administered three 8-week cycles of estramustine combined with vinblastine (vinblastine 6 mg/m^2 per week for 6 weeks with a 2-week rest) combined with high-dose conformal three-dimensional external beam radiation therapy (65–70 cGy) to high-risk prostate cancer patients (Gleason score ≥ 8, PSA > 10 ng/ml; Gleason ≥ 7, PSA > 20 ng/ml; clinical T3N0M0 with PSA > 20 ng/ml; any T4N0M0 disease or TxN1M0 disease). The 2-year PSA relapse-free survival rate was 60%, with acceptable rates of genitourinary and gastrointestinal toxicity[38]. Although a higher rate of proctitis and diarrhea were observed by Khil and colleagues with a 7-week course of estramustine–vinblastine combined with radiation therapy[37], the greatest improvement in PSA control appeared to be found in those high-risk patients with pretreatment PSA levels ranging from 30 to 50 ng/dl. Thus, combined radiotherapy–chemotherapy seems to be a safe and effective treatment strategy for evaluation in future phase III trials.

Adjuvant therapy

Although mitoxantrone combined with a corticosteroid is effective in palliating patients with metastatic prostate cancer, no survival advantage can be detected when mitoxantrone is compared with corticosteroids alone. Ninety-six locally advanced or metastatic patients were randomized to receive androgen blockade alone or in combination with mitoxantrone. The most striking difference in survival was seen in those patients with locally advanced disease, with patients receiving mitoxantrone achieving a median survival of 80 months compared with those treated with androgen blockade alone surviving a median of 36 months. Although these results are impressive, further confirmation in larger studies is necessary. The SWOG and CALGB are collaborating on a study which will compare 2 years of adjuvant hormone therapy plus six cycles of mitoxantrone chemotherapy with androgen blockade in patients post-radical prostatectomy. Thirteen hundred and sixty patients at high risk for relapse (Gleason score ≥ 8, pT3b or T4 disease, N1, Gleason 7 with extracapsular extension and positive margins) will be randomized; the study is designed to detect a 30% increase in survival at 10–13 years. Of note, early chemotherapy was not found to prolong survival in the Wang trial in patients with established metastatic disease[39].

References

1. Yagoda A, Petrylak D. Cytotoxic chemotherapy for advanced hormone-resistant prostate cancer. *Cancer* 1993;71:1098–109
2. Tannock IF, Osoba D, Stockler MR, *et al.* Chemotherapy with mitoxantrone plus prednisone or prednisone alone for symptomatic hormone-resistant prostate cancer: a Canadian randomized trial with palliative end points. *J Clin Oncol* 1996;14:1756–64
3. Kantoff PW, Halabi S, Conaway M, *et al.* Hydrocortisone with or without mitoxantrone in men with hormone-refractory prostate cancer: results of the Cancer and Leukemia Group B 9182 study. *J Clin Oncol* 1999;17:2506–13

4. Hudes GR, Greenberg R, Krigel RL, *et al.* Phase II study of estramustine and vinblastine, two microtubule inhibitors, in hormone-refractory prostate cancer. *J Clin Oncol* 1992;10:1754–61

5. Kreis W, Budman DR, Calabro A. Unique synergism or antagonism of combinations of chemotherapeutic and hormonal agents in human prostate cancer cell lines. *Br J Urol* 1997;79:196–202

6. Seidman AD, Scher HI, Petrylak D, Dershaw DD, Curley T. Estramustine and vinblastine: use of prostate specific antigen as a clinical trial end point for hormone refractory prostate cancer. *J Urol* 1992;147:931–4

7. Hudes G, Einhorn L, Ross E, Balsham A. Vinblastine versus vinblastine plus oral estramustine phosphate for patients with hormone-refractory prostate cancer: a Hoosier Oncology Group and Fox Chase Network phase III trial. *J Clin Oncol* 1999;17:3160–6

8. Hudes G, Ross E, Roth B, *et al.* Improved survival for patients with hormone-refractory prostate cancer receiving estramustine-based antimicrotubule therapy: final report of a Hoosier Oncology Group and Fox Chase Network phase III trial comparing vinblastine and vinblastine plus oral estramustine phosphate. *Proc Am Soc Clin Oncol* 2002;21:177a(abstr 704)

9. Roth BJ, Yeap BY, Wilding G, Kasimis B, McLeod D, Loehrer PJ. Taxol in advanced, hormone-refractory carcinoma of the prostate. *Cancer* 1993;72:2457–60

10. Trivedi C, Redman B, Flaherty LE, *et al.* Weekly 1-hour infusion of paclitaxel. Clinical feasibility and efficacy in patients with hormone-refractory prostate carcinoma. *Cancer* 2000;89:431–6

11. Hudes GR, Nathan F, Khater C, *et al.* Phase II trial of 96-hour paclitaxel plus oral estramustine phosphate in metastatic hormone-refractory prostate cancer. *J Clin Oncol* 1997;15:3156–63

12. Hudes GR, Manola J, Conroy J, Habermann T, Wilding G. Phase II study of weekly paclitaxel (P) by 1-hour infusion plus reduced-dose oral estramustine (EMP) in metastatic hormone-refractory prostate carcinoma (HRPC): a trial of the Eastern Cooperative Oncology Group. *Proc Am Soc Clin Oncol* 2001;20:175a(abstr 697)

13. Haas N, Roth B, Garay C, *et al.* Phase I trial of weekly paclitaxel plus oral estramustine phosphate in patients with hormone-refractory prostate cancer. *Urology* 2001;58:59–64

14. Picus J, Schultz M, Cochrane J. A phase II trial of docetaxel in patients with hormone refractory prostate cancer (HRPC): long term results. *Proc Am Soc Clin Oncol* 1999;18:314a(abstr 1206)

15. Berry W, Rohrbaugh T, the American Oncology Resources Clinical Research Task Force. Phase II trial of single-agent, weekly (Wk) Taxotere® (T) in symptomatic, hormone-refractory prostate cancer (HRPC). *Proc Am Soc Clin Oncol* 1999; 18:335a(abstr 1290)

16. Petrylak DP, Macarthur RB, O'Connor J, *et al.* Phase I trial of docetaxel with estramustine in androgen-independent prostate cancer. *J Clin Oncol* 1999;17:958–67

17. Weitzman AL, Shelton G, Zuech N, *et al.* Dexamethasone does not significantly contribute to the response rate of docetaxel and estramustine in androgen independent prostate cancer. *J Urol* 2000;163:834–7

18. Kreis W, Budman DR, Fetten J, Gonzales AL, Barile B, Vinciguerra V. Phase I trial of the combination of daily estramustine phosphate and intermittent docetaxel in patients with metastatic hormone refractory prostate carcinoma. *Ann Oncol* 1999;10:33–8

19. Petrylak DP, Shelton GB, England-Owen C, *et al.* Response and preliminary survival results of a phase II study of docetaxel (D) + estramustine (E) in patients (Pts) with androgen-independent prostate cancer (AIPC). *Proc Am Soc Clin Oncol* 2000;19:334a(abstr 1312)

20. Savarese DM, Halabi S, Hars V, *et al.*, for the Cancer and Leukemia Group B. Phase II study of docetaxel, estramustine, and low dose hydrocortisone in men with hormone-refractory prostate cancer: a final report of CALGB 9780. Cancer and Leukemia Group B. *J Clin Oncol* 2001;19:2509–16

21. Kosty MP, Ferreira A, Bryntesen T. Weekly docetaxel and low-dose estramustine phosphate in hormone refractory prostate cancer: a phase II study. *Proc Am Soc Clin Oncol* 2001;20;152b(abstr 2360)

22. Raffo AJ, Perlman H, Chen MW, Day ML, Streitman JS, Buttyan R. Overexpression of Bcl-2 protects prostate cancer cells from apoptosis *in vitro* and confers resistance to androgen depletion *in vivo*. *Cancer Res* 1995; 55:4438–45

23. Leung S, Miyake H, Zellweger T, Tolcher A, Gleave ME. Synergistic chemosensitization and inhibition of progression to androgen independence by antisense Bcl-2 oligodeoxynucleotide and paclitaxel in the LNCaP prostate tumor model. *Int J Cancer* 2001;91:846–5

24. Friedland D, Cohen J, Miller R, *et al.* A phase II trial of docetaxel (Taxotere) in hormone-refractory prostate cancer: correlation of antitumor effect to phosphorylation of Bcl-2. *Semin Oncol* 1999;26(Suppl):19–23

25. Tolcher AW. Preliminary phase I results of G3139 (Bcl-2 antisense oligonucleotide) therapy in combination with docetaxel in hormone-refractory prostate cancer. *Semin Oncol* 2001;28 (4 Suppl 15):67–70

26. Brown K, Park S, Kanno T, *et al.* Mutual regulation of the transcriptional activator NF-κB

and its inhibitor IκB-α. *Proc Natl Acad Sci USA* 1993;90:2532–6

27. Palayoor ST, Youmell MY, Calderwood SK. Constitutive activation of IκB kinase α and NF-κB in prostate cancer cell is inhibited by ibuprofen. *Oncogene* 1999;18:7389–94

28. Patel NM, Nozaki S, Shortle NH, *et al.* Paclitaxel sensitivity of breast cancer cells with constitutively activated NF-κB is enhanced by IκBα super-repressor parthenolide. *Oncogene* 2000;19: 4159–69

29. Herrmann JL, Beham AW, Sarkiss M, *et al.* Bcl-2 suppresses apoptosis resulting from the disruption of the NF-κB survival pathway. *Exp Cell Res* 1997;237:101–9

30. Gasparian AV, Yao YJ, Kowalczyk D, *et al.* The role of IKK in constitutive activation of NF-κB transcription factor in prostate carcinoma cells. *J Cell Sci* 2002;115:141–51

31. Suh J, Payvandi F, Edelstein LC, *et al.* Mechanisms of constitutive NF-κB activation in human prostate cancer cell lines. *Prostate* 2002;52:183–200

32. Johnson CS, Hershberger PA, Bernardi RJ, Mcguire TF, Trump DL. Vitamin D receptor: a potential target for intervention. *Urology* 2002; 60(3 Suppl 1):123–30

33. Hershberger PA, Yu WD, Modzelewski RA, Rueger RM, Johnson CS, Trump DL. Calcitriol (1,25-dihydroxycholecalciferol) enhances paclitaxel antitumor activity *in vitro* and *in vivo* and accelerates paclitaxel-induced apoptosis. *Clin Cancer Res* 2001;7:1043–51

34. Beer CM, Eilers KM, Garzotto M, Lowe BA, Henner WD. Androgen-independent prostate cancer (AIPC) treatment with weekly high-dose calcitriol and docetaxel. *Proc Ann Soc Clin Oncol* 2002;21:abstr 707

35. Pettaway CA, Pisters LL, Troncoso P, *et al.* Neoadjuvant chemotherapy and hormonal therapy followed by radical prostatectomy: feasibility and preliminary results. *J Clin Oncol* 2000;18:1050–7

36. Clark P, Peerboom DM, Dreicer R, *et al.* Phase II trial of neoadjuvant estramustine and etoposide plus radical prostatectomy for locally advanced prostate cancer. *Urology* 2001;57:281–6

37. Khil MS, Kim JH, Bricker LJ, Cerny JC. Tumor control of locally advanced prostate cancer following combined estramustine, vinblastine, and radiation therapy. *Cancer J Sci Am* 1997;3: 289–96

38. Zelefsky MJ, Kelly WK, Scher HI, *et al*. Results of a phase II study using estramustine phosphate and vinblastine in combination with high-dose three-dimensional conformal radiotherapy for patients with locally advanced prostate cancer. *J Clin Oncol* 2000;18:1936–41

39. Wang J, Halford S, Rigg A, Roylance R, Lynch M, Waxman J. Adjuvant mitoxantrone chemotherapy in advanced prostate cancer. *BJU Int* 2000;86:675–80

The role of bisphosphonates in prostate cancer

47

D. S. Ernst

Introduction

Bone metastases are a very common manifestation of advanced carcinoma of the prostate. In all, 85–100% of patients who die of prostate carcinoma will have bone metastases[1]. The development of bone pain, pathological fractures, hypercalcemia, and spinal cord and nerve compression syndromes contribute significantly to the morbidity of advanced bone disease[2]. The primary therapy for bone disease has been androgen deprivation. Although initial response to medical or surgical castration is 85%, the median duration of response is 2 years. For the clinician, the number of potential therapeutic options narrows as hormone resistance develops[3]. For the patient, irrespective of interventions, the median survival is limited to 10–12 months[4]. Palliation of these patients is optimized through the subsequent use of opioids, adjunct analgesic and anti-inflammatory agents, external beam radiation and chemotherapy. Unfortunately, much of the morbidity of hormone-refractory prostate cancer (HRPC) stems from the complications of the advancing skeletal disease. New strategies to prevent and manage the metastatic disease and its complications are needed.

Bisphosphonates

The bisphosphonates are a family of pyrophosphate analogs characterized by a stable phosphorus–carbon–phosphorus bond[5]. They bind with high affinity to hydroxyapatite crystal in bone, and peak concentrations in bone appear within hours on intravenous administration[6]. Accumulation is 2–3 times greater in trabecular bone than in cortical bone. The activity of the individual bisphosphonates is extremely variable. Many different bisphosphonates have been manufactured and are distinguishable in the nature of the central carbon side-chain[5]. Etidronate was the first bisphosphonate utilized in clinical practice. Although etidronate has relatively weak antiresorptive capabilities, bone mineralization is also impaired. Alternative agents were developed which do not interfere with normal bone mineralization but also have up to 10 000-fold increase in antiresorptive activity. Agents which have an amino group at the end of the side-chain, such as pamidronate or alendronate, have enhanced antiresorptive activity. Other modifications extending the length of the side-chain's carbon backbone, or inserting a methyl and pentyl group, greatly enhance biological effects on bone resorption.

Many bisphosphonates have been assessed in the management of human disease, including etidronate, pamidronate, clodronate, alendronate, ibandronate and zoledronate. Pamidronate, clodronate, zoledronate and ibandronate have been the most extensively studied bisphosphonates in malignant disease, and were first assessed in the treatment of malignant hypercalcemia[5]. Owing to the bisphosphonates' potent antiresorption activity, they remain the agents of choice in managing hypercalcemia of malignancy, a relatively rare occurrence in prostate cancer because of the predominence of osteoblastic stimulation[7,8].

Pharmacology

The bisphosphonates are resistant to endogenous phosphatases and have a relatively low bioavailability following oral ingestion, reduced further with concurrent food, particularly dairy products[9,10]. Two to three days following an intravenous dose, 20–50% of the bisphosphonate remains in the bones, and is slowly released over several weeks or months. Intravenous bisphosphonates must be given slowly, since insoluble aggregates may be formed and deposited in renal tissue, which can lead to transient proteinuria and impaired renal function. Although oral bisphosphonates can be given in a setting of renal insufficiency, dose modifications are required. Oral bisphosphonates such as clodronate and alendronate may cause upper gastrointestinal effects, including gastric erosions and ulcerations, and, on occasion, diarrhea[5].

Mechanism of action

The bisphosphonates appear to exert their biological activity through a variety of mechanisms[11]. The bisphosphonates have a direct effect on osteoclast function. In many models of rodent and human osteoclasts in vivo, bisphosphonates appear to cause osteoclast degeneration, and are recognized histologically by retraction and cellular fragmentation. Furthermore, the bisphosphonates at low concentrations ($\geq 10^{-7}$ mol/l) have been shown to induce apoptotic cell death in osteoclasts[12]. In addition, bisphosphonates can alter the appearance and function of the convoluted region of the osteoclast, which interacts with the bone surface and which is essential for the resorption process[13].

The bisphosphonates can also influence the function of osteoblasts and other connective tissue cells within bone[11]. The osteoblast may be the initial target cells for some bisphosphonates. Osteoblasts through paracrine mechanisms are instrumental in recruiting and activating osteoclastic bone resorption. Particularly in prostate cancer, tumor cells have been shown to stimulate osteoblastic bone formation and osteoclast activity through the release of a variety of cell mediators, such as transforming growth factor-β, insulin growth factors, urokinase plasminogen and endothelin-1[14].

At the molecular level, bisphosphonates can be classified into two broad groups: nitrogen-containing and non-nitrogen-containing. These two groups have different molecular mechanisms of action. Nitrogen-containing bisphosphonates, such as pamidronate and alendronate, inhibit the mevalonate signalling pathway, which is a biosynthetic process for the production of cholesterol and isoprenoid lipids. The cell consequently loses the ability to activate critical signalling proteins required for osteoclast function, including cell morphology, integrin signalling and membrane ruffling[15]. Non-nitrogen-containing bisphosphonates, such as clodronate, are incorporated into adenosine triphosphate, forming non-hydrolyzable analog and thereby inhibiting acidification and generation of the resorption lacuna at the osteoclast–bone interface[16].

The development of bone metastases is a complex process which ultimately results from direct interaction between the tumor cells and the constituents of bone[17]. Most tumors which metastasize to bone promote osteolysis. In prostate cancer, metastases are typically sclerotic, indicative of osteoblastic stimulation[18]. However, in studies utilizing sensitive biochemical markers of bone resorption, such as pyridinoline cross-links, marked bone resorption occurs, resulting in net bone loss[19]. The sclerotic lesions, often evident on radiographs, result from osteoblastic activation around nests of tumor cells. However, the new bone does not add to the architectural integrity of either cortical or trabecular bone, and patients remain at risk for fractures and pain.

Antitumor effects

In addition to affecting osteoclast and osteoblast function, the bisphosphonates appear to have a direct effect on prostate cancer tumor cells[20,21]. Several studies of prostate cancer cell lines have shown that following bisphosphonate administration, cellular adhesion to non-mineralized bone is reduced. Furthermore, aminobisphosphonate administration has been shown to induce apoptosis and to inhibit metalloproteinase production in human PC3 ML prostate cancer cells *in vitro*[22,23].

Clinical use in prostate cancer

Studies of patients with bone metastases due to breast cancer and multiple myeloma have shown an improvement in pain and decreased risk of skeletal events (fractures, hypercalcemia, need for intervention with surgery, radiation therapy) with bisphosphonates such as clodronate and pamidronate[24,25]. However, investigation of bisphosphonates in prostate cancer is more limited.

Bone pain

In an uncontrolled trial of patients with metastatic prostate cancer, Adami and colleagues first described a reduction in analgesic consumption and in the severity of bone pain in 16 of 17 patients within 10 days of receiving daily intravenous clodronate[26]. In a subsequent open series of studies using various oral and parenteral clodronate schedules, Adami and Mian additionally observed that pain reduction was more pronounced following parenteral administration[27]. Two other uncontrolled studies of daily infusions of clodronate indicated a symptomatic benefit in 60–70% of patients[28,29].

In 1996, Ernst and colleagues reported on a placebo-controlled, double-blind cross-over study of 59 patients with significant bone pain resulting from metastatic bone disease in a variety of primary tumor sites, including prostate cancer[30]. Patients were randomized to receive 600 mg, or 1500 mg, or placebo. Blinded patient selection of the more effective agent was the primary end-point of the trial. Of the 46 evaluable patients, 26 (57%) chose the clodronate; 12 (26%) chose placebo; and eight (17%) could not detect a difference in their pain control ($p < 0.002$).

Elomaa and Tammela conducted a double-blind, placebo-controlled trial in 57 patients with HRPC in which the patients were randomized to receive either clodronate 300 mg intravenously, daily for 5 days, followed by clodronate 1600 mg orally for 3 months, or placebo[31]. Some 34% of the clodronate group and 18% of the controls were pain-free after 1 month. After 3 months, 29% of the clodronate group continued to have no pain, in contrast to 4% of the control group. Several uncontrolled studies in metastatic bone disease with intravenous pamidronate have suggested a pain effect with minimal toxicity[32,33].

Palliation

An increasing number of cytotoxic agents have been shown to have activity in HRPC. The anthracyclines, estramustine, vincalkaloids and, most recently, the taxanes have been increasingly subject to clinical trials in HRPC and have been associated with encouraging rates of response[34]. Unfortunately, no single agent or combination has significantly impacted on overall survival in randomized, controlled trials. Nevertheless, some chemotherapeutic agents appear to play a role in improving palliation of patients with symptomatic progression. In 1996, Tannock and colleagues reported that, in a randomized trial with prednisone alone, the combination of mitoxantrone and prednisone significantly increased the palliative response: 29% vs. 12%[35]. The palliative response was determined utilizing validated patient-administered pain scores and analgesic diaries. The benefit of the combination was also evident using the PROSQOLI quality of life assessment tool. In a similar trial of mitoxantrone and hydrocortisone versus hydrocortisone alone, conducted by the Cancer and Leukemia Group B (CALGB 9132), survival was the primary end-point and no difference was found in either arm[36]. However, in the quality of life assessments, pain was reduced with mitoxantrone.

In order to confirm the findings of the Canadian study of Tannock, and to determine whether the bisphosphonate, clodronate, would further enhance the palliative response, the National Cancer of Canada Clinical Trials Group conducted a clinical trial in 211 symptomatic patients with HRPC. Patients were to receive clodronate 1500 mg intravenously or placebo randomized in a double-blind fashion[37]. Identical primary end-points of palliative response and quality of life assessment were adopted. The palliative response in the clodronate arm was 45% and in the placebo arm 39% ($p = 0.44$). In the pain domain of the PROSQOLI assessment, a statistically significant difference was seen in the median change from baseline as well as best response. The patients had been stratified according to degree of bone pain. In the 75% of patients whose baseline pain was categorized as mild, no difference in palliative response between the two arms was observed. However, in the remaining 25% of patients with moderate pain, the palliative response was 58% and 26% in the clodronate and placebo arms, respectively. These findings offer additional evidence that, in patients who are experiencing significant bone pain, the bisphosphonates may contribute to improving pain and overall palliation without untoward additional toxicity. However, this indication requires further clinical evaluation, particularly in determining the optimal agent, dose, frequency and mode of administration.

Delay in progression

Mounting clinical evidence in breast cancer and multiple myeloma would support the hypothesis that bisphosphonates may indeed prevent or delay the development of bone metastases. In breast cancer, several large randomized studies using chronic bisphosphonate therapy in addition to standard treatment have resulted in reductions of fractures, hypercalcemia, radiotherapy treatments and symptomatic progression[38–40]. Both oral clodronate and intravenous pamidronate have been utilized in these trials. In 1996, Berenson and colleagues reported not only a significant delay in progression but also a survival advantage in patients with multiple myeloma who received monthly pamidronate infusions[41]. In prostate cancer, evidence has been forthcoming more recently.

In a controlled study of the UK Medical Research Council, Dearnaley and Sydes reported early findings in 311 patients with advanced prostate cancer who were randomized to receive oral clodronate 2080 mg or placebo from the time when bone metastases were identified[42]. The primary end-point was symptomatic progression. In the initial analysis, when half the patients had progressed, there appeared to be a 6-month delay in progression in those patients who had received clodronate. Also, median survival was 34 months for the clodronate arm and 27 months for the placebo arm. Although these findings are preliminary, the potential for positively impacting upon the outcome of bone disease exists with early, chronic administration of bisphosphonates.

Zoledronate represents one of the most potent bisphosphonates under clinical development[43]. Unlike previous bisphosphonates, it can be safely administered using foreshortened infusional times, and has marked and sustained antiresorptive activity. In the largest clinical trial of bisphosphonates in prostate cancer to date, Saad and colleagues recently reported on a double-blind, placebo-controlled trial of 643 patients with metastatic disease[44]. Patients were initially randomized to zoledronate 4 mg, or 8 mg, or placebo. The primary end-point of the trials was the proportion of patients who sustained a skeletal-related event (SRE), which included pathological fractures, spinal cord compression, radiotherapy for bone pain, surgery to bone, or change of chemotherapy to manage bone pain. Because of problems with renal dysfunction, the 8-mg arm was halted, and all patients receiving zoledronate subsequently received 4 mg only. The primary analysis was modified accordingly to compare the 4-mg arm with the placebo arm. A statistically significant difference in SRE incidence was observed between the zoledronate 4 mg and placebo arms: 33.2% vs. 44.2%, respectively ($p = 0.02$). Furthermore difference in median time to first SRE was significant: 420 days vs. 321 days ($p = 0.01$). The SRE incidence and time to first SRE in the 8/4-mg arm were 38.5% and 363 days, respectively. In comparison with the placebo arm, these differences were not significantly different. Secondary end-points such as time to disease progression and quality of life were not improved in the zoledronate arm.

Osteoporosis

Osteoporosis is increasingly recognized as a significant complication of prolonged androgen-deprivation therapy. Such therapy could lead to decreased bone mineral density and increasing risks of fractures. In an open-label study of 47 men receiving leuprolide, with or without pamidronate, Smith and associates reported a reduction of mineralization by 3.3% in those patients who did not receive bisphosphonate therapy, and no significant decrease in bone density in those receiving bisphosphonates[45]. Further prospective clinical trials evaluating the bisphosphonates in preventing or retarding osteoporosis are ongoing.

Conclusion

Bisphosphonates continue to show promise in the management of metastatic bone disease. In the few randomized, controlled trials available, their effect in altering the actual course appears to be modest; however, in conjunction with conventional therapies, they can improve the morbidity of skeletal metastases. The role of bisphosphonates in preventing bone metastases is a subject of ongoing research. The development of new bisphosphonates with different toxicity profiles may well serve to increase the therapeutic index of these compounds.

Acknowledgement

I would like to thank Colleen Emerson for her invaluable assistance in the preparation of the manuscript.

References

1. Mundy GR. Mechanisms of bone metastasis. *Cancer* 1997;80:1546–56
2. Scher HI, Steineck G, Kelly WK. Hormone-refractory prostate cancer: refining the concept. *Urology* 1995;46:142–8
3. Harris KA, Reese D. Treatment options – hormone-refractory prostate cancer. *Drugs* 2001; 61:2177–92
4. Mahler C, Denis CJ. Hormone-refractory disease. *Semin Surg Oncol* 1995;11:77–83
5. Fleish H. Bisphosphonates. Pharmacology and use in the treatment of tumor-induced hypercalcemia and metastatic bone disease. *Drugs* 1991;42:919–44
6. Patel S, Lyons AR, Hosking DJ. Drugs used in the treatment of metabolic bone disease. *Drugs* 1993;46:594–617
7. Papapoulos SE, Hamdy NAT, Van der Pluijm G. Bisphosphonates in the management of prostate carcinoma metastatic to the skeleton. *Cancer* 2000;88:3047–53
8. Purohit OP, Radstone CR, Anthony C, *et al.* A randomised double-blind comparison of intra-venous pamidronate and clodronate in the hypercalcaemia of malignancy. *Br J Cancer* 1995; 72:1289–93
9. Plosker GL, Goa KL. Clodronate: a review of its pharmacological properties and therapeutic efficacy in resorptive bone disease. *Drugs* 1994;47:945–82
10. Fitton A, McTavish D. Pamidronate: a review. *Drugs* 1991;41:289–318
11. Rogers MJ, Gordon S, Benford HL, *et al.* Cellular and molecular mechanisms of action of bisphosphonates. *Cancer* 2000;88:2961–78
12. Breuil V, Cosman F, Stein L, *et al.* Human osteoclast formation and activity *in vitro*: effects of alendronate. *J Bone Miner Res* 1998;13:1721–9
13. Sato M, Grasser W. Effects of bisphosphonates on isolated rat osteoclasts as examined by reflected light microscopy. *J Bone Miner Res* 1990;5:31–40
14. Guise TA, Mundy GR. Cancer and bone. *Endocr Rev* 1998;19:18–54
15. Ridley AJ, Hall A. The small GTP-binding protein rho regulates the assembly of focal adhesions and

actin stress fibers in response to growth factors. *Cell* 1992;70:401–10

16. David P, Baron R. The vacuolar H+ ATPase: a potential target for drug development in bone disease. *Exp Opin Invest Drugs* 1995;4:725–39

17. Goltzman D. Mechanisms of the development of osteoblastic metastases. *Cancer* 1997;80:1581–7

18. Adami S. Bisphosphonates in prostate carcinoma. *Cancer* 1997;80:1674–9

19. Percival RC, Urwin GH, Watson ME, et al. Biochemical and histological evidence that carcinoma of the prostate is associated with increased bone resorption. *Eur J Surg Oncol* 1987;13:41–9

20. Lee MV, Fong EM, Singer FR, Guenette RS. Bisphosphonate treatment inhibits the growth of prostate cancer cells. *Cancer Res* 2001;61:2602–8

21. Boissier S, Magnetto S, Frappart L, et al. Bisphosphonates inhibit prostate and breast carcinoma cell adhesion to unmineralized and mineralized bone extracellular matrices. *Cancer Res* 1997; 57:3890–4

22. Stearns ME, Wang M. Alendronate blocks metalloproteinase secretion and bone collagen I release by PC3 ML cells in SCID mice. *Clin Exp Metastases* 1998;16:693–704

23. Boissier S, Ferraras L, Magnetto S, et al. Bisphosphonates inhibit breast and prostate carcinoma cell invasion, an early event in the formation of bone metastases. *Cancer Res* 2000;60:2949–54

24. Diel IJ, Solomayer EF, Bastert G. Bisphosphonates and the prevention of metastases. *Cancer* 2000;88:3080–8

25. Paterson AHG. Bisphosphonates: biological response modifiers in breast cancer. *Clin Breast Cancer* 2002;3:206–16

26. Adami S, Salvagno G, Guarrera G, et al. Dichloromethylene-diphosphonate in patients with prostatic carcinoma metastatic to the skeleton. *J Urol* 1985;134:1152–4

27. Adami S, Mian M. Clodronate therapy of metastatic bone disease in patients with prostatic cancer. *Rec Res Cancer Res* 1989;116:67–72

28. Luzzani M, Vidili MG, Rissotto R, et al. Disodium clodronate in the treatment of pain due to bone metastases. *Int J Clin Pharm Res* 1990;10:243–6

29. Vorreuther R. Bisphosphonates as a adjunct to palliative therapy of bone metastases from prostatic carcinoma. A pilot study on clodronate. *Br J Urol* 1993;72:792–5

30. Ernst DS, Brasher P, Hagen N, et al. A randomized, controlled trial of intravenous clodronate in patients with metastatic bone disease and pain. *J Pain Symptom Manage* 1997;13:319–26

31. Elomaa ET, Tammela T. Effect of oral clodronate on bone pain: a controlled study in patients with metastatic prostatic cancer. *Int Urol Nephrol* 1992;42:159–66

32. Thurlimann B, Morant R, Jungi WF, Radziwill A. Pamidronate for pain control in patients with malignant osteolytic bone disease: a prospective dose–effect study. *Support Care Cancer* 1994;2: 61–5

33. Purohit OP, Anthony C, Radston CR, et al. High dose IV pamidronate for metastatic bone pain. *Br J Cancer* 1994;70:554–8

34. Small EJ, Reese DM, Vogelzang NJ. Hormone refractory prostate cancer: an evolving standard of care. *Semin Oncol* 1999;26(Suppl 17):61–7

35. Tannock IF, Osoba D, Stockler MR, et al. Chemotherapy with mitoxantrone plus prednisone or prednisone alone for symptomatic hormone-resistant prostate cancer: a Canadian randomized trial with palliative end points. *J Clin Oncol* 1996;14:1756–64

36. Kantoff PW, Halabi S, Conaway MR, et al. Hydrocortisone with or without mitoxantrone in men with hormone-refractory prostate cancer: results of Cancer and Leukemia Group B 9182 study. *J Clin Oncol* 1999;17:2506–13

37. Ernst DS, Tannock IF, Venner PM, et al. Randomized placebo controlled trial of mitoxantrone/prednisone and clodronate versus mitoxantrone/prednisone alone in patients with hormone refractory prostate cancer and pain: National Cancer Institute of Canada Clinical Trials Group study. *Proc Am Soc Clin Oncol* 2002;21:abstr 705

38. Hortobagyi GN, Theriault RL, Porter L, et al. Efficacy of pamidronate in reducing skeletal complications in patients with breast cancer and lytic bone metastases. Protocol 19 Aredia Breast Cancer Study Group. *N Engl J Med* 1996;335: 1785–91

39. Paterson AHG, Powles TJ, Kanis JA. Double-blind controlled trial of oral clodronate in patients with bone metastases from breast cancer. *J Clin Oncol* 1993;11:59–65

40. Diel IJ, Solomayer EF, Costa SD, et al. Reduction in new metastases in breast cancer with adjuvant clodronate treatment. *N Engl J Med* 1998;339: 357–63

41. Berenson JR, Lichtenstein A, Porter L, et al. Efficacy of pamidronate in reducing skeletal events in patients with advanced multiple myeloma. *N Engl J Med* 1996;334:448–93

42. Dearnaley DP, Sydes MR, on behalf of the MRC PR5 Collaborators. Preliminary evidence that oral clodronate delays symptomatic progression of bone metastases from prostate cancer: first results of the MRC PR5 trial. *Proc Am Soc Clin Oncol* 2001;20:abstr 693

43. Green JR, Muller K, Jaeggi KA. Preclinical pharmacology of CGP 42'446, a new, potent heterocyclic bisphosphonate compound. *Bone Miner Res* 1994;9:745–51

44. Saad F, Gleason D, Murray R, *et al.* Zometa is effective in the treatment of bone metastases from prostate cancer. Results of a large phase III, double blind randomised trial. Presented at the *SUO Meeting*, 2002:abstr

45. Smith MR, McGovern FJ, Zietman AL, *et al.* Pamidronate to prevent bone loss during androgen-deprivation therapy for prostate cancer. *N Engl J Med* 2001;345:948–55

Direct from the pipeline: results of phase I and II studies of new drugs

48

C. N. Sternberg

Increased insight into the biology of prostate cancer coupled with the emergence of new therapeutic strategies has altered the nihilist approach that has often been adopted for patients with advanced prostate cancer.

Newer hormonal manipulations

The gonadotropin-releasing hormone (GnRH) antagonists are a new therapeutic class of agents that directly block pituitary GnRH receptors. Two phase II trials and three phase III trials have been conducted with Abarelix™[1-5]. These antagonists induce a rapid decrease in prostate volume and prostate-specific antigen (PSA), without testosterone surge and with swift testosterone recovery upon suspension.

Selective androgen receptor modulators (SARMs) can achieve androgen receptor (AR) blockade without causing the increased testosterone levels that are seen with non-steroidal antiandrogens.

After secondary hormonal manipulations, new approaches include: chemotherapy, gene therapy, immunotherapy, inhibition and/or blockade of growth factor receptors or growth factor receptor pathways, inhibition of invasion and metastases and inhibition of neoangiogenesis.

Chemotherapy

No chemotherapeutic regimen has thus far demonstrated an improvement in survival[6]. Two randomized studies have shown an advantage for mitoxantrone plus corticosteroids compared with corticosteroids alone in terms of quality of life end-points[7,8].

The taxanes, docetaxel and paclitaxel, have been increasingly used in hormone-refractory prostate cancer (HRPC). Docetaxel, in two phase II studies, produced a 50% decrease in PSA in 42–45%, with objective responses in 28–42%[9,10]. Other weekly phase II trials have demonstrated PSA responses rates of 34–60%[11-14], similar to the 3-weekly schedule. An international industry-sponsored trial will randomize 804 patients with HRPC to mitoxantrone and prednisone or docetaxel (weekly or every 3 weeks) and prednisone. The Southwest Oncology Group (SWOG) phase III trial compares Estracyt and docetaxel with mitoxantrone and prednisone in 620 patients with HRPC.

Epothilones are semisynthetic analogs of natural epothilones B and D with a mode of action similar to that of the taxanes (microtubular stabilization). They have activity in both paclitaxel-sensitive and -refractory tumors, and are twice as potent as paclitaxel in inducing tubulin polymerization *in vitro*. Cytotoxicity is mediated through induction of Bax conformational changes[15]. Phase I trials show activity in HRPC. The epothilone B analog BMS-247550 combined with estramustine has shown activity in 11/12 patients thus far[16].

Other new taxanes in clinical trials include: BMS 184476, BMS 188797, BMS 275183, IDN 5109/BAY 598862, RPR 109881A and RPR 116258. These new agents have a common characteristic, decreased recognition by p170, the product of the *MDR1* gene. This confers innovative properties such as *in vitro* and *in vivo* activities in tumors expressing p170, along with the advantage of oral administration[17].

Immunotherapy

Until recently, prostate cancer was considered to be a non-immunogenic tumor. This paradigm has changed, and the role of immunotherapy has been explored[18,19].

One approach is the use of granulocyte-macrophage colony-stimulating factor (GM-CSF) either alone or in combination. There were small reported differences in PSA doubling time and slope with GM-CSF in 36 patients[20]. Changes in PSA could not readily be attributed to direct or indirect effects of GM-CSF, the PSA assay or down-regulation of PSA expression by GM-CSF. Toxicity was mild, consisting primarily of transient constitutional symptoms and reactions at the injection site.

Dreicer and colleagues also reported PSA responses with GM-CSF in a phase II trial in less heavily pretreated patients[21]. This led to a more recent trial combining GM-CSF 350 mg three times a week with thalidomide (an antiangiogenic agent) 100–200 mg/day, in HRPC[22].

Dendritic cells (DCs) are the only cells in the body that stimulate naive T cells, and can activate B cells to trigger antibody formation. DCs can be isolated by leukophoresis with the use of GM-CSF and cytokines such as interleukin-4. In a phase I trial[23], DCs were loaded with prostate-specific membrane antigen (PSMA) and given intravenously. Partial remission, defined as a 50% decrease in PSA or improvement on ProstaScint scan was seen in 14% (7/51). In a second series, 37 patients were treated with weekly (× 6) peptide-pulsed DC infusions. One complete remission and ten partial remissions were observed[24].

Autologous DCs have been harvested and pulsed with prostatic acid phosphatase–sargramostim (GM-CSF) fusion protein to produce APC8015 (Provenge). In one trial, patients received a combination of APC8015 and bevacizumab (anti-vascular endothelial growth factor (VEGF) monoclonal antibody). Treatment was repeated every 14 days for three courses. Patients continue to receive bevacizumab every 14 days in the absence of disease progression or unacceptable toxicity[25]. Other trials with autologous DCs are ongoing at Duke University and at other centers.

Gene therapy

Prostate cancer is most likely a consequence of at least five cumulative genetic changes, making it difficult to correct these mutations with gene therapy. Gene therapy is complicated because current vector technology does not give stable integration of genes into 100% of the cancer cells *in vivo*[26]. None the less, in preclinical *in vitro* and *in vivo* models, encouraging results have been observed[27]. Attempts at restoration of normal gene function include insertion of suppressor genes such as *p53*, *Rb*, *p21* and *p16* and attempts to counteract the effects of tumor-promoting oncogenes such as *ras*, *myc*, *erb*B2 and *bcl-2*.

Several gene therapy trials have been initiated. Strategies include vaccine therapy with various cytokines such as interleukin-2 (IL-2) or GM-CSF, suicide cytotoxic therapy such as herpes simplex virus (HSV)–thymidine kinase or toxins, suppressor genes such as *p53* or *Rb*, oncolytic viruses specifically designed to replicate preferentially in prostate cancer cells (CV787 or CN-706) and antisense therapy such as *bcl-2* and c-*myc*[28–31].

The first phase I trial of GM-CSF autologous gene therapy vaccination was an *ex vivo* trial at Johns Hopkins University[28]. In 7/8 patients a positive delayed-type hypersensitivity (DTH) response was seen (2/8 positive prior to vaccination), and antibodies were detected in the sera of these patients recognizing polypeptides from prostate cells. Both T and B cell immune responses were generated. Toxicity was negligible. Although the techniques required are quite complicated, there may be a role for this type of treatment. A number of phase II trials have already been initiated, but no randomized data are available.

In vivo gene therapy is more cost efficient and does not have to be tailored to the individual patient. Disadvantages are that gene transfer efficiency is poor and stimulation of host immunity may have untoward toxicities. There are many methods for DNA gene transfer including viral, liposomal and other novel methods. Adenoviral and retroviral methodologies have been the major focus of attention[32].

Development of genetically engineered, conditionally replication-competent adenoviruses via prostate-specific promoters has led to trials of CN706 (prostate specific oncolytic virus)[30] and to a preliminary phase I/II dose-finding trial in HRPC with CV787[31].

Bcl-2 is a critical regulator of apoptosis in many tissues and is part of a growing family of apoptosis-regulatory gene products. Antisense oligodeoxynucleotides such as Genasense™ therapeutically target genes that play a role in the progression to androgen independence[33]. Genasense has been combined with docetaxel in two phase I/II studies with interesting preliminary results[34,35]. It has also been combined with mitoxantrone[36]. A phase II randomized trial of docetaxel and Genasense compared with docetaxel alone is beginning in the European Organization for Radiation Therapy in Cancer (EORTC, protocol 30021).

Meanwhile, direct gene therapy for bone metastases (Ad50C-E1a) is yet another strategy under development[37].

Growth factor inhibition

Growth factors are required for cell proliferation. Transfection of growth factors or their receptors can convert normal cells to the malignant phenotype. The epidermal growth factor receptor (EGFR) regulates angiogenesis, tumor growth and progression in HRPC.

Inhibition of growth factor receptor kinase-dependent signalling pathways is one of the most promising therapeutic approaches for the treatment of cancer. Aberrant signal transduction plays an important role in the pathophysiology of cancer. Kinases are key enzymes involved in signalling pathways (targets for chemotherapeutic intervention). Growth factor-induced signalling is implicated in the activation of antiapoptotic cell survival pathways[38].

Therapeutic approaches used to target the EGFR and its signal transduction cascade include: anti-EGFR monoclonal antibodies directed against the extracellular binding-domain including IMC-C225 (cetuximab, erbitux), EMD 55900, ICR 62 and ABX-EGF, and others that directly block the EGFR[39]. In an in vitro study of HRPC, blockade of EGFR by the anti-EGFR antibody ImClone C225 inhibited tumor growth and metastasis by inhibiting angiogenesis. Paclitaxel combined with C225 enhanced the results[40].

Other low-molecular-weight inhibitors of the EGFR tyrosine kinase include: Iressa (ZD 1839), OSI-774 (Tarceva), PD182905, PKI-166 and CI-1033. Iressa has shown encouraging results in prostate cancer in a phase I trial[39], and phase II trials have been initiated.

HER-2 protein overexpression and its prognostic value have not been well characterized in prostate cancer[41]. Trastuzumab (Herceptin), a monoclonal antibody binding to the HER-2 receptor, evaluated at MSKCC, was not found to be an effective single agent[42]. In another phase I study, trastuzumab was combined with docetaxel and estramustine. HER-2 positivity was not required and (33%) 2/6 of patients with measurable disease had objective responses[43].

Other monoclonal antibodies

Immunotoxin conjugates may use an antibody directed against EGFR or PSMA joined to a cell toxin. ^{90}Yttrium-dota-HUJ591 (^{90}Y-J591) is a radioisotope-labelled humanized monoclonal antibody (MAb) to the extracellular domain of PSMA[44]. In 20 patients who had failed hormonal therapy or chemotherapy, no patients developed HAHA. Toxicity was dose-related. PSA responses and objective responses were observed.

Another phase I study of ^{90}Yttrium Y MAb m170, paclitaxel and cyclosporin followed by autologous peripheral blood stem cell transplantation is in progress.

Antiangiogenic agents

Increased vascularization has been associated with an aggressive phenotype[45] that may not express high levels of fibroblast growth factor (FGF) or VEGF during tumor progression[46]. Antiangiogenic therapy is thought to be primarily cytostatic rather than cytotoxic, and prolonged intake is probably required. Natural antagonists to angiogenesis such as endostatin, thrombospondin and angiostatin, synthetic analogs, receptor antibodies and small-molecule receptor inhibitors have been evaluated. Prostate cancer is an interesting target for this form of therapy. Studies with thalidomide and with anti-VEGF monoclonal antibodies are in progress.

Vitamin D

Clinical activity of vitamin D (calcitriol, 1,25-dihydroxycholecalciferol) has been reported in HRPC with PSA response rates of around 28%[47,48]. The *in vitro* cytotoxic activity of vitamin D seems to be dose-dependent; however, its clinical hypercalcemic effect limits clinical dose escalation of calcitriol. Several agents such as bisphosphonates, cortisone and chemotherapeutic agents such as carboplatin and paclitaxel can block the hypercalcemia of vitamin D.

Bisphosphonates are important in the palliation of pain due to osseous metastases. The combination of newer, more potent biphosphonates such as zoledronic acid, perhaps in combination with vitamin D, is the subject of ongoing trials[49].

Endothelin-A antagonists

In a randomized study in 288 patients with HRPC, Altrasentan (ABT-627), a selective endothelin-A receptor antagonist, demonstrated a significant delay in time to PSA and clinical progression compared with placebo, although no survival benefit was seen in an intent-to treat analysis[50,51]. This is an interesting new compound which deserves further evaluation.

Exisulind

Exisulind (Aptosyn™) is the first of a new class of targeted agents that induce apoptosis in a broad range of precancerous and cancerous tissues without affecting normal cells[52]. In a randomized, placebo-controlled study, exisulind, a sulfone metabolite of the non-steroidal anti-inflammatory drug sulindac, lengthened the median PSA doubling time in men who had increasing PSA levels after radical prostatectomy[53,54].

Because preclinical studies have suggested synergistic interactions between docetaxel and exisulind, a phase I/II clinical trial combining these agents has been initiated in patients with HRPC[55].

Bisphosphonates

Bisphosphonates are potent inhibitors of bone resorption. Zoledronic acid (Zometa™) has also been shown to be effective in metastatic blastic disease from prostate cancer, as it decreases osteoclast activity in malignant bone. Randomized studies have now shown that this therapy treats both osteoblastic and osteolytic bone metastases, and clearly decreases the frequency of skeletal complications resulting from bone metastases[56–59]. An added beneficial effect appears to be direct antitumor activity. Several studies with Zometa are ongoing, such as a phase I study at MSKCC in combination with calcitriol and a phase II randomized study at the Mayo Clinic of zoledronate with or without BMS-275291 in HRPC.

Conclusions

Molecular targeted small-molecule therapy, monoclonal antibodies, antiangiogenic and immune therapy trials have burst onto the clinical horizon. Several new chemotherapeutic agents that work at different points in the cell cycle also seem promising. Bisphosphonates can alleviate bone pain and may have direct antitumor activity. With the caveat that the results must be corroborated in phase III trials, prospects for the future are hopeful.

References

1. Debruyne F, McLeod D, Ben-Soussen P, Campion M, Garnick MB, for the Abarelix Study Group. Abarelix depot, a pure GnRH antagonist, compared to LHRH agonist in patients with prostate cancer. *Eur Urol* 2000;37(Suppl 2):128 (abstr)

2. Garnick MB, Campion M. Abarelix depot, a GnRH antagonist, v. LHRH superagonists in prostate cancer: differential effects on follicle-stimulating hormone. Abarelix Depot Study Group. *Mol Urol* 2000;4:275–7

3. McLeod D, Trachtenberg J. Abarelix depot (AD) versus leuprolide (L) with and without bicalutamide (Casodex) (C) for prostate cancer; results of two multicenter, randomized phase III studies. *Eur Urol* 2001;39(Suppl 5):78(abstr)

4. Selvaggi F, Khoe GSS, Van Cangh P, *et al.*, for the ABACAS 1 study group. Comparison of Abarelix depot (A-D) and goserelin (G) plus bicalutamide (B) in advanced prostate cancer; results of a multicentre, open-label, randomised, phase III study. *Eur Urol* 2001;39(Suppl 5):78(abstr)

5. Fisher H, Barzell W, Gittelman M, *et al.* for the Abarelix Study Group. Abarelix depot (A-D) monotherapy reduces PSA levels comparable to leuprolide acetate (L) plus bicalutamide (B): results of a multicenter trial of rising PSA, advanced (D1/D2), neoadjuvant hormonal therapy (NHT), and intermittant hormonal therapy (IHT) prostate cancer (PC) patients. *Proc Am Soc Clin Oncol* 2001;20:152b(abstr)

6. Sternberg CN. Systemic treatment and new developments in advanced prostate cancer. *Eur J Cancer* 2001;37(Suppl 7):S147–57

7. Tannock IF, Osoba D, Stochler MR, *et al.* Chemotherapy with mitoxantrone plus prednisone or prednisone alone for symptomatic hormone resistant prostate cancer: a Canadian randomized trial with palliative end-points. *J Clin Oncol* 1996;14:1756–64

8. Kantoff PW, Halabi S, Conaway M, *et al.* Hydrocortisone with or without mitoxantrone in men with hormone refractory prostate cancer: results of Cancer and Leukemia Group B 9182 study. *J Clin Oncol* 1999;17:2506–13

9. Friedland D, Cohen J, Miller R Jr. A phase II trial of docetaxel (Taxotere) in hormone-refractory prostate cancer: correlation of antitumor effect to phosphorylation of Bcl-2. *Semin Oncol* 1999; 26(5 Suppl 17):19–23

10. Picus J, Schultz M. Docetaxel (Taxotere) as a monotherapy in the treatment of hormone-refractory prostate cancer: preliminary results. *Semin Oncol* 1999;26(5 Suppl 17):14–18

11. Berry W, Gregurich M, Dakhil S, Hathorn J, Asmar L. Phase II randomized trial of weekly paclitaxel (Taxol) with or without estramustine phosphate in patients with symptomatic, hormone-refractory, metastatic carcinoma of the prostate (HRMCP). *Proc Am Soc Clin Oncol* 2001;20:175a(abstr)

12. Beer TM, Pierce WC, Lowe BA, Henner WD. Phase II study of weekly docetaxel (Taxotere) in hormone refractory metastatic prostate cancer (HRPC). *Proc Am Soc Clin Oncol* 2000;19:348a(abstr)

13. Gravis G, Bladou F, Salem N, *et al.* Efficacy, quality of life (QOL) and tolerance with weekly docetaxel (D) in metastatic hormone refractory prostate cancer (HRPC) patients. *Proc Annu Meet Am Soc Clin Oncol* 2001;20:171b(abstr)

14. Scholz MC, Guess B, Barrios F, Strum S, Leibowitz R. Low-dose single-agent weekly docetaxel (Taxotere) is effective and well tolerated in elderly men with prostate cancer. *Proc Annu Meet Am Soc Clin Oncol* 2001;20:173b(abstr)

15. Yamaguchi H, Paranawithana SR, Lee MW, Huang Z, Bhalla KN, Wang HG. Epothilone B analogue (BMS-247550)-mediated cytotoxicity through induction of Bax conformational change in human breast cancer cells. *Cancer Res* 2002;62:466–71

16. Smaletz O, Kelly WK, Horse-Grant D, *et al.* Epothilone B analogue (BMS-247550) with estramustine phosphate (EMP) in patients (pts) with progressive castrate-metastatic prostate cancer (PC). *Proc Annu Meet Am Soc Clin Oncol* 2002;21:184a(abstr)

17. Lavelle F. New taxanes and epothilone derivatives in clinical trials. *Bull Cancer* 2002;89:343–50

18. Rini BI, Small EJ. Immunotherapy for prostate cancer. *Curr Oncol Rep* 2001;3:418–23

19. Harris DT, Matyas GR, Gomella LG, *et al.* Immunologic approaches to the treatment of prostate cancer. *Semin Oncol* 1999;26:439–47

20. Small EJ, Reese DM, Um B, Whisenant S, Dixon SC, Figg WD. Therapy of advanced prostate cancer with granulocyte macrophage colony-stimulating factor. *Clin Cancer Res* 1999;5:1738–44

21. Dreicer R, See WA, Klein EA. Phase II trial of GM-CSF in advanced prostate cancer. *Invest New Drugs* 2001;19:261–5

22. Dreicer R, Elson P, Klein EA, Peereboom D, Byzova T, and Plow E. Phase II trial of GM-CSF + thalidomide in patients with androgen-independent metastatic prostate cancer. *Proc Annu Meet Am Soc Clin Oncol* 2002;21:196a(abstr)

23. Murphy G, Tjoa B, Radge H, *et al*. Phase I clinical trial: T-cell therapy for prostate cancer using autologous dendritic cells pulsed with HLA-A0201 specific peptides from prostate specific membrane antigen. *Prostate* 1996;29:371–80

24. Murphy GP, Tjoa BA, Simmons SJ, *et al*. Phase II prostate cancer vaccine trial: report of a study involving 37 patients with disease recurrence following primary treatment. *Prostate* 1999;39: 54–9

25. Rosen LS. Clinical experience with angiogenesis signaling inhibitors: focus on vascular endothelial growth factor (VEGF) blockers. *Cancer Control.* 2002;9(Suppl 2):36–44

26. Harrington K, Spitzweg C, Bateman A, *et al*. Gene therapy for prostate cancer: current status and future prospects. *J Urol* 2001;166:1220–33

27. Martiniello-Wilks R, Tsatralis T, Russell P, *et al*. Transcription-targeted gene therapy for androgen-independent prostate cancer. *Cancer Gene Ther* 2002;9:443–52

28. Simons JW, Mikhak B, Chang JF, *et al*. Induction of immunity to prostate cancer antigens: results of a clinical trial of vaccinaion with irradiated autologous prostate tumor cells engineered to secrete granulocyte-macrophage colony-stimulating factor using *ex vivo* gene transfer. *Cancer Res* 1999;59:5160–8

29. Pantuck AJ, Matherly J, Zisman A, *et al*. Optimizing prostate cancer suicide gene therapy using herpes simplex virus thymidine kinase active site variants. *Hum Gene Ther* 2002;13: 777–89

30. Rodriguez R, Schuur ER, Lim HY, Henderson GA, Simons JW, Henderson DR. Prostate attenuated replication competent adenovirus (ARCA) CN706: a selective cytotoxic agent for prostate-specific antigen-positive prostate cancer cells. *Cancer Res* 1997;57:2559–63

31. Small EJ, Carducci MA, Wilding G. A phase I/II dose finding trial of the intravenous injection of CV787, a prostate specific antigen-dependent cytolytic adenovirus in patients with advanced hormone refractory prostate cancer (HRPC). *Eur J Cancer* 2001;37(Suppl 6):S217 (abstr)

32. Belldegrun A, Bander NH, Lerner SP, Wood DP, Pantuck AJ. Society of Urologic Oncology Biotechnology Forum: new approaches and targets for advanced prostate cancer. *J Urol* 2001;166:1316–21

33. Tamm I, Dorken B, Hartmann G. Antisense therapy in oncology: new hope for an old idea? *Lancet* 2001;000:489–97

34. Morris MJ, Tong WP, Cordon-Cardo C, *et al*. Bcl-2 antisense (G3139) plus docetaxel for treatment of progressive androgen-independent prostate cancer. *Eur J Cancer* 2001;37(Suppl 6)S218 (abstr)

35. Tolcher AW. Preliminary phase I results of G3139 (Bcl-2 antisense oligonucleotide) therapy in combination with docetaxel in hormone-refractory prostate cancer. *Semin Oncol* 2001;28 (4 Suppl 15):67–70

36. Chi KN, Gleave ME, Klasa R, *et al*. A phase I dose-finding study of combined treatment with an antisense Bcl-2 oligonucleotide (Genasense) and mitoxantrone in patients with metastatic hormone-refractory prostate cancer. *Clin Cancer Res* 2001;7:3920–7

37. Scaduto AA, Lieberman JR. Gene therapy for osteoinduction. *Orthop Clin North Am* 1999;30: 625–33

38. Renhowe PA. Inhibitors of growth factor receptor kinase-dependent signaling pathways in anticancer chemotherapy – clinical progress. *Curr Opin Drug Discov Dev* 2002;5:214–24

39. Barton J, Blackledge G, Wakeling A. Growth factors and their receptors: new targets for prostate cancer therapy (1). *Urology* 2001;58 (2 Suppl 1):114–22

40. Karashima T, Sweeney P, Slaton JW, *et al*. Inhibition of angiogenesis by the antiepidermal growth factor receptor antibody ImClone C225 in androgen-independent prostate cancer growing orthotopically in nude mice. *Clin Cancer Res* 2002;8:1253–64

41. Agus DB, Akita RW, Fox WD, *et al*. A potential role for activated HER-2 in prostate cancer. *Semin Oncol* 2000;27(6 Suppl 11):76–83

42. Morris MJ, Reuter VE, Kelly WK, *et al*. HER-2 profiling and targeting in prostate carcinoma. *Cancer* 2002;94:980–6

43. Small EJ, Bok R, Reese DM, Sudilovsky D, Frohlich M. Docetaxel, estramustine, plus trastuzumab in patients with metastatic androgen-independent prostate cancer. *Semin Oncol* 2001; 28(4 Suppl 15):71–6

44. Yao D, Sandhu JS, Trabulsi EJ, *et al*. Phase I trial of ^{90}Yttrium-dota-HUJ591 (^{90}Y-J591), a radioisotope labeled humanized monoclonal (MAB) antibody to the extracellular domain of prostate specific membrane antigen (PSMA$_{EXT}$), in the treatment of advanced prostate cancer (PCA). *J Urol* 2002;167:175(abstr)

45. Weidner N, Carrol P, Flax J, *et al*. Tumor angiogenesis correlates with metastasis in invasive prostate carcinoma. *Am J Pathol* 1993; 143:401–9

46. Duque JL, Loughlin KR, Adam RM, *et al*. Plasma levels of vascular endothelial growth factor are increased in patients with metastatic prostate cancer. *Urology* 1999;54:523–7

47. Trump DL, Rueger RM, Herschberger PA, *et al*. Preclinical and phase I studies of the combination of calcitriol (1,25(OH)2 vitamin D3) and paclitaxel: synergistic antitumor activity and

reduced toxicity. *Proc Annu Meet Am Soc Clin Oncol* 1999;18:231a(abstr)

48. Smith DC, Johnson CS, Freeman CC, Muindi J, Wilson JW, Trump DL. A phase I trial of calcitriol (1,25-dihydroxycholecalciferol) in patients with advanced malignancy. *Clin Cancer Res* 1999;5: 1339–45

49. Major P, Lortholary A, Hon J, *et al.* Zoledronic acid is superior to pamidronate in the treatment of hypercalcemia of malignancy: a pooled analysis of two randomized, controlled clinical trials. *J Clin Oncol* 2001;19:558–67

50. Singh A, Padley RJ, Ashraf T. The selective endothelin-A receptor antagonist improves quality of life (QOL) weighted time to progression in hormone refractory prostate cancer patients. *Eur J Cancer* 2001;37(Suppl 6):S220 (abstr)

51. Schulman C, Nelson JB, Weinberg MA, Humerickhouse RA, Schmitt JL, Nabulsi AA. Altrasentan delayed PSA progression in a phase II trial of men with hormone refractory prostate cancer. *J Urol* 2002;167:176(abstr)

52. Goluboff ET. Exisulind, a selective apoptotic antineoplastic drug. *Expert Opin Invest Drugs* 2001;10:1875–82

53. Goluboff ET, Prager D, Rukstalis D, *et al.* Safety and efficacy of exisulind for treatment of recurrent prostate cancer after radical prostatectomy *J Urol* 2001;166:882–6

54. Goluboff ET, Prager D, Rukstalis D. *et al.* Long-term use of exisulind in men with prostate cancer following radical prostatectomy. *J Urol* 2002;167:176(abstr)

55. Ryan CW, Stadler WM, Vogelzang NJ. Docetaxel and exisulind in hormone-refractory prostate cancer. *Semin Oncol* 2001;28(4 Suppl 15):56–61

56. Coleman RE, Seaman JJ. The role of zoledronic acid in cancer: clinical studies in the treatment and prevention of bone metastases. *Semin Oncol* 2001;28(2 Suppl 6):11–16

57. Lee MV, Fong EM, Singer FR, Guenette RS. Bisphosphonate treatment inhibits the growth of prostate cancer cells. *Cancer Res* 2001;61:2602–8

58. Boissier S, Ferreras M, Peyuchaud O, *et al.* Bisphosphonates inhibit breast and prostate carcinoma cell invasion, an early event in the formation of bone metastases. *Cancer Res* 2000; 60:2954

59. Berenson JR. Zoledronic acid in cancer patients with bone metastases: results of phase I and II trials. *Semin Oncol* 2001;28(2 Suppl 6):25–34

Chemotherapy in the management of prostate cancer

C. Logothetis and R. E. Millikan

49

'The salutary effects of androgen deprivation for patients with advanced prostate cancer were already well appreciated in the first half of this century. By the early 1970s, when cytotoxic agents began to dramatically alter the natural history of some hematologic and germ cell malignancies, the War on Cancer brought chemotherapy even to patients with adenocarcinoma of the prostate. Although flawed by modern standards, a series of clinical trials completed by the National Prostate Cancer Project (NPCP) provided evidence of biologic activity (such as palliation of symptoms) but in the end failed to convincingly establish the role of chemotherapy[1]'

Despite this interpretation of the early experience, another generation has passed since the NPCP trials were initiated, without cytotoxic therapy earning a place in the routine management of patients with metastatic prostate cancer. Recent modification of chemotherapy and the introduction of prostate-specific antigen (PSA) testing that permits efficient assessment of 'response' have changed this perception.

It is instructive to consider some of the factors contributing to this perception. First, evaluation of clinical response has been difficult. Second, the fact that even patients with disseminated prostate cancer are commonly managed exclusively by urologists has attenuated the experience of medical oncologists in this disease, and very likely has contributed to the slow development of cytotoxic paradigms. Third, there has been an ironic distraction produced by the advent of medical testicular suppression. For some time, clinical research in advanced prostate cancer has seen disproportionate resources expended on randomizing many thousands of patients to variants of hormonal therapies[2]. More than a decade of such experience has demonstrated that no matter how complex or expensive we make androgen deprivation, its therapeutic impact is still limited. Finally, the palliative impact of cytotoxic drugs is underappreciated. As pointed out by Slack and Murphy in the quotation above, cytotoxic therapy carefully applied can often provide symptom relief with less morbidity than that associated with narcotics or other palliative interventions.

Progress towards more routine assessment of the role of chemotherapy has been made because of a number of factors that have been addressed:

(1) Establishment of standardized response criteria;

(2) Closer ties between medical oncologists and urologists in 'academic centers of excellence';

(3) Recognition of the toxicity and therapeutic limitations of androgen ablation;

(4) Inclusion of quality-of-life end-points in clinical research.

One of the clear trends in recent clinical investigation is the use of PSA as a 'response' end-point, despite appropriate scepticism about the clinical relevance of tumor marker fluctuations[3]. In addition to the potential pitfall of altered PSA expression unrelated to an antitumor effect, it is reported[4] that PSA levels in androgen-independent disease do not correlate well with disease volume, and can, in extreme circumstances, decrease even as tumors are progressing but becoming more undifferentiated. Despite these limitations, it is consistently observed that 'PSA decline' correlates with improved survival, and with markers of clinical benefit such as improved pain, increased hemoglobin, normalization of bone-derived alkaline phosphatase, weight gain and improved performance status. Examination of published data reveals that patients with a 75–80% PSA decline, maintained for at least 8 weeks, are very likely to show unequivocal clinical benefit. For the present, this should serve as a useful benchmark for comparing therapies, and represents a readily applied, objective standard for clinical research.

Despite these challenges related to the disease and its clinical evaluation, there are some useful tools already at hand for treating patients with androgen-independent prostate cancer, including some options other than chemotherapy.

Although 'second-line' hormonal therapies have a poor reputation in prostate cancer, this notion is being challenged[5]. There are now well-documented withdrawal responses for several hormonal agents, including agents interfering with adrenal function. Although there have been conflicting reports over many years, it is now established that high-dose ketoconazole (taken with care to ensure an acidic gastric environment) can produce clinically relevant responses, even in the setting of confirmed castrate testosterone levels and progression despite the use, and withdrawal, of anti-androgens[6]. This activity is offset by the observations that ketoconazole at the usually employed dose of 400 mg three times a day is quite expensive and associated with non-trivial morbidity. In our experience, consonant with that of Mahler and colleagues[7], about 20% of patients started on ketoconazole are unable to continue the drug owing to expense, gastrointestinal upset or hepatic toxicity.

A recent report from the Mayo Clinic[8] on the use of 'low-dose' dexamethasone, which is inexpensive and generally well tolerated, confirms the sometimes dramatic effects seen with glucocorticoids. At the slightly supra-physiological dose of 0.75 mg twice a day, this retrospective study identified symptomatic improvement in 63% of treated patients. Interestingly, 23 of 38 patients (61%) showed a PSA decline of $\geq 80\%$, and the median time to progression in this group was just over 10 months, probably reflecting a clinically relevant biological activity, since most published series put median survival in this range. Despite the obvious limitations of such a retrospective chart review study, these results, taken together with the reports on ketoconazole, unequivocally demonstrate that 'second-line' hormone responses do occur in prostate cancer, and highlight the importance of controlling for these effects in trials of chemotherapy.

Systemic irradiation, as with bone-homing strontium-89, is another approach to treatment that is useful for up to 80% of patients[9]. Although sometimes associated with an initial pain flare, eventual pain relief is often substantial. In general, one can expect about 10% of treated patients to have complete pain relief, which in some cases can be durable for up to several months. Unfortunately, there is only weak evidence that such treatment alters the natural history of the disease. For example, treatment with strontium-89 rarely results in significant PSA decline. Furthermore, in patients with reduced hematological reserves engendered by widespread marrow involvement or previous cytotoxic therapy (including previous exposures to strontium-89), this agent has real potential for prolonged myelosuppression, especially thrombocytopenia. While rarely of life-threatening proportion, Sr-89-related thrombocytopenia could certainly limit other treatment options. None the less, for many patients with multifocal bone involvement, strontium-89 is a useful way of controlling bone pain. In an effort to boost the antitumor effect of Sr-89, combinations with 'radiosensitizing' agents such as doxorubicin[10], cisplatin[11] or gemcitabine[12] have been investigated. Investigations along this line continue, but so far this interesting concept has not produced an apparent clinical advance.

Single-agent cytotoxic therapy

Numerous excellent reviews on single-agent chemotherapy are available[13–15]. More recent results are presented in Table 1. The salient points of the single-agent experience can be summarized:

(1) No single cytotoxic agent has an objective response rate exceeding 30%.

(2) Weekly exposure to a modest dose seems more promising than higher doses given with a longer drug-free interval.

(3) Consistent, palliative relevant activity is seen with anthracyclines and cyclophosphamide, with provocative activity also seen with infusional cisplatin and infusional mitomycin C, although the toxicity of these last two agents in patients with advanced prostate cancer can be both substantial and unpredictable.

Recently, Tannock and colleagues[23] have investigated the use of mitoxantrone in combination with prednisone. In a phase III trial, significantly better symptom palliation was demonstrated for the combination than was achieved with prednisone alone. Although survival was not seen, this work is significant in two respects. First, the study illustrates the use of quality-of-life end-points in an exemplary way. Second, it demonstrates that even modest doses delivered every 21 days provide clinically relevant symptom relief.

Cytotoxic combinations

Estramustine phosphate was originally synthesized based on the premise that it would deliver a nitrogen mustard-alkylating activity selectively to cells expressing estrogen receptors. As it turns out, the mustard function is not labile to hydrolysis as had been supposed, and the agent actually acts by interacting with nuclear matrix microtubules[24]. Although the single-agent activity of estramustine phosphate is insignificant[25], it remains of interest in combination with other agents, especially those with 'antimicrotubule' effects. In fact, preclinical models demonstrate synergy with several agents. The groups at Fox Chase[26] and Michigan[27] have contributed both preclinical and clinical studies of estramustine combinations. Based on this work, it has emerged that paclitaxel–estramustine and etoposide (VP-16)–estramustine have clinically relevant activity. Several combinations of these agents in various schedules are currently being investigated in the clinic. Early clinical results seem promising in this area, and many more phase II results are anticipated within the next year.

Estramustine phosphate and vinblastine have been used together in the clinic for several years[28]. However, there is no hint of improved survival with this regimen. Moreover, weekly exposure to estramustine–vinblastine can be associated with significant myelosuppression, constipation and peripheral neuropathy.

In a different vein, the combination of ketoconazole with doxorubicin has been of

Table 1 Single agents in advanced prostate cancer

Agent	Dose/schedule	Response	TTP*	Survival†	Palliation	Reference
Gemcitabine	1000 mg/m² day 1, day 8, day 15 every 28 days	1/20	< 4	NR	NR	16
Carboplatin	150 mg/m² weekly	4/25	7	NR	NR	17
Carboplatin	400 mg/m² every 21 days	3/28	NR	NR	NR	18
Mitomycin C	12 mg/m² every 4 weeks	7/26	2.1	10.6	10/26	19
VP-16	50 mg/m²/day × 21 days every 28 days	2/22	NR	7.1	NR	20
Vinorelbine	25 mg/m² weekly	3/47	2.8	7.4	NR	21
Paclitaxel‡	135–150 mg/m² over 24 h every 21 days	1/23	NR	9	no	22

*Median time to progression (months); †median survival (months); ‡patients with bone-only disease were excluded from this trial; NR, not reported; VP-16, etoposide

interest at the University of Texas M. D. Anderson Cancer Center. Preclinical studies[29] suggested a synergistic effect of combining ketoconazole with cytotoxics, an effect quite apart from its role as a hormonal therapy mediated by inhibiting steroid biosynthesis. A phase II trial[30] reported significant PSA responses in up to 40% of patients. This regimen was fraught with significant accrual toxicity: nail loss and severe infections, often with positive blood cultures for gram-positive organisms, were commonly encountered. A randomized phase II trial of this combination versus ketoconazole alone has recently been completed (unpublished results of Millikan and Logothetis). This multicenter, community-based trial showed no difference in response rates or median survival. Remarkably, the two arms showed very similar toxicities. Of note, fully 20% of patients in *both* arms discontinued therapy owing to unacceptable toxicity, which we feel reflects the very real morbidity of high-dose ketoconazole. Further work on p450-targeted therapy is expected[31], and it seems likely that additional regimens based on this theme will be forthcoming.

We have studied a four-drug combination obtained by alternating, on a weekly basis, ketoconazole–doxorubicin and estramustine–vinblastine[32]. As anticipated, this alternating strategy was less toxic than either component given week after week. In addition, the regimen produced a 52% response rate based on a PSA reduction of $\geq 80\%$, while 12 of 16 patients (75%) with measurable soft tissue lesions responded according to standard criteria. Overall, 76% of patients reported symptomatic improvement. The median survival for all patients was 19 months, and among the responders, median survival was well in excess of 2 years. While only randomized trials will definitively establish the value of this regimen, the large number of phase II trials reporting a median survival in the range of 10–11 months raises hope that this regimen actually may alter the natural history of androgen-independent prostate cancer. A confirmatory trial is under way.

In order to evaluate toxicity further and confirm the activity reported from trials conducted at tertiary centers, a multicenter randomized phase II trial of ketoconazole–doxorubicin alternating with estramustine–vinblastine versus Pienta's regimen of paclitaxel–VP-16–estramustine has been initiated at M. D. Anderson and its Community Clinical Oncology Program (CCOP) affiliates.

Taking a different tack from these chronic, low-dose regimens, Small and colleagues[33] reported a 'dose-escalated' regimen of doxorubicin ($40 \, \text{mg/m}^2$) and cyclophosphamide ($1200 \, \text{mg/m}^2$ with prior pelvic irradiation or $1600 \, \text{mg/m}^2$ without prior radiotherapy). This was well tolerated and produced a 29% response rate based on $\geq 75\%$ PSA decline. Overall, the median survival was 11 months. As usual, responders fared better, showing a median survival of 23 months.

Results from a number of recently reported regimens are summarized in Table 2.

The National Comprehensive Cancer Network (NCCN) guidelines for the management of prostate cancer clearly support a role for chemotherapy in prostate cancer management. As recently updated[42], the NCCN guidelines endorse two successive trials of systemic cytotoxic therapy (including Sr-89 in this category) as a standard approach to the palliation of advanced, androgen-independent prostate cancer.

Although there is currently no 'gold standard' regimen or treatment algorithm, there are some generalizations that can be offered. Before a trial of chemotherapy, it is appropriate to confirm that patients have received optimal hormonal therapy (i.e. testosterone levels in range of 20 ng/dl or less), including anti-androgen withdrawal. Since chemotherapy in this setting is palliative, the temptation to 'treat the PSA' should be resisted.

Small cell carcinoma

'Neuroendocrine' features are well described in a subset of patients with prostate cancer. The expression of neuroendocrine markers

Table 2 Selected combination regimens in advanced prostate cancer

Regimen	Response by NPCP criteria	≥ 80% PSA reduction	Median survival (months)	Symptom palliation	Reference
VP-16–epirubicin–carboplatin	11/12	3/12	11	yes	34
VP-16–infusional carboplatin	6/7	NR	9	yes	35
Mitomycin C–doxorubicin–5-fluorouracil	NR	11/68	9	no	36
VP-16 50 mg/m²/day × 21 days–estramustine 140 mg t.i.d. × 21 days	40/56	(58%)*	13	NR	37
VP-16 50 mg/m²/day × 21 days–estramustine 15 mg/kg/day × 21 days	NR	12/42	9.9	NR	38
VP-16 50 mg/m²/day × 21 days–estramustine 10 mg/kg/day × 21 days	NR	(24/62)*	12.9	NR	39
VP-16 (p.o.)–estramustine–vinorelbine	NR	32%	NR	yes	40
VP-16 50 mg/day(p.o.)–cyclophosphamide 100 mg/day (p.o.)	NR	7/20	11	yes	41
Ketoconazole–doxorubicin alternating with estramustine–vinblastine	NR	24/46	19	yes	32
Cyclophosphamide–doxorubicin	NR	10/35	11	yes	33

*These authors reported only prostate-specific antigen (PSA) reductions of ≥ 50%.; VP-16, etoposide; NPCP, National Prostate Cancer Project; NR, not reported; t.i.d., three times a day; p.o., by mouth

correlates with relative insensitivity to hormonal therapy and a more aggressive clinical course[43]. At the extreme of this phenotypic spectrum is 'small cell' carcinoma[44]. Usually encountered in the evolution of pre-existing high-grade adenocarcinoma, the small cell phenotype can rarely arise de novo. Small cell carcinoma is characterized by lytic bone disease, visceral involvement (especially liver) and hypercalcemia, the last feature being conspicuously absent from the natural history of adenocarcinoma of the prostate. Although uncommon, this variant is important to recognize, since it usually responds well to VP-16–cisplatin or other conventional regimens for small cell carcinomas[45]. Even though such therapy is not curative, it usually results in worthwhile palliation. As with other small cell carcinomas, it is likely that the prognosis will substantially improve with early-integrated therapy. This last point has not been critically tested.

Future directions

The response rates being reported for treatment of androgen-independent prostate cancer rival those for other diseases in which chemotherapy applied in an adjuvant setting has improved both survival and cure fraction. This suggests that chemotherapy applied earlier in the natural history of prostate cancer is an important topic for clinical research. This is not a new concept of course[46]. Non-randomized data from Japan[47] strongly support the concept, and the authors claim that a phase III trial has been initiated on the basis of these data. Recently, mature follow-up of a randomized trial of total androgen blockade (TAB; accomplished in this trial by surgical castration plus flutamide) versus TAB plus 18 weeks of epirubicin (25 mg/m²/week) has been reported by Pummer and colleagues[48]. This study of 145 patients demonstrated statistically significant improvement in time to progression (from 12 to 18 months) and a strong trend ($p = 0.12$) in overall survival (from 22 to 30 months) favoring the combination treatment. A quality-of-life instrument showed favorable results for those with the prolonged disease-free interval, despite the acute effects of weekly chemotherapy. There are no trials yet reported using the more recently identified combination regimens. A phase III trial of TAB versus TAB plus 18 weeks of ketoconazole–doxorubicin alternating with estramustine–vinblastine has been initiated at M. D. Anderson. This trial is accruing well. Similar trials of front-line chemohormonal therapy are also under way at other centers. If these trials are positive, as the report of Pummer suggests they will be, this will constitute the first conceptual advance in the treatment of non-localized prostate cancer in more than 50 years.

In addition to applying therapy earlier in the course of the disease, there is also interest in applying chemotherapy perioperatively in patients at risk for a non-curative resection. 'Neoadjuvant' hormonal therapy has not produced tangible clinical benefit in terms of relapse-free or overall survival. Of note, neoadjuvant hormonal therapy never produces a surgical specimen free of cancer. Whether or not neoadjuvant chemotherapy will fare better remains to be seen. Such trials are now in progress at M. D. Anderson.

Finally, it is likely that the activity of currently available chemotherapy justifies conducting a landmark trial comparing the best currently available combination regimens with an algorithm of palliative interventions (such as mitoxantrone–prednisone and strontium-89). Palliative use of cytotoxic therapy should be considered as 'standard'. Physicians treating prostate cancer should be encouraged to embrace the view that optimized and selective use of cytotoxic therapy may contribute to the welfare of patients with prostate cancer. It should also be emphasized that the impact on survival has not yet been critically tested.

References

1. Slack NH, Murphy GP. A decade of experience with chemotherapy for prostate cancer. *Urology* 1983;22:1–7
2. Caubet JF, Tosteson TD, Dong EW, *et al.* Maximum androgen blockade in advanced prostate cancer: a meta-analysis of published randomized controlled trials using nonsteroidal antiandrogens. *Urology* 1997;49:71–8
3. Eisenberger MA, Nelson WG. How much can we rely on the level of prostate-specific antigen as an end-point for evaluation of clinical trials? A word of caution! *J Natl Cancer Inst* 1996;88:779–80
4. Wood CG, Finn L, Logothetis CJ. Prostate specific antigen (PSA) to tumor burden ratio: a prognostic variable in androgen-independent prostate cancer (AIPC). *J Urol* 1997;157:297
5. Small EJ, Vogelzang NJ. Second-line hormonal therapy for advanced prostate cancer: a shifting paradigm. *J Clin Oncol* 1997;15:382–8
6. Small EJ, Baron AD, Fippin L, *et al.* Ketoconazole retains activity in advanced prostate cancer patients with progression despite flutamide withdrawal. *J Urol* 1997;157:1204–7
7. Mahler C, Verhelst J, Denis L. Ketoconazole and liarozole in the treatment of advanced prostatic cancer. *Cancer* 1993;71:1068–73
8. Storlie JA, Buckner JC, Wiseman GA, *et al.* Prostate specific antigen levels and clinical response to low dose dexamethasone for hormone-refractory metastatic prostate carcinoma. *Cancer* 1995;76:96–100
9. Robinson RG, Preston DF, Schiefelbein M, *et al.* Strontium 89 therapy for the palliation of pain due to osseous metastases. *J Am Med Assoc* 1995;274:420–4
10. Tu S-M, Delpassand ES, Jones D, *et al.* Strontium-89 combined with doxorubicin in the treatment of patients with androgen-independent prostate cancer. *Urol Oncol* 1996;2:191–7
11. Mertens WC, Porter AT, Reid RH, *et al.* Strontium-89 and low-dose infusion cisplatin for

patients with hormone refractory prostate carcinoma metastatic to bone: a preliminary report. *J Nucl Med* 1992;33:1437–43

12. Pagliaro L, *et al.* Protocol DM 96–216. Houston, TX: M. D. Anderson Cancer Center

13. Yagoda A, Petrylak D. Cytotoxic chemotherapy for advanced hormone-resistant prostate cancer. *Cancer* 1993;71:1098–109

14. Kreis, W. Current chemotherapy and future directions in research for the treatment of advanced hormone-refractory prostate cancer. *Cancer Invest* 1995;13:296–312

15. Raghavan D, Koczwara B, Javle M. Evolving strategies of cytotoxic chemotherapy for advanced prostate cancer. *Eur J Cancer* 1997;33: 566–74

16. Morant R, Ackermann D, Trinkler F, *et al.* Gemcitabine in hormone refractory metastatic prostatic carcinoma, a phase II study of the SAKK. *Proc Annu Meet Am Soc Clin Oncol* 1997; 16:A1109

17. Canobbio L, Guarneri D, Miglietta L, *et al.* Carboplatin in advanced hormone refractory prostatic cancer patients. *Eur J Cancer* 1993;29A: 2094–6

18. Junoi WF, Hanselmann S, Schmitz SF, *et al.* Carboplatin in advanced hormone refractory prostate cancer. *Proc Annu Meet Am Soc Clin Oncol* 1995;14:A616

19. Coppin C, Murray N, Bryce C, *et al.* Mitomycin C revisited for androgen-independent prostate cancer (AIPC). *Proc Annu Meet Am Soc Clin Oncol* 1997;16:A1180

20. Hussain MH, Pienta KJ, Redman BG, *et al.* Oral etoposide in the treatment of hormone-refractory prostate cancer. *Cancer* 1994;74:100–3

21. Caty A, Oudard S, Humblet Y, *et al.* Phase II study of vinorelbine in patients with hormone refractory prostate cancer. *Proc Annu Meet Am Soc Clin Oncol* 1997;16:A1106

22. Roth BJ, Yeap BY, Wilding G, *et al.* Taxol in advanced, hormone-refractory carcinoma of the prostate. *Cancer* 1993;72:2457–60

23. Tannock IF, Osoba D, Stockler MR, *et al.* Chemotherapy with mitoxantrone plus prednisone or prednisone alone for symptomatic hormone-resistant prostate cancer: a Canadian randomized trial with palliative end points. *J Clin Oncol* 1996;14:1756–64

24. Tew KD, Stearns ME. Estramustine – a nitrogen mustard/steroid with antimicrotubule activity. *Pharmacol Ther* 1989;43:299–319

25. Iversen P, Rasmussen F, Asmussen C, *et al.* Estramustine phosphate versus placebo as second line treatment after orchiectomy in patients with metastatic prostate cancer: DAPROCA Study 9002. *J Urol* 1997;157:929–34

26. Hudes GR, Obasaju C, Chapman A, *et al.* Phase I study of paclitaxel and estramustine: preliminary

activity in hormone-refractory prostate cancer. *Semin Oncol* 1995;22(Suppl 6):S6–11

27. Pienta KJ, Naik H, Lehr JE. Effect of estramustine, etoposide, and taxol on prostate cancer cell growth *in vitro* and *in vivo*. *Urology* 1996; 48:164–70

28. Seidman AD, Scher HI, Petrylak D, *et al.* Estramustine and vinblastine: use of prostate specific antigen as a clinical trial end point for hormone refractory prostate cancer. *J Urol* 1992;147:931–4

29. Eichenberger T, Trachtenberg J, Chronis P, *et al.* Synergistic effect of ketoconazole and antineoplastic agents on hormone-independent prostatic cancer cells. *Clin Invest Med – Med Clin Exp* 1989;12:363–6

30. Sella A, Kilbourn R, Amato R, *et al.* Phase II study of ketoconazole combined with weekly doxorubicin in patients with androgen-independent prostate cancer. *J Clin Oncol* 1994;12:683–8

31. De Coster R, Wouters W, Bruynseels J. P450-dependent enzymes as targets for prostate cancer therapy. *J Steroid Biochem Mol Biol* 1996;56:133–43

32. Ellerhorst JA, Tu S-M, Amato RJ, *et al.* Phase II trial of alternating weekly chemohormonal therapy for patients with androgen-independent prostate cancer. *Clin Cancer Res* 1997;3:2371–6

33. Small EJ, Srinivas S, Egan B, *et al.* Doxorubicin and dose-escalated cyclophosphamide with granulocyte colony-stimulating factor for the treatment of hormone-resistant prostate cancer. *J Clin Oncol* 1996;14:1617–25

34. Fuse H, Muraishi Y, Fujishiro Y, *et al.* Etoposide, epirubicin and carboplatin in hormone-refractory prostate cancer. *Int Urol Nephrol* 1996; 28:79–85

35. Olver IN, Goulding J, Stephenson J, *et al.* A phase I study of prolonged ambulatory infusion carboplatin with oral etoposide showing activity in prostate cancer. *Proc Annu Meet Am Soc Clin Oncol* 1995;14:A677

36. Blumenstein B, Crawford ED, Saiers JH, *et al.* Doxorubicin, mitomycin C and 5-fluorouracil in the treatment of hormone refractory adenocarcinoma of the prostate: a Southwest Oncology Group study. *J Urol* 1993;150:411–13

37. Dimopoulos MA, Panopoulos C, Bamia C, *et al.* Oral estramustine and oral etoposide for hormone-refractory prostate cancer. *Urology* 1997; 50:754–8

38. Pienta KJ, Redman B, Hussain M, *et al.* Phase II evaluation of oral estramustine and oral etoposide in hormone-refractory adenocarcinoma of the prostate. *J Clin Oncol* 1994;12: 2005–12

39. Pienta KJ, Redman BG, Bandekar R, *et al.* A phase II trial of oral estramustine and oral etoposide in hormone refractory prostate cancer. *Urology* 1997;50:401–7

40. Colleoni M, Graiff C, Vicario G, *et al.* Phase II study of estramustine, oral etoposide, and vinorelbine in hormone-refractory prostate cancer. *Am J Clin Oncol* 1997;20:383–6

41. Maulard-Durdux C, Dufour B, Hennequin C, *et al.* Phase II study of the oral cyclophosphamide and oral etoposide combination in hormone-refractory prostate carcinoma patients. *Cancer* 1996;77:1144–8

42. Millikan RE, Logothetis C. Update of the NCCN guidelines for treatment of prostate cancer. *Oncology* 1997;11:180–93

43. di Sant'Agnese PA. Neuroendocrine differentiation in carcinoma of the prostate. *Cancer* 1992;70:254–68

44. Oesterling JE, Hauzeur CG, Farrow GM. Small cell anaplastic carcinoma of the prostate: a clinical, pathological and immunohistological study of 27 patients. *J Urol* 1992;147:804–7

45. Amato RJ, Logothetis CJ, Hallinan R, *et al.* Chemotherapy for small cell carcinoma of prostatic origin. *J Urol* 1992;147:935–7

46. Murphy GP, Becklye S, Brady MF, *et al.* Treatment of newly diagnosed metastatic prostate cancer patients with chemotherapy agents in combination with hormones versus hormones alone. *Cancer* 1983;51:1264–72

47. Kubota Y, Nakada T, Imai K, *et al.* Chemo-endocrine therapy in patients with stage D2 prostate cancer. *Prostate* 1995;26:50–4

48. Pummer K, Lehnert M, Stettner H, *et al.* Randomized comparison of total androgen blockade alone versus combined with weekly epirubicin in advanced prostate cancer. *Eur Urol* 1997;32(Suppl 3):81–5

Index